Movement Disorders in Psychiatry

Movement Disorders in Psychiatry

Edited by

Antonio L. Teixeira, Erin Furr Stimming,
and William G. Ondo

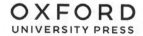

OXFORD
UNIVERSITY PRESS

OXFORD
UNIVERSITY PRESS

Oxford University Press is a department of the University of Oxford. It furthers
the University's objective of excellence in research, scholarship, and education
by publishing worldwide. Oxford is a registered trade mark of Oxford University
Press in the UK and certain other countries.

Published in the United States of America by Oxford University Press
198 Madison Avenue, New York, NY 10016, United States of America.

Library of Congress Cataloging-in-Publication Data
Names: Teixeira, Antonio L., editor. | Furr Stimming, Erin, editor. |
Ondo, William G., editor.
Title: Movement disorders in psychiatry /
edited by Antonio L. Teixeira, Erin Furr Stimming, and William G. Ondo.
Description: New York, NY : Oxford University Press, [2023] |
Includes bibliographical references and index.
Identifiers: LCCN 2022018783 (print) | LCCN 2022018784 (ebook) |
ISBN 9780197574317 (paperback) | ISBN 9780197574331 (epub) |
ISBN 9780197574348 (online)
Subjects: MESH: Movement Disorders—psychology |
Movement Disorders—complications | Mental Disorders—complications
Classification: LCC RC376.5 (print) | LCC RC376.5 (ebook) | NLM WL 390 |
DDC 616.8/3—dc23/eng/20220803
LC record available at https://lccn.loc.gov/2022018783
LC ebook record available at https://lccn.loc.gov/2022018784

DOI: 10.1093/med/9780197574317.001.0001

1 3 5 7 9 8 6 4 2

Printed by Marquis, Canada

Contents

Preface

Psychiatric disorders are among the main causes of disability worldwide. While pharmacological strategies remain at the forefront of the management of these conditions, they are not devoid of side effects. Movement disorders are frequent complications of psychiatric medications. The use of antipsychotics can induce acute dystonic reactions, akathisia, and parkinsonism, while chronic use can cause tardive dyskinesia. Antidepressants and mood stabilizers also cause neurological side effects. These movement disorders can add a significant burden to patients with psychiatric disorders.

Additionally, primary movement disorders are commonly accompanied by psychiatric syndromes, such as Parkinson's disease, Huntington's disease, Tourette's syndrome to name a few.

There are other intersections between neurology and psychiatry, such as epilepsy and dementia, but the field of movement disorders is probably the most robust and fascinating. The heterogeneity of movement disorders, their complex pathophysiology, and the comorbid conditions pose continuous challenges for clinicians. Bearing these concepts in mind, we proposed this book to provide a broad up-to-date overview of the interaction and overlap between psychiatry and movement disorders. While previous manuscripts and books have addressed specific movement disorders in psychiatry, mostly tardive dyskinesia, no previous single volume has been entirely dedicated to the complex interface of "movement disorders and psychiatry."

Our book has four parts. In Part 1 presents, an overview of the pathophysiology and different phenotypes of movement disorders is presented. Part 2 discusses movement disorders due to acute and chronic use of different classes of psychotropic drugs, including dopamine antagonists, selective serotonin antagonist inhibitors, mood stabilizers, and amphetamines. Part 3 addresses movement disorders seen in primary psychiatric conditions, such as developmental disorders and schizophrenia. Finally, Part 4 discusses conditions simultaneously marked by psychiatric and movement disorders like Parkinson's disease, Huntington's disease, Tourette's disorders, among others.

The book was written by neurologists and psychiatrists with clinical and research experience, allowing for an integrated and updated view of this ever-changing area. We hope that not only new clinicians but also "seasoned" professionals will enjoy the reading of the book.

Contributors

Albert Y. Amran
Research Assistant and Medical Student
Department of Neurology
McGovern Medical School, University of Texas
Health Science Center at Houston
Houston, TX, USA

Karen Anderson, MD
Professor of Psychiatry
Georgetown University Medical Center
Washington, DC, USA

Melody Badii, MD
Resident Physician
Stanley H Appel Department of Neurology
Houston Methodist Hospital
Houston, TX, USA

Carla Bejjani, MD
Assistant Professor
Department of Psychiatry and Behavioral
Sciences
Baylor College of Medicine
Houston, TX, USA

Daniel R. Benke, MS
Researcher
Cell and Molecular Biology
Federal University of Paraná
Curitiba, PR, BR

Moira Black, MD
Chief Resident
Department of Pediatrics, Division of Child and
Adolescent Neurology
McGovern Medical School, University of Texas
Health Science Center Houston
Houston, TX, USA

Avram S. Bukhbinder, BA
Research Coordinator and Medical Student
Department of Neurology
McGovern Medical School, University of Texas
Health Science Center at Houston
Houston, TX, USA

Francisco Cardoso, MD, PhD
Professor of Neurology
Department of Internal Medicine
Universidade Federal de Minas Gerais
Belo Horizonte, BR

Claudio Da Cunha, PhD
Professor
Department of Pharmacology
Universidade Federal do Parana
Curitiba, BR

Emmanuel H. During, MD
Associate Professor
Department of Psychiatry and Behavioral
Sciences
Stanford University
Palo Alto, CA, USA

Abdulmunaim M. Eid, MD
Resident Physician
Stanley H Appel Department of Neurology
Houston Methodist Neurological Institute
Houston, TX, USA

Alberto J. Espay, MD
Professor of Neurology
Chair, James J. and Joan A. Gardner
Family Center for Parkinson's Disease, and
Movement Disorders
University of Cincinnati
Cincinnati, OH, USA

Brittany Finocchio, PharmD, BCPP
Clinical Pharmacist
Department of Pharmacy
Harris County Psychiatric Center, University of
Texas Health Science Center at Houston
Houston, TX, USA

Carlos Manuel Guerra Galicia, MD, MS
Director, Advanced Center for Parkinson,
Movement Disorders and Dementia
Professor, Departments of Physical Medicine and
Rehabilitation and Neurology
Autonomous University of San Luis Potosi
San Luis Potosi, MX

Jordi Gandini, MD
Neurologist
Department of Neurology
CHU-Charleroi, Belgium

Michael D. Geschwind, MD, PhD
Professor of Neurology
Michael J. Homer Chair in Neurology
University of California, San Francisco (UCSF)
Memory and Aging Center
San Francisco, CA, USA

Jennifer G. Goldman, MD, MS
Section Chief and Professor
Parkinson's Disease and Movement Disorders,
Shirley Ryan Ability Lab
Departments of Physical Medicine and
Rehabilitation and Neurology
Northwestern University Feinberg School of
Medicine
Chicago, IL, USA

Christina J. Herold, PhD
Post-doctoral Research Assistant
Department of General Psychiatry
University Hospital Heidelberg
Heidelberg, DE

Joseph Jankovic, MD
Professor of Neurology, Distinguished Chair in
Movement Disorders
Department of Neurology
Baylor College of Medicine
Houston, TX, USA

Joohi Jimenez-Shahed, MD
Associate Professor of Neurology
Department of Neurology
Icahn School of Medicine at Mount Sinai
New York, NY, USA

Mary Kay Koenig, MD
Professor of Pediatrics, Division of Child &
Adolescent Neurology
McGovern Medical School, University of Texas
Health Science Center at Houston
Houston, TX, USA

Abhishek Lenka, MD, PhD
Neurology Resident
Department of Neurology
Medstar Georgetown University Hospital
Washington, DC, USA

Andy Liu, BS
Medical Student
Department of Psychiatry
Georgetown University Medical Center
Washington, DC, USA

Ricardo Maciel, MD
Neurologist
Movement Disorders Clinic
Universidade Federal de Minas Gerais
Belo Horizonte, BR

Débora Palma Maia, MD
Neurologist
Movement Disorders Clinic
Universidade Federal de Minas Gerais
Belo Horizonte, BR

Mario Manto, MD
Professor of Neuroanatomy and Neurological
Semiology at University of Mons, Belgium
Head of the Department of Neurology
CHU-Charleroi, Belgium

Laura Marsh, MD
Professor and Executive Director of Mental
Health Care
Departments of Psychiatry and Neurology
Baylor College of Medicine and Michael
E. DeBakey Veterans Affairs Medical Center
Houston, TX, USA

Raja Mehanna, MD
Associate Professor of Neurology
Director of Movement Disorder Curriculum
Assistant Movement Disorder Fellowship
Director
Department of Neurology
McGovern Medical School, University of Texas
Health Science Center at Houston
Houston, TX, USA

Nidaullah Mian, MD
Neurologist
Our Lady of Lourdes Regional Medical Center
Lafayatte, LA, USA

Satyajit Mohite, MD, MPH
Assistant Professor, Senior Associate Consultant
Department of Psychiatry and Psychology
Mayo Clinic Health System
Mankato, MN, USA

William G. Ondo, MD
Director, Methodist Neurological Institute
Movement Disorders Clinic
Professor of Neurology, Weill Cornell
Medical School
Adjunct Professor of Neurology, Texas A&M
Medical School
Houston, TX, USA

Ossama T. Osman, MD
Professor of Psychiatry
Department of Psychiatry and Behavioral
Sciences
McGovern Medical School, University of Texas
Health Science Center at Houston
Houston, TX, USA

Bradley T. Peet, MD
Neuropsychiatrist
Memory and Aging Center
Department of Neurology
Weill Institute for Neurosciences
University of California, San Francisco
San Francisco, California, USA

Vinicius Sousa Pietra Pedroso, MD, PhD
Associate Professor
Department of Medicine
Pontifical Catholic University of Minas Gerais
Betim, BR

Teresa Pigott, MD
Professor of Psychiatry
Director, Psychopharmacology
Harris County Psychiatry Center
Department of Psychiatry and Behavioral
Sciences
McGovern Medical School, University of Texas
Health Science Center at Houston
Houston, TX, USA

José Augusto Pochapski, PhD
Post-Doctoral Researcher
Department of Pharmacology and Department
of Biochemistry
Universidade Federal do Paraná
Curitiba, BR

Julia Ridgeway-Diaz, MD, MS
Assistant Professor
Menninger Department of Psychiatry
Baylor College of Medicine
Houston, TX, USA

James F. Rini, MD
Neurologist
Memory and Aging Center
Department of Neurology
Weill Institute for Neurosciences
University of California, San Francisco
San Francisco, California, USA

Natalia Pessoa Rocha, PharmD, MSc, PhD
Assistant Professor
Mitchell Center for Alzheimer's Disease & Brain
Disorders
Department of Neurology
McGovern Medical School, University of Texas
Health Science Center at Houston
Houston, TX, USA

Sam Nicholas Russo, MD
Assistant Professor
Department of Pediatrics, Division of Pediatric
Neurology
McGovern Medical School, University of Texas
Health Science Center at Houston
Houston, TX, USA

Haitham Salem, MD, PhD
Assistant Professor
Department of Psychiatry and Human Behavior
The Warren Alpert Medical School of Brown
University
Providence, RI, USA

João Vinícius Salgado, MD, PhD
Associate Professor
Department of Morphology
Federal University of Minas Gerais
Belo Horizonte, BR

William Sánchez-Luna, PhD
Visiting Research Fellow
National Institute on Drug Abuse, Integrative
Neurobiology Section
National Institutes of Health
Baltimore, MD, USA

Johannes Schröder, MD
Professor and Head, Section of Geriatric
Psychiatry
University of Heidelberg
Heidelberg, DE

Paul E. Schulz, MD
Rick McCord Professor in Neurology
Umphrey Family Professor of Neurodegenerative
Disorders
Director, Memory Disorders and
Dementia Clinic
Director, Neuropsychiatry and Behavioral
Neurology Fellowship
McGovern Medical School, University of Texas
Health Science Center at Houston
Houston, TX, USA

Lokesh Shahani, MD
Associate Professor
Chief Medical Officer, Harris County
Psychiatric Center
Department of Psychiatry and Behavioral
Sciences
McGovern Medical School, University of Texas
Health Science Center at Houston
Houston, TX, USA

Jennifer S. Sharma, MD
Neurologist
Department of Neurology and Rehabilitation
Medicine
Gardner Family Center for Parkinson's Disease
and Movement Disorders
University of Cincinnati
Cincinnati, OH, USA

Erin Furr Stimming, MD, FAAN
Professor of Neurology
Director, HDSA Center of Excellence
Director, Neurology Clerkship
Department of Neurology
McGovern Medical School, University of Texas
Health Science Center at Houston
Houston, TX, USA

Antonio L. Teixeira, MD, PhD
Professor of Psychiatry and Neurology
Director, Neuropsychiatry Program
McGovern Medical School, University of Texas
Health Science Center at Houston
Houston, TX, USA
Professor, Faculdade Santa Casa BH
Belo Horizonte, BR

Nivedita Thakur, MD
Associate Professor of Clinical Neurology
Department of Neurology
Perelman School of Medicine at the University of
Pennsylvania
Philadelphia, PA, USA

Luiz Paulo Vasconcelos, MD, MSc
Associate Professor
Department of Internal Medicine
Três Rios Faculty of Medical Science
(SUPREMA)
Três Rios, BR

John W. Winkelman, MD, PhD
Professor of Psychiatry
Chief, Sleep Disorders Clinical Research
Program
Massachusetts General Hospital
Harvard Medical School
Boston, MA, USA

Fernando Henrique Teixeira Zonzini, MSc
Pharmacist
Department of Pharmacology
Universidade Federal do Paraná
Curitiba, PR, BR

PART I
MOVEMENT DISORDERS OVERVIEW

1

Introduction to the Movement Disorders

Definition and Clinical Phenotypes

Erin Furr Stimming and William G. Ondo

Introduction

Movement disorders are a group of clinically, pathologically, and genetically heterogeneous neurological conditions that clinically manifest as a perturbation in normal motor function. These disorders are mostly characterized by an abnormal function of the basal ganglia, but other central nervous anatomy, and even peripheral nervous system structures, can be involved.[1,2] Even though advances in imaging, electrophysiology, and genetics have improved the diagnostic process in movement disorders, an accurate recognition based on their phenotype is paramount for proper identification and treatment.[1]

Over the years, efforts have been made to establish a definitive classification for movement disorders, taking into consideration novel research findings and recognition of clinical characteristics. The first descriptions of movement disorders included detailed patterned descriptions of abnormal movement patterns associated with some diseases, and they initially recognized disorders such as tremor, chorea, athetosis, myoclonus, and asterixis.[3] Initially, the term "extrapyramidal" was coined to refer to movement disorders, but it was later recognized that the basal ganglia have connections with the pyramidal tract system, so that they were not truly extrapyramidal and this term is now discouraged.[4,5] As the semiology of these neurological diseases evolved, a conventional categorization has divided movement disorders into two major groups: hyperkinetic movement disorders and hypokinetic movement disorders.[6] Once the phenotype of movement is identified properly, the diagnostic evaluation and treatment become more focused.[7]

Novel approaches and recent advances in genetics and molecular techniques have also suggested different classifications according to pathology, physiology, or genetic etiology. Pathologic based divisions include (1) synucleinopathies, caused by a misfolded alpha-synuclein (α-Syn) protein that forms amyloid-like filamentous inclusions, e.g., Lewy body disorders such as Parkinson's disease (PD), dementia with Lewy bodies (DLB), pure autonomic failure, and multiple system atrophy (MSA);[8–10] (2) tauopathies, caused by neurofibrillary tau pathology (i.e., progressive supranuclear palsy (PSP), corticobasal degeneration (CBD); (3) genetic polyglutamine disorders linked to CAG repeats (i.e., Huntington's disease [HD]) and other specific genes for many forms of ataxia, dystonia, and parkinsonism; and (4) paraneoplastic forms with antibodies against receptors and other proteins.[10–13] Overall however, there is no widely accepted unified classification system for all "movement disorders."

To better understand the psychiatric manifestations associated with movement disorders, we present this initial chapter to present some consensus regarding their terminology and phenotypical descriptions.

Hyperkinetic Movement Disorders

The different types of movement disorders are described based on their phenomenology, i.e., their clinical appearance. Hyperkinetic movement disorders are determined by excessive and involuntary movements that intrude into the normal flow of motor activity. This category includes chorea, dystonia, myoclonus, athetosis, tics, and tremor.[6]

Chorea

Chorea can be defined as "dancelike" involuntary movements, with an unpredictable and nonrhythmic pattern resulting from random flow of muscle contractions that appear to flow from one body part to the next.[6,7] Interestingly, patients with chorea can develop a phenomenon called *parakinesia*, in which they learn to merge the movements into a purposeful action, such as running their finger through their hair or adjusting glasses, hampering the identification of chorea.[6,7,14,15] Other typical signs are motor impersistence, defined as an inability to perform sustained motor activities,[15] as in the "milkmaid's grip" (the fluctuating strength of the grip), nonsustained tongue protrusion and hung-up reflexes (variable muscle contraction and choreatic movements of the leg after the knee-jerk reflex).[6,7,15] Chorea can be observed in various disease states, a few of which include Huntington's disease, benign hereditary chorea, endocrine-mediated disorders (i.e., hyperthyroidism), or autoimmune-mediated disorders (i.e., Sydenham's chorea and lupus). Chorea can also be observed in patients with Parkinson's disease who experience levodopa-induced dyskinesias and in patients with tardive dyskinesia induced by neuroleptic use.[16]

As ballism shares the same pathophysiology of chorea, it is considered part of the same spectrum. Ballistic movements are often unilateral and classically occur after a lesion near the contralateral subthalamic nucleus, although other locations such as the thalamus, contralateral basal ganglia or corona radiata may be culpable.[15,17] These movements are uncontrollable, severe, mainly proximal, large-amplitude choreatic movements, sometimes with a flinging or flailing quality.[6,7,14]

Dystonia

Dystonia is defined by abnormal, sustained or intermittent, involuntary, patterned muscle contraction, causing twisting and repetitive movements around one or multiple joints.[2,4,7,16,18,19] This movement disorder can be idiopathic or genetic but may also be associated with injury to the basal ganglia, in particular the putamen and globus pallidus.[14] Nevertheless, recent evidence has linked most cases of dystonia with other brain areas including the cerebellum, brainstem, and sensory cortex.

Epidemiological reports of prevalence vary markedly, with numbers ranging from 15–30/100,000[20] to 732/100,000,[21] raising concern about the difficulty to ascertain the diagnosis given the lack of objective biomarkers for most cases of dystonia.[22] Women have twice the prevalence compared to men, and a family history is reported in about 20% of patients with dystonia.[23,24]

Dystonia can involve agonist-antagonist pairs of axial and appendicular muscles, producing postures that cannot be suppressed and that classically worsen with voluntary movement.[6] These contractions are usually sustained at the peak of the movement, which helps differentiate them from the transient contractions seen in chorea and myoclonus.[2]

Different classification systems have been used for dystonia, which traditionally included divisions according to age of onset, distribution of body regions, genetics. and etiology.[2,7,25] However, a more recent classification has divided dystonia into two axes according to the clinical characteristics and etiology (Table 1.1).[26]

Although dystonia is classified as a hyperkinetic movement disorder, the apparent muscle contraction can result in slowed volitional movement and can also be rhythmic enough to be considered tremor. As the dystonia evolves, a phenomenon called overflow dystonia can occur and actions in one body region can induce dystonic movements in another region.[2] An interesting feature is the sensory trick (*geste antagoniste*) in which patients can improve the dystonia by touching specifically an affected body part (i.e., touching the cheek to correct torticollis or chewing gum to reduce oromandibular dystonia).[7]

Myoclonus

Myoclonic movements are brief, sudden, jerk-like involuntary movements. These gestures can be positive due to a muscle contraction, or negative due to a brief inhibition of muscular tone, e.g., asterixis in hepatic or uremic encephalopathy.[3,7] Based on the pattern of contraction, myoclonus can be synchronous (muscles contract simultaneously), spreading (muscles contract in a predictable sequence), or asynchronous (muscles contract with varying and unpredictable timing).[14] Lifetime prevalence of myoclonus was 8.6 per 100,000 population in a study in Minnesota, increasing after the age of 50.[27] It can result from pathology in the cerebral cortex, subcortical regions, spinal cord, and even peripheral nerves.[6] Symptomatic or secondary myoclonus, which is a symptom of an identifiable underlying disorder, is the most common type (72%), followed by epileptic (17%) and essential myoclonus (11%).[28] Secondary myoclonus mostly results from cerebral hypoxia. According to the damaged structure, myoclonus can present with different characteristics. For example, cortical myoclonus occurs mostly in response to distal touch or stretch, and occasionally can be triggered by visual stimuli, it tends to be focal. In contrast, brainstem myoclonus is provoked mostly by auditory stimuli, or by tactile stimuli around the face or mouth, and it has a tendency to be more generalized. Startle reactions, characterized by a bilaterally synchronous shock-like set of movements, are also provoked by external stimuli, most often by auditory triggers, surprise, alarm, or acute pain.[7] Although in many cases myoclonus is associated with catastrophic neurological injury, in some situations, such as sleep,[14] exercise, or anxiety, and especially in children, myoclonus can be considered physiologic.[6,16] For example, hiccups (singultus) is a form of myoclonus.

Table 1.1 Classification of Dystonia According to Clinical Characteristics and Etiology

Axis I. Clinical characteristics	
Clinical characteristics of dystonia	
Age of onset	Infancy (birth to 2 years) Childhood (3–12 years) Adolescence (13–20 years) Early adulthood (21–40 years) Late adulthood (>40 years)
Body distribution	Focal Segmental Multifocal Generalized (with or without leg involvement) Hemidystonia
Temporal pattern	Disease course (static, progressive) Variability (persistent, action-specific, diurnal, paroxysmal)
Associated features	
Isolated or combined with another movement disorder	Isolated dystonia Combined dystonia
Other neurological or systemic manifestations	
Axis II. Etiology	
Nervous system pathology	Evidence of degeneration Evidence of structural lesions No evidence of degeneration or structural lesions
Inherited or acquired	Inherited (AD, AR, X-linked, mitochondrial) Acquired Perinatal brain injury Infection Drug Toxic Vascular Neoplastic Brain injury Psychogenic Idiopathic (sporadic or familial)

AD = autosomal dominant; AR = autosomal recessive

Source: Reprinted from Albanese, A., Bhatia, K., Bressman, S., DeLong, M., Fahn, S., Fung, V., . . . Teller, J. (2013). Phenomenology and classification of dystonia: a consensus update. Movement Disorders, 28(7), 863–873. https://doi.org/10.1002/mds.25475

The rhythmicity of the myoclonus can be regular or irregular, which is important to identify since rhythmic myoclonus can be mistaken as a tremor. For example, spinal segmental myoclonus and hereditary cortical myoclonus are rhythmic and could be erroneously labeled as "cortical tremor." Similarly, when myoclonus is arrhythmic (i.e., polyminimyoclonus, fine myoclonic individual jerks in outstretched hands, in patients with multiple system atrophy) can be mistaken for irregular tremor.[7] Palatal myoclonus usually results from lesions within Molleret's triangle between the inferior olive, cerebellum, and red nucleus, is very rhythmic, and is alternatively called palatal tremor.

Athetosis

This movement disorder has been described as slow, writhing, sinuous and irregular movements especially marked in the digits and extremities, and even the perioral muscles,[15,18] often accompanied by abnormal posturing.[3,7,14] The ongoing movement is not composed of discrete movements but a continuously flowing, random pattern. It is a relatively rare movement disorder, with a prevalence calculated as 15/100000 in a population study in Egypt.[29] It can be distinguished from tremor because of its lack of rhythmicity and repeatability, and from myoclonus because it does not have rapid jerk-like movements.[14] Athetosis can sometimes occur in combination with chorea, therefore the term "choreoathetosis" has been coined to refer to this phenomenon.[6] Pseudoathetosis can be seen with peripheral denervation, especially if visual fixation is withdrawn (closed eyes).

Tics

Tics are intermittent, purposeless, repeated, and recognizable sudden movements or sounds, out of a normal background, that can be triggered by suggestion, stress, or excitement and can be partially suppressed. Their prevalence in school-age children can be as high as 21%– 24%, and they may last from several weeks or persist for many years into adulthood.[7,18] Patients report that these movements are usually associated with a rising discomfort or urge to perform the movement[14] and are followed by a sense of relief after the tic. They can be divided into simple (i.e., eye blinking, shoulder shrugging, throat clearing), complex (i.e., touching things, smelling objects, echopraxia, jumping) and by whether they are pure motor or phonic (including simple, brief phonations or vocalizations). Complex motor tics may have a component of dystonia, other complex movements, or even obscene gestures (copropraxia). Complex vocal tics can include words or phrases, repeating other's sounds (echolalia), and profanity (coprolalia), although copralalia is actually an uncommon tic.[16] Even though tics are partially suppressible, they inevitably return and may be more severe after a period of suppression (rebound phenomenon).[6] Tic disorders are somewhat arbitrarily classified by age of onset, duration, and whether or not both motor and vocal tics are present, which is needed for a formal diagnosis of Tourette's syndrome.

Tremor

Based on its general phenotypical characteristics, tremor is defined as involuntary, hyperkinetic, rhythmic, and sinusoidal alternating movements of one or more body parts, usually resulting from the contractions of antagonistic muscle groups.[3,18] Tremor can be classified as resting, in that it occurs when the muscles are not volitionally actively contracted (usually seen in Parkinson's disease), or action, which is seen when those muscles are volitionally contracting. Action tremor may occur while apparently still but countering gravity (postural) or where the body part is volitionally moved (kinetic). Other categories include intentional (where the tremor is most seen as the body part approaches a target as in cerebellar outflow syndromes) and dystonic (accompanying or part of dystonia).[1] A new classification for tremors was released in 2018, which divided them according to their clinical features and etiology (Table 1.2).[30]

The prevalence of essential tremor (ET), the most common form of tremor, is 4% in people aged over 40 years, increasing up to 14% in people over 65 years of age,[7] and may occur in up to 5% in the general population. Its recognition is of importance since many patients with essential tremor are misdiagnosed with other tremor disorders, including Parkinson's disease (PD). Advancing age is a risk factor for its development, but a positive family history, seen in about 60% of subjects, correlates with a younger age of onset.[31] Clear differences for sex-dependent prevalence have not been identified.[2,32] This type of tremor is commonly seen in the upper extremities, head, and voice, and classically has a frequency from 4–12 Hz.[2] Even though it has been traditionally considered as a mono-symptomatic disease, patients with essential tremor have shown higher rates of hearing loss,[33,34] cognitive impairment,[35] and gait abnormalities.[2] The course of ET is usually progressive, with increased amplitude, decreased frequency, and proximal spreading over years.[2,36]

Intention tremor comprises a progressive increase in amplitude as the intended target is reached,[7] classically seen in the setting of cerebellar dysfunction from many different causes.[2] When the tremor affects a body part that has signs characteristic of dystonia, it is classified as a dystonic tremor.[7] Resting tremor is one of the hallmarks of PD. Tremor is the presenting symptom in PD in 50% to 70% patients and is seen in more than 80% of PD cases. Resting tremor occurs when a limb is relaxed, is typically asymmetric, characterized by a pill-rolling (supination-pronation) movement and with a frequency of 3–6 Hz. It improves with volitional movement. Rest tremor can be seen in severe cases of ET but not in the absence of severe action tremor.

Stereotype

Stereotype is the least clearly codified hyperkinetic phenotype and has some features of tremor, tics, and chorea. The movements are loose, patterned, and repetitive but not simple or oscillatory enough to be tremor. They are often suppressible like tics and may or may not have a subjective urge. One subtype of stereotype is seen in the setting of autistic spectrum disorder or normal children, which include such actions as rocking or hand waving. The other subtype of stereotype is less well structured and most commonly seen in the setting of tardive dyskinesia, such as repetitive tongue or mouth movements.[37]

Hypokinetic Movement Disorders

This group of disorders comprises a reduction in the movement capacity of the patients and they may be categorized based on the severity of the symptoms. According to this, hypokinetic movement disorders have been defined as akinesia (meaning lack of movement), hypokinesia (a reduction in the amplitude/size of movement), bradykinesia (slow movement),

Table 1.2 Classification of Tremor According to Clinical Features and Etiology

Axis I. Clinical features	
Historical features	
Age at onset	Infancy (birth to 2 years)
	Childhood (3–12 years)
	Adolescence (13–20 years)
	Early adulthood (21–45 years)
	Middle adulthood (46–60 years)
	Late adulthood (>60 years)
Temporal onset and evolution	
Past medical history	
Family history	
Alcohol and drug sensitivity	
Tremor characteristics	
Body distribution	Focal
	Segmental
	Hemitremor
	Generalized
Activation conditions	Postural
	Kinetic (simple and intention)
	Task-specific
	Isometric tremors
Tremor frequency	<4 Hz
	4–8 Hz
	8–12 Hz
	>12 Hz
Associated signs	
Isolated	
Combined	Signs of systemic illness
	Neurologic signs
	Soft signs
Additional laboratory tests	
Electrophysiological tests	
Structural imaging	
Receptor imaging	
Serum and tissue biomarkers	
Axis II. Etiology	
Acquired	
Genetically defined	
Idiopathic	Familial
	Sporadic

Source: Adapted from Bhatia, K., Bain, P., Bajaj, N., Elble, R., Hallett, M., Louis, E.... Tremor Task Force of the International Parkinson and Movement Disorder Society. (2018). Consensus Statement on the Classification of Tremors. From the Task Force on Tremor of the International Parkinson and Movement Disorder Society. Movement Disorders, 33(1), 75–87. https://doi.org/10.1002/mds.27121

and rigidity.[6] "Akinesia" is an umbrella term for a symptoms complex that includes brady-kinesia and hypokinesia. Additionally, akinesia characteristically has progressive fatiguing and amplitude decrement of repetitive movements.[7] These disorders have also been referred to as *parkinsonism* since they are seen in PD.[16,38] True weakness is not part of parkinsonism, although patients often report "weakness". The clinical diagnosis of parkinsonism relies on three key elements: bradykinesia, tremor, and rigidity, with bradykinesia being essential among them.[39,40]

The most common cause of parkinsonism is PD; however, some parkinsonian syn-dromes present with atypical features such as early dementia, recurrent falls, ocular motor impairment, significant dysautonomia, ataxia, or poor or absent response to levodopa. These other idiopathic syndromes involve degeneration in multiple systems and include PSP, MSA, CBD, and DLB (Table 1.3). Secondary causes of parkinsonism may be vas-cular, infectious, metabolic, neoplastic, or hereditary.[40] Parkinsonism is also commonly medication-induced.

PD is the second most frequent neurodegenerative disorder (prevalence 100–572/100,000; incidence 4.5–21/100,000), after Alzheimer's disease.[2,10,41] It is characterized by pathologic intraneuronal alpha-synuclein-positive Lewy bodies and neuronal loss.[2] The clinical features of PD, which commonly present asymmetrically, are bradykinesia, resting tremor, and ri-gidity, along with numerous nonmotor features.[42] Cognitive dysfunction may occur, with dementia being common in later stages, while mood symptoms, psychosis, and depression can appear at any time in the disease.[10,43,44] Even though the pathological studies have fo-cused mainly on substantia nigra–basal ganglia damage, evidence shows that the disease process involves almost the entire central nervous system and autonomic peripheral nervous system, often explaining nonmotor features that have nothing to do with dopamine and may

Table 1.3 Key Differentiating Parkinsonian Signs and Symptoms Seen Relatively Early in the Disease Course

	PD	DLB	MSA	PSP	CBD
Unilateral Features	+++	+	+	+	+++
Rest Tremor	+++	++	+	+	–
Myoclonus	+	++	++	+	+++
Bulbar Symptoms	+	++	++	+++	+
Oculomotor Dysfunction	+	+	+	+++	++
Balance	+	+	++	+++	++
Early Orthostatic Hypotension and other Autonomic Symptoms	+	++	+++	+	+
Hallucinations	++	+++	++	+	+
Dementia	+	+++	+	++	++
Response to Dopaminergics	+++	++	++	+	–

PD = Parkinson's disease; DLB = Lewy body dementia; MSA = multiple system atrophy; PSP = progressive supranu-clear palsy; CBD = corticobasal degeneration occur prior to dopaminergic motor manifestations.[2,45] Clinical examination is the standard for diagnosing PD, thus the importance of learning about its characteristics and diagnostic criteria according to the UK Parkinson's Disease Society Brain Bank.[46] In general, the diagnostic accuracy by general neurologists has been estimated to be 70% and by movement disorders specialists approaches 90%.[47]

Clinical Features in PD and Other Hypokinetic Movement Disorders

Previously, bradykinesia was identified to be the feature in PD that correlated best with dopamine deficiency,[48–50] although recent studies on brain metabolism have shown a better correlation with rigidity.[51] Bradykinesia is subjectively reported as many different symptoms depending on anatomy. Patients may report difficulty with fine motor tasks, an increase in saliva because of infrequent swallowing, micrographia (small handwriting), hypomimia (loss of facial expression), or hypophonia (quiet, monotonous speech).[2,39] In addition, PD patients can exhibit a decreased blink rate, shortened stride length, and diminished arm swing when walking.[48] Bradykinesia and hypokinesia can be provoked on examination using repeated movements such as finger tapping or pronation/supination, observing not only slowness but also decrementing amplitude.[39,48] Interestingly, a phenomenon called *kinesia paradoxica* has been described in patients with PD, where emotional status can influence the motor programming in these patients. For example, patients with PD may be able to suddenly run if someone screams "fire."[48]

Resting tremor in PD is typically of low frequency (3–5 Hz) and usually characterized by a pill-rolling (pronation/supination) movement. It can involve the extremities and face. Hand tremor is best seen while walking, and patients can suppress it with concentration or with volitional action of the affected region. Tremor does not need to be present for a diagnosis of PD; however, 69% of patients have it at disease onset and 80% have tremor at some point in their disease course.[39,52]

Rigidity is the increased resistance to passive movement across a joint. It could be reported as unilateral pain or stiffness, commonly in the shoulder, and some people get an initial diagnosis of frozen shoulder.[48,53] When evaluating rigidity in patients, the examination often displays it better at the wrist and its severity could be enhanced with the patient performing an action on the contralateral side (i.e., opening and closing the fingers), which is known as the Froment's maneuver.[48]

Patients with PD may also suffer from postural instability, although presentation with postural instability is more associated with other parkinsonian conditions. It could be assessed during the physical examination by performing the pull test, in which the patient is pulled backward or forward by the shoulders, evaluating retropulsion or propulsion, respectively.[48] Postural instability increases the risk of falls and hip fractures, and its latency from symptom onset to the first fall helps differentiate PD from PSP and MSA, in which falls occur sooner compared to PD.[48,54]

Freezing is another phenomenon in patients with PD, in which they present with transient (<10 s) motor blocks.[55,56] It usually occurs at later stages of the disease, being more frequent in men and most seen while attempting walking.[57,58] It has been classified into five subtypes according to the impaired action: start hesitation, turn hesitation, hesitation in tight quarters, destination hesitation, and open space hesitation but most patients have multiple types.[59] This phenomenon is variably responsive to dopaminergic medications, and is called "on" freezing when seen in the *on* period,[48] the period when motor symptoms are otherwise improved by levodopa.

Nonmotor features in PD are very common and include autonomic dysfunction, cognitive and neurobehavioral abnormalities, and sensory and sleep abnormalities.[48] Autonomic failure in PD manifests as orthostatic hypotension (in 30%–50%, with only 16% being symptomatic), sweating dysregulation, and urinary and erectile dysfunction. Cardiovascular autonomic dysfunction can cause lightheadedness, blurry vision, tiredness, dyspnea, and neck and shoulder pain ("coat hanger pain").[60] Gastrointestinal issues such as esophageal dysmotility, delayed gastric emptying, and prolonged stool transit, can also occur, which are of importance since they can alter the absorption capacity for medications to treat the disease.[61,62] Also, L-dopa can further slow gastrointestinal motility on dopaminergic enteric receptors.[60,63]

Neuropsychiatric symptoms in patients with PD can be very disabling, 84% may manifest cognitive decline and 48% can develop dementia,[64] which may also be accompanied by depression, apathy, anxiety, and psychosis.[65] Hallucinations are very common and typically visual. Delusions are usually persecutory or infidelity related. Additional psychiatric manifestations will be addressed in the chapter "Parkinson's Disease and Atypical Parkinsonian Syndromes." Sleep disorders are a prominent part of PD, with REM sleep behavior disorder (RBD) occurring in many patients, often prior to PD diagnosis. This is characterized by acting out violent dream content, talking, swearing, punching, kicking, and other potentially injurious motor activity. Restless legs syndrome is common, but sleep apnea may actually be less common in PD than the general population.

Sensory symptoms include pain,[66] akathisia, and olfactory dysfunction, which is another early marker of the disease preceding motor symptoms. Olfactory dysfunction could be related to neuronal loss in the corticomedial amygdala or decreased dopaminergic neurons in the olfactory bulb.[48,67]

The etiology of idiopathic Parkinson's disease is incompletely understood and likely multifactorial with both genetic and environmental contributions. Secondary parkinsonian conditions including drug-induced, vascular, infectious, and structural parkinsonism should be considered in order to make a correct diagnosis and management.

Conclusion

Patient history and the neurological examination remain the most important factors when approaching movement disorders. Once a phenotype is established, subsequent imaging, genetic and serologic testing can elucidate the exact diagnosis and optimize treatments. Motor symptoms and psychiatric symptoms are highly integrated. Psychiatric manifestations are very common in diseases that are recognized as movement disorders, movement disorder manifestations are very common in psychiatric conditions, and the treatment of either can result in side effects of the other. Subsequent chapters will review movement disorders that may occur as a side effect of psychiatric medications, evaluate movement disorders in primary psychiatric diagnoses, and review the psychiatric symptoms seen in a number of phenotypical movement disorders.

References

1. Klein, C. (2005). Movement disorders: Classifications. Journal of Inherited Metabolic Disease, 28(3), 425–439. https://doi.org/10.1007/s10545-005-7495-8

2. Ostrem, J. L., & Galifianakis, N. B. (2010). Overview of common movement disorders. CONTINUUM Lifelong Learning in Neurology, 16(1), 13–48. https://doi.org/10.1212/01.CON.0000348899.02339.9d

3. Walker, H. (1990). Involuntary movements. In H. Walker, D. Hall, & J. Hurst (Eds.), Clinical Methods (3rd Edition, pp. 360–362). Boston: Butterworths.

4. Fahn, S. (2011). Classification of movement disorders. Movement Disorders, 26(6), 947–957. https://doi.org/10.1002/mds.23759

5. Walker, R. H. (2013). Thoughts on selected movement disorder terminology and a plea for clarity. Tremor and Other Hyperkinetic Movements (New York, N.Y.), 3, 1–3. https://doi.org/10.7916/D8R49PG6

6. Youssef, P., Mack, K., & Flemming, K. (2015). Classification and approach to movement disorders. In K. Flemming & L. Jones Jr. (Eds.), Mayo Clinic Neurology Board Review Clinical Neurology for Initial Certification and MOC (pp. 183–187). New York: Oxford University Press.

7. Abdo, W. F., Van De Warrenburg, B. P. C., Burn, D. J., Quinn, N. P., & Bloem, B. R. (2010). The clinical approach to movement disorders. Nature Reviews Neurology, 6(1), 29–37. https://doi.org/10.1038/nrneurol.2009.196

8. Alafuzoff, I., & Hartikainen, P. (2018). Alpha-synucleinopathies. Handbook of Clinical Neurology, 145, 339–353. https://doi.org/10.1016/B978-0-12-802395-2.00024-9

9. Goedert, M., Jakes, R., & Spillantini, M. G. (2017). The synucleinopathies: twenty years on. Journal of Parkinson's Disease, 7(s1), S53–S71. https://doi.org/10.3233/JPD-179005

10. Jellinger, K. A. (2019). Neuropathology and pathogenesis of extrapyramidal movement disorders: a critical update—I. Hypokinetic-rigid movement disorders. Journal of Neural Transmission, 126(8), 933–995. https://doi.org/10.1007/s00702-019-02028-6

11. Dash, D., & Pandey, S. (2019). Movement disorders associated with neuronal antibodies. Acta Neurologica Scandinavica, 139(2), 106–117. https://doi.org/10.1111/ane.13039

12. Chirra, M., Marsili, L., Gallerini, S., Keeling, E. G., Marconi, R., & Colosimo, C. (2019). Paraneoplastic movement disorders: phenomenology, diagnosis, and treatment. European Journal of Internal Medicine, 67(April), 14–23. https://doi.org/10.1016/j.ejim.2019.05.023

13. Popławska-Domaszewicz, K., Florczak-Wyspiańska, J., Kozubski, W., & Michalak, S. (2018). Paraneoplastic movement disorders. Reviews in the Neurosciences, 29(7), 745–755. https://doi.org/10.1515/revneuro-2017-0081

14. Sanger, T. D., Chen, D., Fehlings, D. L., Hallett, M., Lang, A. E., Mink, J. W., . . . Childhood, M. I. N. (2011). Definition and classification of hyperkinetic. Movement Disorders, 25(11), 1538–1549. https://doi.org/10.1002/mds.23088

15. Termsarasab, B. P. (2019). Chorea. CONTINUUM Lifelong Learning in Neurology, 25(4), 1001–1035.

16. Samii, A., & Ransom, B. R. (2005). Movement disorders: overview and treatment options. P and T, 30(4), 228–238.

17. Postuma, R., & Lang, A. (2003). Hemiballism: revisiting a classic disorder. Lancet Neurology, 2(11), 661–668. https://doi.org/10.1016/S1474-4422(03)00554-4

18. Delgado, M. R., & Albright, A. L. (2003). Movement disorders in children: definitions, classifications, and grading systems. Journal of Child Neurology, 18(Suppl. 1), 1–8. https://doi.org/10.1177/0883073803018001s0301

19. De Koning, T. J., & Tijssen, M. A. J. (2015). Movement disorders in 2014: genetic advances spark a revolution in dystonia phenotyping. Nature Reviews Neurology, 11(2), 78–79. https://doi.org/10.1038/nrneurol.2014.254

20. ESDE. (2000). A prevalence study of primary dystonia in eight European countries. Journal of Neurology, 247(10), 787–792. https://doi.org/10.1007/s004150070094

21. Müller, J., Kiechl, S., Wenning, G., Seppi, K., Willeit, J., Gasperi, A., … Poewe, W. (2002). The prevalence of primary dystonia in the general community. Neurology, 59(6), 941–943. https://doi.org/10.1212/01.WNL.0000026474.12594.0D

22. Albanese, A., Di Giovanni, M., & Lalli, S. (2019). Dystonia: diagnosis and management. European Journal of Neurology, 26(1), 5–17. https://doi.org/10.1111/ene.13762

23. Schmidt, A., Jabusch, H., Altenmüller, E., Hagenah, J., Brüggemann, N., Lohmann, K., … Klein, C. (2009). Etiology of musician's dystonia: Familial or environmental? Neurology, 72(14), 1248–1254. https://doi.org/10.1212/01.wnl.0000345670.63363.d1

24. Williams, L., McGovern, E., Kimmich, O., Molloy, A., Beiser, I., Butler, J., … Hutchinson, M. (2017). Epidemiological, clinical and genetic aspects of adult onset isolated focal dystonia in Ireland. European Journal of Neurology, 24(1), 73–81. https://doi.org/10.1111/ene.13133

25. Tarsy, D., & Simon, D. (2006). Dystonia. New England Journal of Medicine, 355, 818–829.

26. Albanese, A., Bhatia, K., Bressman, S., DeLong, M., Fahn, S., Fung, V., . . . Teller, J. (2013). Phenomenology and classification of dystonia: a consensus update. Movement Disorders, 28(7), 863–873. https://doi.org/10.1002/mds.25475

27. Lozsadi, D. (2012). Myoclonus: a pragmatic approach. Practical Neurology, 12(4), 215–224. https://doi.org/10.1136/practneurol-2011-000107

28. Borg, M. (2006). Symptomatic myoclonus. Neurophysiologie Clinique, 36(5–6), 309–318. https://doi.org/10.1016/j.neucli.2006.12.006

29. Badry, R., Abdelhamed, M. A., Sayed, M. A. M., ElHady, A. A., & Mostafa, M. (2019). Epidemiology of dystonia, chorea, and athetosis in Al Quseir City (Red Sea Governorate), Egypt. Egyptian Journal of Neurology, Psychiatry and Neurosurgery, 55(1), 0–3. https://doi.org/10.1186/s41983-019-0109-4

30. Bhatia, K., Bain, P., Bajaj, N., Elble, R., Hallett, M., Louis, E., . . . Tremor Task Force of the International Parkinson and Movement Disorder Society. (2018). Consensus Statement on the Classification of Tremors. From the Task Force on Tremor of the International Parkinson and Movement Disorder Society. Movement Disorders, 33(1), 75–87. https://doi.org/10.1002/mds.27121

31. Louis, E. D., & Ottman, R. (2006). Study of possible factors associated with age of onset in essential tremor. Movement Disorders, 21(11), 1980–1986. https://doi.org/10.1002/mds.21102

32. Das, S. K., Banerjee, T. K., Roy, T., Raut, D. K., Chaudhuri, A., & Hazra, A. (2009). Prevalence of essential tremor in the city of Kolkata, India: a house-to-house survey. European Journal of Neurology, 16(7), 801–807. https://doi.org/10.1111/j.1468-1331.2009.02589.x

33. Benito-León, J., Louis, E., & Bermejo-Pareja, F. (2007). Reported hearing impairment in essential tremor: a population-based case-control study. Neuroepidemiology, 29(3–4), 213–217. https://doi.org/10.1159/000112463

34. Ondo, W. G., Sutton, L., Dat Vuong, K., Lai, D., & Jankovic, J. (2003). Hearing impairment in essential tremor. Neurology, 61(8), 1093–1097. https://doi.org/10.1212/01.WNL.0000086376.40750.AF

35. Benito-León, J., Louis, E., & Bermejo-Pareja, F. (2006). Elderly-onset essential tremor is associated with dementia [6]. Neurology, 66, 1500–1505.

36. Putzke, J. D., Whaley, N. R., Baba, Y., Wszolek, Z. K., & Uitti, R. J. (2006). Essential tremor: predictors of disease progression in a clinical cohort. Journal of Neurology, Neurosurgery & Psychiatry, 77(11), 1235–1237. https://doi.org/10.1136/jnnp.2006.086579

37. Ondo, W. G. (2012). Tetrabenazine treatment for stereotypies and tics associated with dementia. Journal of Neuropsychiatry and Clinical Neuroscience, 24(2), 208–214. https://doi.org/10.1176/appi.neuropsych.11030077

38. Borrell, E. (2000). Hypokinetic Movement Disorders. Journal of Neuroscience Nursing, 32(5), 254–255.

39. Greenland, J., & Barker, R. (2018). The differential diagnosis of Parkinson's disease. In T. Stoker & J. Greenland (Eds.), Parkinson's Disease Pathogenesis and Clinical Aspects (pp. 109–128). Brisbane, Australia: Codon Publications.

40. McFarland, N. (2016). Diagnostic approach to atypical parkinsonian syndromes. CONTINUUM Lifelong Learning in Neurology, 22(4), 1117–1142. https://doi.org/10.1212/CON.0000000000000348

41. Marras, C., Beck, J., Bower, J., Roberts, E., Ritz, B., Ross, G., . . . Tanner, C. (2018). Prevalence of Parkinson's disease across North America. NPJ Parkinson's Disease, 4(1), 1–7. https://doi.org/10.1038/s41531-018-0058-0

42. Marsili, L., Rizzo, G., & Colosimo, C. (2018). Diagnostic criteria for Parkinson's disease: From James Parkinson to the concept of prodromal disease. Frontiers in Neurology, 9(MAR), 1–10. https://doi.org/10.3389/fneur.2018.00156

43. Lees, A. J., Hardy, J., & Revesz, T. (2009). Parkinson's disease. Lancet, 373(9680), 2055–2066. https://doi.org/10.1016/S0140-6736(09)60492-X

44. Emre, M., Aarsland, D., Brown, R., Burn, D. J., Duyckaerts, C., Mizuno, Y., . . . Dubois, B. (2007). Clinical diagnostic criteria for dementia associated with Parkinson's disease. Movement Disorders, 22(12), 1689–1707. https://doi.org/10.1002/mds.21507

45. Braak, H., Del Tredici, K., Bratzke, H., Hamm-Clement, J., Sandmann-Keil, D., & Rüb, U. (2002). Staging of the intracerebral inclusion body pathology associated with idiopathic Parkinson's disease (preclinical and clinical stages). Journal of Neurology, Supplement, 249(3), 1–5. https://doi.org/10.1007/s00415-002-1301-4

46. Hughes, A. J., Daniel, S. E., Kilford, L., & Lees, A. J. (1992). Accuracy of clinical diagnosis of idiopathic Parkinson's disease: a clinico-pathological study of 100 cases. Journal of Neurology Neurosurgery and Psychiatry, 55(3), 181–184. https://doi.org/10.1136/jnnp.55.3.181

47. Hughes, A., Daniel, S., Ben-Shlomo, Y., & Lees, A. (2002). The accuracy of diagnosis of parkinsonian syndromes in a specialist movement disorder service. Brain, 125(4), 861–870.   http://www.embase.com/search/results?subaction=viewrecord&from=export&id=L34279780

48. Jankovic, J. (2008). Parkinson's disease: CLINICAL features and diagnosis. Journal of Neurology, Neurosurgery and Psychiatry, 79(4), 368–376. https://doi.org/10.1136/jnnp.2007.131045

49. Vingerhoets, F., Schulzer, M., Calne, D., & Snow, B. (1997). Which clinical sign of Parkinson's disease best reflects the nigrostriatal lesion? Annals of Neurology, 41(1), 58–64. https://doi.org/10.1002/ana.410410111

50. Lozza, C., Marié, R., & Baron, J. (2002). The metabolic substrates of bradykinesia and tremor in uncomplicated Parkinson's disease. NeuroImage, 17(2), 688–699. https://doi.org/10.1006/nimg.2002.1245

51. Liu, F. T., Ge, J. J., Wu, J. J., Wu, P., Ma, Y., Zuo, C. T., & Wang, J. (2018). Clinical, dopaminergic, and metabolic correlations in Parkinson disease: a dual-tracer PET study. Clinical Nuclear Medicine, 43(8), 562–571. https://doi.org/10.1097/RLU.0000000000002148

52. Hughes, A., Daniel, S., Blankson, S., & Lees, A. (1993). A clinicopathologic study of 100 cases of Parkinson's disease, Archives of Neurology, 50, 140–148. http://archneur.jamanetw ork.com/

53. Riley, D., Lang, A., Blair, R., Birnbaum, A., & Reid, B. (1989). Frozen shoulder and other shoulder disturbances in Parkinson's disease. Journal of Neurology, Neurosurgery, and Psychiatry, 52(6), 63–66. https://doi.org/10.1136/ jnnp.52.1.63

54. Williams, D., Watt, H., & Lees, A. (2006). Predictors of falls and fractures in bradykinetic rigid syndromes: a retrospective study. Journal of Neurology, Neurosurgery and Psychiatry, 77(4), 468–473. https://doi.org/10.1136/jnnp.2005.074070

55. Giladi, N., McDermott, M. P., Fahn, S., Przedborski, S., Jankovic, J., Stern, M., & Tanner, C. (2001). Freezing of gait in PD: prospective assessment in the DATATOP cohort. Neurology, 56(12), 1712–1721. https://doi.org/10.1212/WNL.56.12.1712

56. Bloem, B., Hausdorff, J., Visser, J., & Giladi, N. (2004). Falls and freezing of gait in Parkinson's disease: a review of two interconnected, episodic phenomena. Movement Disorders, 19(8), 871–884. https://doi.org/10.1002/mds.20115

57. Macht, M., Kaussner, Y., Möller, J., Stiasny-Kolster, K., Eggert, K., Krüger, H., & Ellgring, H. (2007). Predictors of freezing in Parkinson's disease: a survey of 6,620 patients. Movement Disorders, 22(7), 953–956. https://doi.org/10.1002/mds.21458

58. Boghen, D. (1997). Apraxia of lid opening: a review. Neurology, 48(6), 1491–1494. https://doi. org/10.1212/WNL.48.6.1491

59. Schaafsma, J., Balash, Y., Gurevich, T., Bartels, A., Hausdorff, J., & Giladi, N. (2003). Characterization of freezing of gait subtypes and the response of each to levodopa in Parkinson's disease. European Journal of Neurology, 10(4), 391–398. https://doi.org/10.1046/ j.1468-1331.2003.00611.x

60. Palma, J., & Kaufmann, H. (2018). Treatment of autonomic dysfunction in Parkinson disease and other synucleinopathies. Movement Disorders, 33(3), 372–390. https://doi.org/10.1002/ mds.27344.

61. Suttrup, I., Suttrup, J., Suntrup-Krueger, S., Siemer, M., Bauer, J., Hamacher, C., . . . Warnecke, T. (2017). Esophageal dysfunction in different stages of Parkinson's disease. Neurogastroenterology and Motility, 29(1), 1–7. https://doi.org/10.1111/nmo.12915

62. Su, A., Gandhy, R., Barlow, C., & Triadafilopoulos, G. (2017). Clinical and manometric characteristics of patients with Parkinson's disease and esophageal symptoms. Diseases of the Esophagus, 30(4), 1–6. https://doi.org/10.1093/dote/dow038

63. Bestetti, A., Capozza, A., Lacerenza, M., Manfredi, L., & Mancini, F. (2017). Delayed gastric emptying in advanced Parkinson disease. Clinical Nuclear Medicine, 42(2), 83–87. https:// doi.org/10.1097/RLU.0000000000001470

64. Hely, M., Morris, J., Reid, W., & Trafficante, R. (2005). Sydney multicenter study of Parkinson' s disease: non-L-dopa-responsive problems dominate at 15 years. Movement Disorders, 20(2), 190–199. https://doi.org/10.1002/mds.20324

65. Aarsland, D., Ehrt, U., Deyn, P., Tekin, S., Emre, M., & Cummings, J. (2007). Neuropsychiatric symptoms in patients with Parkinson's disease and dementia: frequency, profile and associated care giver stress. Journal of Neurology, Neurosurgery & Psychaitry, 36–42. https://doi. org/10.1136/jnnp.2005.083113

66. Stamey, W., Davidson, A., & Jankovic, J. (2008). Shoulder pain: a presenting symptom of Parkinson disease. Journal of Clinical Rheumatology, 14(4), 253.

67. Harding, A., Stimson, E., Henderson, J., & Halliday, G. (2002). Clinical correlates of selective pathology in the amygdala of patients with Parkinson's disease. Brain, 125, 2431–2445.

2

Pathophysiology of Primary and Secondary Movement Disorders

*Claudio Da Cunha, William Sánchez-Luna,
Fernando Henrique Teixeira Zonzini, Daniel R. Benke,
and José Augusto Pochapski*

Introduction

Traditionally neurologist doctors treat movement disorders and the psychiatry doctors treat behavioral and mental disorders. However, motor impairments are common side effects of psychiatric drugs and behavioral and mental symptoms are present in most, if not all, movement disorders. Parkinson's disease (PD) and schizophrenia are good examples. Bradykinesia, rigidity, and rest tremor are cardinal motor signs of PD[1] and are also side effects of antipsychotic drugs.[2] Conversely, psychotic and impulse control symptoms are commonly found in medicated PD patients.[3] In addition, cognitive impairment, depression, and sleep problems are common in PD.[4] Two forms of dyskinesia are side effects of the medications for both PD and schizophrenia.[5] Several other examples of overlapping symptoms in psychiatric and movement disorders exist. Akathisia, defined as a subjective feeling of restlessness and urgent need to move, is a core symptom of the restless legs syndrome[6] and a side effect of neuroleptics.[7] Is it a movement disorder sign or a psychiatric symptom? Several other motor signs and psychiatric symptoms that occur in both movement disorders and psychiatric disorders are examined in details in this book. What most of them have in common is a malfunctioning of the corticobasal ganglia circuitry. Therefore, the goal of this chapter is to describe the normal functioning and the dysfunctions of the basal ganglia that are implicated in the pathophysiology of primary and secondary movement disorders.

Physiology of the basal ganglia

The basal ganglia are formed by: (a) an input station—the corpus striatum; (b) intermediate nuclei—the external parts of the globus pallidus (GPe) and the subthalamic nucleus (STN), which can also work as an input nucleus; (c) the output nuclei—the internal part of the globus pallidus (GPi) and the reticulate part of the substantia nigra (SNr), and the ventral pallidum (VP); (d) associated modulatory nuclei—the compact part of the substantia nigra (SNc), and the ventral tegmental area (VTA) (Figure 2.1).

Because the degeneration of components of the basal ganglia was early discovered to be the cause of the motor impairments of PD and Huntington's disease, the basal ganglia were initially taken as a system involved only in motor control.[8–10] However, the internal circuitry

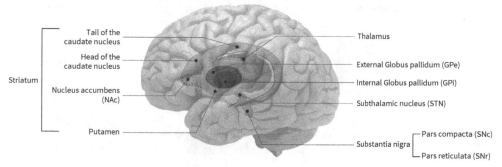

Figure 2.1 Anatomy of the basal ganglia.
See Parent and Hazrati (1995a, 1995b) for anatomical details.

that exists in the motor parts of the basal ganglia is very similar to the circuitry found in the associative and limbic parts (Figure 2.2), which are associated with executive aspects of decision-making, motivation, and other emotional states. In the last three decades a growing body of studies has been reporting nonmotor symptoms in these movement disorders. These findings changed the classic view of the basal ganglia as a system dedicated only to motor control. Nowadays the basal ganglia are mostly seen as a subcortical system that helps the frontal cortex in selection-related functions.[11,12]

The basal ganglia are functionally divided into three major loops that make reciprocal connections with the frontal lobe, forming the so-called motor loop, limbic loop, and associative loop[13] (Figure 2.3). The motor loop receives inputs from the sensorimotor cortex and sends outputs to the premotor and motor cortex.[14] It is proposed that the motor loop influences the selection of automatic responses based solely on sensorial information.[15] Therefore, this kind of action-selection receives no influence from cognitive and emotional processes.[16,17] On the other hand, the limbic loop is uploaded by contextual information coming from the

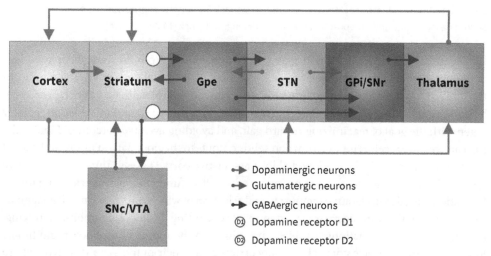

Figure 2.2 Basic cortical-basal ganglia circuitry.
GPe, external globus pallidus; GPi, internal globus pallidus; SNc, substantia nigra pars compacta; SNr, substantia nigra pars reticulata; STN, subthalamic nuclei; VTA, ventral tegmental area.
Source: Based on the model proposed by Alexander et al. (1986).

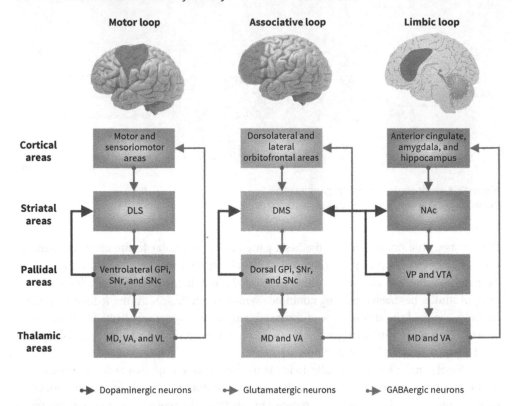

Figure 2.3 Schematic illustrations of the three functional loops between the motor, limbic, and associative cortices with the basal ganglia.

For the sake of simplicity, the indirect pathway and the oculomotor loop are not represented in this diagram. DLS, dorsolateral striatum; DMS, dorsomedial striatum; GPi, internal globus pallidus; NAc nucleus accumbens; MD, medial dorsal thalamic nucleus; SNc, substantia nigra pars compacta; SNr, substantia nigra pars reticulata; VA ventral anterior thalamic nucleus; VP, ventral pallidum; VL, ventrolateral thalamic nucleus, VTA, ventral tegmental area.

Source: Based on the model proposed by Alexander, Delong, and Strick (1986).

hippocampal formation and emotional information coming from the amygdala, hypothalamus, anterior cingulate prefrontal cortex, and medial prefrontal cortex.[18,19] The outputs of the limbic loop limbic are areas of the neocortex and the ventral pallidum, which projects to brainstem motor nuclei. Thus, the influence of the limbic loop in action-selection is likely taken with the goal of maximizing reward gain and avoiding aversive outcomes. Finally, the associative loop receives inputs from and sends outputs to the dorsolateral prefrontal, lateral orbitofrontal, parietal lobe, and medial lobe associative cortical areas. Thus, the associative loop likely participates in selection processes of cognitive functions such as searching for information stored as declarative memories, and selection of which information will be temporarily stored in the working memory, attentional set-shifting, behavioral inhibition, judging, and other executive functions.[20,21] Note that, although the inputs of the motor and limbic loops come from diverse cortical and subcortical areas, their outputs are directed only to the frontal lobe of the neocortex and to motor nuclei of the brainstem. This suggests that the motor and limbic loops are dedicated to action-selection. The outputs of the associative loop are not motor areas of the frontal cortex but cortical areas involved in planning future actions based on higher order feelings, consciously evoked memories, and reasoning. In summary, the motor loop plays a role in automatic motor responses to sensory cues, the limbic loop participates in the selection of actions that maximize rewards, and the associative loop is part of a system that selects future action to be taken. Seen this way it is easy to understand why the basal ganglia play critical roles in motor, behavioral, and psychiatric aspects of movement disorders.

The basal ganglia best understood function is action-selection.[4,12,15,22] Motor actions related to manipulation of objects and other automatic movements (stimulus-response habits, unconditioned responses, and conditioned responses) and voluntary movements of the arms and head are encoded by parts of the motor and premotor cortices that project to the motor pattern generators in the spinal cord and brainstem. According to the model illustrated in Figure 2.4, a motor action can be initiated by excitatory (glutamatergic) projections from the ventrolateral oralis nuclei (VLo) and ventrolateral media (VLm) nuclei of the thalamus. The VLo and VLm are under tonic inhibition of the output station of the basal ganglia formed by SNr and GPi. Therefore, initiation of a motor action depends on selective disinhibition of output station neurons. This disinhibition is made by a subpopulation of GABAergic neurons in the striatum known as neurons of the direct pathway. They were named this way because they make direct projections to the output stations, thus causing disinhibition of subpopulations of output station neurons, resulting in the initiation of a

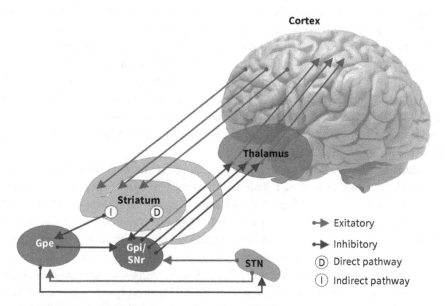

Figure 2.4 Corticobasal ganglia circuitry for action-selection.
Inhibitory (GABA) neurons are printed in red, and excitatory (glutamate) neurons are printed in green. Thalamic neurons can activate motor actions in the motor cortex, but these thalamic neurons are under tonic inhibition of the output station of the basal ganglia. Activation of the direct pathway can selectively disinhibit the initiation of an action, while the indirect pathway can prevent action initiation. The hyperdirect pathway increases the inhibitory action of the indirect pathway. GPe, external globus pallidus; GPi, internal globus pallidus; SNr, substantia nigra pars reticulata, STN, subthalamic nuclei.
Source: Based on anatomical and physiological findings and in computational modeling (Albin et al., 1990; Alexander et al., 1986; Da Cunha et al., 2009; Frank et al., 2016; Mink, 1996; Nambu et al., 2002).

motor action. Another subpopulation of GABAergic neurons in the striatum is named indirect pathway neurons. They project to the output stations in an indirect way that makes it to increase the inhibition over the thalamus, thus inhibiting or halting motor actions. The no-go neurons synapse GABAergic neurons of the GPe. The GPe neurons are tonically active and make projections to the output stations. Therefore, when they are inhibited by the no-go neurons, they increase the inhibition over the thalamus. GPe neurons also project to the STN, which in turn sends glutamatergic projections to the output nuclei. Therefore, the activation of the STN increases the inhibition of the output station over the thalamus. The STN also receives excitatory inputs from neocortex neurons that form the hyperdirect pathway.[23,24] Computational simulations suggest that the activation of the STN by the hyperdirect pathway plays an important role in preventing impulsive responses.[25] Another important input onto the striatum are projections from the thalamus. The thalamic centromedian-parafascicular complex (CM/Pf) of the thalamus is the source of a major excitatory glutamatergic input to the striatum, but there are thalamostriatal inputs from other intralaminar and other thalamic nuclei.[26,27]

The action-selection model illustrated in Figure 2.4 proposes that the motor programs of the motor cortex compete for the control of behavior. The winner will be the motor program that overtakes the threshold needed to disinhibit the thalamus-cortical neurons from the output basal ganglia inhibition. Increased activity of the motor cortex increases this threshold by activation of the hyperdirect pathway.[23] A cortical motor program can overtake this threshold by activating the direct pathway neurons that can selectively disinhibit this motor program. The cortical neurons of this program can also prevent the other motor programs from initiate alternative motor actions by activation of the indirect pathway. Therefore, action-selection depends on the strength of the synapses between the neurons that input information into the striatum and the striatal neurons of the direct and indirect pathways. The strength of these synapses will determine the influence of the different stimuli, memories, and affective states over behavior. Malfunctioning or nonadaptive connections in the neural network are the most common cause of motor signs and behavioral symptoms of most neuropsychiatric diseases.

The main modulator of the corticostriatal synapses is the neurotransmitter dopamine released in the striatum by midbrain neurons. There are two families of dopamine receptors. The D2, D3, and D4 receptors form the D2 family of dopamine receptors (D2Rs), and the D1 and D5 receptors form the D1 family (D1Rs). D1Rs and D2Rs are mostly segregated into different neurons. D1Rs are mostly expressed in the dendrites of the direct pathway neurons and D2Rs in the dendrites of the indirect pathway neurons. In the striatum, D2Rs are also expressed in the presynaptic membrane of dopamine neurons. Co-expression of D1Rs and D2Rs in the dorsal striatum occurs in only 6% of the medium spiny neurons. D1-D2 heteromers bind to the Gq/11 protein resulting in the release of Ca^{2+} from intracellular stores.[28] D1-D3 heteromers have also been reported.[29]

Activated D1 and D2 receptors bind to the Gs and Gi/o proteins resulting in the activation or (D1) inhibition (D2) of the adenylyl cyclase enzyme (Figure 2.5). Activated D1Rs also bind to the Gq proteins, which activate the phospholipase C enzyme causing an increase of the second messengers diacylglycerol (DAG), inositol triphosphate (IP3), and Ca^{2+}. Activation of D2Rs can also activate the beta-arrestin 2/akt pathway and inhibit the phospholipase C enzyme. Therefore, binding of dopamine into the D1Rs increases intracellular levels of cyclic adenosine monophosphate (cAMP, 3′,5′-cyclic adenosine monophosphate) while binding

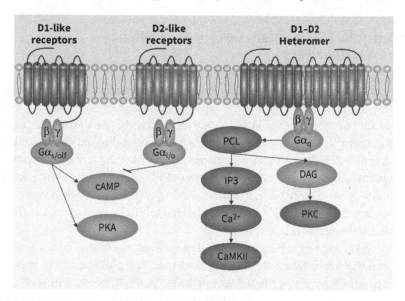

Figure 2.5 Signaling pathways regulated by dopamine D1 and D2 receptor families.

cAMKII, Ca²⁺/calmodulin-dependent protein kinase II; cAMP, cyclic adenosine monophosphate; DAG, diacylglycerol; Gαβγ, G protein (guanine nucleotide-binding protein); IP3, inositol triphosphate; PKA, protein kinase A; PKC, protein kinase C; PLC, phospholipase C.

of dopamine into the D2Rs causes the opposite effect. The second messengers cAMP and Ca²⁺ are cofactors needed to activate the protein kinase A (PKA) and the Ca²⁺/calmodulin-dependent protein kinase II (CaMKII), respectively, which phosphorylates voltage-gated K⁺ and Ca²⁺ channels.

The classical view established by anatomists and pathologists nearly 30 years ago proposes that dopamine favors the activation of the striatal neurons of the direct pathway and reduces the excitability of the neurons of the indirect pathway.[30] However, a growing body of evidence showed a more complicated picture, which we try to summarize in a simplified manner. The resting membrane of the striatal projection neurons, namely the medium spiny neurons, flips between under the more hyperpolarized "down state" and the subthreshold "up state." Activation of D1 receptors promotes synaptic integration and spike firing while increasing the threshold for upward transitions, effectively acting to enhance contrast between up and down states. On the other hand, the excitability of the medium spiny neurons of the indirect pathway is reduced by D2Rs by decreasing the influx of Ca²⁺ through CaV1 somatic channels and by reducing the duration of the up state.[31]

Most, if not all, motor dysfunctions observed in movement disorders can be divided in one of two categories: hypokinetic and hyperkinetic. Hypokinetic signs include bradykinesia (slow movement), hypokinesia (reduced amplitude of movements), akinesia (inability to initiate movements), and rigidity. Hyperkinetic movement disorders are characterized by excessive involuntary movements, including dyskinesias and tremors. In the next topics we report what is actually known about the mechanisms of the hypokinetic and hyperkinetic movement disorders. What these movement disorders have in common is that most of them can be explained as hyper- or hypofunctioning of the basal ganglia direct and indirect pathways.

Basal Ganglia Mechanisms of Hypokinetic Movement Disorders

The understanding of the role of the basal ganglia in motor control greatly changed in the last 40 years. The first big change was the replacement of the extrapyramidal model of the basal ganglia for the go/no-go model. Voluntary motor control signals originate in the motor cortex and are sent to the motor neurons in the spinal cord through the pyramidal tracts. Because the motor deficits of PD, such as tremor and hypokinesia, are involuntary, the term "extrapyramidal symptoms" has been used to refer to PD-like motor dysfunctions. The term "extrapyramidal system" can be found in scientific publications published since the late 1940s. Nowadays the expression "extrapyramidal side-effects" is used to refer to the effects of drugs that block dopamine D2 receptors.[32]

The go/no-go model proposes that the basal ganglia and the frontal cortex form a system dedicated to initiate voluntary actions by means of the direct pathway and to prevent or halt voluntary actions by means of the indirect pathway. In other words, this model proposes that the dichotomy action (go) vs. no-action (no-go) are mediated by the direct and indirect pathway, respectively.[13] This go/no-go concept has also been used to explain the role of the basal ganglia in psychiatric disorders.[33] Recent studies have shown that the implications of the direct and indirect pathways are not so simple as proposed by the go/no-go model. Adding the selection function to the basal ganglia greatly increases the capacity of the go/no-go model to explain the accumulated data about the basal ganglia functioning during normal movement and about the mechanisms of current treatments of movement disorders.[4,12,15] Adding selection to the go/no-go model is equivalent to saying that the neurons of the direct pathway are not massively activated to initiate any kind of movement. Instead, selective subpopulations of direct pathway neurons are activated to initiate specific movements.

The other modernization of the go/no-go model was the addition of the hyperdirect pathway to the corticobasal ganglia circuitry. It was proposed that when motor programs encoded in the neocortex are competing for the solution of an action demand, the hyperdirect projection of the cortical neurons to the STN increases the threshold that the neurons of the direct pathway need to overtake to initiate an action.[23] This prevents impulsive actions, a function analytically called "hold your horses."[25] Finally, the concept that the direct and indirect pathways have opposite effects has been challenged by the finding that both are active by the time voluntary actions initiate.[34] This finding was conciliated with the selection hypothesis by the understanding that at the same time those specific neurons of the direct pathway are activated to trigger the initiation of a specific action, several neurons of the indirect pathway are concomitantly activated to prevent initiation of concurrent actions.

These concepts of the roles of the direct, indirect, and hyperdirect pathways functions are the framework used to explain most of the hypokinetic and hyperkinetic dysfunctions that occur in several movement disorders.

Hypokinetic Deficits in PD

Probably the oldest and best known pathophysiological mechanism related to the basal ganglia are the hypokinetic signs observed in PD patients. They include bradykinesia, akinesia, and rigidity. Hypokinesia is used to describe the reduction of movements, bradykinesia is movement slowness, and akinesia is the inability to initiate movements. Rigidity is associated with a feeling of stiffness and may be estimated by examining muscle resistance against passive stretching. Other motor deficits such as gait disturbance, micrographia, precision grip impairment, and speech problems are also common in PD.[35–37]

Most of these deficits are caused by degeneration of the dopaminergic neurons of the substantia nigra pars compacta. Neurodegeneration occurs after the intracellular accumulation of the protein α-synuclein, which forms Lewy neurites and Lewy bodies.[38] However, there is evidence that nonmotor symptoms could begin in many instances 10 to 20 years before, not in the dopamine neurons but more likely in the lower brainstem and the olfactory bulb, or even in the peripheral autonomic nervous system.[39] Early premotor symptoms include constipation, hyposmia, pain, genitourinary problems, and sleep disorders.[3,11,40] Braak et al. divided PD into five stages.[41] In stages 1 and 2, Lewy bodies are restricted to the medulla oblongata/pontine tegmentum, olfactory bulb, and olfactory nucleus. Attention and working memory deficits and depression usually arise before motor signs become evident, which happens only in stages 3 and 4, when severe pathological changes occur in the substantia nigra and other midbrain nuclei. All symptomatic motor aspects of the disease occur only in stages 5 with the progressive spreading of the α-synuclein inclusions in the neocortex. At this time, in addition to the worsening of motor impairment, apathy, dementia, visual hallucinations, and other psychotic symptoms are more commonly observed.[41]

These hypokinetic deficits are well explained by the Alexander, DeLong, and Crutcher model of the basal ganglia (Figure 2.4). When the concentration of dopamine is below the threshold needed to activate D2Rs, the indirect pathway will be overactive, thus reducing initiation, frequency, and vigor of movements. This hypothesis is supported by several preclinical studies. Muscle rigidity, akinesia, and bradykinesia are observed after the loss of dopamine neurons of the substantia nigra induced by the neurotoxin 1-methyl-4-phenyl 1,2,3,6-tetrahydropyridine (MPTP) in monkeys and by the neurotoxin 6-hydroxydopamine (6-OHDA) in rodents.[42] Electrophysiological recording in the striatum of 6-OHDA treated rats also showed a reduction in the spontaneous activity of the direct pathway neurons and a hyperactivation of the neurons of the indirect pathway.[43,44] Thus, it has been proposed that the onset of the hypokinetic signs of PD is caused by the absence of stimulation of striatal D1Rs and D2Rs in the neurons of the direct and indirect pathways, respectively. The sum of these events results in excessive thalamic inhibition, making it difficult to initiate movements.[45] This explains the success of the restoration of basal levels of dopamine with the treatment with the dopamine precursor L-3,4-dihydroxyphenylalanine (L-DOPA), which improve these symptoms. Indeed, most drugs used to mitigate the motor deficits of PD result in increased levels of striatal dopamine (e.g., L-DOPA, opicapone, entacapone, opicapone, selegiline, rasagiline) or are direct agonists of dopamine receptors (e.g., pramipexole, ropinirole).[46] The imbalance between the direct and indirect pathway caused by reduced activation of DRs can also be mitigated by blocking the output of the basal ganglia with lesions in the motor thalamus or GPi. High frequency stimulation of the GPi or STN by deep brain stimulation (DBS) also alleviates the motor deficits of PD. It is possible that the DBS causes a reversible inhibition of the GPi and STN. As shown in Figures 2.2 and 2.4, the STN receives inputs from the motor cortex (hyperdirect pathway) and further activates the indirect pathway by excitatory projections to the GPe.[23] This way, the STN DBS can counteract the hyperactivity of the indirect pathway caused by the dopamine depletion and it is one of the most successful treatments available to improve the motor signs of PD.[47] It has also been proposed that the STN DBS causes a retrograde activation of the motor cortex.

Rigidity in PD is associated with increased activity in the STN and functional connectivity among the cerebellum, and the motor cortex, temporal cortex, occipital cortex, and the caudate nucleus in off-medicated patients.[48] Beta wave, or beta rhythm, is a neural oscillation (brainwave) in the brain with a frequency range of between 12.5 and 30 Hz (12.5 to 30 cycles per second). Cyclic oscillations in local electric field potentials at the range of 12–30 Hz (beta-band) that occur in the motor cortex and in the basal ganglia nuclei are correlated with PD rigidity, bradykinesia, and tremor.[49,50] Rigidity improvement is correlated with a decrease in the sharpness of the beta-band ratio.[51–53] Rigidity, tremor, and bradykinesia are improved with L-DOPA treatment and high frequency STN DBS concomitant modulation of abnormal oscillations during rest and movement.[54]

Hypokinetic Dysfunctions of Other Movement Disorders

Catatonia

Catatonia was described by Karl Kahlbaum in the 1870s as an independent syndrome characterized by motor, affective, and behavioral abnormalities.[55] Nowadays, catatonia is taken as a nosologically unspecific syndrome associated with schizophrenia spectrum disorder, mood disorders, as well as various neurological and other medical conditions.[56,57] The word "catatonia" appears 116 times in the DSM-5 as part of multiple conditions. Catatonia consists of a hypokinetic state (stupor, akinesia, catalepsy, rigor, resistance to passive movements) alternating with hyperkinetic signs (stereotypies, dyskinesia) in addition to emotional and affective symptoms (flat affect or affect incontinence, anxiety), and behavioral symptoms (mutism, echolalia, impulsivity, etc.). There is a clear overlap between PD and catatonia symptoms that makes the differential diagnostic difficult. The implication of the basal ganglia in catatonia and PD, as confirmed by multimodal RMN imaging studies, explains the occurrence of akinesia in both disorders.[57,58] Northoff et al. proposed that similar akinetic signs observed in PD and catatonia may be explained by altered bottom-up modulation of the cortico-basal ganglia motor loop mediated by dopamine deficits.[58] This hypothesis is supported by the fact that the likelihood of developing a drug-induced neuroleptic malignant syndrome, which symptomatically overlaps with catatonia, is directly proportional to the degree of D2 receptor antagonism.[59,60] However, NMDA (N-methyl-D-aspartate) receptor partial antagonists, and electroconvulsive therapies are efficient treatments for both catatonia and neuroleptic malignant syndrome.[58,61–63] This implicates the GABAergic, glutamatergic, and serotonergic neurotransmitter systems in the pathophysiology of catatonia. In a recent review of imaging studies, Hirjak et al. compared catatonia patients with diagnoses based on motor and behavioral parameters with those in which the Northoff Catatonia Rating Scale (NCRS) was used.[64] The NCRS also includes the affective symptoms that were present in the Kahlbaum's definition of catatonia. The Hirjak's review proposes that while the motor signs of catatonia result from altered bottom-up modulation between the dopamine system and the premotor/motor cortex, the emotional/affective symptoms result from a horizontal orbitofrontal/parietal abnormal modulation.

Hyperkinetic Dysfunctions

Tremors in PD

Resting tremor (which occurs at musclular rest) is much more frequent in PD than kinetic tremor (which occurs during voluntary movements) and postural tremor (which results in inaptitude to sustain a posture). Unlike PD rigidity, akinesia, and bradykinesia, which are strongly related to dopamine depletion in the basal ganglia, many studies did not find a correlation between increased activity in the GPi and PD resting tremors.[36,65] Although tremor often ameliorates with L-DOPA and STN DBS, some authors claim that the resting tremor is less related to dopamine depletion. While some studies reported greater dopamine depletion in the striatum and pallidum of PD patients with dominant akinesia,[66,67] another study has found more dopamine loss in the tremor dominant compared to akinesia dominant patients.[68] Qanhawi et al. also reported decreased raphe serotonin transporter in PD patients with greater tremor.[68] In the past, PD tremor was treated with anticholinergics drugs, but the mechanism of the improvement remains nuclear.[69]

An alternative model proposes that the beta-band oscillations are caused by transfer of information among the neuronal networks that are abnormal in PD.[54,70,71] Nevertheless, neurons in the basal ganglia, motor thalamus nuclei, and cortex fire at a rate of 3–6 Hz, which is close to the rate in which the resting tremors occur and the activity of these neurons occurs in concomitance with the tremors occurrence.[72,73] In addition, increases in single unit firing and in the power of beta-band oscillations in the STN and primary motor cortex of PD patients have been proposed to be related to the PD tremors.[50,74,75]

Essential Tremor

Essential tremor is among the most common movement disorders, affecting at least 1% of the global population.[76] It is a chronic and progressive disease characterized by the presence of involuntary, rhythmic, oscillatory movement of a body member.[77] Essential tremor is usually observed in the hands and arms. However, it can also be observed in the head, jaw, and other regions.[76,78] Tremor is a sign that can be observed in other hyperkinetic movement disorders.[79] However, different from the rhythm of the tremors that occur in other diseases, essential tremor occurs characteristically at 4–12 Hz.[80]

The main risk factors for essential tremor are age, genetic, and possibly environmental factors.[77,81] Usually, essential tremor is associated with advanced age patients and studies described that the incidence progressively increases with age.[82,83] Approximately 5% of patients older than 65 years present essential tremor. The incidence can reach about 20% of subjects older than 95 years.[83] A polymorphism in the protein LINGO1 was associated with a familiar history of essential tremor.[76,78,84] In normal people, this protein plays an important role in synaptic plasticity and neuronal development.

An ongoing debate remains for the definition of the essential tremor physiopathology. However, structural, molecular, and neuroimaging evidence pointed to an important involvement of the cerebellum.[85–87] Functional abnormalities, volume decrease, and neuronal loss in the cerebellum of essential tremor patients have been reported, and the decrease in Purkinje cells density, dendritic arborization, and axonal morphology were also observed.[88,89] Purkinje cells are the major inhibitory neuronal population in the cerebellum, and Purkinje cells loss associated with morphological and functional changes in its activity may result in cerebellar hyperactivity of the deep cerebellar nuclei.[77,90] Essential tremor has also been associated with changes in the rhythmic activity on the cortico-ponto-cerebello-thalamo-cortical loop.[76] However, the origin of this oscillation is still not elucidated. Lewy bodies have also been reported in patients with essential tremor.[91] However, the Lewy bodies distribution pattern was different from that observed in PD.[85]

In the early stages of essential tremor the motor impairments may not cause significant impairments in daily activities and no intervention may be needed.[92] However, in more advanced stages, propranolol or primidone treatment are commonly applied. Also, surgical approaches, such as DBS, are described to promote a considerable decrease in tremor levels.[92,93]

Levodopa-Induced Dyskinesia in PD

After 1 year of levodopa administration, nearly 7% of the PD patients demonstrate dyskinesia signs. This prevalence escalates to 40% after 4 years and 87% after 9–15 years of levodopa treatment.[94] The clinical manifestations of levodopa-induced dyskinesia are diverse, including chorea, akathisia, ballism, dystonia, and myoclonus.[95] Nevertheless, the more commonly observed levodopa-induced dyskinesia manifestation is chorea/choreoathetoid movements.[96]

Even after extensive investigation, the etiology of levodopa-induced dyskinesia is still not completely known. Currently, it is described that levodopa administration is necessary for levodopa-induced dyskinesia development. The duration of levodopa treatment, severity of the PD dysfunctions, female sex, and genetic polymorphisms are the main risk factors for levodopa-induced dyskinesia.[97] The degeneration of the dopaminergic nigrostriatal pathway and consequent decrease in dopamine levels that occur in PD result in hypersensitivity of dopaminergic receptors, which can result in hyperactivation of the direct pathway and hyperinhibition of the indirect pathway, thus causing involuntary movements.[97,98] In addition, PD patients lack the functional long-term potentiation that adapts the degree of activation of voluntary movement to their effects and develop a "nonplastic" form of striatal long-term potentiation that is not sensitive to neuronal input changes.[99]

Prolonged D1R stimulation can result in changes in synaptic plasticity mechanisms, including increased activity of the extracellular signal-regulated kinase (ERK) pathway.[100–102] This increased ERK activity can result in abnormal phosphorylation of histone-3 by the mitogen- and stress-activated kinase 1 (MSK1) and subsequent increase in striatal ΔFosB levels, a marker of neuronal activity, in the direct pathway neurons.[102] PD rodent models demonstrated that the specific stimulation of D1-MSN (medium spiny neurons expressing D1R) resulted in improved motor function but also in development of dyskinesia. In contrast, D2-MSN stimulation had no similar effect.[103] Interestingly, morphological changes are also observed in levodopa-induced dyskinesia models.[96] Preclinical models described that in denervated striatum, levodopa treatment enhanced neuronal spine density on D2-MSN (medium spiny neurons expressing D2R). However, no change was observed on D1-MSN.[104] Nevertheless, even though an increased spiny density is observed in D2-MSN, the hyperexcitability of the neurons of the indirect pathway observed in levodopa-induced dys-kinesia is also dependent on D1R activity.[104] These changes promote a decrease in the inhib-itory activity of the pallidum/SNr over the thalamus, resulting in a subsequent increase in motor cortex activation.[96] Preclinical studies also observed in levodopa-induced dyskinesia models an association between the prefrontal cortex and basal ganglia neuronal activity.[105] In addition to the glutamatergic system, nondopaminergic, serotonergic, and adenosinergic systems are also involved in levodopa-induced dyskinesia physiopathology.[98]

The motor impairments promoted by levodopa remain one of the most concerning prob-lems in PD treatment. Currently, amantadine, an NMDA receptor antagonist, is a common therapeutic strategy for dyskinesia treatment. However, limited treatment efficacy and con-siderable side effects are observed.[106] Also, DBS is described to promote significant improve-ment.[107] Delaying the onset and lowering the doses of levodopa has been proposed to prevent or manage dyskinesia in PD patients.[108]

Tardive Dyskinesia

Nearly 25% of patients using antipsychotic drugs develop tardive dyskinesia.[109–110] However, tardive dyskinesia can be promoted by several other pharmacologic agents, if they block dopa-mine receptors.[111] Therefore, tardive dyskinesia is not only a side effect of psychotropic drugs but a motor disorder that develops during the treatment with these drugs.[110] Motor symp-toms can appear a few weeks to many years after the beginning of treatment.[112] They consist in repetitive and involuntary movements in the oral-buccal-lingual area.[113] Choreic-athetoid movements are also observed in muscles of the body extremities.[114] These motor impairments can be long-lasting, continuing even after the end of the treatment, and in many cases are irre-versible, resulting in considerable disability and poor life quality for the patients.[115,116]

Factors that increase tardive dyskinesia development risk are classified into modified and nonmodified. Modified factors include the type of the pharmacologic agent, dosage and treat-ment duration, and existence of previous motor or mood disorders.[109,117] Older age, female sex, and African and Caucasian ethnicity are examples of nonmodified risk factors.[112,118,119] Genetic polymorphism can also play a role. Genetic mutations on cytochrome P450 genes can induce changes in antipsychotic metabolism and changes in genes involved in dopamine metabolism and signaling can increase the risk of developing tardive dyskinesia.[120–122]

Tardive dyskinesia is a complex and multifactorial disorder, and its complete patho-physiology is not completely elucidated.[112] D2-like dopamine receptors overexpression in consequence of prolonged exposition of dopamine receptor antagonists is the most likely cause of tardive dyskinesia.[123,124] This results in hypersensitization of the D2R in the striatal neurons, thus reducing the inhibitory control of the indirect pathway under nonfunctional movements.[125] However, this hypothesis cannot explain all clinical observations.[126] Analysis of D2R expression on tardive dyskinesia patients by positron emission tomography (PET) showed no difference in D2R expression compared to control patients and an animal model more implicated D3 receptors.[125] Other hypotheses for tardive dyskinesia pathophysiology propose mechanisms related to possible disturbance of dopaminergic and cholinergic sys-tems, the presence of noradrenergic dysfunction, imbalance on GABA signaling, glutama-tergic excitotoxicity,[113,127–130] neurodegeneration and oxidative stress.[131,132]

Recently, the Food and Drug Administration has approved the use of vesicular monoamine transporter type 2 (VMAT2) inhibitors, which inhibit the release of dopamine to treat tardive dyskinesia, but the development of more efficient drugs is still a challenge.[133]

Akathisia

Akathisia is a hyperkinetic movement disorder described as a mental and physical restlessness resulting in an inability to stay still. Akathisic patients with mild conditions may just report an uneasy feeling, primarily on the lower limbs, but in more severe cases, also on the upper limbs and trunk. In severe cases, the inner discomfort can be so distressful and unbearable that may result in aggressive, hostile behaviors and suicide ideation. The compelling urge to move gets some relief as soon as the movement starts but promptly resumes to the prior agitated state when the patient returns to rest. Besides the subjective feeling of restlessness, patients objectively demonstrate behaviors of repeated movements like fidgeting, pacing or rocking back and forth, and persistent swinging or shaking legs.[134,135] Different from a dyskinesia, which is involuntary, in akathisia, there is an uncontrollable desire or compulsion that leads to voluntary movements. Therefore, more than just a movement disorder, akathisia has an sensory and emotional component.[136]

The etiology of the drug-induced akathisia is mainly associated with typical antipsychotics extrapyramidal side effects but also, with minor incidence, associated with atypical antipsychotics, selective serotonin reuptake inhibitors antidepressants, and antiemetics.[137]

Clinically it can be defined, without any strict distinction, in different types: acute akathisia, when symptoms appear soon or a few days after first drug administration, tardive akathisia, when symptoms onset after three months from drug treatment initiation, withdrawal akathisia, when symptoms manifest upon discontinuation or decrease of anticholinergics, antipsychotics and other psychotropic drugs. Chronic akathisia can last for more than six months after changes in medication prescriptions.[137,138] Furthermore, akathisia can even last for many years after antipsychotic treatment discontinuing.[139]

There is evidence that akathisia pathogenesis may be related to unbalanced iron homeostasis.[140] Low plasma levels of iron and ferritin are associated with akathisia in patients with chronic psychotic disorder.[141] Low CNS iron is also strongly implicated in restless legs syndrome, which is an akathisia, but thought to represent a distinct syndrome. Early evidence based on animal models shows that low iron diets imitate dopamine receptor D2 blocking.[142] Since iron is a cofactor of tyrosine hydroxylase, an enzyme acting on the dopamine synthesis pathway, low iron levels may downregulate dopamine synthesis, although there is no human data supporting this. This finding does agree with recent results from an experiment that concluded that loss of transferrin receptor caused the death of dopaminergic neurons in the substantia nigra and depletion of dopaminergic projections to the striatum in mice.[143] Furthermore, an increase in dopamine concentration and a decrease in dopamine transporter and D2R activities in the striatum has been found in iron-deficient rats.[144] In addition, antidopaminergic drugs and lesions on the ventral tegmental area may result in akathisia.[135,138] Since anticholinergics, benzodiazepines, and beta-blockers are used in akathisia treatment, it has been proposed that GABA, acetylcholine, and norepinephrine are possibly also involved in the pathophysiology of akathisia.

Another study suggests that the decreased activity in the ventral striatum results in an unbalanced activity between the nucleus accumbens (NAc) due to a compensatory effect of the adrenergic projections from the locus coeruleus. A relative overstimulation of the NAc shell would be responsible for the urge in displaying averting or curious behaviors and dysphoric feelings. The blockade of norepinephrine firing neurons in the locus coeruleus could be an explanation for the mitigation of akathisia symptoms by beta blockers.[136]

Chorea

Chorea is a hyperkinetic dysfunction characterized by abrupt involuntary contraction of muscles caused by dysfunctions in motor areas of the cortex and their communications with the basal ganglia. Chorea varies from subtle choreiform movements of the eyes or face to severe generalized contractions of the trunk and limbs muscles.[145] The signs can be accentuated by emotions and stress and occur mostly in awake patients, being rarely reported in sleepy persons. Chorea is one of the main dysfunctions observed in Huntington's disease, but can also be induced by levodopa and can occur as a consequence of lesions in the subthalamic nucleus.[65,146] In addition to chorea, Huntington's disease patients also present progressive motor incoordination, gait imbalance, speech and swallowing impairment, bradykinesia, and rigidity. Huntington's disease is an inherited autosomal dominant neurodegenerative disease caused by a CAG trinucleotide repeat expansion in the huntingtin gene.[147] This expansion causes protein aggregation in the cytosol and nucleus of neurons causing neuronal loss observed mostly in the neocortex and striatum. Striatal neurons of the indirect pathway are most vulnerable, particularly in the early phase of the disease.

Deficient inhibition of improper movements by the indirect pathway is the most likely cause for chorea in Huntington's disease. Loss of cortical and direct pathway neurons explains the hypokinetic deficits that occur in later phases of the disease (Figure 2.6). Another mechanism proposed for chorea is the imbalance of GABAergic projection from GPi to the thalamus.[146] It was initially reported that loss of striatal neurons or loss of dopamine receptors D1 and D2 explained chorea episodes in Huntington's patients.[148–150] Increased levels of GABA were found in the subthalamic nucleus and thalamus of Huntington's disease patients with chorea, compared to patients that presented only rigidity.[151] Chorea has been most consistently associated with lesions in the caudate nucleus or putamen, resulting in disinhibition of the external globus pallidus. Other systemic potential causes of chorea are ischemia-hypoxia, toxins, drugs, and metabolic disorders.[151]

Because the basal ganglia indirect pathway is compromised in Huntington's disease chorea, treatment with DBS of the internal globus pallidus has been used with good results. High frequency (130–180 Hz) demonstrates better benefits, and low frequency (40 Hz) worsens chorea.[152] DBS has been successful for treating chorea that occurs in other diseases, like chorea-acanthocytosis and cerebral palsy.[153–155]

In 2020, tetrabenazine and deutetrabenazine were the only pharmacological treatment for chorea approved by FDA. Tetrabenazine is a human VMAT2 inhibitor that rapidly is converted to α-dihydrotetrabenazine (also a VMAT2 inhibitor) that decreases extracellular dopamine concentration, showing good results in improving chorea in Huntington's patients.[156] Deutetrabenazine is a tetrabenazine modified by the 6 hydrogen substitution with deuterium, which increases the drug half-life time.[152,157,158]

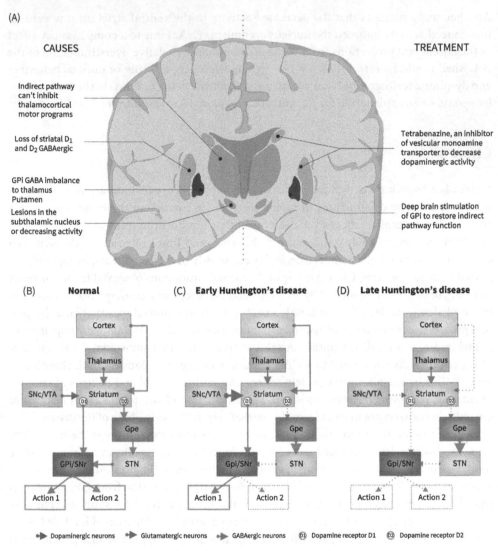

Figure 2.6 Causes and treatment of choreic movement disorders.

(A) The corticostriatal circuit (B) is compared with the alterations observed in the early (C) and late (D) stages of Huntington's disease (HD). GPe, globus pallidus external segment; GPi, globus pallidus internal segment; SNc, substantia nigra pars compacta; SNr, substantia nigra pars reticulate, STN, subthalamic nucleus; VTA, ventral tegmental area.

Source: Modified from Sepers and Raymond, 2014.

Nonmotor symptoms of PD

Most, but not all symptoms of PD are related to the dramatic decrease of dopamine in the dorsal striatum. In the early phases, the extracellular concentrations of dopamine are still enough to activate D2Rs. However, even in the early phases of PD, reinforcement learning is impaired because it depends on higher levels of dopamine to activate D1Rs in the corticostriatal synapses.

The dopamine neurons of the midbrain are phasically activated by better than expected rewards.[159] When a voluntary motor action results in something better than expected, the extracellular concentration of dopamine is high enough to activate the D1Rs expressed in the medium spiny neurons of the direct pathway that were active. D1Rs activation reinforces the synapses between the prefrontal neurons that encode the action goal and the medium spiny neurons of the anterior part of the caudate that encoded the rewarded action. Phasic release of dopamine in the putamen also reinforces the synapses between the sensory cortex neurons that encode environmental stimuli and the medium spiny neurons that initiate the reinforced response.[4] The failure of these learning processes makes the behavior of PD patients more rigid, based more on the outcomes of experiences that occurred before the severe loss of midbrain neurons. PD patients are particularly bad at learning from mistakes than from rewarding experiences.[160] One lab tested rats that were made parkinsonian by injecting them with a neurotoxin that destroys the dopamine neurons of the substantia nigra. Next, a group of rats was placed in two compartments of a box, one in which they found sucrose pellets and the other that was empty. Both the control and parkinsonian rats later preferred to spend more time in the compartment paired with sucrose than in the neutral compartment. Another group of parkinsonian rats was trained by paring a compartment in which they are given a bitter solution, contrasted with a neutral compartment. Different from control rats that showed aversion for the compartment paired with the bitter solution, the parkinsonian rats spend nearly the same time in both the aversive and neutral compartment.[161]

The part of the striatum that is mostly depleted of dopamine is the putamen nuclei, which is a key place for habit learning. Therefore, habit learning is impaired in Parkinson's disease. A habit is a behavioral response that is automatically evoked by an environmental stimulus that has been cued that this response will be rewarded. It is learned slowly and is not performed in expectation of reward. Instead, it is evoked unconsciously, even in situations when the reward is no longer wanted.[162] On the other hand, except for cases that progress to dementia, declarative (conscious) memories are largely preserved in most PD patients. A classical study[163] used a probabilistic task in which the participants are asked to guess whether sun or rain will appear on the computer screen. There was a probability of the outcome to be "sun" or "rain" associated with each card, but it is not said to the participants. Amnestic patients and healthy people improved their right choice ratio after several days of training. However, they could not say why they made each choice. The amnesic patients could not even remember to have been in the testing room in the previous days. On the other hand, the PD patients remembered having participated in this game, but their score never improved above the chance level. One lab tested parkinsonian rats in a spatial and a visually cued version of the Morris water maze, which was proposed as animal models of declarative and stimulus-response learning and memory tasks, respectively. As observed in human studies, rats with lesions in the substantia nigra pars compacta could learn the spatial task but learned the cued task much more slowly.[164–167] They also tested substantia nigra pars compacta lesioned rats in more than one working memory task. Consistent with studies that tested PD patients in this kind of memory,[168,169] the rats failed to keep in the working memory an information that they learned a few seconds before.[167,170,171]

Conclusion

This chapter discussed several pathophysiological mechanisms of primary and secondary movement disorders. The corticobasal ganglia system was shown to play key roles in both hyperkinetic and hypokinetic signs of several movement and psychiatric disorders. Important advances have been made to clarify the normal and pathological activity of the basal ganglia in the past decades. However, several questions remain unanswered and new questions are constantly emerging from recent advances in molecular, structural, and functional aspects of the basal ganglia. What can be said for sure is that separation of movement disorders from behavioral/mental disorders no longer makes sense. Motor signs, cognitive, mental, and behavioral symptoms are present in most neurological diseases and psychiatric disorders, and many of them arise from malfunctioning of the motor, associative, and limbic loops of the corticobasal ganglia circuit.

References

1. Postuma, R. B., Berg, D., Stern, M., Poewe, W., Olanow, C. W., Oertel, W., Obeso, J., Marek, K., Litvan, I., Lang, A. E., Halliday, G., Goetz, C. G., Gasser, T., Dubois, B., Chan, P., Bloem, B. R., Adler, C. H., & Deuschl, G. (2015). MDS clinical diagnostic criteria for Parkinson's disease. *Movement Disorders*, *30*(12), 1591–1601. https://doi.org/10.1002/mds.26424

2. Tarsy, D., Baldessarini, R. J., & Tarazi, F. I. (2002). Effects of newer antipsychotics on extrapyramidal function. *CNS Drugs*, *16*(1), 23–45. https://doi.org/10.2165/00023210-200216 010-00003

3. Zahodne, L. B., & Fernandez, H. H. (2008). Pathophysiology and treatment of psychosis in parkinson's disease: A review. *Drugs & Aging*, *25*(8), 665–682. https://doi.org/10.2165/00002 512-200825080-00004

4. Da Cunha, C., Wietzikoski, E. C., Dombrowski, P., Bortolanza, M., Santos, L. M., Boschen, S. L., & Miyoshi, E. (2009). Learning processing in the basal ganglia: A mosaic of broken mirrors. *Behavioural Brain Research*, *199*(1), 157–170. https://doi.org/10.1016/j.bbr.2008.10.001

5. Vijayakumar, D., & Jankovic, J. (2016). Drug-induced dyskinesia, Part 2: Treatment of tardive dyskinesia. *Drugs*, *76*(7), 779–787. https://doi.org/10.1007/s40265-016-0568-1

6. Ferré, S., García-Borreguero, D., Allen, R. P., & Earley, C. J. (2019). New insights into the neurobiology of restless legs syndrome. *Neuroscientist*, *25*(2), 113–125. https://doi.org/10.1177/1073858418791763

7. *Diagnostic and statistical manual of mental disorders: DSM-5*. (2013). (5th ed.). American Psychiatric Association.

8. Carlsson, A. (1964). Evidence for a role of dopamine in extrapyramidal functions. *Acta Neurovegetativa*, *26*(4), 484–493. https://doi.org/10.1007/BF01252144

9. Hassler, R. (1937). Zur Normalanatomie der Substantia nigra. Versuch einer architektonischen Gliederung. *Journal of Psychology and Neurology*, *48:1–55*.

10. Reiner, A., Albin, R. L., Anderson, K. D., D'Amato, C. J., Penney, J. B., & Young, A. B. (1988). Differential loss of striatal projection neurons in Huntington disease. *Proceedings of the National Academy of Sciences*, *85*(15), 5733–5737. https://doi.org/10.1073/pnas.85.15.5733

11. Cunha, C., Wietzikoski, E. C., Bortolanza, M., Dombrowski, P. A., Santos, L. M. d., Boschen, S. L., Miyoshi, E., Vital, M. A. B. F., Boerngen-Lacerda, R., & Andreatini, R. (2009). Nonmotor function of the midbrain dopaminergic neurons. In G. Giovanni, V. Di Matteo, & E. Esposito (Eds.), *Birth, life and death of dopaminergic neurons in the substantia nigra. Journal of Neural Transmission. Supplementa*, *73*, Springer. http://link.springer.com/10.1007/978-3-211-92660-4_12

12. Redgrave, P., Prescott, T. J., & Gurney, K. (1999). The basal ganglia: A vertebrate solution to the selection problem? *Neuroscience, 89*(4), 1009–1023. https://doi.org/10.1016/S0306-4522(98)00319-4

13. Alexander, G. E., DeLong, M. R., & Strick, P. L. (1986). Parallel organization of functionally segregated circuits linking basal ganglia and cortex. *Annual Review of Neuroscience, 9*(1), 357–381. https://doi.org/10.1146/annurev.ne.09.030186.002041

14. DeLong, M. R., & Wichmann, T. (2015). Basal ganglia circuits as targets for neuromodulation in Parkinson disease. *JAMA Neurology, 72*(11), 1354. https://doi.org/10.1001/jamaneurol.2015.2397

15. Mink, J. W. (1996). The basal ganglia: Focused selection and inhibition of competing motor programs. *Progress in Neurobiology, 50*(4), 381–425. https://doi.org/10.1016/S0301-0082(96)00042-1

16. Balleine, B. W., Delgado, M. R., & Hikosaka, O. (2007). The role of the dorsal striatum in reward and decision-making. *Journal of Neuroscience, 27*(31), 8161–8165. https://doi.org/10.1523/JNEUROSCI.1554-07.2007

17. Balleine, B. W., & Dezfouli, A. (2019). Hierarchical action control: Adaptive collaboration between actions and habits. *Frontiers in Psychology, 10*, 2735. https://doi.org/10.3389/fpsyg.2019.02735

18. Haber, S. N., & Knutson, B. (2010). The reward circuit: Linking primate anatomy and human imaging. *Neuropsychopharmacology, 35*(1), 4–26. https://doi.org/10.1038/npp.2009.129

19. Ikemoto, S., Yang, C., & Tan, A. (2015). Basal ganglia circuit loops, dopamine and motivation: A review and enquiry. *Behavioural Brain Research, 290*, 17–31. https://doi.org/10.1016/j.bbr.2015.04.018

20. O'Reilly, R. C., & Frank, M. J. (2006). Making working memory work: A computational model of learning in the prefrontal cortex and basal ganglia. *Neural Computation, 18*(2), 283–328. https://doi.org/10.1162/089976606775093909

21. Seo, R., Stocco, A., & Prat, C. S. (2018). The bilingual language network: Differential involvement of anterior cingulate, basal ganglia and prefrontal cortex in preparation, monitoring, and execution. *Neuroimage, 174*, 44–56. https://doi.org/10.1016/j.neuroimage.2018.02.010

22. Grillner, S., & Robertson, B. (2016). The basal ganglia over 500 million years. *Current Biology, 26*(20), R1088–R1100. https://doi.org/10.1016/j.cub.2016.06.041

23. Nambu, A., Tokuno, H., & Takada, M. (2002). Functional significance of the cortico-subthalamo–pallidal "hyperdirect" pathway. *Neuroscience Research, 43*(2), 111–117. https://doi.org/10.1016/S0168-0102(02)00027-5

24. Polyakova, Z., Chiken, S., Hatanaka, N., & Nambu, A. (2020). Cortical control of subthalamic neuronal activity through the hyperdirect and indirect pathways in monkeys. *Journal of Neuroscience, 40*(39), 7451–7463. https://doi.org/10.1523/JNEUROSCI.0772-20.2020

25. Frank, M. J. (2006). Hold your horses: A dynamic computational role for the subthalamic nucleus in decision making. *Neural Networks, 19*(8), 1120–1136. https://doi.org/10.1016/j.neunet.2006.03.006

26. Johansson, Y., & Silberberg, G. (2020). The functional organization of cortical and thalamic inputs onto five types of striatal neurons is determined by source and target cell identities. *Cell Reports, 30*(4), 1178–1194.e1173. https://doi.org/10.1016/j.celrep.2019.12.095

27. Smith, Y., Raju, D., Nanda, B., Pare, J.-F., Galvan, A., & Wichmann, T. (2009). The thalamostriatal systems: Anatomical and functional organization in normal and parkinsonian states. *Brain Research Bulletin, 78*(2–3), 60–68. https://doi.org/10.1016/j.brainresbull.2008.08.015

28. Rashid, A. J., So, C. H., Kong, M. M. C., Furtak, T., El-Ghundi, M., Cheng, R., O'Dowd, B. F., & George, S. R. (2007). D1-D2 dopamine receptor heterooligomers with unique pharmacology are coupled to rapid activation of Gq/11 in the striatum. *Proceedings of the National Academy of Sciences*, *104*(2), 654–659. https://doi.org/10.1073/pnas.0604049104

29. Ferré, S. (2015). The GPCR heterotetramer: Challenging classical pharmacology. *Trends in Pharmacological Sciences*, *36*(3), 145–152. https://doi.org/10.1016/j.tips.2015.01.002

30. Gerfen, C. R., & Surmeier, D. J. (2011). Modulation of striatal projection systems by dopamine. *Annual Review of Neuroscience*, *34*(1), 441–466. https://doi.org/10.1146/annurev-neuro-061010-113641

31. Tritsch, Nicolas X., & Sabatini, Bernardo L. (2012). Dopaminergic modulation of synaptic transmission in cortex and striatum. *Neuron*, *76*(1), 33–50. https://doi.org/10.1016/j.neuron.2012.09.023

32. Ohno, Y., Kunisawa, N., & Shimizu, S. (2019). Antipsychotic treatment of behavioral and psychological symptoms of dementia (BPSD): Management of extrapyramidal side effects. *Frontiers in Pharmacology*, *10*, 1045. https://doi.org/10.3389/fphar.2019.01045

33. Maia, T. V., & Frank, M. J. (2017). An integrative perspective on the role of dopamine in schizophrenia. *Biological Psychiatry*, *81*(1), 52–66. https://doi.org/10.1016/j.biopsych.2016.05.021

34. Cui, G., Jun, S. B., Jin, X., Pham, M. D., Vogel, S. S., Lovinger, D. M., & Costa, R. M. (2013). Concurrent activation of striatal direct and indirect pathways during action initiation [Report]. *Nature*, *494*, 238+. https://doi.org/10.1038/nature11846

35. Marsden, C. D. (1989). Slowness of movement in Parkinson's disease. *Movement Disorders*, *4*(S1), S26–S37. https://doi.org/10.1002/mds.870040505

36. Moustafa, A. A., Chakravarthy, S., Phillips, J. R., Gupta, A., Keri, S., Polner, B., Frank, M. J., & Jahanshahi, M. (2016). Motor symptoms in Parkinson's disease: A unified framework. *Neuroscience & Biobehavioral Reviews*, *68*, 727–740. https://doi.org/10.1016/j.neubiorev.2016.07.010

37. Poewe, W., Seppi, K., Tanner, C. M., Halliday, G. M., Brundin, P., Volkmann, J., Schrag, A. E., & Lang, A. E. (2017). Parkinson disease. *Nature Reviews Disease Primers*, *3*, 17013. https://doi.org/10.1038/nrdp.2017.13

38. Dickson, D. W., Braak, H., Duda, J. E., Duyckaerts, C., Gasser, T., Halliday, G. M., Hardy, J., Leverenz, J. B., Del Tredici, K., Wszolek, Z. K., & Litvan, I. (2009). Neuropathological assessment of Parkinson's disease: Refining the diagnostic criteria. *Lancet Neurol*, *8*(12), 1150–1157. https://doi.org/10.1016/S1474-4422(09)70238-8

39. Postuma, R. B., Gagnon, J.-F., Pelletier, A., & Montplaisir, J. (2013). Prodromal autonomic symptoms and signs in Parkinson's disease and dementia with Lewy bodies: Prodromal autonomic changes in Parkinson's. *Movement Disorders*, *28*(5), 597–604. https://doi.org/10.1002/mds.25445

40. Simuni, T., Caspell-Garcia, C., Coffey, C. S., Weintraub, D., Mollenhauer, B., Lasch, S., Tanner, C. M., Jennings, D., Kieburtz, K., Chahine, L. M., & Marek, K. (2018). Baseline prevalence and longitudinal evolution of non-motor symptoms in early Parkinson's disease: The PPMI cohort. *Journal of Neurology, Neurosurgery & Psychiatry*, *89*(1), 78–88. https://doi.org/10.1136/jnnp-2017-316213

41. Braak, H., Tredici, K. D., Rüb, U., de Vos, R. A. I., Jansen Steur, E. N. H., & Braak, E. (2003). Staging of brain pathology related to sporadic Parkinson's disease. *Neurobiology of Aging*, *24*(2), 197–211. https://doi.org/10.1016/S0197-4580(02)00065-9

42. Burns, R. S., Chiueh, C. C., Markey, S. P., Ebert, M. H., Jacobowitz, D. M., & Kopin, I. J. (1983). A primate model of parkinsonism: Selective destruction of dopaminergic neurons in the pars compacta of the substantia nigra by N-methyl-4-phenyl-1,2,3,6-tetrahydropyridine. *Proceedings of the National Academy of Sciences, 80*(14), 4546–4550. https://doi.org/10.1073/pnas.80.14.4546

43. Mallet, N. (2006). Cortical inputs and GABA interneurons imbalance projection neurons in the striatum of parkinsonian rats. *Journal of Neuroscience, 26*(14), 3875–3884. https://doi.org/10.1523/JNEUROSCI.4439-05.2006

44. Parker, J. G., Marshall, J. D., Ahanonu, B., Wu, Y.-W., Kim, T. H., Grewe, B. F., Zhang, Y., Li, J. Z., Ding, J. B., Ehlers, M. D., & Schnitzer, M. J. (2018). Diametric neural ensemble dynamics in parkinsonian and dyskinetic states. *Nature, 557*(7704), 177–182. https://doi.org/10.1038/s41586-018-0090-6

45. Galvan, A., Devergnas, A., & Wichmann, T. (2015). Alterations in neuronal activity in basal ganglia-thalamocortical circuits in the parkinsonian state. *Frontiers in Neuroanatomy, 9*(5). https://doi.org/10.3389/fnana.2015.00005

46. Armstrong, M. J., & Okun, M. S. (2020). Diagnosis and treatment of Parkinson disease: A review. *JAMA, 323*(6), 548. https://doi.org/10.1001/jama.2019.22360

47. Halje, P., Brys, I., Mariman, J. J., da Cunha, C., Fuentes, R., & Petersson, P. (2019). Oscillations in cortico-basal ganglia circuits: implications for Parkinson's disease and other neurologic and psychiatric conditions. *Journal of Neurophysiology, 122*(1), 203–231. https://doi.org/10.1152/jn.00590.2018

48. Baradaran, N., Tan, S. N., Liu, A., Ashoori, A., Palmer, S. J., Wang, Z. J., Oishi, M. M. K., & McKeown, M. J. (2013). Parkinson's disease rigidity: Relation to brain connectivity and motor performance. *Frontiers in Neurology, 4*, 67. https://doi.org/10.3389/fneur.2013.00067

49. Pogosyan, A., Yoshida, F., Chen, C. C., Martinez-Torres, I., Foltynie, T., Limousin, P., Zrinzo, L., Hariz, M. I., & Brown, P. (2010). Parkinsonian impairment correlates with spatially extensive subthalamic oscillatory synchronization. *Neuroscience, 171*(1), 245–257. https://doi.org/10.1016/j.neuroscience.2010.08.068

50. Tinkhauser, G., Pogosyan, A., Little, S., Beudel, M., Herz, D. M., Tan, H., & Brown, P. (2017). The modulatory effect of adaptive deep brain stimulation on beta bursts in Parkinson's disease. *Brain, 140*(4), 1053–1067. https://doi.org/10.1093/brain/awx010

51. Brown, P., & Williams, D. (2005). Basal ganglia local field potential activity: Character and functional significance in the human. *Clinical Neurophysiology, 116*(11), 2510–2519. https://doi.org/10.1016/j.clinph.2005.05.009

52. Cole, S. R., van der Meij, R., Peterson, E. J., de Hemptinne, C., Starr, P. A., & Voytek, B. (2017). Nonsinusoidal beta oscillations reflect cortical pathophysiology in Parkinson's disease. *Journal of Neuroscience, 37*(18), 4830–4840. https://doi.org/10.1523/JNEUROSCI.2208-16.2017

53. Kühn, A. A., Tsui, A., Aziz, T., Ray, N., Brücke, C., Kupsch, A., Schneider, G.-H., & Brown, P. (2009). Pathological synchronisation in the subthalamic nucleus of patients with Parkinson's disease relates to both bradykinesia and rigidity. *Experimental Neurology, 215*(2), 380–387. https://doi.org/10.1016/j.expneurol.2008.11.008

54. David, F. J., Munoz, M. J., & Corcos, D. M. (2020). The effect of STN DBS on modulating brain oscillations: Consequences for motor and cognitive behavior. *Experimental Brain Research, 238*(7), 1659–1676. https://doi.org/10.1007/s00221-020-05834-7

55. Kahlbaum, K. (1874). Die Katatonie oder das Spannungsirresein. *Vertex (Buenos Aires, Argentina), 23*, 312–320.

56. Fink, M. (2013). Rediscovering catatonia: The biography of a treatable syndrome. *Acta Psychiatrica Scandinavica*, *127*, 1–47. https://doi.org/10.1111/acps.12038

57. Hirjak, D., Kubera, K. M., Wolf, R. C., & Northoff, G. (2020). Going Back to Kahlbaum's psychomotor (and GABAergic) origins: Is catatonia more than just a motor and dopaminergic syndrome? *Schizophrenia Bulletin*, *46*(2), 272–285. https://doi.org/10.1093/schbul/sbz074

58. Northoff, G., Eckert, J., & Fritze, J. (1997). Glutamatergic dysfunction in catatonia? Successful treatment of three acute akinetic catatonic patients with the NMDA antagonist amantadine. *Journal of Neurology, Neurosurgery & Psychiatry*, *62*(4), 404–406. https://doi.org/10.1136/jnnp.62.4.404

59. Fink, M. (1996). Neuroleptic malignant syndrome and catatonia: One entity or two? *Biological Psychiatry*, *39*(1), 1–4. https://doi.org/10.1016/0006-3223(95)00552-8

60. Graham, K., & Carroll, B. (2002). Dopamine in Catatonia. *Journal of Clinical Psychopharmacology*, *21*, 624–625. https://doi.org/10.1097/00004714-200112000-00019

61. Guzman, C. S. M., Myung, V. H., & Wang, Y.P. (2008). Treatment of periodic catatonia with atypical antipsychotic, olanzapine. *Psychiatry and Clinical Neurosciences*, *62*(4), 482–482. https://doi.org/10.1111/j.1440-1819.2008.01819.x

62. Lloyd, J. R., Silverman, E. R., Kugler, J. L., & Cooper, J. J. (2020). Electroconvulsive therapy for patients with catatonia: Current perspectives. *Neuropsychiatric Disease and Treatment*, *16*, 2191–2208. https://doi.org/10.2147/NDT.S231573

63. Van Den Eede, F., Van Hecke, J., Van Dalfsen, A., Van den Bossche, B., Cosyns, P., & Sabbe, B. G. C. (2005). The use of atypical antipsychotics in the treatment of catatonia. *European Psychiatry*, *20*(5-6), 422–429. https://doi.org/10.1016/j.eurpsy.2005.03.012

64. Hirjak, D., Rashidi, M., Kubera, K., Northoff, G., Fritze, S., Schmitgen, M., Sambataro, F., Calhoun, V., & Wolf, R. (2020). Multimodal magnetic resonance imaging data fusion reveals distinct patterns of abnormal brain structure and function in catatonia. *Schizophrenia Bulletin*, *46*(1), 202–210. https://doi.org/10.1093/schbul/sbz042

65. Berardelli, A., Noth, J., Thompson, P. D., Bollen, E. L., Currà, A., Deuschl, G., van Dijk, J. G., Töpper, R., Schwarz, M., & Roos, R. A. (1999). Pathophysiology of chorea and bradykinesia in Huntington's disease. *Movement Disorders*, *14*(3), 398–403.

66. Rajput, A. H., Voll, A., Rajput, M. L., Robinson, C. A., & Rajput, A. (2009). Course in Parkinson disease subtypes: A 39-year clinicopathologic study. *Neurology*, *73*(3), 206–212. https://doi.org/10.1212/WNL.0b013e3181ae7af1

67. Schillaci, O., Chiaravalloti, A., Pierantozzi, M., Di Pietro, B., Koch, G., Bruni, C., Stanzione, P., & Stefani, A. (2011). Different patterns of nigrostriatal degeneration in tremor type versus the akinetic-rigid and mixed types of Parkinson's disease at the early stages: Molecular imaging with 123I-FP-CIT SPECT. *International Journal of Molecular Medicine*, *28*(5), 881–886. https://doi.org/10.3892/ijmm.2011.764

68. Qamhawi, Z., Towey, D., Shah, B., Pagano, G., Seibyl, J., Marek, K., Borghammer, P., Brooks, D. J., & Pavese, N. (2015). Clinical correlates of raphe serotonergic dysfunction in early Parkinson's disease. *Brain*, *138*(10), 2964–2973. https://doi.org/10.1093/brain/awv215

69. Sahoo, L. K., Holla, V. V., Batra, D., Prasad, S., Bhattacharya, A., Kamble, N., Yadav, R., & Pal, P. K. (2020). Comparison of effectiveness of trihexyphenidyl and levodopa on motor symptoms in Parkinson's disease. *Journal of Neural Transmission*, *127*(12), 1599–1606. https://doi.org/10.1007/s00702-020-02257-0

70. Ashby, F. G., Turner, B. O., & Horvitz, J. C. (2010). Cortical and basal ganglia contributions to habit learning and automaticity. *Trends in Cognitive Sciences, 14*(5), 208–215. https://doi.org/10.1016/j.tics.2010.02.001

71. Wichmann, T. (2019). Changing views of the pathophysiology of Parkinsonism. *Movement Disorders, 34*(8), 1130–1143. https://doi.org/10.1002/mds.27741

72. Alonso-Frech, F. (2006). Slow oscillatory activity and levodopa-induced dyskinesias in Parkinson's disease. *Brain, 129*(7), 1748–1757. https://doi.org/10.1093/brain/awl103

73. Lenz, F., Tasker, R., Kwan, H., Schnider, S., Kwong, R., Murayama, Y., Dostrovsky, J., & Murphy, J. (1988). Single unit analysis of the human ventral thalamic nuclear group: Correlation of thalamic "tremor cells" with the 3-6 Hz component of parkinsonian tremor. *Journal of Neuroscience, 8*(3), 754–764. https://doi.org/10.1523/JNEUROSCI.08-03-00754.1988

74. Guan, X., Zeng, Q., Guo, T., Wang, J., Xuan, M., Gu, Q., Wang, T., Huang, P., Xu, X., & Zhang, M. (2017). Disrupted functional connectivity of basal ganglia across tremor-dominant and akinetic/rigid-dominant Parkinson's disease. *Frontiers in Aging Neuroscience, 9*, 360. https://doi.org/10.3389/fnagi.2017.00360

75. Hirschmann, J., Hartmann, C. J., Butz, M., Hoogenboom, N., Özkurt, T. E., Elben, S., Vesper, J., Wojtecki, L., & Schnitzler, A. (2013). A direct relationship between oscillatory subthalamic nucleus–cortex coupling and rest tremor in Parkinson's disease. *Brain, 136*(12), 3659–3670. https://doi.org/10.1093/brain/awt271

76. Haubenberger, D., & Hallett, M. (2018). Essential Tremor. *New England Journal of Medicine, 378*(19), 1802–1810. https://doi.org/10.1056/NEJMcp1707928

77. Louis, E. D., Gerbin, M., & Galecki, M. (2013). Essential tremor 10, 20, 30, 40: Clinical snapshots of the disease by decade of duration. *European Journal of Neurology, 20*(6), 949–954. https://doi.org/10.1111/ene.12123

78. Clark, L. N., & Louis, E. D. (2018). Essential tremor. *Handbook of Clinical Neurology* (Vol. 147, pp. 229–239). Elsevier. https://linkinghub.elsevier.com/retrieve/pii/B9780444632333000154

79. Hallett, M. (2016). Functional (psychogenic) movement disorders—Clinical presentations. *Parkinsonism & Related Disorders, 22*, S149–S152. https://doi.org/10.1016/j.parkreldis.2015.08.036

80. Reich, S. G. (2019). Essential tremor. *Medical Clinics of North America, 103*(2), 351–356. https://doi.org/10.1016/j.mcna.2018.10.016

81. Bain, P. G. (2003). Essential tremor and primary writing tremor. *Handbook of Clinical Neurophysiology* (Vol. 1, pp. 365–376). Elsevier. https://linkinghub.elsevier.com/retrieve/pii/S1567423109701716

82. Deuschl, G., Petersen, I., Lorenz, D., & Christensen, K. (2015). Tremor in the elderly: Essential and aging-related tremor. *Movement Disorders, 30*(10), 1327–1334. https://doi.org/10.1002/mds.26265

83. Louis, E. D., & Ferreira, J. J. (2010). How common is the most common adult movement disorder? Update on the worldwide prevalence of essential tremor. *Movement Disorders, 25*(5), 534–541. https://doi.org/10.1002/mds.22838

84. Stefansson, H., Steinberg, S., Petursson, H., Gustafsson, O., Gudjonsdottir, I. H., Jonsdottir, G. A., Palsson, S. T., Jonsson, T., Saemundsdottir, J., Bjornsdottir, G., Böttcher, Y., Thorlacius, T., Haubenberger, D., Zimprich, A., Auff, E., Hotzy, C., Testa, C. M., Miyatake, L. A., Rosen, A. R., . . . Stefansson, K. (2009). Variant in the sequence of the LINGO1 gene confers risk of essential tremor. *Nature Genetics, 41*(3), 277–279. https://doi.org/10.1038/ng.299

85. Mavroudis, I., Petridis, F., & Kazis, D. (2019). Neuroimaging and neuropathological findings in essential tremor. *Acta Neurologica Scandinavica*, *139*(6), 491–496. https://doi.org/10.1111/ane.13101

86. Pagan, F. L., Butman, J. A., Dambrosia, J. M., & Hallett, M. (2003). Evaluation of essential tremor with multi-voxel magnetic resonance spectroscopy. *Neurology*, *60*(8), 1344–1347. https://doi.org/10.1212/01.WNL.0000065885.15875.0D

87. Shin, H., Lee, D.-K., Lee, J.-M., Huh, Y.-E., Youn, J., Louis, E. D., & Cho, J. W. (2016). Atrophy of the cerebellar vermis in essential tremor: Segmental volumetric MRI analysis. *Cerebellum*, *15*(2), 174–181. https://doi.org/10.1007/s12311-015-0682-8

88. Choe, M., Cortés, E., Vonsattel, J.-P. G., Kuo, S.-H., Faust, P. L., & Louis, E. D. (2016). Purkinje cell loss in essential tremor: Random sampling quantification and nearest neighbor analysis: Loss of Purkinje Cells in ET. *Movement Disorders*, *31*(3), 393–401. https://doi.org/10.1002/mds.26490

89. Kuo, S.-H., Wang, J., Tate, W. J., Pan, M.-K., Kelly, G. C., Gutierrez, J., Cortes, E. P., Vonsattel, J.-P. G., Louis, E. D., & Faust, P. L. (2017). Cerebellar pathology in early onset and late onset essential tremor. *Cerebellum*, *16*(2), 473–482. https://doi.org/10.1007/s12311-016-0826-5

90. Paris-Robidas, S., Brochu, E., Sintes, M., Emond, V., Bousquet, M., Vandal, M., Pilote, M., Tremblay, C., Di Paolo, T., Rajput, A. H., Rajput, A., & Calon, F. (2012). Defective dentate nucleus GABA receptors in essential tremor. *Brain*, *135*(1), 105–116. https://doi.org/10.1093/brain/awr301

91. Shill, H., Adler, C., & Beach, T. (2016). Lewy bodies are incidental in essential tremor. *Parkinsonism & Related Disorders*, *26*, 81. https://doi.org/10.1016/j.parkreldis.2016.02.025

92. Miskin, C., & Carvalho, K. S. (2018). Tremors: Essential tremor and beyond. *Seminars in Pediatric Neurology*, *25*, 34–41. https://doi.org/10.1016/j.spen.2018.02.002

93. Zesiewicz, T. A., Elble, R. J., Louis, E. D., Gronseth, G. S., Ondo, W. G., Dewey, R. B., Okun, M. S., Sullivan, K. L., & Weiner, W. J. (2011). Evidence-based guideline update: Treatment of essential tremor: Report of the Quality Standards Subcommittee of the American Academy of Neurology. *Neurology*, *77*(19), 1752–1755. https://doi.org/10.1212/WNL.0b013e318236f0fd

94. Ahlskog, J. E., & Muenter, M. D. (2001). Frequency of levodopa-related dyskinesias and motor fluctuations as estimated from the cumulative literature: Levodopa Motor Complication Frequency. *Movement Disorders*, *16*(3), 448–458. https://doi.org/10.1002/mds.1090

95. Brotchie, J. M. (2005). Nondopaminergic mechanisms in levodopa-induced dyskinesia. *Movement Disorders*, *20*(8), 919–931. https://doi.org/10.1002/mds.20612

96. Espay, A. J., Morgante, F., Merola, A., Fasano, A., Marsili, L., Fox, S. H., Bezard, E., Picconi, B., Calabresi, P., & Lang, A. E. (2018). Levodopa-induced dyskinesia in Parkinson disease: Current and evolving concepts: Dyskinesia in PD. *Annals of Neurology*, *84*(6), 797–811. https://doi.org/10.1002/ana.25364

97. Thanvi, B., Lo, N., & Robinson, T. (2007). Levodopa-induced dyskinesia in Parkinson's disease: Clinical features, pathogenesis, prevention and treatment. *Postgraduate Medical Journal*, *83*(980), 384–388. https://doi.org/10.1136/pgmj.2006.054759

98. Tran, T. N., Vo, T. N. N., Frei, K., & Truong, D. D. (2018). Levodopa-induced dyskinesia: Clinical features, incidence, and risk factors. *Journal of Neural Transmission*, *125*(8), 1109–1117. https://doi.org/10.1007/s00702-018-1900-6

99. Morgante, F., Espay, A. J., Gunraj, C., Lang, A. E., & Chen, R. (2006). Motor cortex plasticity in Parkinson's disease and levodopa-induced dyskinesias. *Brain*, *129*(4), 1059–1069. https://doi.org/10.1093/brain/awl031

100. Fasano, S., Bezard, E., D'Antoni, A., Francardo, V., Indrigo, M., Qin, L., Dovero, S., Cerovic, M., Cenci, M. A., & Brambilla, R. (2010). Inhibition of Ras-guanine nucleotide-releasing factor 1 (Ras-GRF1) signaling in the striatum reverts motor symptoms associated with L-dopa-induced dyskinesia. *Proceedings of the National Academy of Sciences, 107*(50), 21824–21829. https://doi.org/10.1073/pnas.1012071107

101. Pavón, N., Martín, A. B., Mendialdua, A., & Moratalla, R. (2006). ERK phosphorylation and FosB expression are associated with L-DOPA-induced dyskinesia in hemiparkinsonian mice. *Biological Psychiatry, 59*(1), 64–74. https://doi.org/10.1016/j.biopsych.2005.05.044

102. Santini, E., Alcacer, C., Cacciatore, S., Heiman, M., Hervé, D., Greengard, P., Girault, J.-A., Valjent, E., & Fisone, G. (2009). L-dopa activates ERK signaling and phosphorylates histone H3 in the striatonigral medium spiny neurons of hemiparkinsonian mice. *Journal of Neurochemistry, 108*(3), 621–633. https://doi.org/10.1111/j.1471-4159.2008.05831.x

103. Alcacer, C., Andreoli, L., Sebastianutto, I., Jakobsson, J., Fieblinger, T., & Cenci, M. A. (2017). Chemogenetic stimulation of striatal projection neurons modulates responses to Parkinson's disease therapy. *Journal of Clinical Investigation, 127*(2), 720–734. https://doi.org/10.1172/JCI90132

104. Suarez, L. M., Solis, O., Aguado, C., Lujan, R., & Moratalla, R. (2016). L-dopa oppositely regulates synaptic strength and spine morphology in D1 and D2 striatal projection neurons in dyskinesia. *Cerebral Cortex, 26*(11), 4253–4264. https://doi.org/10.1093/cercor/bhw263

105. Picconi, B., Centonze, D., Håkansson, K., Bernardi, G., Greengard, P., Fisone, G., Cenci, M. A., & Calabresi, P. (2003). Loss of bidirectional striatal synaptic plasticity in L-DOPA-induced dyskinesia. *Nature Neuroscience, 6*, 501–506. https://doi.org/10.1038/nn1040

106. Prashanth, L. K., Fox, S., & Meissner, W. G. (2011). L-dopa-induced dyskinesia—Clinical presentation, genetics, and treatment. *International Review of Neurobiology, 98*, 31–54. Elsevier. https://linkinghub.elsevier.com/retrieve/pii/B978012381328200002X

107. Odekerken, V. J. J., van Laar, T., Staal, M. J., Mosch, A., Hoffmann, C. F. E., Nijssen, P. C. G., Beute, G. N., van Vugt, J. P. P., Lenders, M. W. P. M., Contarino, M. F., Mink, M. S. J., Bour, L. J., van den Munckhof, P., Schmand, B. A., de Haan, R. J., Schuurman, P. R., & de Bie, R. M. A. (2013). Subthalamic nucleus versus globus pallidus bilateral deep brain stimulation for advanced Parkinson's disease (NSTAPS study): A randomised controlled trial. *Lancet Neurology, 12*(1), 37–44. https://doi.org/10.1016/S1474-4422(12)70264-8

108. Kempster, P. (2020). Predicting levodopa-induced dyskinesia. *Arquivos de Neuropsiquiatria,78*, 185–186. https://doi.org/10.1590/0004-282x20200023

109. Carbon, M., Hsieh, C.-H., Kane, J., & Correll, C. (2017). Tardive dyskinesia prevalence in the period of second-generation antipsychotic use: A meta-analysis. *Journal of Clinical Psychiatry, 78*(3), e264–e278. https://doi.org/10.4088/JCP.16r10832

110. Lerner, P., & Miodownik, C. (2015). Tardive dyskinesia (syndrome): Current concept and modern approaches to its management: Modern approaches to tardive dyskinesia. *Psychiatry and Clinical Neurosciences, 69*(6), 321–323. https://doi.org/10.1111/pcn.12270

111. Ortí-Pareja, M., Jiménez-Jiménez, F. J., Vázquez, A., Catalan, M.-J., Zurdo, M., Burguera, J., Martinez-Martin, P., & Molina, J. (1999). Drug-induced tardive syndromes. *Parkinsonism & Related Disorders, 5*, 59–65. https://doi.org/10.1016/S1353-8020(99)00015-2

112. D'Abreu, A., Akbar, U., & Friedman, J. (2018). Tardive dyskinesia: Epidemiology. *Journal of the Neurological Sciences, 389*, 17–20. https://doi.org/10.1016/j.jns.2018.02.007

113. Frei, K., Truong, D., Fahn, S., Jankovic, J., & Hauser, R. (2018). The nosology of tardive syndromes. *Journal of the Neurological Sciences, 389*, 17–20. https://doi.org/10.1016/j.jns.2018.02.008

114. Correll, C., Kane, J., & Citrome, L. (2017). Epidemiology, prevention, and assessment of tardive dyskinesia and advances in treatment. *Journal of Clinical Psychiatry, 78*(8), 1136–1147 https://doi.org/10.4088/JCP.tv17016ah4c

115. Arya, D., Khan, T., Margolius, A., & Fernandez, H. (2019). Tardive dyskinesia: Treatment update. *Current Neurology and Neuroscience Reports, 19*(9), 69. https://doi.org/10.1007/s11 910-019-0976-1

116. Meyer, J. (2016). Forgotten but not gone: New developments in the understanding and treatment of tardive dyskinesia. *CNS Spectrums, 21*, 13–24. https://doi.org/10.1017/S109285291 6000730

117. Morgenstern, H. (1993). Identifying risk factors for tardive dyskinesia among long-term outpatients maintained with neuroleptic medications. *Archives of General Psychiatry, 50*, 723. https://doi.org/10.1001/archpsyc.1993.01820210057007

118. Souza, R., Remington, G., Chowdhury, N., Lau, M., Voineskos, A., Lieberman, J., Meltzer, H., & Kennedy, J. (2010). Association study of the GSK-3B gene with tardive dyskinesia in European Caucasians. *European Neuropsychopharmacology, 20*, 688–694. https://doi.org/ 10.1016/j.euroneuro.2010.05.002

119. Woerner, M., Correll, C., Alvir, J., Greenwald, B., Delman, H., & Kane, J. (2011). Incidence of tardive dyskinesia with risperidone or olanzapine in the elderly: Results from a 2-year, prospective study in antipsychotic-naive patients. *Neuropsychopharmacology, 36*, 1738–1746. https://doi.org/10.1038/npp.2011.55

120. Miksys, S., Wadji, F., Tolledo, C., Remington, G., Nobrega, J., & Tyndale, R. (2017). Rat brain CYP2D enzymatic metabolism alters acute and chronic haloperidol side-effects by different mechanisms. *Progress in Neuro-Psychopharmacology and Biological Psychiatry, 78*, 140–148. https://doi.org/10.1016/j.pnpbp.2017.04.030

121. Zai, C., de Luca, V., Hwang, R., Voineskos, A., Mueller, D. J., Remington, G., & Kennedy, J. (2007). Meta-analysis of two dopamine D-2 receptor gene polymorphisms with tardive dyskinesia in schizophrenia patients. *Molecular Psychiatry, 12*, 794–795. https://doi.org/ 10.1038/sj.mp.4002023

122. Zai, C., Lee, F., Tiwari, A., Lu, J., de Luca, V., Maes, M., Herbert, D., Sh, A., Cheema, S., Zai, G., Atukuri, A., Sherman, M., Shaikh, S., Tampakeras, M., Freeman, N., King, N., Mueller, D. J., Greenbaum, L., Lerer, B., & Kennedy, J. (2018). Investigation of the HSPG2 gene in tardive dyskinesia—New data and meta-analysis. *Frontiers in Pharmacology, 9*, 974. https://doi.org/ 10.3389/fphar.2018.00974

123. Hauser, R., & Truong, D. (2018). Tardive dyskinesia: Out of the shadows. *Journal of the Neurological Sciences, 389*, 1–3. https://doi.org/10.1016/j.jns.2018.02.009

124. Margolese, H., Chouinard, P., Kolivakis, T., Beauclair, L., & Miller, R. (2005). Tardive dyskinesia in the era of typical and atypical antipsychotics. Part 1: Pathophysiology and mechanisms of induction. *Canadian Journal of Psychiatry. Revue Canadienne de Psychiatrie, 50*, 541–547. https://doi.org/10.1177/070674370505000907

125. Mahmoudi, S., Lévesque, D., & Blanchet, P. (2014). Upregulation of dopamine D3, not D2, receptors correlates with tardive dyskinesia in a primate model. *Movement Disorders, 29*(9), 1125–1133. https://doi.org/10.1002/mds.25909

126. Kulkarni, S., & Pattipati, S. (2003). Pathophysiology and drug therapy of tardive dyskinesia: Current concepts and future perspectives. *Drugs of Today (Barcelona, Spain: 1998), 39*, 19–49. https://doi.org/10.1358/dot.2003.39.1.799430

127. Bhidayasiri, R., Fahn, S., Weiner, W., Gronseth, G., Sullivan, K., & Zesiewicz, T. (2013). Evidence-based guideline: Treatment of tardive syndromes: Report of the Guideline Development Subcommittee of the American Academy of Neurology. *Neurology, 81*, 463–469. https://doi.org/10.1212/WNL.0b013e31829d86b6

128. Salem H, Pigott T, Zhang XY, Zeni CP, Teixeira AL (2017). Antipsychotic-induced Tardive dyskinesia: from biological basis to clinical management. *Expert Rev Neurother, 17*(9), 883–894. https://doi.org/10.1080/14737175.2017.1361322.

129. Bishnoi, M., Chopra, K., & Kulkarni, S. (2007). Possible anti-oxidant and neuroprotective mechanisms of zolpidem in attenuating typical anti-psychotic-induced orofacial dyskinesia—A biochemical and neurochemical study. *Progress in Neuro-Psychopharmacology & Biological Psychiatry, 31*, 1130–1138. https://doi.org/10.1016/j.pnpbp.2007.04.007

130. Casey, D. (1980). γ-Acetylenic GABA in tardive dyskinesia. *Archives of General Psychiatry, 37*, 1376. https://doi.org/10.1001/archpsyc.1980.01780250062007

131. Cho, C.-H., & Lee, H.-J. (2013). Oxidative stress and tardive dyskinesia: Pharmacogenetic evidence. *Progress in Neuro-Psychopharmacology & Biological Psychiatry, 46*, 207–213.

132. Waln, O., & Jankovic, J. (2013). An update on tardive dyskinesia: From phenomenology to treatment. *Tremor and Other Hyperkinetic Movements (New York, N.Y.), 3*, 03-161-4138-1. https://doi.org/10.7916/D88P5Z71

133. Bashir, H., & Jankovic, J. (2020). Treatment of tardive dyskinesia. *Neurologic Clinics, 38*(2), 379–396. https://doi.org/10.1016/j.ncl.2020.01.004

134. Adler, L., Angrist, B., Reiter, S., & Rotrosen, J. (1989). Neuroleptic-induced akathisia: A review. *Psychopharmacology, 97*, 1–11. https://doi.org/10.1007/BF00443404

135. Sachdev, P., & Longragan, C. (1991). The present status of akathisia. *Journal of Nervous and Mental Disease, 179*, 381–391. https://doi.org/10.1097/00005053-199107000-00001

136. Loonen, A., & Stahl, S. (2011). The mechanism of drug-induced akathisia. *CNS Spectrums, 16*, 7.

137. Tachere, R., & Modirrousta, M. (2017). Beyond anxiety and agitation: A clinical approach to akathisia. *Australian Family Physician, 46*, 296–298.

138. Sachdev, P. (1995). *Akathisia and restless legs.* Cambridge University Press, p. 425. https://doi.org/10.1017/CBO9780511530203

139. Burke, R., Kang, U., Jankovic, J., Miller, L., & Fahn, S. (1989). Tardive akathisia: An analysis of clinical features and response to open therapeutic trials. *Movement Disorders: Official Journal of the Movement Disorder Society, 4*, 157–175. https://doi.org/10.1002/mds.870040208

140. Schoretsanitis, G., Nikolakopoulou, A., Guinart, D., Correll, C., & Kane, J. (2020). Iron homeostasis alterations and risk for akathisia in patients treated with antipsychotics: A systematic review and meta-analysis of cross-sectional studies. *European Neuropsychopharmacology, 35*, 1–11. https://doi.org/10.1016/j.euroneuro.2020.04.001

141. Barton, A., Bowie, J., & Ebmeier, K. (1990). Low plasma iron status & akathisia. *Journal of Neurology, Neurosurgery, and Psychiatry, 53*, 671–674. https://doi.org/10.1136/jnnp.53.8.671

142. Brown, K., Glen, S., & White, T. (1987). Low serum iron status and akathisia. *Lancet, 1*, 1234–1236. https://doi.org/10.1016/S0140-6736(87)92687-0

143. Matak, P., Matak, A., Moustafa, S., Aryal, D., Benner, E., Wetsel, W., & Andrews, N. (2016). Disrupted iron homeostasis causes dopaminergic neurodegeneration in mice. *Proceedings of the National Academy of Sciences, 113*, 201519473. https://doi.org/10.1073/pnas.1519473113

144. Unger, E., Bianco, L., Jones, B., Allen, R., & Earley, C. (2014). Low brain iron effects and reversibility on striatal dopamine dynamics. *Experimental Neurology*, *261*, 462–468. https://doi.org/10.1016/j.expneurol.2014.06.023

145. Jankovic, J., & Roos, R. A. C. (2014). Chorea associated with Huntington's disease: To treat or not to treat? *Movement Disorders*, *29*(11), 1414–1418. https://doi.org/10.1002/mds.25996

146. Cardoso, F., Seppi, K., Mair, K. J., Wenning, G. K., & Poewe, W. (2006). Seminar on choreas. *Lancet Neurology*, *5*(7), 589–602. https://doi.org/10.1016/S1474-4422(06)70494-X

147. Estevez-Fraga, C., Flower, M. D., & Tabrizi, S. J. (2020). Therapeutic strategies for Huntington's disease. *Current Opinion in Neurology*, *33*(4), 508–518. https://doi.org/10.1097/WCO.0000000000000835

148. Albin, R. L., Reiner, A., Anderson, K. D., Penney, J. B., & Young, A. B. (1990). Striatal and nigral neuron subpopulations in rigid Huntington's disease: Implications for the functional anatomy of chorea and rigidity-akinesia. *Annals of Neurology*, *27*(4), 357–365. https://doi.org/10.1002/ana.410270403

149. Coyle, J. T., & Schwarcz, R. (1976). Lesion of striatal neurons with kainic acid provides a model for Huntington's chorea. *Nature*, *263*(5574), 244–246. https://doi.org/10.1038/263244a0

150. Perry, T. L., Hansen, S., & Kloster, M. (1973). Huntington's chorea: Deficiency of γ-aminobutyric acid in brain. *New England Journal of Medicine*, *288*(7), 337–342. https://doi.org/10.1056/NEJM197302152880703

151. Janavs, J. L., & Aminoff, M. J. (1998). Dystonia and chorea in acquired systemic disorders. *Journal of Neurology, Neurosurgery & Psychiatry*, *65*(4), 436–445. https://doi.org/10.1136/jnnp.65.4.436

151. Storey, E., & Beal, M. F. (1993). Neurochemical substrates of rigidity and chorea in Huntington's disease. *Brain*, *116*(5), 1201–1222. https://doi.org/10.1093/brain/116.5.1201

152. Frank, S., Stamler, D., Kayson, E., Claassen, D. O., Colcher, A., Davis, C., Duker, A., Eberly, S., Elmer, L., Furr-Stimming, E., Gudesblatt, M., Hunter, C., Jankovic, J., Kostyk, S. K., Kumar, R., Loy, C., Mallonee, W., Oakes, D., Scott, B. L., . . . Testa, C. M., for the Huntington Study Group/Alternatives for Reducing Chorea in Huntington Disease, I. (2017). Safety of converting from tetrabenazine to deutetrabenazine for the treatment of chorea. *JAMA Neurology*, *74*(8), 977. https://doi.org/10.1001/jamaneurol.2017.1352

153. Apetauerova, D., Schirmer, C. M., Shils, J. L., Zani, J., & Arle, J. E. (2010). Successful bilateral deep brain stimulation of the globus pallidus internus for persistent status dystonicus and generalized chorea: Report of 2 cases. *Journal of Neurosurgery*, *113*(3), 634–638. https://doi.org/10.3171/2010.1.JNS091127

154. Li, P., Huang, R., Song, W., Ji, J., Burgunder, J.-M., Wang, X., Zhong, Q., Kaelin-Lang, A., Wang, W., & Shang, H.-F. (2012). Deep brain stimulation of the globus pallidus internal improves symptoms of chorea-acanthocytosis. *Neurological Sciences*, *33*(2), 269–274. https://doi.org/10.1007/s10072-011-0741-y

155. Miquel, M., Spampinato, U., Latxague, C., Aviles-Olmos, I., Bader, B., Bertram, K., Bhatia, K., Burbaud, P., Burghaus, L., Cho, J. W., Cuny, E., Danek, A., Foltynie, T., Garcia Ruiz, P. J., Giménez-Roldán, S., Guehl, D., Guridi, J., Hariz, M., Jarman, P., . . . Tison, F. (2013). Short and long term outcome of bilateral pallidal stimulation in chorea-acanthocytosis. *PLoS ONE*, *8*(11), e79241. https://doi.org/10.1371/journal.pone.0079241

156. Scott, L. J. (2011). Tetrabenazine: For chorea associated with Huntington's disease. *CNS Drugs*, *25*(12), 1073–1085. https://doi.org/10.2165/11208330-000000000-00000

157. Frank, S., Testa, C. M., Stamler, D., Kayson, E., Davis, C., Edmondson, M. C., Kinel, S., Leavitt, B., Oakes, D., O'Neill, C., Vaughan, C., Goldstein, J., Herzog, M., Snively, V., Whaley, J., Wong, C., Suter, G., Jankovic, J., Jimenez-Shahed, J., . . . Christopher, E. (2016). Effect of deutetrabenazine on chorea among patients with Huntington disease: A randomized clinical trial. *JAMA*, *316*(1), 40. https://doi.org/10.1001/jama.2016.8655

158. Schneider, F., Bradbury, M., Baillie, T., Stamler, D., Hellriegel, E., Cox, D., Loupe, P., Savola, J. M., & Rabinovich-Guilatt, L. (2020). Pharmacokinetic and metabolic profile of deutetrabenazine (TEV-50717) compared with tetrabenazine in healthy volunteers. *Clinical and Translational Science*, *13*(4), 707–717. https://doi.org/10.1111/cts.12754

159. Schultz, W., & Dickinson, A. (2000). Neuronal coding of prediction errors. *Annual Review of Neuroscience*, *23*(1), 473–500. https://doi.org/10.1146/annurev.neuro.23.1.473

160. Frank, M. J. (2004). By carrot or by stick: Cognitive reinforcement learning in parkinsonism. *Science*, *306*(5703), 1940–1943. https://doi.org/10.1126/science.1102941

161. Lima, B. F. C., Ramos, D. C., Barbiero, J. K., Pulido, L., Redgrave, P., Robinson, D. L., Gómez-A, A., & Da Cunha, C. (2017). Partial lesion of dopamine neurons of rat substantia nigra impairs conditioned place aversion but spares conditioned place preference. *Neuroscience*, *349*, 264–277. https://doi.org/10.1016/j.neuroscience.2017.02.052

162. Yin, H. H., & Knowlton, B. J. (2006). The role of the basal ganglia in habit formation. *Nature Reviews Neuroscience*, *7*(6), 464–476. https://doi.org/10.1038/nrn1919

163. Knowlton, B. J., Mangels, J. A., & Squire, L. R. (1996). A neostriatal habit learning system in humans. *Science*, *273*(5280), 1399–1402. https://doi.org/10.1126/science.273.5280.1399

164. Cunha, C., Silva, M., Wietzikoski, S., Wietzikoski, E., Ferro, M., Kouzmine, I., & Canteras, N. (2007). Place learning strategy of substantia nigra pars compacta-lesioned rats. *Behavioral Neuroscience*, *120*, 1279–1284. https://doi.org/10.1037/0735-7044.120.6.1279

165. Cunha, C., Wietzikoski, S., Wietzikoski, E., Miyoshi, E., Ferro, M., Anselmo-Franci, J., & Canteras, N. (2003). Evidence for the substantia nigra pars compacta as an essential component of a memory system independent of the hippocampal memory system. *Neurobiology of Learning and Memory*, *79*, 236–242. https://doi.org/10.1016/S1074-7427(03)00008-X

166. Ferro, M., Bellissimo, M., Anselmo-Franci, J., Angellucci, M., Canteras, N., & Cunha, C. (2005). Comparison of bilaterally 6-OHDA- and MPTP-lesioned rats as models of the early phase of Parkinson's disease: Histological, neurochemical, motor and memory alterations. *Journal of Neuroscience Methods*, *148*, 78–87. https://doi.org/10.1016/j.jneum eth.2005.04.005

167. Miyoshi, E., Wietzikoski, S., Camplessei, M., Silveira, R., Takahashi, R., & Cunha, C. (2002). Impaired learning in a spatial working memory version and in a cued version of the water maze in rats with MPTP-induced mesencephalic dopaminergic lesions. *Brain Research Bulletin*, *58*, 41–47. https://doi.org/10.1016/S0361-9230(02)00754-2

168. Lee, E., Cowan, N., Vogel, E., Rolan, T., Valle-Inclán, F., & Hackley, S. (2010). Visual working memory deficits in patients with Parkinson's disease are due to both reduced storage capacity and impaired ability to filter out irrelevant information. *Brain*, *133*, 2677–2689. https://doi. org/10.1093/brain/awq197

169. Papagno, C., & Trojano, L. (2018). Cognitive and behavioral disorders in Parkinson's disease: An update. I: Cognitive impairments. *Neurological Sciences*, *39*(2), 215–223. https:// doi.org/10.1007/s10072-017-3154-8

170. Bellissimo, M., Kouzmine, I., Ferro, M., Oliveira, B., Canteras, N., & Cunha, C. (2004). Is the unilateral lesion of the left substantia nigra pars compacta sufficient to induce working

memory impairment in rats? *Neurobiology of Learning and Memory, 82,* 150–158. https://doi.org/10.1016/j.nlm.2004.06.006

171. Braga, R., Kouzmine, I., Canteras, N., & Cunha, C. (2005). Lesion of the substantia nigra, pars compacta impairs delayed alternation in a Y-maze in rats. *Experimental Neurology, 192,* 134–141. https://doi.org/10.1016/j.expneurol.2004.11.006

PART II
MOVEMENT DISORDERS ASSOCIATED WITH PSYCHOTROPICS

3

Dopamine Antagonist-Induced Parkinsonism

Abdulmunaim M. Eid and William G. Ondo

Definitions

"Secondary parkinsonism" is a term that is often used to describe parkinsonism that is not of a neurodegenerative disorder. Arguably, the most important and frequent form of secondary parkinsonism is drug-induced parkinsonism (DIP). DIP is the occurrence of parkinsonism in relationship to an offending drug treatment. This should be distinguished from more permanent parkinsonism resulting from environmental toxins or illicit drugs. The list of drugs that can induce or exacerbate parkinsonism is long, but we can divide it into two major groups; those drugs that interfere directly with dopaminergic system and those that don't. Because the term "neuroleptics" appear variably in literature, it may be useful to define it here as used in the rest of this chapter. Neuroleptic is a Greek word that literally means "that which takes hold of the neuron/nerve." The term was coined by Deniker to denote a class of "major tranquilizers." However, its use in contemporary neuropsychiatry has evolved to denote antidopaminergic drugs, mainly antipsychotics and to a lesser extent antiemetics.[2]

Classically, the diagnosis of DIP requires the presence of parkinsonism (defined as a syndrome of two of four cardinal signs (resting tremor, bradykinesia, rigidity, and impaired postural reflexes) plus all three of the following criteria: symptom onset while on neuroleptic or other culpable drug, no parkinsonism symptoms before drug treatment, and resolution of symptoms within 6 months of withdrawal of drug treatment, if applicable (i.e., for patients who never discontinued the drug, the first two criteria were sufficient for diagnosis).[3,4] Not surprisingly, however, there are exceptions to these criteria that wouldn't disqualify a patient from carrying the diagnosis of DIP. Another term, "reversible antipsychotic-induced parkinsonism" (AIP), has been proposed for parkinsonism that resolves within 6 months of drug withdrawal, however, some cases of AIP have symptoms that extend beyond 6 months (up to longer than a year) but eventually recover.[5]

The *Diagnostic and Statistical Manual of Mental Disorders*, fifth edition (DSM-5) defines DIP (both neuroleptic-induced parkinsonism and other medication-induced parkinsonism) as follows: resting tremor, muscular rigidity, akinesia (i.e., loss of movement or difficulty initiating movement), or bradykinesia (i.e., slowing movement) developing within a few weeks of starting or raising the dosage of a medication (e.g., a neuroleptic) or after reducing the dosage of a medication used to treat extrapyramidal symptoms.[6] This definition has two problems; the first is the determination of time of onset by "a few weeks" after initiating/

increasing the dose of the medication which makes intuitive sense but is not data driven. Time from drug exposure to onset of symptoms has been as low as 3 weeks, but may occur after many years. [7] Also, the inclusion of reduction of dosage of a medication used to treat extrapyramidal symptoms is not clear. Almost all idiopathic Parkinson's disease (IPD) patients who have benefited from levodopa, for example, will have re-emergence of parkinsonian signs upon reduction of the dose to a relatively less effective level, but those patients wouldn't qualify for the diagnosis of DIP.

DIP most commonly results from dopamine receptor antagonists/inverse agonists and less commonly dopamine release inhibitors targeting vesicular monoamine transporter-1 and -2 (VMAT inhibitors) such as reserpine, tetrabenazine, and valbenazine. Almost no systematic studies of DIP from VMAT inhibitors exist. Other agents, including the calcium-channel blockers cinnarizine and flunarizine, antidepressants, lithium, and valproate account for a large minority of DIP and will be discussed separately.[8] In addition, up to 25% of DIP cases (8%–13% of antipsychotic-induced parkinsonism) remain symptomatic beyond 6 months of withdrawing the offending drug.[9] About 11% of patients who initially recovered from DIP went on to subsequently develop PD.[10,11] In a French cohort, the risk of PD was increased by over threefold after exposure to antipsychotics.[12] Therefore, it appears that DIP is a risk for idiopathic parkinsonism. This has three potential explanations. The first is that these drugs unmask a subclinical neurodegenerative parkinsonian syndrome that was already present but had yet to clinically manifest. It is important to realize that clinical parkinsonism starts many years after onset of PD pathology, only after about 60% of dopamine innervation is lost.[13,14] Also, many asymptomatic brain autopsies show evidence of Lewy body pathology, suggesting they would have developed idiopathic parkinsonism if they lived long enough. The unmasking of degenerative parkinsonism possibility is generally supported by studies of dopamine imaging.[15,16] The second explanation is that drug-induced toxicity from dopamine antagonists to the dopaminergic system leads to neurodegeneration.[17] A limited number of studies have investigated some aspects of this theory with evidence suggesting that antidopaminergics affect mitochondrial respiratory chain, increase dopamine turnover, enhance production of neurotoxic free radicals, and cause neuroinflammation, as reviewed by Erro et al.[17] A third explanation is that diseases associated with the use of dopamine antagonists (schizophrenia, bipolar disorder, etc.) are also risk factors for idiopathic parkinsonism.

Using diffusion tensor imaging (DTI) to compare patients with DIP with patients with IPD and healthy controls, Lee et al. showed that DIP patients had significantly lower fractional anisotropy (FA) and higher mean diffusivity (MD) values over widespread white matter (WM) areas than control subjects and similar values to those of IPD patients.[18] FAs were negatively correlated with the severity of motor symptoms and cognitive dysfunction.[18] Interestingly, neither exposure time to the offending drugs nor duration of parkinsonism showed an association with FAs or MDs,[18] which suggests that DIP may be reflective of underlying microstructural WM abnormalities and not necessarily causing them. Evaluating for an association between DTI measures and exposure time/dose to offending drugs in the GI prokinetic subgroup and the psychotherapy group would be interesting to see in order to further understand the relationship between potential microstructural abnormalities associated with psychiatric disease and risk of DIP.

Epidemiology and Risk Factors

DIP is estimated to be the second-most-common cause of parkinsonism after IPD. Unfortunately, accurate epidemiological data of DIP in general, and DIP secondary to specific groups of medications in particular, is limited by variable definitions and the possibility of underdiagnosis. In addition, difficulties in differentiating between mild DIP and motor retardation of depression or catatonic schizophrenic symptoms may have made it more difficult to make a clear diagnosis, especially when DIP was relatively new to medicine.[19] Many drugs that can cause parkinsonism are prescribed by nonneurologist medical professionals, which may also exacerbate the problem of underdiagnosis.

DIP prevalence varies widely from 2% to more than 50% of cases of parkinsonism.[20] In one report, 22% of all cases with parkinsonism were attributed to antipsychotics and similar medications.[21] In another report from Olmsted County, Minnesota, the prevalence was 20% of all parkinsonism cases between 1976- and 1990.[3] Interestingly, another study from the same population reported antipsychotics to be responsible for 11% of cases between 1976 and 2005.[4] In a report from the Canton of Geneva, DIP was the most frequent of all nondegenerative parkinsonism (43.4%), which was about 9% of all parkinsonism cases, with a crude all-age prevalence of $21.7/10^5$.[22] It's worth noting that DIP in this study, and many others, was defined based on the classical definition (see "Introduction"), i.e., it essentially meant reversible antipsychotic-induced parkinsonism. Munhoz et al. reported 10% of all parkinsonism cases in a prospective study to be secondary to drugs, 50% of which cases were attributed to neuroleptics.[9] In another study by Munhoz et al. similar results were published accounting 7.9% of parkinsonism cases to drugs, 52% of which were neuroleptics.[23]

Studies on risk factors of DIP are abundant, but they have variable, sometimes contradictory results. One unequivocal fact is that there's a remarkable influence of individual susceptibility for developing DIP.[24] An early survey exploring the presence of DIP in close relatives of patients with DIP found a two- to threefold increase in parkinsonism in subjects with DIP vs. a control group of patients on similar medicines, but without DIP, suggesting a hereditary susceptibility.[25] Candidate gene studies looking at dopamine receptors and metabolism, and Parkinson's disease genes have not shown a consistent association. A genome-wide association study found several single-nucleotide polymorphisms especially of the genes *EPF1*, *NOVA1*, and *FIGN* are associated with DIP severity.[26] *EPF1* and *NOVA1* are involved with dopamine cell development. HLA-B44 (an HLA antigen) was significantly more prevalent in the subset of a group of inpatient schizophrenic white men with DIP compared to those without DIP, with a relative risk of 7.16 for the presence of the antigen.[27] However, this has not been replicated.

Age of onset of DIP ranges between 10 months and 96 years, with 50% of patients between 60 and 79 years of age.[8] VigiBase®, the WHO Global Individual Case Safety Report database, DIP reports between 2000 and 2017 were significantly more frequent in patients aged 75 and over (ROR = 2.12; 95% CI 1.98–2.26) and older age appears to be the most robust risk for DIP.[20] Normal age-related loss of nigral dopaminergic neurons and increased Lewy body-like neuronal inclusions in the elderly, even in asymptomatic people, may cause higher insult susceptibility and explain the increased risk of DIP in elderly.[24,28] In addition, polypharmacotherapy and treatment with antipsychotics for behavior-related disorders and dopamine antagonist antiemetics/promotility drugs for GI symptoms may add to this risk.[24] It should be noted, however, that idiopathic parkinsonism is also much rarer in younger patients, therefore the relative prevalence of DIP, as opposed to IPD, is actually higher in the young. Savica et al. found DIP to be the most common cause for parkinsonism in patients under 40, accounting for 73.3% of cases, although this would very much depend on the population studied.[4]

Classically, risk of developing DIP is thought to be moderately higher in females compared males, in contrast to degenerative parkinsonism.[4,8,22] A similar conclusion was initially reached by a de Germay et al. descriptive study using VigiBase® database. However, when they then performed a comparative analysis factoring in the fact that adverse drug reactions (ADRs) are more frequently reported in women than in men in general and in VigiBase® in particular, they found that DIP was actually significantly more reported in men than in women (ROR = 1.39; 95% CI 1.31–1.47).[20] They concluded that the sex difference between DIP prevalence and DIP reporting could be explained, at least partly, by a difference in DIP reporting between men and women.[20] This, however, goes against most studies that found higher prevalence in women, and thus needs more investigation. The reason for the difference in prevalence between two sexes, assuming it exists, is not well understood, but possible explanations include higher dosage per kilogram in female patients, more compliance with treatment, or a higher consumption of drugs by women.[8] A contributory role of estrogen is also possible. For example, the difference of incidence rates of DIP between the two sexes increases with older age groups (directed toward higher risk in women),[4] suggesting a role of menopause and decreased level of estrogen after a certain age. However, in general this is not compatible with several studies suggesting an antiparkinsonian role of estrogen in IPD.[29] In summary, there is not sufficient data to explain with reasonable certainty the difference in incidence rates between the two sexes and the role of estrogens in DIP.

Other risk factors include antidopaminergic potency, dose, and duration, and the co-occurrence of other extrapyramidal symptoms (EPS) which include akathisia, tardive dyskinesia (TD), and neuroleptic malignant syndrome in addition to parkinsonism, and dementia.[5] It's important to note that many patients with dementia are prescribed antipsychotics to control behavior-related symptoms, which will increase the risk of DIP even further. Moreover, IPD and dementia with Lewy body (DLB) are understandably risk factors for DIP, which in this case would represent a worsening in parkinsonism.[24] Subclinical nigral degeneration is common in HIV infection and could possibly explain the heightened susceptibility of HIV patients to DIP in one study.[30]

The relationship of cigarette smoking to DIP in a group of 111 chronic institutionalized schizophrenic patients was investigated, with smokers found to have a lower prevalence of DIP compared to nonsmokers.[31] This is especially interesting given the extensive epidemiologic data showing an inverse association between smoking and IPD.[32]

Pathophysiology

Central dopamine receptor families include D1-like receptors (D1 and D5) and D2-like receptors (D2, D3, and D4). Most CNS antidopaminergic medications have been designed to block D2 family receptors in mesocortical, mesolimbic, nigrostriatal, and tuberoinfundibular systems, and variably block D1 family receptors. By blocking D2 receptors in mesocortical and mesolimbic system, they exert their main therapeutic antipsychotic effect.[33] However, exerting the same effects on the nigrostriatal system is thought to be the main mechanism of DIP.[33] In addition, blocking dopamine transmission in the mesocortical and mesolimbic systems can cause behavioral and cognitive side effects beyond the therapeutic benefit desired.[33] By blocking dopamine transmission, GABA- and enkephalin-containing neurons in the striatum becomes disinhibited, decreasing the tonic inhibition of the globus pallidus pars interna and substantia nigra pars reticulata (GPi/SNr) of the thalamic ventral anterior and ventral lateral nuclei (indirect pathway), followed by disinhibition of the subthalamic nucleus facilitating the tonic inhibition of GPi/SNr to the thalamocortical projections.[34] Therefore, there are many "downstream" impacts of dopamine receptor inhibition.

Occupancy of D2 receptors in the basal ganglia was found to be related to the risk of DIP, as patients with DIP were found to have higher occupancy, usually greater than 70%–80%.[35] It is generally thought that 80% occupancy causes DIP in most people, and decades ago DIP was actually clinically used to determine the dose of first-generation antipsychotics, which would be titrated up to that point. This explains why drugs with higher D2 affinity, e.g., haloperidol, pose a higher risk for DIP compared to drugs with relatively lower D2 affinity, e.g., clozapine, or drugs with virtually no affinity, e.g., pimavanserin (see Table 3.1). The role of D1 antagonism is less understood, as there are no pure D1 antagonists approved for any indication. Ecopipam, a pure D1 family antagonist, has not been reported to cause DIP in several clinical trials to date.[36] [73–83]

The long duration of DIP symptoms following drug withdrawal is poorly understood. Although some subjects improve after about five half-lives of the drug, most take months to fully recover. Some percentage of these may have unmasked IPD, but the majority do not. The reason for this recovery delay in those without evidence of neurodegeneration requires further study. Clearly there is some change in the dopamine receptor, change in endogenous dopamine release, secondary messenger change, or system impact that requires additional time to resolve.

The pathophysiology of DIP from VMAT inhibitors seems much less complicated. The reduced release of dopamine causes the parkinsonism and anecdotally almost always improves within days of drug reduction.

Clinical Manifestations: Motor Features

By definition, the diagnosis of DIP is based on a consistent drug intake history and clinical symptoms and signs of parkinsonism (rest tremor, hypokinesia, rigidity, and postural instability).

One Olmsted County, Minnesota, investigation of DIP between 1976 and 2005 reported the DIP was tremor-predominant in 57.4% of patients and akinetic rigid in 42.6%.[4] Symmetry was a major characteristic, as only about 17% of patients presented with asymmetric parkinsonism.[4] Among adverse drug reactions with parkinsonian feature(s) reported to the Midi-Pyrenees French Pharmacovigilance Center between 1993 and 2009, the most frequently reported sign was rigidity (78.7%), followed by resting tremor (61.9%) and akinesia (56.8%).[8] It's worth noting, however, that 40% of those patients only had one cardinal feature and that the neurological examination was not necessarily done by a neurologist. This high prevalence of tremor in patients with DIP, in contrast to older reports, was confirmed

Table 3.1 Drugs That Induce Parkinsonism through a Dopaminergic Mechanism and Their Affinities to Dopamine Receptors

Drug*	Class**	Dopamine receptor affinity / alternative mechanism***				
		D1	D2	D3	D4	D5
α-methyldopa	AH, phenylpropanoic acid	dopamine synthesis inhibitor				
amisulpride	AA, benzamide	–	+++	++++	++	+
aripiprazole	AA, piperazine	++	++++	+++	++	+
asenapine[73]	AA, dibenzoxepine	++++	++++	++++	++++	
benperidol	TA, butyrophenone	+	++++		++++	
brexpiprazole	AA, piperazine		++++	++++		
bromperidol	TA, butyrophenone	++	++++	++++	+++	
bromopride	PK, aminophenyl ether	potent antidopaminergic; specific affinity-related information wasn't found				
cariprazine	AA, piperazine		++++	++++		
clebopride	PK, benzylpiperidine	++	++++	++++		
chlorpromazine	TA, phenothiazine	+++	++++	++++	+++	++
chlorprothixene	TA, thixanthene	+++	++++	++++	++++	++++
cinitapride[74]	PK, nitrobenzene	5-HT receptor antagonist and agonist activity				
cinnarizine[75]	CCB, diphenylmethane		+++			
clopenthixol	TA, thixanthene	++	++++			
clothiapine	TA, dibenzepine		+++			
clozapine	AA, dibenzodiazepine	++	++	++	+++	++
cyamemazine	TA, phenothiazine	++++	++++	++++	++++	
deutetrabenazine	DD, tetrahydroisoquinoline	vesicular monoamine transporter 2 inhibitor				
domperidone	PK, benzimidazole	+	++++	++++		
droperidol	TA, butyrophenone	++	++++		++++	
ecopipam[76]	AA, benzazepines	++++	–		–	++++
flunarizine[75]	CCB, diphenylmethane		+++			
flupenthixol	TA, thixanthene	++++	++++	++++	+++	
fluphenazine	TA, phenothiazine	+++	++++	++++	+++	+++
fluspirilene	TA, diphenylbutylpiperidine	++	++++	++++	++++	
haloperidol	TA, butyrophenone	+++	++++	+++	++++	++
iloperidone	AA, carbonyl compound	++	++++	+++	++++	++
itopride[77]	PK, N-benzylbenzamide	potent antidopaminergic; specific affinity-related information wasn't found				

Table 3.1 Continued

Drug*	Class**	Dopamine receptor affinity / alternative mechanism***				
		D1	D2	D3	D4	D5
levomepromazine	TA, phenothiazine		+++			
levosulpiride	AA, benzamide		+++	++		
loxapine	TA, dibenzepine	+++	+++	+++	++++	+++
lumateperone[78]	AA, carbonyl compound		+++			
lurasidone	AA, piperazine		++++			
melperone	AA, carbonyl compound	++++	++	++	++	
mesoridazine	TA, phenothiazine	+++	+++	++++	+++	
metoclopramide	PK, aminophenyl ether	–	+++	+++		
molindone	TA, dihydroindolone	+	+++	+++	+	
olanzapine	AA, benzodiazepine	+++	+++	+++	+++	
paliperidone	AA, pyridopyrimidine		++++	++++	+++	
pericyazine	TA, phenothiazine	++++	++++	++++	++++	
perphenazine	TA, phenothiazine	+++	++++	++++	+++	
pimavanserin[79]	AA, phenol ether	mainly inverse agonist at 5-HT2A				
			+	+		
pimozide	TA, diphenylbutylpiperidine	++++	++++	++++	++++	
pipotiazine	TA, phenothiazine		++++	++++		
prochloperazine	TA, phenothiazine	++	++++	++++	++++	
promazine	TA, phenothiazine	+	+++	+++		
quetiapine	AA, dibenzodiazepine	+	++	++	+	+
raclopride	TA, benzamide	+	++++	++++	+	
remoxipride	TA, benzamide	+	++	+	+	
reserpine	DD, yohimbine alkaloid	vesicular monoamine transporter 1 and 2 inhibitor				
		+	++	++		
risperidone	AA, pyridopyrimidine	++	++++	++++	++++	
sertindole	AA, pyrrole	+++	++++	++++	+++	
sulpiride	TA, benzamide	+	+++	+++	+	
sultopride	TA, benzamide		++++	++++		
tetrabenazine	DD, tetrahydroisoquinoline	vesicular monoamine transporter 2 inhibitor				
			+			

(continued)

Table 3.1 Continued

Drug*	Class**	Dopamine receptor affinity / alternative mechanism***				
		D1	D2	D3	D4	D5
tiapride	TA, Benzenesulfonyl		++	++	+++	
thiethylperazine[80]	PK/AV, phenothiazine		++++			
thioproperazine	TA, phenothiazine		++++	++++	+++	
thioridazine	TA, phenothiazine	+++	+++	++++	+++	++
thiothixene	TA, thixanthene	+++	++++	++++	+++	++
trifluperazine	TA, phenothiazine	+++	++++	++++	++	
valbenazine[81]	DD, alpha amino acid ester	vesicular monoamine transporter 2 inhibitor				
		+	+			
ziprasidone	AA, piperazine	+++	++++	++++	+++	++
zuclopenthixol[82]	TA, benzothiopyran	++++	++++			

* National Institute of Mental Health's Psychoactive Drug Screening Program (PDSP) Ki Database is used to search and obtain the Ki values (averaged values for cloned human or alternatively cloned rat, only if the former isn't available, are used) that are used to generate this affinity table; https://pdsp.unc.edu/databases/kidb.php.[83] When information isn't found in the PDSP Ki database, other sources are used and accordingly cited.

** Clinical class is mentioned followed by chemical class/subclass. Note that some medications are clinically categorized in more than one category; we used the most common categorization.

AH: antihypertensive, TA: typical antipsychotic, AA: atypical antipsychotic, DD: dopamine depleter, PK: prokinetic, CCB: calcium channel blocker, AV: antivertiginous

***minimal if any affinity; + very low; ++ low; +++ moderate; ++++ high

by Morley et al. upon comparing patients with DIP to age-matched patients with IPD in a Veterans Affairs (VA) population in Pennsylvania with near-identical prevalence of tremor; 79% in IPD and 78% in DIP.[37] It's worth noting that a stratified analysis based on reversibility of DIP after discontinuing or, more commonly, changing the offending drug (usually substituting with quetiapine because of its association with low incidence of DIP) found that in reversible DIP, tremor was present in 74% of patients, compared to 92% in those with DIP persistent for at least three months, suggesting some of those may have unmasked IP. [37] Interestingly, although tremor prevalence was similar, higher tremor scores were recorded in patients with DIP compared to those with IPD. Although the definition of DIP in this study included patients who were concurrently taking other medications associated with DIP, all but one took at least one dopamine antagonist, the other took lithium. Morley et al. also reported loss of facial expressiveness in 43% of IPD patients compared with 28% in DIP patients, and higher postural instability gait disorder scores in the IPD group.[37] Overall, although DIP is generally more symmetric and may have a mildly higher tremor frequency,[38] it cannot be reliably distinguished from IPD based on examination alone.

Another phenotype associated with DIP is rabbit syndrome. Rabbit syndrome is classically a neuroleptic-induced disorder that's usually acute in onset and is characterized by rapid vertical perioral movements imitating a rabbit's rapid chewing movements. This movement has a frequency of 2.5–5.5 Hz and is almost exclusively vertical with no horizontal or rotatory movements, which is important to differentiate it from TD.[39] Although there are exceptions, rabbit syndrome doesn't usually involve the tongue, which also helps differentiate it from TD. Rabbit syndrome may be a variant of simple jaw tremor seen in DIP, but is distinguished by its acute onset, long persistence after drug withdrawal, and response to amantadine. Although the majority of rabbit syndrome cases are associated with DIP, some cases are reported with IPD and more recently associated with other medications without parkinsonism e.g., there's an interesting report of an 11-year-old child with OCD who developed rabbit syndrome with fluoxetine at a therapeutic dose which was reversible with lower doses.[40]

DIP and TD have contrasting phenotypes and treatments, however, their concomitant presence in many patients at least suggests certain similar intrinsic and extrinsic factors are associated with both, or possibly that they are directly related. Gardos and Cole summarized older epidemiological studies and found that concomitant TD was present in up to 27.3% of patients with DIP.[41] Other studies have found higher percentages in specific populations e.g., those older than 65 years.[41] Kane et al. found in their prospective study a statistically significant association between DIP and subsequent development of TD confirming the idea that DIP can be a forerunner of TD.[42] In our experience and as found by Crane, discontinuation of the neuroleptic medication(s) in a patient with DIP is a risk factor for then developing withdrawal emergent dyskinesia as the parkinsonism resolves.[43] The DSM-5 differentiates withdrawal emergent dyskinesia from TD, however similar phenotype and treatment response suggest they have identical pathophysiology.[6] DIP is also a common side effect in patients with TD who receive dopamine-depleting (VMAT-2 inhibitors) agents as a treatment for their TD, and is seen more commonly than when those agents are used for chorea or tics, although this may be due to older age in the TD population.[44] This can confuse patients and clinicians, especially when DIP presents with prominent perioral tremor, which to the untrained observer may look like persistent TD. DIP can also be associated with akathisia or neuroleptic malignant syndrome among other forms of drug-induced movement disorders.

Clinical Manifestations: Nonmotor Features

IPD is characterized by many nonmotor features that make it among the most complex diseases in clinical medicine. These nonmotor features include but are not limited to autonomic dysfunction, constipation, hyposmia, REM behavioral disorder (RBD), cognitive dysfunction, psychosis, and depression. An important question would be whether or not DIP has the same or a similar nonmotor profile and could we distinguish between the two conditions based on the nonmotor features, since we can't differentiate based on motor features alone.

Several studies have found similar nonmotor features in patients with DIP, including RBD, dysautonomia including urinary symptoms, constipation, and impotence, and orthostatic hypotension, cognitive dysfunction, and mood symptoms.[45–51] Depression is a very common symptom in patients with DIP, but because it's also common in the elderly, a population at special risk for DIP, and in many conditions that require treatment with antidopaminergics, attributing its presence to DIP itself is difficult.[49] Similarly, cognitive deficits, though present in many patients with DIP, are also common in concomitant diseases.[49] Despite these difficulties, some studies have tried to differentiate between neuropsychological deficits secondary to DIP from those secondary to a concomitant disease. A cross-sectional study found higher scores of subjective cognitive-perceptual dysfunction in schizophrenic patients treated with antipsychotics complicated by DIP than those without DIP.[46] Another study of 13 patients with DIP (most were on antidopaminergics for functional dyspepsia and a minority with depression, one had orolingual dyskinesia, one had delusion) described neuropsychological scores worse than controls and similar to a group with IPD.[47]

Although hyposmia is prevalent in patients with presumed DIP, differentiation between those with underlying dopamine deficits and those without yields important distinctions.[45] In a retrospective review of DIP patients seen in one center, hyposmia was significantly more common among subjects with IPD compared to DIP and olfactory testing correctly predicted whether DIP subjects would recover after drug withdrawal in 11/13 cases.[50] Whether the olfactory dysfunction in patients with DIP is exclusively secondary to dopaminergic loss rather than dopaminergic loss and/or dopaminergic receptor blockade is debatable. Several studies have found that patients with DIP and abnormal DaTscan (see "Imaging: Dopamine Imaging," below) had worse olfactory function than patients with DIP and normal DaTscan; the latter group typically not distinguishable from normal subjects.[45–50] In one of study 10.7% of DIP patients with a normal DaTscan had hyposmia, whereas 46.2% of patients with an abnormal scan had hyposmia; a negative predictive value of hyposmia was calculated at 78.1% and a positive predictive value at 66.7% to predict DaTscan status.[48,52] Therefore, worse olfaction seems more common in IPD and DIP that unmasks IPD.

In summary, although population-based differences between clinical features of IPD and those of DIP exist, in an individual patient, it is probably not possible to definitively differentiate between the two conditions.

Imaging: Dopamine Imaging

There are several ways to image dopamine in the human brain with either single photon emission computed tomography (SPECT) or positron emission tomography (PET), using ligands targeting dopamine transporter (DAT) protein (many ligands), dopamine receptors (many ligands), dopamine storage vesicles (C^{11}-dihydrotetrabenazine), and dopamine precursors (L-6-[F18] fluoro-3,4-dihydroxyphenylalnine). The most widely available ligand is $[^{123}I]$N-ω-fluoropropyl-2β-carbomethoxy-3β-(4-iodophenyl)nortropane ($[^{123}I]$FP-CIT), which binds to presynaptic dopamine transporters that are located most abundantly in the striatum (DaTscan). Neurodegeneration involving the nigrostriatal system will cause decreased uptake of this ligand by the dopamine transporters and thus decreased signal on SPECT. This occurs in all degenerative parkinsonian syndromes, which can't be accurately differentiated from each other based on this modality alone.[53,54]

In theory, a drug binding to dopamine receptors should not alter DAT binding, so this could be used to differentiate DIP from primary parkinsonism. A comprehensive review of involvement of DaTscan in differentiating between IPD and DIP was performed by Brigo et al. in 2014.[55] Overall, they found that DaTscan can be a reliable technique to differentiate the two conditions with relatively good sensitivity and specificity values,[55] however results of individual studies were moderately variable (see Table 3.2).[56–61] Tinazzi et al. among other groups explored the theory that those patients with DIP and abnormal DaTscan may have underlying degenerative parkinsonism and found that motor symptoms of this subgroup of patients tend not to resolve after withdrawal of the offending drug(s).[56–61] Furthermore, one study found that this abnormal DaTscan subgroup tends to respond better to levodopa,

Table 3.2 Imaging for Suspected Drug-Induced Parkinsonism

Modality	DIP suspected	Normal	Abnormal	Clinical outcomes after drug withdrawal (unless another intervention is otherwise specified)
18F-dopa PET	13 patients[62]	9	4	8 of 9 with normal study improved. 3 of 4 with abnormal study had persistent parkinsonism.
DaT-SPECT	57 patients[84]	28	29	28 of 32 with normal scan improved by 18 months. 25 of 25 with abnormal scans had persistent parkinsonism at 18 months.
DaT-SPECT	20 patients[56]	9	11	not evaluated
DaT-SPECT	19 patients[7]	15	4	13 of 15 with normal scan recovered by 6–34 months. 2 of 15 with normal scan and all 4 with abnormal scan had persistent parkinsonism by 14-–27 months.
DaT-SPECT	19 patients[58]	10	9	3 of 10 patients with normal scan and in 8 of 9 patients with abnormal scan had improvement of motor symptoms by 19–39 months by use of L-dopa.
DaT-SPECT	97 patients[59,60]	56	41	L-dopa trial in 35 patients showed a deeper reduction of motor UPDRS in the abnormal scan group compared to the normal scan group (11.42 versus 3.56 points, $p = 0.002$).
DaT-SPECT	32 patients[61]	18	14	not evaluated
DaT-SPECT	20 patients[85]	16	2 (another 2 with equivocal results)	16 of 16 patients with normal scan and the 2 patients with equivocal scan had remission within 3 months. However, the 2 patients with equivocal scan had reappearance of parkinsonism within 1–2 years, and then improved with L-dopa. The 2 patients with abnormal scans had persistent parkinsonism, and then improved with L-dopa.
MIBG cardiac scintigraphy	20 patients[15]	18	2	18 of 18 patients with normal imaging recovered. 2 of 2 with abnormal imaging had persistent parkinsonism, and then responded dramatically to L-dopa.
MIBG cardiac scintigraphy	15 patients[68]	14	1	14 of 14 patient with normal imaging recovered. The only patient with abnormal imaging had persistent parkinsonism, and then responded to L-dopa.

(continued)

Table 3.2 Continued

Modality	DIP suspected	Normal	Abnormal	Clinical outcomes after drug withdrawal (unless another intervention is otherwise specified)
MIBG cardiac scintigraphy	20 patients[85]	16	4	16 of 16 patients with normal scan and 2 of 4 patients with abnormal scan had remission within 3 months. However, the 2 patients with abnormal scan had reappearance of parkinsonism within 1–2 years, and then improved with L-dopa.
				2 of 4 patients with abnormal scan had persistent parkinsonism, and then improved with L-dopa.
TCS of SN	20 patients[66]	14	6	12 of 14 with normal scan improved at 6 months.
				2 of 6 with abnormal scans improved. Rest of patients had scans that correlated with final clinical diagnosis.
TCS of SN	69 patients[63]	45	24	41 of 45 with normal scan and 6 of 24 with abnormal scan had resolution of parkinsonism at 6 months.
				4 of 45 with normal scan and 18 of 24 with abnormal scan had persistent parkinsonism at 6 months.

unlike typical DIP and more like IPD behavior.[58] The latter two observations were confirmed in a prospective study by the same group declaring that abnormal initial DaTscan was the only predictor of motor progression and better response to levodopa treatment in presumed DIP.[60] Collectively these observations suggest that DaTscan, although useful in the differentiation between DIP and IPD, can be abnormal in a subgroup of DIP with concurrent underlying degenerative pathology. A normal DaTscan strongly suggests they do not have concurrent IPD. A small study using the dopamine precursor F^{18}-Dopa also showed good predictive value.[62]

Imaging: Transcranial Sonography (TCS)

TCS is a noninvasive, relatively easy to use, non-time-consuming, and relatively cheap imaging modality that can be used to help explore various neurological conditions; including IPD. TCS of the midbrain in patients with IPD typically identifies an enlarged hyperechogenic signal representing increased iron in the substantia nigra. This finding is present in 68%–99% of patients with IPD and lacking in 85%–90% of healthy subjects and in the majority of patients with other degenerative parkinsonian conditions, giving it a good diagnostic value.[63,64]

Many studies have found this technique useful in differentiating DIP from IPD, with the typical finding of normal echogenicity in patients with DIP.[63,65,66] One study found no statistically significant difference in echogenicity of substantia nigra between the two groups, however a limitation of small sample size (N = 40; half of them with DIP and half with PD) was acknowledged by the authors as the likely reason for not reaching significance.[66] This could also suggest that increased brain iron is a risk factor for DIP, which has not otherwise been explored. Several studies found that DIP patients with persistent symptoms after withdrawal of the offending drug had TCS findings similar to those of patients with IPD; a finding of the same significance of a similar finding using DaTscan as discussed above.[63,67]

Imaging: Cardiac Sympathetic Imaging (CSI)

Reduced uptake of the radiotracer sympathetic analogue [^{123}I]metaiodobenzylguanidine (^{123}I-MIBG) as measured by heart/mediastinum ratio on cardiac scintigraphy reflects postganglionic cardiac autonomic (sympathetic) denervation, which is proposed as a marker for early detection of IPD and differentiates it from multiple systems atrophy, which has clinically greater autonomic symptoms but lacks postsynaptic autonomic degeneration.[53] Contraindications such as diabetes mellitus, ischemic heart disease, heart failure, thyroid dysfunction, and multiple medications can limit the routine use of this modality.[53]

There are several studies that investigated the use of CSI in patients with DIP. In one study, 93% of patients with DIP had normal MIBG uptake, normal olfaction (by Cross Cultural Smell Identification test), and resolution or significant improvement of parkinsonism with withdrawal of the offending drugs, whereas the only patient with abnormal uptake was found to have impaired olfaction and persistent parkinsonism after drug withdrawal. Interestingly enough, this patient responded well to levodopa, showing 63% improvement in Unified Parkison's Disease Rating Scale (UPDRS).[68] This data, again, suggest that patients with evidence of degenerative changes in the dopaminergic system and not just isolated and reversible dopamine receptor blockade, represent a subgroup with clinical features more similar to IPD.

Table 3.2 summarizes various imaging modalities and data relevant to their role in the diagnosis of DIP.

Prevention

Avoiding drugs that are known to cause parkinsonism when not indicated or when there's a reasonable alternative that hasn't been tried for the patient would be the first preventive strategy. This is especially true for patients with risk factors for DIP, such as older age. If these drugs are necessary, using the lowest effective dose for the shortest time possible can lower risk of DIP. Continuous monitoring of manifestations of DIP is required. This necessitates that primary care physicians and other practitioners who frequently prescribe antipsychotics, prokinetics, and other dopamine antagonists have the essential knowledge and skills to identify possible DIP and refer the patient to a neurologist if needed.

In the past, anticholinergics were used for prophylaxis, but their use at least before onset of disease remains controversial especially given their many side effects. We generally don't recommend routine prophylactic anticholinergic use.[69]

Management

Some authorities suggest treating patients with DIP only if the symptoms are severe enough to interfere with daily activities. This may be generally sound, however the possibility that long-term use of antidopaminergics may cause neurotoxicity and inflammatory response that lead to irreversible degenerative parkinsonism argues for more aggressive withdrawal. Also, DIP may be a risk, or at least a warning sign, for developing TD, which is mostly irreversible. The first management option for a patient with DIP would be to stop, or at least reduce, the offending drug if possible. This often requires detailed communication between physicians and of course depends on the absolute necessity of the drug. For example, we usually switch metoclopramide to domperidone, which has lesser risk for DIP in patients who still need a gastroenteric prokinetic. Changing typical antipsychotics to atypical antipsychotics follows the same concept, although only clozapine and quetiapine truly lack meaningful dopamine receptor affinity at typical doses. If these options aren't possible, adding pharmacologic therapy may be needed. Various anticholinergics (most commonly trihexyphenidyl and benztropine in the United States), and the N-methyl-D-aspartate antagonist amantadine (100 mg BID up to 200 mg TID) have been tried for DIP. Importantly, these medicines can help even if the offending dopamine antagonist is continued. Although early studies have found that amantadine may be more effective than anticholinergics, this may have been attributable to dosage differences.[38] A double-blind placebo-controlled cross-over study compared amantadine to the M1-selective anticholinergic biperiden and found both similarly significantly effective.[70] Amantadine typically has less memory-related and peripheral side effects than antimuscarinics and thus may be a safer option to try first.[71] On the other hand, amantadine may exacerbate psychosis, which is a common indication for antidopaminergics, possibly due to its dopaminergic reuptake inhibition properties or glutamate antagonist properties.[38] Amantadine also causes livedo reticularis in most people with chronic use. L-dopa and dopamine agonists do not offer as much benefit unless there is an underlying intrinsic dopamine deficit. In one study, only 2 out of 12 patients who were initially suspected to have primary parkinsonism and thus received levodopa while potentially still on the offending drug (the final diagnosis of those 12 patients was DIP) had some benefit of L-dopa.[4] Nevertheless, dopaminergics could be tried. In our experience they can be effective if the dopamine antagonist is stopped but not if the offending drug is continued.

There's some evidence that electroconvulsive therapy (ECT) may be effective as an antiparkinsonian modality in patients with DIP.[72] Possible mechanism of action includes potentiating dopamine transmission and increasing the sensitivity of dopamine receptors.[69] ECT can help indirectly as well by using it for treatment of psychosis, which may reduce the need for antipsychotics or at least allow for reduction of the dose.

Conclusion

DIP is still a common condition that requires monitoring for all patients on dopamine antagonists and VMAT-2 inhibitors. In most cases of dopamine receptor blockade induced DIP, the symptoms gradually improve over weeks to months. A subset of subjects never completely improves, but most of these likely had unmasked IPD. Risk factors for DIP include older age, possibly female sex, possibly genetic factors, and duration and potency of the offending agent. First line treatment involves removal or reduction of the drug when possible, and amantadine and/or anticholinergics.

References

1. Dunnett, S. B., Bentivoglio, M., Björklund, A., & Hökfelt, T. (2004). *Dopamine*. Elsevier.
2. Miller, L. G., & Jancovic, J. (1999). Drug-induced dyskinesias: an overview. In A. B. Joseph & R. R. Young (Eds.), *Movement Disorders in Neurology and Neuropsychiatry* (Second ed.). Blackwell Science, Inc.
3. Bower, J. H., Maraganore, D. M., McDonnell, S. K., & Rocca, W. A. (1999). Incidence and distribution of parkinsonism in Olmsted County, Minnesota, 1976–1990. *Neurology, 52*(6), 1214–1220. https://doi.org/10.1212/wnl.52.6.1214
4. Savica, R., Grossardt, B. R., Bower, J. H., Ahlskog, J. E., Mielke, M. M., & Rocca, W. A. (2017). Incidence and time trends of drug-induced parkinsonism: A 30-year population-based study. *Mov Disord, 32*(2), 227–234. https://doi.org/10.1002/mds.26839
5. Caligiuri, M. R., Jeste, D. V., & Lacro, J. P. (2000). Antipsychotic-induced movement disorders in the elderly: Epidemiology and treatment recommendations. *Drugs Aging, 17*(5), 363–384. https://doi.org/10.2165/00002512-200017050-00004
6. American Psychiatric Association. (2013). *Diagnostic and Statistical Manual of Mental Disorders (DSM-5*®*)*. American Psychiatric Pub.
7. Chung, S. J., Yoo, H. S., Moon, H., et al. (2018). Early-onset drug-induced parkinsonism after exposure to offenders implies nigrostriatal dopaminergic dysfunction. *J Neurol Neurosurg Psychiatry, 89*(2), 169–174. https://doi.org/10.1136/jnnp-2017-315873
8. Bondon-Guitton, E., Perez-Lloret, S., Bagheri, H., Brefel, C., Rascol, O., & Montastruc, J.-L. (2011). Drug-induced parkinsonism: A review of 17 years' experience in a regional pharmacovigilance center in France. *Mov Disord, 26*(12), 2226–2231. https://doi.org/10.1002/mds.23828
9. Munhoz, R. P., Bertucci Filho, D., & Teive, H. A. (2017). Not all drug-induced parkinsonisms are the same: The effect of drug class on motor phenotype. *Neurol Sci, 38*(2), 319–324. https://doi.org/10.1007/s10072-016-2771-y
10. Peabody, C. A., Warner, M. D., Whiteford, H. A., & Hollister, L. E. (1987). Neuroleptics and the elderly. *Journal of the American Geriatrics Society, 35*(3), 233–238. https://doi.org/10.1111/j.1532-5415.1987.tb02315.x
11. Rajput, A. H., Rozdilsky, B., Hornykiewicz, O., Shannak, K., Lee, T., & Seeman, P. (1982). Reversible drug-induced parkinsonism: Clinicopathologic study of two cases. *Arch Neurol, 39*(10), 644–646. https://doi.org/10.1001/archneur.1982.00510220042009
12. Foubert-Samier, A., Helmer, C., Perez, F., et al. (2012). Past exposure to neuroleptic drugs and risk of Parkinson disease in an elderly cohort. *Neurology, 79*(15), 1615–1621. https://doi.org/10.1212/WNL.0b013e31826e25ce
13. Bridi, J. C., & Hirth, F. (2018). Mechanisms of α-synuclein induced synaptopathy in Parkinson's disease. *Front Neurosci, 12*, 80. https://doi.org/10.3389/fnins.2018.00080
14. Mahlknecht, P., Iranzo, A., Högl, B., et al. (2015). Olfactory dysfunction predicts early transition to a Lewy body disease in idiopathic RBD. *Neurology, 84*(7), 654–658. https://doi.org/10.1212/wnl.0000000000001265

15. Lee, P. H., Kim, J. S., Shin, D. H., Yoon, S. N., & Huh, K. (2006). Cardiac 123I-MIBG scintigraphy in patients with drug induced parkinsonism. *J Neurol Neurosurg Psychiatry, 77*(3), 372–374. https://doi.org/10.1136/jnnp.2005.073999

16. Yomtoob, J., Koloms, K., & Bega, D. (2018). DAT-SPECT imaging in cases of drug-induced parkinsonism in a specialty movement disorders practice. *Parkinsonism Relat Disord, 53*, 37–41. https://doi.org/10.1016/j.parkreldis.2018.04.037

17. Erro, R., Bhatia, K. P., & Tinazzi, M. (2015). Parkinsonism following neuroleptic exposure: A double-hit hypothesis? *Mov Disord, 30*(6), 780–785. https://doi.org/10.1002/mds.26209

18. Lee, Y., Ho Choi, Y., Lee, J. J., et al. (2017). Microstructural white matter alterations in patients with drug induced parkinsonism. *Hum Brain Mapp, 38*(12), 6043–6052. https://doi.org/10.1002/hbm.23809

19. Prosser, E. S., Csernansky, J. G., Kaplan, J., Thiemann, S., Becker, T. J., & Hollister, L. E. (1987). Depression, parkinsonian symptoms, and negative symptoms in schizophrenics treated with neuroleptics. *J Nerv Ment Dis, 175*(2), 100–105. https://doi.org/10.1097/00005053-198702000-00006

20. de Germay, S., Montastruc, F., Carvajal, A., Lapeyre-Mestre, M., & Montastruc, J.-L. (2020). Drug-induced parkinsonism: Revisiting the epidemiology using the WHO pharmacovigilance database. *Parkinsonism Relat Disord, 70*, 55–59. https://doi.org/10.1016/j.parkreldis.2019.12.011

21. Benito-León, J., Bermejo-Pareja, F., Rodríguez, J., Molina, J. A., Gabriel, R., & Morales, J. M. (2003). Prevalence of PD and other types of parkinsonism in three elderly populations of central Spain. *Mov Disord, 18*(3), 267–274. https://doi.org/10.1002/mds.10362

22. Fleury, V., Brindel, P., Nicastro, N., & Burkhard, P. R. (2018). Descriptive epidemiology of parkinsonism in the canton of Geneva, Switzerland. *Parkinsonism Relat Disord, 54*, 30–39. https://doi.org/10.1016/j.parkreldis.2018.03.030

23. Munhoz, R. P., Werneck, L. C., & Teive, H. A. G. (2010). The differential diagnoses of parkinsonism: Findings from a cohort of 1528 patients and a 10 years comparison in tertiary movement disorders clinics. *Clinical Neurology and Neurosurgery, 112*(5), 431–435. https://doi.org/https://doi.org/10.1016/j.clineuro.2010.03.003

24. López-Sendón, J. L., Mena, M. A., & de Yébenes, J. G. (2012). Drug-induced parkinsonism in the elderly. *Drugs & Aging, 29*(2), 105–118. https://doi.org/10.2165/11598540-000000000-00000

25. Myrianthopoulos, N. C., Kurland, A. A., & Kurland, L. T. (1962). Hereditary predisposition in drug-induced parkinsonism. *Arch Neurol, 6*, 5–9. https://doi.org/10.1001/archneur.1962.00450190007002

26. Alkelai, A., Greenbaum, L., Rigbi, A., Kanyas, K., & Lerer, B. (2009). Genome-wide association study of antipsychotic-induced parkinsonism severity among schizophrenia patients. *Psychopharmacology (Berl), 206*(3), 491–499. https://doi.org/10.1007/s00213-009-1627-z

27. Metzer, W. S., Newton, J. E., Steele, R. W., et al. (1989). HLA antigens in drug-induced parkinsonism. *Mov Disord, 4*(2), 121–128. https://doi.org/10.1002/mds.870040203

28. Thal, D. R., Del Tredici, K., & Braak, H. (2004). Neurodegeneration in normal brain aging and disease. *Sci Aging Knowledge Environ, 2004*(23), pe26. https://doi.org/10.1126/sageke.2004.23.pe26

29. Lee, Y. H., Cha, J., Chung, S. J., et al. (2019). Beneficial effect of estrogen on nigrostriatal dopaminergic neurons in drug-naïve postmenopausal Parkinson's disease. *Scientific Reports, 9*(1), 10531. https://doi.org/10.1038/s41598-019-47026-6

30. Reyes, M. G., Faraldi, F., Senseng, C. S., Flowers, C., & Fariello, R. (1991). Nigral degeneration in acquired immune deficiency syndrome (AIDS). *Acta Neuropathologica, 82*(1), 39–44.
https://doi.org/10.1007/BF00310921

31. Sandyk, R. (1993). Cigarette smoking: Effects on cognitive functions and drug-induced
parkinsonism in chronic schizophrenia. *Int J Neurosci, 70*(3-4), 193–197. https://doi.org/
10.3109/00207459309000574

32. Li, X., Li, W., Liu, G., Shen, X., & Tang, Y. (2015). Association between cigarette smoking and
Parkinson's disease: A meta-analysis. *Arch Gerontol Geriatr, 61*(3), 510–516. https://doi.org/
10.1016/j.archger.2015.08.004

33. Seeman, P. (2010). Historical overview: Introduction to the dopamine receptors. In: Kim A.
Neve (Ed.). *The Dopamine Receptors* (pp. 1–21). Springer.

34. Shin, H. W., & Chung, S. J. (2012). Drug-induced parkinsonism. *J Clin Neurol, 8*(1), 15–21.
https://doi.org/10.3988/jcn.2012.8.1.15

35. Farde, L., Nordström, A. L., Wiesel, F. A., Pauli, S., Halldin, C., & Sedvall, G. (1992). Positron
emission tomographic analysis of central D1 and D2 dopamine receptor occupancy in patients
treated with classical neuroleptics and clozapine: Relation to extrapyramidal side effects. *Arch
Gen Psychiatry, 49*(7), 538–544. https://doi.org/10.1001/archpsyc.1992.01820070032005

36. Maguire, G. A., LaSalle, L., Hoffmeyer, D., et al. (2019). Ecopipam as a pharmacologic treatment of stuttering. *Ann Clin Psychiatry, 31*(3), 164–168.

37. Morley, J. F., Pawlowski, S. M., Kesari, A., Maina, I., Pantelyat, A., & Duda, J. E. (2014).
Motor and non-motor features of Parkinson's disease that predict persistent drug-induced
Parkinsonism. *Parkinsonism Relat Disord, 20*(7), 738–742. https://doi.org/10.1016/j.parkrel
dis.2014.03.024

38. Osser, D. N. (1998). Neuroleptic-induced pseudoparkinsonism. In A. B. Joseph & R. R.
Young (Eds.), *Movement Disorders in Neurology and Neuropsychiatry*. Blackwell Science
Publications.

39. Casey, D. E. (1998). Rabbit syndrome. In A. B. Joseph & R. R. Young (Eds.), *Movement
Disorders in Neurology and Neuropsychiatry*. Blackwell Science Publications.

40. Naguy, A., Moodliar-Rensburg, S., Elsori, D. H., & Alamiri, B. (2022). Fluoxetine-induced
"rabbit syndrome" in a child with juvenile obsessive-compulsive disorder. *Am J Ther, 29*(3),
e363–e364. https://doi.org/10.1097/mjt.0000000000001195

41. Gardos, G., & Cole, J. O. (1998). Drug-induced parkinsonism and concomitant tardive
dyskinesia. In A. B. Joseph & R. R. Young (Eds.), *Movement Disorders in Neurology and
Neuropsychiatry*. Blackwell Science Publications.

42. Kane, J. M., Woerner, M., Weinhold, P., Wegner, J., & Kinon, B. (1982). A prospective study of
tardive dyskinesia development: Preliminary results. *J Clin Psychopharmacol, 2*(5), 345–349.

43. Crane, G. E. (1972). Pseudoparkinsonism and tardive dyskinesia. *Arch Neurol, 27*(5), 426–
430. https://doi.org/10.1001/archneur.1972.00490170058008

44. Jankovic, J., & Beach, J. (1997). Long-term effects of tetrabenazine in hyperkinetic movement
disorders. *Neurology, 48*(2), 358–362. https://doi.org/10.1212/wnl.48.2.358

45. Bovi, T., Antonini, A., Ottaviani, S., et al. (2010). The status of olfactory function and the
striatal dopaminergic system in drug-induced parkinsonism. *J Neurol, 257*(11), 1882–1889.
https://doi.org/10.1007/s00415-010-5631-3

46. Kim, J. H., & Byun, H. J. (2009). Non-motor cognitive-perceptual dysfunction associated
with drug-induced parkinsonism. *Hum Psychopharmacol, 24*(2), 129–133. https://doi.org/
10.1002/hup.1009

47. Kim, Y. D., Kim, J. S., Chung, S. W., et al. (2011). Cognitive dysfunction in drug induced parkinsonism (DIP). *Arch Gerontol Geriatr*, *53*(2), e222–226. https://doi.org/10.1016/j.arch ger.2010.11.025

48. Lee, S. H., Kim, H. K., Lee, Y. G., Lyoo, C. H., Ahn, S. J., & Lee, M. S. (2017). Clinical features indicating nigrostriatal dopaminergic degeneration in drug-induced parkinsonism. *J Mov Disord*, *10*(1), 35–39. https://doi.org/10.14802/jmd.16045

49. Mena, M. A., & de Yébenes, J. G. (2006). Drug-induced parkinsonism. *Expert Opin Drug Saf*, *5*(6), 759–771. https://doi.org/10.1517/14740338.5.6.759

50. Morley, J. F., & Duda, J. E. (2014). Use of hyposmia and other non-motor symptoms to distinguish between drug-induced parkinsonism and Parkinson's disease. *J Parkinson's Disease*, *4*, 169–173. https://doi.org/10.3233/JPD-130299

51. Stacy, M., & Jankovic, J. (1992). Tardive tremor. *Mov Disord*, *7*(1), 53–57. https://doi.org/10.1002/mds.870070110

52. Höllerhage, M. (2019). Chapter fifteen—Secondary parkinsonism due to drugs, vascular lesions, tumors, trauma, and other insults. In M. Stamelou & G. U. Höglinger (Eds.), *International Review of Neurobiology* (Vol. 149, pp. 377–418). Academic Press.

53. Cousins, O., Yousaf, T., Wilson, H., Pagano, G., & Politis, M. (2019). Chapter three—Molecular imaging of dementia with Lewy bodies. In M. Politis (Ed.), *International Review of Neurobiology* (Vol. 144, pp. 59–93). Academic Press.

54. Rossi, C., Volterrani, D., Nicoletti, V., et al. (2009). Parkinson-dementia diseases: A comparison by double tracer SPECT studies. *Parkinsonism Relat Disord*, *15*(10), 762–766. https://doi.org/10.1016/j.parkreldis.2009.05.012

55. Brigo, F., Erro, R., Marangi, A., Bhatia, K., & Tinazzi, M. (2014). Differentiating drug-induced parkinsonism from Parkinson's disease: An update on non-motor symptoms and investigations. *Parkinsonism Relat Disord*, *20*(8), 808–814. https://doi.org/10.1016/j.parkrel dis.2014.05.011

56. Lorberboym, M., Treves, T. A., Melamed, E., Lampl, Y., Hellmann, M., & Djaldetti, R. (2006). [123I]-FP/CIT SPECT imaging for distinguishing drug-induced parkinsonism from Parkinson's disease. *Mov Disord*, *21*(4), 510–514.

57. Romero, J. O., & Padillo, A. A. (2013). Diagnostic accuracy of 123I-FP-CIT SPECT in diagnosing drug-induced parkinsonism: A prospective study. *Neurología (English Edition)*, *28*(5), 276–282.

58. Tinazzi, M., Antonini, A., Bovi, T., et al. (2009). Clinical and [123 I] FP-CIT SPET imaging follow-up in patients with drug-induced parkinsonism. *J Neurol*, *256*(6), 910–915.

59. Tinazzi, M., Cipriani, A., Matinella, A., et al. (2012). [123I] FP-CIT single photon emission computed tomography findings in drug-induced Parkinsonism. *Schizophr Res*, *139*(1–3), 40–45.

60. Tinazzi, M., Morgante, F., Matinella, A., et al. (2014). Imaging of the dopamine transporter predicts pattern of disease progression and response to levodopa in patients with schizophrenia and parkinsonism: A 2-year follow-up multicenter study. *Schizophr Res*, *152*(2–3), 344–349.

61. Tinazzi, M., Ottaviani, S., Isaias, I. U., et al. (2008). [123I] FP-CIT SPET imaging in drug-induced parkinsonism. *Mov Disord*, *23*(13), 1825–1829.

62. Burn, D. J., & Brooks, D. J. (1993). Nigral dysfunction in drug-induced parkinsonism: An 18F-dopa PET study. *Neurology*, *43*(3 Pt 1), 552–556. https://doi.org/10.1212/wnl.43.3_par t_1.552

63. Oh, Y. S., Kwon, D. Y., Kim, J. S., Park, M. H., & Berg, D. (2018). Transcranial sonographic findings may predict prognosis of gastroprokinetic drug-induced parkinsonism. *Parkinsonism Relat Disord, 46*, 36–40. https://doi.org/10.1016/j.parkreldis.2017.10.011

64. Poewe, W., & Seppi, K. (2013). Diagnosis of drug-induced parkinsonism: Can transcranial sonography make the difference? *Eur J Neurol, 20*(11), 1429–1430. https://doi.org/10.1111/ene.12189

65. Joseph, A. B., & Young, R. R. (1992). *Movement Disorders in Neurology and Neuropsychiatry.* Blackwell Scientific Publications.

66. Olivares Romero, J., Arjona Padillo, A., Barrero Hernández, F. J., Martín González, M., & Gil Extremera, B. (2013). Utility of transcranial sonography in the diagnosis of drug-induced parkinsonism: A prospective study. *Eur J Neurol, 20*(11), 1451–1458. https://doi.org/10.1111/ene.12131

67. Berg, D., Jabs, B., Merschdorf, U., Beckmann, H., & Becker, G. (2001). Echogenicity of substantia nigra determined by transcranial ultrasound correlates with severity of parkinsonian symptoms induced by neuroleptic therapy. *Biological Psychiatry, 50*(6), 463–467. https://doi.org/https://doi.org/10.1016/S0006-3223(01)01190-8

68. Lee, P. H., Yeo, S. H., Yong, S. W., & Kim, Y. J. (2007). Odour identification test and its relation to cardiac 123I-metaiodobenzylguanidine in patients with drug induced parkinsonism. *J Neurol Neurosurg Psychiatry, 78*(11), 1250–1252. https://doi.org/10.1136/jnnp.2007.121285

69. Estevez-Fraga, C., Zeun, P., & López-Sendón Moreno, J. L. (2018). Current methods for the treatment and prevention of drug-induced parkinsonism and tardive dyskinesia in the elderly. *Drugs & Aging, 35*(11), 959–971. https://doi.org/10.1007/s40266-018-0590-y

70. Silver, H., Geraisy, N., & Schwartz, M. (1995). No difference in the effect of biperiden and amantadine on parkinsonian- and tardive dyskinesia-type involuntary movements: A double-blind crossover, placebo-controlled study in medicated chronic schizophrenic patients. *J Clin Psychiatry, 56*(4), 167–170.

71. McEvoy, J. P. (1987). A double-blind crossover comparison of antiparkinson drug therapy: Amantadine versus anticholinergics in 90 normal volunteers, with an emphasis on differential effects on memory function. *J Clin Psychiatry, 48*(9, Suppl), 20–23.

72. Goswami, U., Dutta, S., Kuruvilla, K., Papp, E., & Perenyi, A. (1989). Electroconvulsive therapy in neuroleptic-induced parkinsonism. *Biol Psychiatry, 26*(3), 234–238. https://doi.org/10.1016/0006-3223(89)90035-8

73. McIntyre, R. S. (2010). Pharmacology and efficacy of asenapine for manic and mixed states in adults with bipolar disorder. *Expert Rev Neurother, 10*(5), 645–649. https://doi.org/10.1586/ern.10.49

74. Wishart, D. S., Knox, C., Guo, A. C., et al. (2006). DrugBank: A comprehensive resource for in silico drug discovery and exploration. *Nucleic Acids Res, 34*(Database issue), D668–672. https://doi.org/10.1093/nar/gkj067

75. Brücke, T., Wöber, C., Podreka, I., et al. (1995). D2 receptor blockade by flunarizine and cinnarizine explains extrapyramidal side effects. A SPECT study. *J Cereb Blood Flow Metab, 15*(3), 513–518. https://doi.org/10.1038/jcbfm.1995.63

76. Qiang, L., Sasikumar, T. K., Burnett, D. A., et al. (2010). Discovery of new SCH 39166 analogs as potent and selective dopamine D1 receptor antagonists. *Bioorganic & Medicinal Chemistry Letters, 20*(3), 836–840. https://doi.org/https://doi.org/10.1016/j.bmcl.2009.12.100

77. Shin, H. W., Kim, J. S., Oh, M., et al. (2015). Clinical features of drug-induced parkinsonism based on [18F] FP-CIT positron emission tomography. *Neurol Sci, 36*(2), 269–274. https://doi.org/10.1007/s10072-014-1945-8

78. Davis, R. E., & Correll, C. U. (2016). ITI-007 in the treatment of schizophrenia: From novel pharmacology to clinical outcomes. *Expert Rev Neurother, 16*(6), 601–614. https://doi.org/10.1080/14737175.2016.1174577

79. Kitten, A. K., Hallowell, S. A., Saklad, S. R., & Evoy, K. E. (2018). Pimavanserin: A novel drug approved to treat Parkinson's disease psychosis. *Innov Clin Neurosci, 15*(1–2), 16–22.

80. Ison, P. J., & Peroutka, S. J. (1986). Neurotransmitter receptor binding studies predict antiemetic efficacy and side effects. *Cancer Treat Rep, 70*(5), 637–641.

81. Grigoriadis, D. E., Smith, E., Hoare, S. R. J., Madan, A., & Bozigian, H. (2017). Pharmacologic characterization of valbenazine (NBI-98854) and its metabolites. *J Pharmacol Exp Ther, 361*(3), 454–461. https://doi.org/10.1124/jpet.116.239160

82. Hajjo, R., Setola, V., Roth, B. L., & Tropsha, A. (2012). Chemocentric informatics approach to drug discovery: Identification and experimental validation of selective estrogen receptor modulators as ligands of 5-hydroxytryptamine-6 receptors and as potential cognition enhancers. *J Med Chem, 55*(12), 5704–5719. https://doi.org/10.1021/jm2011657

83. Roth, B. L., Lopez, E., Patel, S., & Kroeze, W. K. (2000). The multiplicity of serotonin receptors: Uselessly diverse molecules or an embarrassment of riches? *The Neuroscientist, 6*(4), 252–262. https://doi.org/10.1177/107385840000600408

84. Diaz-Corrales, F. J., Sanz-Viedma, S., Garcia-Solis, D., Escobar-Delgado, T., & Mir, P. (2010). Clinical features and 123I-FP-CIT SPECT imaging in drug-induced parkinsonism and Parkinson's disease. *European Journal of Nuclear Medicine and Molecular Imaging, 37*(3), 556–564. https://doi.org/10.1007/s00259-009-1289-4

85. Kim, J.-S., Oh, Y.-S., Kim, Y.-I., et al. (2013). Combined use of 123I-metaiodobenzylguanidine (MIBG) scintigraphy and dopamine transporter (DAT) positron emission tomography (PET) predicts prognosis in drug-induced Parkinsonism (DIP): A 2-year follow-up study. *Arch Gerontol Geriatr, 56*(1), 124–128. https://doi.org/https://doi.org/10.1016/j.archger.2012.05.001

4

Akathisia

Satyajit Mohite, Ossama T. Osman, Lokesh Shahani, and Antonio L. Teixeira

Introduction

The *Diagnostic and Statistical Manual of Mental Disorders* (DSM-5), describes akathisia as a subjective complaint of restlessness often with objective increase in movements, and in association with antipsychotic drugs.[1] These observed excessive movements include pacing, rocking, an inability to sit or stand still, and fidgety movements of the legs, and can be noticed within days or weeks of either starting or stopping antipsychotic treatment or changing dosage.

The history of akathisia can be broadly divided into two moments: the pre- and postantipsychotic eras. The earliest records of akathisia date back to the 17th century when the British physician Thomas Willis described akathisia-like symptoms: "diseased are no more able to sleep, than if they were in a place of the greatest torture,"[2] although this probably referred to restless legs syndrome. Also referred to as *anxietas tibiarum*[3] and within the *neurasthenia* umbrella,[4] the term "akathisia" was coined in 1901 by Lad Haskovec, and means "not to sit."[5] Akathisia was distinguished from the restlessness related to mood or psychotic disorders, and was seen as "psychogenic" in origin. Over the years, it was further described as *professional abulia, kathisophobia*,[6] *tasikinesia*,[7] *hyperkinesis*,[8] *leg jitters*,[9] *irritable legs*, or *asthenia crurum paraesthetica*.[10]

Drug-induced akathisia was first reported in 1947 with promethazine use.[11] Even during the antipsychotic era, the inconsistencies in the use of term "akathisia" continued, the condition being referred to as *turbulent reactions* with reserpine[12] and *paradoxical reactions* with reserpine-chlorpromazine.[13] Akathisia was finally recognized as an acute antipsychotic-drug-related phenomenon in the late 1950s.[5,14–16]

In this chapter, we will revisit akathisia, a frequently overlooked problem in clinical practice, discussing its pathophysiology, diagnosis, and management.

Clinical Epidemiology and Pathophysiology

The prevalence of akathisia in psychiatric populations has varied widely over the years from 6.3% to 24%.[17–23] The range of prevalence varied according to study design, group of patients studied, and type of antipsychotic drugs. In specific populations, first-episode nonaffective psychosis patients had akathisia prevalence of around 20%,[24] cancer patients had 4%,[25] patients with delirium up to 30%,[26] and adolescent patients up to 10%.[27] Conflicting data have been reported on sex susceptibility, with studies reporting either no difference between men and women, or higher incidence of akathisia in middle aged women.[28]

In comparison to placebo, the odds ratio (OR) of akathisia development with antipsychotics was reported to be 2.43 (95% CI: 1.91–3.10).[22] Akathisia has been mainly associated with first-generation antipsychotics (FGAs).[29] Systematic reviews evaluating akathisia emergence during the use of FGAs and second-generation antipsychotics (SGAs) showed that the lowest rates were seen with paliperidone (3.3%) and iloperidone (3.9%),[22] and highest rates with haloperidol (24.8%).[30] A high risk of akathisia is also seen after the rapid escalation in antipsychotics dosing.[31] Moreover, antipsychotic polypharmacy also had twice the risk of monotherapy.[18] Although SGAs have improved akathisia-related safety and tolerability profiles[32] compared to FGAs,[33,34] the risk of akathisia is still high with the latter,[22,23,35] and SGA polypharmacy has three times the risk of SGA monotherapy.[18]

Akathisia has not been limited to antipsychotic use. Other dopamine antagonists most commonly used to treat nausea, gastric dysmotility, and migraine (prochlorperazine and metoclopramide) cause akathisia.[36] Other psychiatric drugs have also been associated with akathisia, including selective serotonin receptor inhibitors (SSRIs),[37] agomelatine with duloxetine,[38] monoamine oxidase inhibitors (MAOIs),[39] and tricyclic antidepressants.[40] Actually, some authors propose that the phenotype of this SSRI-related "akathisia" is subtly different and more consistent with an overall jitteryness/hyperactivity rather than a pure urge to move. This jitteriness can be interpreted as one feature of the so-called serotonin syndrome. Psychostimulant medications (e.g., amphetamines, methylphenidate) can also cause a jittery hyperactive variation of akathisia.[41,42] Miscellaneous medications associated with akathisia include iazithromycin[43] and amlodipine.[44] Smoking nicotine and cannabis, and alcohol use were hypothesized as protective factors for akathisia, but the evidence is weak.[42,45,46]

Despite the well-established clinical and epidemiological link between antipsychotics and akathisia, the pathophysiology underlying akathisia is still unclear. Based on the mechanisms of action of antipsychotics, dopaminergic pathways, especially related to D2 receptors, were initially considered critical for akathisia.[47,48] The purposeless movement characteristic of akathisia is believed to be the result of the loss of tonic dopaminergic inhibition on the locomotor system. The imbalance of mesocorticolimbic pathways, i.e., projections from the ventral tegmental area (VTA) to prefrontal cortex and ventral striatum, also seems to play a role in the development of akathisia.[49–51] Due to intricate relationships among different neurotransmitter pathways, including dopaminergic, serotonergic, noradrenergic, and cholinergic, different strategies exert beneficial effects on akathisia, implicating multiple pathways in its pathophysiology.[52] Genome-wide association studies (GWAS) reported genetic links and susceptibility for akathisia (e.g., genes regulating motor development: Zic4, Nkx6-1, glutamate receptors: GRIN1, GRIN2a, dopamine receptor: DRD1a), but such genetic information is not further explored in large studies or being currently translated into clinical practice.[53,54]

Types of Akathisia

Medication-induced akathisia has been loosely classified under different categories, but the most consistent one is based on the timing of onset of clinical symptoms (Figure 4.1). Accordingly, akathisia can be divided into four types: acute, chronic, withdrawal emergent, and tardive, although the distinction between acute and chronic is temporally arbitrary.[55]

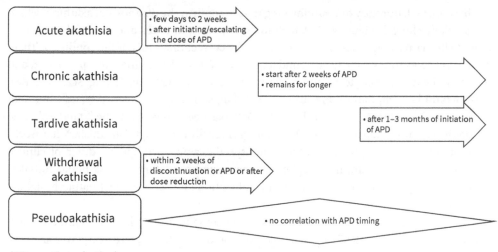

APD = antipsychotic drugs

Figure 4.1 Types of akathisia and their characteristics.

Acute akathisia develops within a few days to 2 weeks of initiating or escalating the dose of a dopamine antagonist (e.g., antipsychotic drug or antinausea medication). If symptoms occur after this 2-week timeframe, some authors consider it a chronic type.[56] Tardive akathisia occurs 1–3 months to years after initiation of an antipsychotic, and such symptoms can be observed long after its discontinuation.[1,35] If symptoms occur within 2 weeks of antipsychotic discontinuation or after dose reduction, they are classified as withdrawal-emergent akathisia. If such withdrawal-emergent akathisia persists for more than 6 weeks, it is recategorized as tardive akathisia.[56] The key distinction is whether symptoms improve with offending drug reduction (acute and chronic) or don't (withdrawal emergent and tardive). The term "pseudoakathisia" has been used in cases with objective motor signs of akathisia without any subjective complaints, commonly seen as a tardive dyskinesia syndrome.[55–57]

Clinical Presentation and Assessment of Akathisia

In the past, akathisia was related to vague somatic restlessness associated with anxiety, and "dramatic exacerbation of psychosis" without an emphasis on motor symptoms.[58] Later, akathisia was conceptualized as the combination of subjective and objective symptoms rather than focusing on only one aspect.[59] Currently, DSM-5 categorizes akathisia as the subjective feeling of restlessness or uneasiness (subjective component) along with increased movements (objective component).[1] Subjective symptoms include sense of inability to sit, stand, or lay still, an irresistible urge to move around, growing sense of tension, compulsive desire to move for relief of the sensation, and overall difficulty in expressing the unease.[60] The observed motor or objective component involves a person making frequent or continuous movements for the relief of subjective feelings. Akathisia primarily involves lower extremities and incorporates distinct repetitive movements or constant shifting, for instance, shifting from one foot to another, leg swinging or crossing, and bouncing.[61,62]

There are no laboratory or neuroimaging tests to confirm the diagnosis of akathisia, which is essentially clinical (Figure 4.2). A high index of suspicion index and a careful consideration of alternative diagnoses are warranted for the correct diagnosis of the condition. There are several tools to assess "extrapyramidal symptoms" (or EPS) in the clinical practice, and many of them incorporate akathisia symptoms: Barnes Akathisia-Rating Scale (BARS), Extrapyramidal Symptom Rating Scale (ESRS), Simpson Angus Scale (SAS), and Abnormal Involuntary Movement Scale (AIMS).[63-65] BARS has been considered the "standard" scale for akathisia, with a global score of ≥2 indicating clinically meaningful akathisia.[60] It is worth mentioning that the expression "EPS" is nonspecific, as it encompasses different clinical syndromes (parkinsonism, neuroleptic malignant syndrome, tardive dyskinesia, and akathisia) that may be seen in isolation or in combination and have distinct pathophysiology and treatments.

The clinical presentation of akathisia resembles some neuropsychiatric conditions, such as restless leg syndrome (RLS), tics, anxiety, psychomotor agitation, tardive dyskinesia (TD),

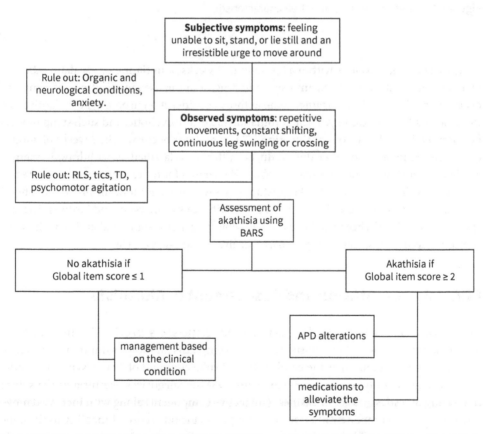

RLS- restless leg syndrome, TD- tardive dyskinesia, BARS- Barnes Akathisia Rating Scale, APD -antipsychotic drugs

Figure 4.2 Clinical diagnosis of akathisia.

Source: Adapted from Salem, H., Nagpal, C., Pigott, T., & Lucio Teixeira, A. (2017). Revisiting antipsychotic-induced akathisia: current issues and prospective challenges. *Current* neuropharmacology, *15*(5), 789–798; and Barnes, T. R. (2003). The Barnes Akathisia rating scale–revisited. *Journal of Psychopharmacology, 17*(4), 365–370.

and also neurologic diseases like neurological stereotypies (commonly autism spectrum disorders and frontotemporal dementia) and Huntington's disease (HD) (Table 4.1).

In akathisia, lower limbs and torso are much more affected than upper limbs and cranial segment, with the persistent feeling of uneasiness and frequent moving or rocking of lower limbs.[66] Such characteristics mimic RLS and anxiety, but distinguish akathisia from TD, tics, and severe psychomotor agitation. Absence of dysesthesia and less association with sleep or night-time worsening of symptoms discriminate akathisia from RLS. Furthermore, akathisia symptoms do not fluctuate in severity with supine position (like RLS) or with external stressors (like tics). Unlike tics and TD, akathisia is not commonly seen in facial or perioral regions, nor does it present with gait impairment like Parkinson's disease (PD) or HD.

Therapeutic Management and Alternatives

Therapeutic management of akathisia mainly consists of three steps: prevention, antipsychotic drug adjustment, and symptomatic management.

Prevention

Before starting any antipsychotics, critical discussion about the pros and cons, weighting the potential risks and benefits of using these drugs is definitely warranted. Antipsychotic side effects, including motor and metabolic ones, are often overlooked, and there has also been a trend to increase the clinical indications of this class of drugs much beyond psychotic disorders.

Close monitoring for early signs of akathisia is the safest preventive approach.[67] While deciding between FGAs and SGAs, careful consideration should be given to the side effect profile of each drug. The risk of akathisia is higher with FGAs (8%–76%) when compared to newer SGAs (3%–17%),[22] therefore, SGAs should be prioritized if possible. Additionally, rapid escalation in antipsychotic dosing and polypharmacy should be avoided. In medical settings, drug combinations should be considered to prevent akathisia (Figure 4.3). For instance, with the use of akathisia-inducing-drugs like metoclopramide, short-term use of an adjuvant such as diphenhydramine was reported to reduce the incidence of akathisia.[68,69]

Antipsychotic Drug Adjustment

In the case of development of akathisia, antipsychotics regarded as the primary causative agents need to be either stopped, reduced, or switched. Monotherapy is preferred to polypharmacy, using the antipsychotic with the lowest akathisia potential. If the antipsychotics are to be rapidly and completely discontinued, careful monitoring for withdrawal emergent akathisia is required for the next two weeks.[56,70] Antipsychotics can be safely tapered down and discontinued in a few days or switched to another drug with lower akathisia risk.[31] Slow versus fast initiation of antipsychotics does not seem to influence the development of akathisia.[71] If the patient is on a high-potency FGA at the time of akathisia emergence, they could be switched to a low-potency FGA, or preferably to an SGA.[56] The CATIE trial (Clinical

Table 4.1 Differential Diagnosis of Akathisia

Condition	Akathisia	RLS	Tics	Anxiety	Psychomotor agitation	Tardive dyskinesia	Neurologic disorders
Prevalence, sex predominance	6.3%–39%, Same in males and females	3%–9%, slightly more common in females, peak in middle age	3%–8%, common in males	17.7%, common in females	19.5%–57%	10%–20% on APD for > 1 year, slightly more common in females, higher in African Americans	Huntington's disease (HD): 10.6–13.7 per 100,000
Associations/ risk factors	Old age, female sex, negative symptoms, cognitive dysfunction, prior akathisia, concomitant parkinsonism, mood disorders	SSRI, Iron deficiency	ADHD	Panic attacks, phobias, OCD, higher socioeconomic status	Mania, schizophrenia, depression, dementia	Antipsychotics, old age, mood disorders, history of acute EPS, dementia	HD, depression, psychosis, anxiety, OCD
Characteristics	- Usually lack of paresthesia, sleep disturbance, and myoclonus - Seen at any time of the day - Lying down decreases the symptoms	- Motor restlessness - Paresthesia seen mostly at night, disappears in the morning - Sleep disturbance - Lying down aggravates the symptoms - Myoclonus in severe cases	- Involuntary, sudden, repetitive, nonrhythmic, partially controllable - Aggravates with stress - Seen in any body parts, mainly eyelids, facial muscles, vocal	- Clumsiness, coordination problems - Lip smacking, picking, along with heart racing, chest discomfort, light-headed/dizziness, sweating, blushing, visual disturbance	- Unintentional, purposeless movements, pacing, wringing the hands, uncontrolled tongue movement, pulling off clothing and putting it back on - Whole body involvement with extreme arousal and tense feeling	- Abnormal, involuntary, irregular, choreoathetoid movements of head, limbs, trunk. - Most common: perioral - Remission rate 5%–40%	- HD- involuntary eye movements, speech, alternating hand movements, dystonia, chorea and gait
Management	Anticholinergic drugs and beta-blockers	Dopamine agonists Other- benzodiazepine, levodopa, propranolol	Antipsychotics, tetrabenazine	Anxiolytics, therapy	Antipsychotics with low akathisia risk or mood stabilizers, based on the clinical condition	Antipsychotics dose reduction or switch to newer SGA	HD- tetrabenazine, sulpiride, APDs

ADHD—Attention deficit hyperactivity disorder, OCD—obsessive compulsive-disorder, RLS—restless leg syndrome, APD—antipsychotic drugs, SSRI—selective serotonin receptor inhibitors, MAO-Bi— monoamine oxidase type B inhibitors, COMTi—catechol-O-methyltransferase inhibitors, NMDAi—NMDA receptor antagonist

Adapted from [28,55,56,67,84–91].

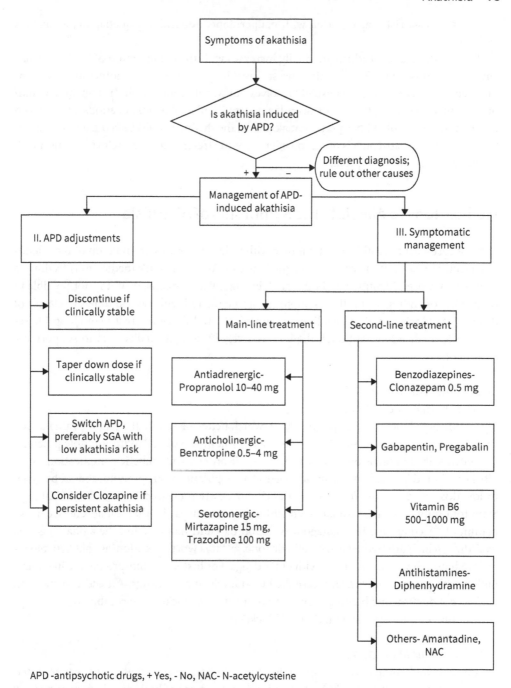

APD -antipsychotic drugs, + Yes, - No, NAC- N-acetylcysteine

Figure 4.3 Management of akathisia.

Antipsychotic Trials of Intervention Effectiveness) indicated that switching from an FGA (perphenazine) to an SGA (risperidone) still carries an elevated risk for akathisia.[72] All the SGAs were considered safer for akathisia historically, but recent evidence suggests otherwise.[30] This is not surprising, as SGAs have markedly different dopamine receptor affinities.

Lowest akathisia risk was reported with paliperidone, iloperidone, quetiapine, asenapine, and clozapine.

Because the risk of akathisia markedly increases with the combination of SGAs and also with higher doses of SGAs,[18,35] the lowest possible dose of SGA monotherapy is recommended. Nontardive akathisia usually resolves quickly after antipsychotic adjustment and/or introduction of symptomatic drugs.[22] If a patient is on a stable dose of antipsychotics with good clinical control but has persistent akathisia, the dosing should be reduced, or alternatives considered. Clozapine is often considered for the treatment of refractory akathisia with persistent psychiatric symptoms.[56]

Medications to Alleviate the Symptoms of Akathisia

In most cases, acute akathisia will improve with reduction or discontinuation of the offending agent. However, if the causative factor (antipsychotics, or other medication) leading to akathisia has been identified and mitigated, but akathisia remains, or if it is not possible to reduce the offending agent, then symptoms can be treated with several different classes of drugs. Beta blockers and anticholinergics are considered first-line treatment alongside serotonergic medications, although there is relatively little high-quality data to support any treatment.

First-Line Treatment
Antiadrenergic Medications
Lipophilic beta blockers (e.g., propranolol), which better penetrate the blood-brain barrier, were considered the gold standard to treat akathisia in the past.[73] With multiple potential side effects like hypotension, bradycardia, sleep disorders, and diabetic complications, beta blockers should be used with caution in geriatric populations. Propranolol should be given in low doses (e.g., 10 mg three times a day) and slowly increased if needed (40–120 mg). Symptom improvement is usually seen within hours to days.[72] Other antiadrenergic drugs commonly used are the beta antagonists metoprolol and nadolol, and the alpha-2 agonist clonidine, which also reduced sympathetic tone.[31,74] It is worth mentioning that beta blockers can have relevant interactions with other drugs. For instance, chlorpromazine in combination with propranolol may increase the blood levels of both drugs. An additive effect on cardiac conduction and blood pressure can occur if beta blockers are combined with drugs with similar effects (e.g., calcium channel blockers).

Anticholinergic Medications
Less established compared to propranolol, the anticholinergic benztropine was reported to be effective against akathisia.[31] Oral and intravenous use of high dose benztropine (4–8 mg) showed neutralizing effect on akathisia, but caused cognitive side effects.[75] Biperiden is another anticholinergic effective against akathisia.[76] Anticholinergic medications are especially effective if akathisia is concomitant with drug-induced parkinsonism, which may also improve. These should be started in low doses (for instance, benztropine 0.5 mg) and slowly titrated upward to avoid peripheral (e.g., constipation, dry mouth) and central (memory impairment, delirium) anticholinergic side effects, especially in geriatric patients.

Serotonin (5HT2a)–Modulating Medications

Medications blocking 5HT2a serotonin receptors and indirectly activating dopaminergic pathways were reported to reduce akathisia symptoms.[77] Improvement in akathisia has been reported with mirtazapine (15 mg for 5–7 days), mianserin (15 mg for 5 days), trazodone (100 mg for 3 days), and cyproheptadine (16 mg for 4 days), with mirtazapine and cyproheptadine showing antiakathisia effects similar to propranolol.[31,56] Mirtazapine may also improve akathisia via its potent histamine-1 antagonist and alpha-2 antagonist properties. A Cochrane Review systematically assessing the effects of mirtazapine as adjunct treatment for people with schizophrenia showed positive effects on mental status and akathisia.[78] In the case of beta blocker contraindication, mirtazapine (15 mg) should be considered while monitoring its main side effect, i.e., drowsiness. Mirtazapine can also worsen restless leg syndrome, which can be misdiagnosed as akathisia, presumably through its antihistamine properties. Zolmitriptan (5HT1d agonist), another serotonin receptor modulating medication, showed propranolol-equivalent action against akathisia.[79]

Second-Line Treatment

Second line treatments include benzodiazepines, vitamin B6, GABA enhancers, and some other medications with limited efficacy data or more problematic side effects. These agents may improve akathisia, but have not shown more efficacy than first-line treatments. Two trials each on clonazepam (0.5–2.5 mg for 7–14 days) and vitamin B6 (pyridoxine) (600–1200 mg for 5 days) showed significant improvement of akathisia symptoms.[31]

Benzodiazepines are known for abuse potential, drowsiness, and cognitive impairments, while vitamin B6 is known to cause peripheral neuropathy with high doses (>1000 mg).[80] Based on the limited data and side effect profile, it is recommended to use clonazepam in a low dose (0.5 mg) and vitamin B6 in a dose below 1000 mg if needed.

The two known alpha-2-delta subunit L-type calcium channel receptor antagonists (gabapentin and pregabalin) may help akathisia.[81] Anecdotal reports and two clinical trials showed their potential to minimize akathisia symptoms without problematic side effects, but more data are needed to support their use.[31,82,83]

Other medications with debatable utility for akathisia include dopamine agonists (ropinirole and apomorphine), the N-methyl-D-aspartate (NMDA) antagonist amantadine, diphenhydramine, and N-acetylcysteine (NAC).[31,56]

Conclusion

Even though akathisia has gained some traction in the field of neuropsychiatry in recent years, it is still an overlooked problem. It is associated with negative clinical outcomes, including treatment nonadherence. The clinical presentation of akathisia can closely mimic some other conditions, especially psychomotor agitation. At times, it may be difficult for a patient to explain their subjective feelings related to akathisia, and the diagnosis can be missed. The symptoms can also be misdiagnosed as anxiety and restless leg syndrome. Therefore, detailed clinical history and examination are needed to clearly establish the diagnosis and plan the management accordingly. Risks and benefits of antipsychotics should always be weighed-in to avoid akathisia in the first place. Even though SGAs were considered to have reduced risk for akathisia, recent data suggest that using SGAs with high risk of akathisia (like risperidone) would be as harmful as using any FGA. Hence, the choice of SGA should be made wisely while starting antipsychotic treatment. Combinations, rapid upward or downward titrations, and sudden discontinuation of antipsychotics should be avoided. Beta blockers, anticholinergics, serotonergic medications, and benzodiazepines can effectively control the symptoms of akathisia. In sum, akathisia demands a careful consideration, prompt monitoring, and treatment.

References

1. American Psychiatric Association. (2013). Medication-induced movement disorders and other adverse effects of medication. *Diagnostic and statistical manual of mental disorders* (5th ed.). American Psychiatric Association.
2. Critchley, M. (1955). The pre-dormitum. *Revue neurologique, 93*(1), 101.
3. Wittmaack, T. (1861). *Lehrbuch der Nervenkrankheiten auf Grundlage physiologischer Begriffsbestimmung des Krankseins und mit steter Berücksichtigung der Untersuchungs-Ergebnisse bis auf die Gegenwart: Pathologie und Therapie der Sensibilität-Neurosen mit Einschluss der primär psychisch bedingten auf Grundlage physiologischer Begriffsbestimmtung des Krankseins und mit steter Berücksichtigung der Untersuchungsergebnisse bis auf die Gegenwart* (Vol. 1). Schäfer.
4. Beard, G. M. (1880). A practical treatise on nervous exhaustion (neurasthenia): its symptoms, nature, sequences, treatment. *American Journal of Psychiatry, 36*(4), 521–526.
5. Sachdev, P. (1995). The development of the concept of akathisia: a historical overview. *Schizophrenia Research, 16*(1), 33–45.
6. Bing, R. (1923). Über einige bemerkenswerte Begleiterscheinungen der "extrapyramidalen Rigidität"(Akathisie-Mikrographie-Kinesia paradoxa). Schweizerische Medizinische Wochenschrift *Schweiz Med Wsch, 53*, 167–171.
7. Sicard, J. (1923). Akathisie and tasikinesie. *Presse Medicale, 31*, 265–266.
8. Mussio Fournier, J., & Rawak, F. (1940). Agitation paresthésique des extrémités. *Revue neurologique (Paris), 79*, 337–341.
9. Allison, F. G. (1943). Obscure pains in the chest, back or limbs. *Canadian Medical Association Journal, 48*(1), 36.
10. Ekbom, K. (1944). Asthenia crurum paraesthetica ("irritable legs"): a new syndrome consisting of weakness, sensation of cold and nocturnal paresthesia in the legs, responding to a certain extent to treatment with priscol and doryl.—a note on paresthesia in general. *Acta Medica Scandinavica, 118*(1–3), 197–209.
11. Sigwald, J. (1947). Le traitement de la maladie de Parkinson et des manifestations extrapyramidalles par le diethylaminoethyl n-thiophyenylamine (2987RP): résultats d'une année d'application. *Revue neurologique, 79*, 683–687.
12. Barsa, J. A., & Kline, N. S. (1956). Use of reserpine in disturbed psychotic patients. *American Journal of Psychiatry, 112*(9), 684–690.
13. Sarwer-Foner, G., & Ogle, W. (1956). Psychosis and enhanced anxiety produced by reserpine and chlorpromazine. *Canadian Medical Association Journal, 74*(7), 526.

14. Freyhan, F. A. (1959). Therapeutic implications of differential effects of new phenothiazine compounds. *American Journal of Psychiatry*, *115*(7), 577–585.

15. Deniker, P. (1960). Experimental neurological syndromes and the new drug therapies in psychiatry. *Comprehensive Psychiatry*, *1*(2), 92–102.

16. Denham, J., & Carrick, D. (1961). Therapeutic value of thioproperazine and the importance of the associated neurological disturbances. *Journal of Mental Science*, *107*(447), 326–345.

17. Jouini, L., Ouali, U., Ouanes, S., Rania, Z., Jomli, R., Zgueb, Y., & Nacef, F. (2017). Akathisia: prevalence and risk factors in patients with psychosis and bipolar disorder. *European Psychiatry*, *41*, S330–S331.

18. Berna, F., Misdrahi, D., Boyer, L., Aouizerate, B., Brunel, L., Capdevielle, D., ... Dubertret, C. (2015). Akathisia: prevalence and risk factors in a community-dwelling sample of patients with schizophrenia. Results from the FACE-SZ dataset. *Schizophrenia Research*, *169*(1–3), 255–261.

19. Halstead, S. M., Barnes, T. R., & Speller, J. C. (1994). Akathisia: prevalence and associated dysphoria in an in-patient population with chronic schizophrenia. *British Journal of Psychiatry*, *164*(2), 177–183.

20. Kim, J.-H., & Byun, H.-J. (2003). Prevalence and characteristics of subjective akathisia, objective akathisia, and mixed akathisia in chronic schizophrenic subjects. *Clinical Neuropharmacology*, *26*(6), 312–316.

21. Janno, S., Holi, M., Tuisku, K., & Wahlbeck, K. (2004). Prevalence of neuroleptic-induced movement disorders in chronic schizophrenia inpatients. *American Journal of Psychiatry*, *161*(1), 160–163.

22. Demyttenaere, K., Detraux, J., Racagni, G., & Vansteelandt, K. (2019). Medication-induced akathisia with newly approved antipsychotics in patients with a severe mental illness: a systematic review and meta-analysis. *CNS Drugs*, *33*(6), 549–566.

23. Kumsa, A., Agenagnew, L., Alemu, B., & Girma, S. (2020). Psychotropic medications induced parkinsonism and akathisia in people attending follow-up treatment at Jimma Medical Center, Psychiatry Clinic. *PloS One*, *15*(7), e0235365.

24. Juncal-Ruiz, M., Ramirez-Bonilla, M., Gomez-Arnau, J., de la Foz, V. O.-G., Suarez-Pinilla, P., Martinez-Garcia, O., ... Crespo-Facorro, B. (2017). Incidence and risk factors of acute akathisia in 493 individuals with first episode non-affective psychosis: a 6-week randomised study of antipsychotic treatment. *Psychopharmacology*, *234*(17), 2563–2570.

25. Kawanishi, C., Onishi, H., Kato, D., Kishida, I., Furuno, T., Wada, M., & Hirayasu, Y. (2007). Unexpectedly high prevalence of akathisia in cancer patients. *Palliative & Supportive Care*, *5*(4), 351–354.

26. Forcen, F. E., Matsoukas, K., & Alici, Y. (2016). Antipsychotic-induced akathisia in delirium: a systematic review. *Palliative & Supportive Care*, *14*(1), 77.

27. Forcen, F. E., Radwan, K., Arauz, A., Ali, J., Syed, S., Brown, M., ... Keenan, K. (2017). Drug-induced akathisia in children and adolescents. *Journal of Child and Adolescent Psychopharmacology*, *27*(1), 102–103.

28. Sadock, V. A. (2014). *Kaplan & Sadock's synopsis of psychiatry: behavioral sciences/clinical psychiatry* (11th ed.). Wolters Kluwer.

29. Oh, G. H., Yu, J.-C., Choi, K.-S., Joo, E.-J., & Jeong, S.-H. (2015). Simultaneous comparison of efficacy and tolerability of second-generation antipsychotics in schizophrenia: mixed-treatment comparison analysis based on head-to-head trial data. *Psychiatry Investigation*, *12*(1), 46.

30. Martino, D., Karnik, V., Osland, S., Barnes, T. R., & Pringsheim, T. M. (2018). Movement disorders associated with antipsychotic medication in people with schizophrenia: an overview of Cochrane reviews and meta-analysis. *Canadian Journal of Psychiatry, 63*(11), 730–739.

31. Pringsheim, T., Gardner, D., Addington, D., Martino, D., Morgante, F., Ricciardi, L., ... Carson, A. (2018). The assessment and treatment of antipsychotic-induced akathisia. *Canadian Journal of Psychiatry, 63*(11), 719–729.

32. Solmi, M., Murru, A., Pacchiarotti, I., Undurraga, J., Veronese, N., Fornaro, M., ... Seeman, M. V. (2017). Safety, tolerability, and risks associated with first-and second-generation antipsychotics: a state-of-the-art clinical review. *Therapeutics and Clinical Risk Management, 13*, 757.

33. Zhang, J.-P., Gallego, J. A., Robinson, D. G., Malhotra, A. K., Kane, J. M., & Correll, C. U. (2013). Efficacy and safety of individual second-generation vs. first-generation antipsychotics in first-episode psychosis: a systematic review and meta-analysis. *International Journal of Neuropsychopharmacology, 16*(6), 1205–1218.

34. Haddad, P. M., Das, A., Keyhani, S., & Chaudhry, I. B. (2012). Antipsychotic drugs and extrapyramidal side effects in first episode psychosis: a systematic review of head–head comparisons. *Journal of Psychopharmacology, 26*(5 suppl), 15–26.

35. Chow, C. L., Kadouh, N. K., Bostwick, J. R., & VandenBerg, A. M. (2020). Akathisia and newer second-generation antipsychotic drugs: a review of current evidence. *Pharmacotherapy: The Journal of Human Pharmacology and Drug Therapy, 40*(6), 565–574.

36. Wright, M. T. (2007). Antiemetics, akathisia, and pregnancy. *Psychosomatics, 48*(6), 461–466.

37. Hawthorne, J. M., & Caley, C. F. (2015). Extrapyramidal reactions associated with serotonergic antidepressants. *Annals of Pharmacotherapy, 49*(10), 1136–1152.

38. Imboden, C., & Hatzinger, M. (2012). Agomelatine-induced akathisia with concomitant duloxetine medication: a case report. *Pharmacopsychiatry, 45*(4), 162–163.

39. Anderson, H. D., Pace, W. D., Libby, A. M., West, D. R., & Valuck, R. J. (2012). Rates of 5 common antidepressant side effects among new adult and adolescent cases of depression: a retrospective US claims study. *Clinical Therapeutics, 34*(1), 113–123.

40. Madhusoodanan, S., Alexeenko, L., Sanders, R., & Brenner, R. (2010). Extrapyramidal symptoms associated with antidepressants—a review of the literature and an analysis of spontaneous reports. *Annals of Clinical Psychiatry, 22*(3), 148–156.

41. Asser, A., & Taba, P. (2015). Psychostimulants and movement disorders. *Frontiers in Neurology, 6*, 75.

42. Zhornitsky, S., Stip, E., Pampoulova, T., Rizkallah, E., Lipp, O., Bentaleb, L. A., ... Potvin, S. (2010). Extrapyramidal symptoms in substance abusers with and without schizophrenia and in nonabusing patients with schizophrenia. *Movement Disorders, 25*(13), 2188–2194.

43. Riesselman, A., & El-Mallakh, R. S. (2015). Akathisia with azithromycin. *Annals of Pharmacotherapy, 49*(5), 609–609.

44. Dressler, D. (2014). Tardive dystonic syndrome induced by the calcium-channel blocker amlodipine. *Journal of Neural Transmission, 121*(4), 367–369.

45. Kern, D., & Lange, A. (2015). Acute akathisia. In: Joseph H. Friedman (Ed.) *Medication-Induced Movement Disorders*, Cambridge University Press, pp. 3–19.

46. de Leon, J., Diaz, F. J., Aguilar, M. C., Jurado, D., & Gurpegui, M. (2006). Does smoking reduce akathisia? Testing a narrow version of the self-medication hypothesis. *Schizophrenia Research, 86*(1–3), 256–268.

47. Farde, L. (1992). Selective D1-and D2-dopamine receptor blockade both induces akathisia in humans—a PET study with [11 C] SCH 23390 and [11 C] raclopride. *Psychopharmacology*, *107*(1), 23–29.

48. Marsden, C., & Jenner, P. (1980). The pathophysiology of extrapyramidal side-effects of neuroleptic drugs. *Psychological Medicine*, *10*(1), 55–72.

49. Basu, B., Gangopadhyay, T., Dutta, N., Mandal, B., De, S., & Mondal, S. (2014). A case of akathisia induced by escitalopram: case report & review of literature. *Current Drug Safety*, *9*(1), 56–59.

50. Bateup, H. S., Santini, E., Shen, W., Birnbaum, S., Valjent, E., Surmeier, D. J., ... Greengard, P. (2010). Distinct subclasses of medium spiny neurons differentially regulate striatal motor behaviors. *Proceedings of the National Academy of Sciences*, *107*(33), 14845–14850.

51. Kim, J.-H., Son, Y.-D., Kim, H.-K., Lee, S.-Y., Cho, S.-E., Kim, Y.-B., & Cho, Z.-H. (2011). Antipsychotic-associated mental side effects and their relationship to dopamine D2 receptor occupancy in striatal subdivisions: a high-resolution PET study with [11C] raclopride. *Journal of Clinical Psychopharmacology*, *31*(4), 507–511.

52. Sachdev, P., & Brüne, M. (2000). Animal models of acute drug-induced akathisia–a review. *Neuroscience & Biobehavioral Reviews*, *24*(3), 269–277.

53. Crowley, J. J., Kim, Y., Szatkiewicz, J. P., Pratt, A. L., Quackenbush, C. R., Adkins, D. E., ... Wang, W. (2012). Genome-wide association mapping of loci for antipsychotic-induced extrapyramidal symptoms in mice. *Mammalian Genome*, *23*(5–6), 322–335.

54. Bakker, P. R., Bakker, E., Amin, N., van Duijn, C. M., van Os, J., & van Harten, P. N. (2012). Candidate gene-based association study of antipsychotic-induced movement disorders in long-stay psychiatric patients: a prospective study. *PloS One*, *7*(5), e36561.

55. Kane, J. M., Fleischhacker, W. W., Hansen, L., Perlis, R., , A., III, & Assuncao-Talbott, S. (2009). Akathisia: an updated review focusing on second-generation antipsychotics. *Journal of Clinical Psychiatry*, *70*(5), 627.

56. Salem, H., Nagpal, C., Pigott, T., & Lucio Teixeira, A. (2017). Revisiting antipsychotic-induced akathisia: current issues and prospective challenges. *Current Neuropharmacology*, *15*(5), 789–798.

57. Shahidi, G., Rohani, M., Munhoz, R. P., & Akhoundi, F. H. (2018). Tardive akathisia with asymmetric and upper-body presentation: report of two cases and literature review. *Tremor and Other Hyperkinetic Movements*, *8*, 563. DOI: http://doi.org/10.5334/tohm.415.

58. Van Putten, T. (1975). The many faces of akathisia. *Comprehensive Psychiatry*, *16*(1), 43–47.

59. Stahl, S. M. (1985). Akathisia and tardive dyskinesia: changing concepts. *Archives of general psychiatry*, *42*(9), 915–917.

60. Barnes, T. R. (2003). The Barnes Akathisia rating scale–revisited. *Journal of Psychopharmacology*, *17*(4), 365–370.

61. Hirjak, D., Kubera, K., Bienentreu, S., Thomann, P., & Wolf, R. (2019). Antipsychotic-induced motor symptoms in schizophrenic psychoses, part 1: dystonia, akathisia und parkinsonism. *Der Nervenarzt*, *90*(1), 1–11.

62. Leucht, S., Komossa, K., Rummel-Kluge, C., Corves, C., Hunger, H., Schmid, F., ... Davis, J. M. (2009). A meta-analysis of head-to-head comparisons of second-generation antipsychotics in the treatment of schizophrenia. *American Journal of Psychiatry*, *166*(2), 152–163.

63. Barnes, T. R. (1989). A rating scale for drug-induced akathisia. *British Journal of Psychiatry*, *154*(5), 672–676.

64. Suzuki, T. (2011). Which rating scales are regarded as "the standard" in clinical trials for schizophrenia? A critical review. *Psychopharmacology Bulletin*, 44(1), 18.

65. Chouinard, G., & Margolese, H. C. (2005). Manual for the extrapyramidal symptom rating scale (ESRS). *Schizophrenia Research*, 76(2–3), 247–265.

66. Forcen, F. E. (2015). Akathisia: is restlessness a primary condition or an adverse drug effect. *Current Psychiatry*, 14(1), 14–18.

67. Caroff, S. N., Hurford, I., Lybrand, J., & Campbell, E. C. (2011). Movement disorders induced by antipsychotic drugs: implications of the CATIE schizophrenia trial. *Neurologic Clinics*, 29(1), 127–148.

68. Erdur, B., Tura, P., Aydin, B., Ozen, M., Ergin, A., Parlak, I., & Kabay, B. (2012). A trial of midazolam vs diphenhydramine in prophylaxis of metoclopramide-induced akathisia. *American Journal of Emergency Medicine*, 30(1), 84–91.

69. Vinson, D. R., & Drotts, D. L. (2001). Diphenhydramine for the prevention of akathisia induced by prochlorperazine: a randomized, controlled trial. *Annals of Emergency Medicine*, 37(2), 125–131.

70. Soundarrajan, G., Chogtu, B., Krishna, V., Kamath, G., & Murugesan, M. (2019). Akathisia induced by abrupt withdrawal of risperidone: a case report. *Psychopharmacology Bulletin*, 49(1), 80–83.

71. Takeuchi, H., Thiyanavadivel, S., Agid, O., & Remington, G. (2018). Rapid vs. slow antipsychotic initiation in schizophrenia: a systematic review and meta-analysis. *Schizophrenia Research*, 193, 29–36.

72. Sienaert, P., van Harten, P., & Rhebergen, D. (2019). The psychopharmacology of catatonia, neuroleptic malignant syndrome, akathisia, tardive dyskinesia, and dystonia. . In: Victor I. Reus, Daniel Lindqvist (Eds) Psychopharmacology of Neurologic Disease. *Handbook of clinical neurology* (Vol. 165, pp. 415–428): Elsevier.

73. Lima, A., Weiser, K. V., Bacaltchuk, J., Barnes, T. R., Lima, A. R., & Soares-Weiser, K. (2002). Anticholinergics for neuroleptic-induced acute akathisia. *Cochrane Database of Systematic Reviews*, 3, CD003727.

74. Poyurovsky, M., Pashinian, A., Weizman, R., Fuchs, C., & Weizman, A. (2006). Low-dose mirtazapine: a new option in the treatment of antipsychotic-induced akathisia. A randomized, double-blind, placebo-and propranolol-controlled trial. *Biological Psychiatry*, 59(11), 1071–1077.

75. Stroup, T. S., & Gray, N. (2018). Management of common adverse effects of antipsychotic medications. *World Psychiatry*, 17(3), 341–356.

76. Baskak, B., Atbasoglu, E. C., Ozguven, H. D., Saka, M. C., & Gogus, A. K. (2007). The effectiveness of intramuscular biperiden in acute akathisia: a double-blind, randomized, placebo-controlled study. *Journal of Clinical Psychopharmacology*, 27(3), 289–294.

77. Poyurovsky, M., & Weizman, A. (2015). Treatment of antipsychotic-related akathisia revisited: the role of serotonin 2a receptor antagonists. *Journal of Clinical Psychopharmacology*, 35(6), 711–714.

78. Perry, L. A., Ramson, D., & Stricklin, S. (2018). Mirtazapine adjunct for people with schizophrenia. *Cochrane Database of Systematic Reviews*, 5, CD011943.

79. Avital, A., Gross-Isseroff, R., Stryjer, R., Hermesh, H., Weizman, A., & Shiloh, R. (2009). Zolmitriptan compared to propranolol in the treatment of acute neuroleptic-induced akathisia: a comparative double-blind study. *European Neuropsychopharmacology*, 19(7), 476–482.

80. Hemminger, A., & Wills, B. K. (2020). Vitamin B6 toxicity. In *StatPearls [Internet]:* StatPearls Publishing. PMID: 32119387.

81. De Berardis, D., Serroni, N., Moschetta, F. S., Martinotti, G., & Di Giannantonio, M. (2013). Reversal of aripiprazole-induced tardive akathisia by addition of pregabalin. *Journal of Neuropsychiatry and Clinical Neurosciences, 25*(2), E09–E10.

82. Naguy, A. (2019). A comment on "successful management of clozapine-induced akathisia with gabapentin enacarbil: a case report." *Clinical Psychopharmacology and Neuroscience, 17*(4), 564.

83. Takeshima, M., Ishikawa, H., Kanbayashi, T., & Shimizu, T. (2018). Gabapentin enacarbil for antipsychotic induced akathisia in schizophrenia patients: a pilot open-labeled study. *Neuropsychiatric Disease and Treatment, 14,* 3179.

84. Mansutti, I., Venturini, M., & Palese, A. (2019). Episodes of psychomotor agitation among medical patients: findings from a longitudinal multicentre study. *Aging Clinical and Experimental Research, 32*(6), 1101–1110.

85. Maj, M., Pirozzi, R., Magliano, L., & Bartoli, L. (2003). Agitated depression in bipolar I disorder: prevalence, phenomenology, and outcome. *American Journal of Psychiatry, 160*(12), 2134–2140.

86. Judd, L. L., Schettler, P. J., Akiskal, H., Coryell, W., Fawcett, J., Fiedorowicz, J. G., . . . Keller, M. B. (2012). Prevalence and clinical significance of subsyndromal manic symptoms, including irritability and psychomotor agitation, during bipolar major depressive episodes. *Journal of Affective Disorders, 138*(3), 440–448.

87. Sacchetti, E., Valsecchi, P., Tamussi, E., Paulli, L., Morigi, R., & Vita, A. (2018). Psychomotor agitation in subjects hospitalized for an acute exacerbation of schizophrenia. *Psychiatry Research, 270,* 357–364.

88. Tysnes, O.-B., & Storstein, A. (2017). Epidemiology of Parkinson's disease. *Journal of Neural Transmission, 124*(8), 901–905.

89. Sveinbjornsdottir, S. (2016). The clinical symptoms of Parkinson's disease. *Journal of Neurochemistry, 139,* 318–324.

90. McColgan, P., & Tabrizi, S. J. (2018). Huntington's disease: a clinical review. *European Journal of Neurology, 25*(1), 24–34.

91. D'Abreu, A., Akbar, U., & Friedman, J. H. (2018). Tardive dyskinesia: epidemiology. *Journal of the Neurological Sciences, 389,* 17–20.

5

Tardive Dyskinesia

Vinicius Sousa Pietra Pedroso, João Vinícius Salgado,
and Antonio L. Teixeira

Introduction

Traditionally, the era of psychopharmacology is considered to have begun in the 1950s with the rise of behavioral pharmacology and the emergence of the first antidepressant and antipsychotic drugs. However, even before the introduction of the first psychiatric drugs, bizarre or odd postures and movements have been associated with mental illness. Evidence from historical records and from contemporary studies points to the existence of movement disorders, catatonic symptoms, and soft neurological signs in patients with schizophrenia, including groups free from pharmacological treatment, such as children at high risk for psychosis, as well as in first psychotic episode patients.[1,2] These findings suggest that psychomotor abnormalities may constitute a central symptomatic dimension in the spectrum of schizophrenia.

However, the first reports of abnormal movements associated with the prescription of antipsychotics were published shortly after its clinical use starting with the seminal reports on the investigation of phenothiazines as pre-anesthetic agents and on the administration of chlorpromazine to psychiatric patients based on the observations of Laborit, Delay, and colleagues.[3,4] In these initial studies, the positive clinical effects described were mainly psychomotor, including sedation, "a calm and distant attitude," reduced excitement, and deceleration that resembled parkinsonian bradykinesia. These movement disorders ended up being called "extrapyramidal side effects" and, thus, were understood to be important for the therapeutic effect, as well as effective dosage markers. This idea persisted until further studies distinguished neurological/motor effects from those antipsychotic effects.[2,5] Although the acute drug-induced motor side effects were recognized, clinicians were reassured by the fact that they would be transient and mitigated by antiparkinsonian agents or by changes in the dose or potency of antipsychotics.

In 1957, Schonecker reported the first cases of involuntary and persistent abnormal movements associated with antipsychotics.[6] He described the appearance of persistent perioral movements with the use of multiple antipsychotic drugs. Since then and during the 1960s, many clinicians received with skepticism the possible association between antipsychotic drugs and dyskinesias. They argued that these involuntary movements could be related to other causes, such as old age or psychotic disorders themselves. Some even argued that spontaneous dyskinesia (SD), an involuntary choreoathetoid movement usually from the orofacial area, were to blame, rather than antipsychotic-induced movement disorders. Most of the arguments were based on a well-known relationship between old age and manifestation of abnormal orofacial movements.[7]

Faurbye and colleagues, in 1964, reviewed their own descriptions of chronic psychotic patients with irreversible masticatory buccolingual dyskinesias, which, in some cases, were also associated with generalized dystonic symptoms or akathisia, and coined the term "tardive dyskinesia" (TD), establishing essential clinical and epidemiological characteristics of the condition.[8] They also noted that some dyskinesias appeared or worsened after withdrawing the medication. The term "tardive" highlights the temporal aspect of symptoms onset and differentiates this type of dyskinesia from other motor syndromes, jointly referred to as "extrapyramidal signs," which includes dystonia, akathisia, and parkinsonism. These latter are, in turn, more frequently associated with acute antipsychotic drugs exposure. According to the original descriptions, TD is characterized by involuntary, nonrhythmic, repetitive, purposeless, hyperkinetic movements. Dyskinetic movements emerging after discontinuation and/or reduction of antipsychotic medication is better known as antipsychotic withdrawal-emergent dyskinesia (WED), which is usually time limited, lasting less than eight weeks. Despite the controversies, an increasing body of research subsequently established the clinical significance of TD, and the entity was officially accepted and sanctioned by the mid-1970s.[9]

This chapter will discuss current knowledge regarding clinical manifestations, differential diagnosis, epidemiology, pathophysiology, treatment strategies, and natural history of TD. However, as we will see in the next sections, some doubts remain to be fully clarified, and these include how often it occurs, the characteristics of the population at higher or lower risk, the possibility of reversibility, its functional impact, and its differentiation from other abnormal movements known to occur among patients long before the use of psychiatric drugs.

Clinical Presentation and Differential Diagnosis

TD has been divided into two distinct subsyndromes based on its topography: orofaciolingual and limb-truncal dyskinesias.[10] Orofaciolingual dyskinesia is the typical or classic presentation of TD. It involves the oromasticatory and facial muscles, leading to abnormal involuntary movements, such as chewing; tongue protrusion, curling, or twisting; lip smacking, puckering, and sucking; mouth retraction, grimacing, bulging of the cheeks; and eye blinking. It can be debilitating and may ultimately impair eating and swallowing. Limb-truncal dyskinesia involves purposeless choreiform movements of trunk and/or limbs, and may cause gait disturbances and falls, along with choreoathetoid movements of the fingers, hands, and toes. There are hypotheses suggesting that these two presentations are, in fact, distinct clinical entities, with their own risk factors. In that sense, there is some evidence that orofaciolingual dyskinesia is more prevalent among elderly patients and is associated with more cognitive and negative symptoms.[11-13]

The onset of TD is usually insidious, appearing after prolonged exposure to dopamine receptor blocking agents (DRBAs), such as antipsychotics and antiemetics. Table 5.1 presents a list of drugs associated with TD. Movements associated with TD are more likely to appear after at least two months of DRBA administration and persist for at least four to six months after discontinuation. The late onset of symptoms may contribute to underestimates of the prevalence of TD in short-term controlled studies and clinical trials.

Table 5.1 Agents That Have Been Associated With Tardive Dyskinesia

Pharmacological class	Example of drugs
1st Generation Antipsychotics	Chlorpromazine, Fluphenazine, Haloperidol, Loxapine, Molindone, Perphenazine, Pimozide, Thioridazine, Thiothixene, Trifluoperazine
2nd Generation Antipsychotics	Aripripazole, Asenapine, Olanzapine, Quetiapine, Risperidone, Ziprasidone
Anticonvulsants	Carbamazepine, Lamotrigine
Antidepressants	Amitriptyline, Amoxepine, Citalopram, Clomipramine, Duloxetine, Doxepin, Fluoxetine, Imipramine, MAOI, Sertraline, Trazodone
Antiemetics	Droperidole, Metoclopramide, Prochlorperazine
Antihistamine	Hydroxyzine
Antimalarial	Chloroquine, Amodiaquine
Anxiolytics	Barbiturates, GABA agonists
Calcium channel blockers	Cinnarizine, Flunarizine
Mood stabilizers	Lithium

The diagnosis of TD is still eminently clinical and is based on the appearance of involuntary movements in the context of recent or past exposure to DRBA. The primary differential diagnosis of TD includes idiopathic spontaneous dyskinesias or stereotype associated with other diseases such as edentulous dyskinesia or frontal-temporal dementia, withdrawal dyskinesias, and other tardive syndromes (e.g., tardive akathisia and tardive dystonia).

In contrast to TD, which usually develops after prolonged exposure to DRBA, spontaneous dyskinesias can be seen in patients never exposed to such drugs. The phenomenology of idiopathic dyskinesias and drug-induced TD has been compared by several authors. Gross neurological signs, such as dystonia, athetosis, or chorea, are found in patients with TD, but are not typical of the spontaneous dyskinesias described in patients with schizophrenia or in normal aging. Thus, they would be indicative of neurological disease. However, the classic manifestation of TD, the so-called bucco-lingual-masticatory syndrome, represents a real challenge to clinical evaluation. This is due to its great similarity with the descriptions of stereotypies and mannerisms that affect the orofacial region in chronic schizophrenia and among the elderly. In the case of withdrawal-emergent dyskinesia (WED), it develops after DRBA discontinuation, or after a change or reduction in its dosage. It is usually time limited, lasting up to three months. Antipsychotic drugs and antiemetic agents, such as metoclopramide and prochlorperazine, have been most implicated. However, if the WED persists beyond eight weeks, the patient would be considered as having TD. Since DRBA use can actively reduce the same movements that they cause, it is not clear that WED does not represent a milder form of TD that is suppressed until the offending agent is removed.

In clinical practice, in addition to these hyperkinetic movement disorders, a situation confused with TD is drug-induced parkinsonism. However, there are important differences between the two conditions. First, parkinsonism is marked by rigidity and bradykinesia (instead of hyperkinesias) alongside resting tremors that are rhythmic and faster (3 to 6 Hz) compared to the slow arrhythmic movements typical of TD. Second, drug-induced parkinsonism often occurs soon after the introduction of an antipsychotic or when the prescribed dose is increased, although it may occur after decades. Importantly, when the dose of the antipsychotic is reduced, the clinical manifestations improve, although this may take months. As suggested by its name, TD usually occurs later after the start of medication. When the dose of the antipsychotic is reduced, symptoms often worsen, at least temporarily. In addition, dyskinetic movements appear to be improved, or masked, when the dose of the antipsychotic is increased, while the opposite happens with drug-induced parkinsonism. Finally, anticholinergic drugs, such as benztropine, are effective in the treatment of drug-induced parkinsonism, but they can worsen TD.

The *Diagnostic and Statistical Manual of Mental Disorders*, fifth edition (DSM-5), defines TD as a medication-induced movement disorder, caused by DRBA, which begins after a few months of medication use (or less in an older patient) and persists for at least one month after changing or discontinuing medication.[14] As mentioned, differentiating TD from other movement disorders, which could even be comorbid, can be challenging. TD is characterized by involuntary, repetitive, and purposeless movements, usually of the tongue, jaw, lips, face, trunk, and upper and lower extremities. They may vary during the day and disappear during sleep. The emotional state can also interfere with the presentation of symptoms, which may worsen with anxiety. The abnormal movements can be associated with significant functional impairment and can be socially stigmatizing.

In this regard, after so much time since the initial debates about the validity and importance of the concept of TD, some reflections still deserve to be made. A set of arguments raised at that time largely reflected a lack of knowledge about the characteristics of movement disorders, which can still be misleading nowadays. Thus, interpretations made by caregivers or uninformed professionals that the abnormal movements would be voluntary behaviors or whose objective would be to attract attention are mistaken. Statements like this are still common in the present day, especially due to certain aspects of the disorder, such as fluctuation with anxiety or distraction, disappearance during sleep and suppression by voluntary control.

Clinical evaluation of patients for TD requires careful observation. It can be reliably assessed with rating scales. Various measuring instruments have been developed to quantify the severity of symptoms. The most used are the Abnormal Involuntary Movement Scale (AIMS), the Simpson Dyskinesia Scale, and the Extrapyramidal Symptoms Rating Scale (ESRS).[15-17] Although useful, these instruments may not actually capture the full extent of the motor and psychological impairment that patients experience in the various presentations of tardive syndromes.

The AIMS is undoubtedly the most used scale. It is a 12-item scale, developed by the US National Institute of Mental Health (NIMH), which evaluates involuntary movements across seven body regions. It is simpler, faster to apply and requires less training than more sophisticated instruments such as ESRS. The AIMS was used as a primary outcome measure in recent studies of agents that have been approved by the US Food and Drug Administration (FDA) for the treatment of TD.[18] The isolated use of the scale is not suitable to diagnose TD, but it can serve as a comprehensive screening tool and can be useful to monitor a patient over time.

According to the Schooler-Kane criteria, as long as other causes of abnormal movements have been ruled out, an AIMS score of at least 2 (i.e., mild) in two or more body regions or a score of 3 (moderate) or 4 (severe) in at least one body region in a patient with at least three months of cumulative antipsychotic drug exposure corresponds to a probable diagnosis of TD.[19] The Glazer-Morgenstern criteria present an alternative definition for the identification of TD.[20] According to them, case detection is based on two applications of the AIMS, one at the beginning and one at the end of each consultation. For the diagnosis of TD, a total AIMS score of 3 or more in both applications in two successive consultations and the identification of at least one body area with a score equal to or greater than 2 in both applications in those same two consecutive consultations are required.

According to the recommendations of the American Psychiatric Association, patients using antipsychotics should be regularly evaluated for movement disorders.[21] In this sense, patients who take a first-generation antipsychotic (FGA) should be screened every six months and those using second-generation antipsychotics (SGA), annually. However, in the presence of additional risk factors for TD, the recommended monitoring should be more frequent, that is, every 3 months for those using FGA and every 6 months for those using SGA.

Clinical Epidemiology

Despite being recognized as an undesirable side effect of the use of DRBAs for more than five decades, the epidemiology of TD is not completely clear. There are several reasons for this, starting with the diagnostic conundrum of TD versus spontaneous dyskinesia (SD). Some authors have already argued that clinicians and researchers should not underestimate the increased prevalence of SD with advanced age and suggested subtracting the prevalence rate of SD from the reported prevalence of TD to find the true prevalence of TD.[7] Gervin and colleagues, for example, reported a 7.6% prevalence rate of SD for first episode schizophrenia or schizophreniform disorder.[22]

The incidence and prevalence of SD are higher in patients diagnosed with schizophrenia or schizophreniform disorder than in healthy controls, even if patients have never been exposed to antipsychotic drugs. The presence of SD in these patients has already been associated with low education and intelligence quotient (IQ). In a study of treatment-naive patients diagnosed with chronic schizophrenia, McCreadie and colleagues reported that 57% of the examined subjects presented SD and parkinsonism at least once during the follow-up period.[23] Accordingly, SD should be seen as an integral part of the schizophrenic process and that the pathology underlying schizophrenia could lead to involuntary movements that would not be associated with the use of antipsychotic drugs.

In the 1980s, the American Psychiatric Association set up a task force to examine epidemiological data related to TD and SD, while seeking to control as many external factors as possible.[24] The results of this endeavor revealed the great difficulty of differentiating antipsychotic-induced TD from SD. The risk factors predisposing to the development of SD and TD are similar, especially with regard to age and the presence of brain injuries. In addition, the clinical presentations of SD are almost identical to the classic presentations of TD. The task force concluded that it is virtually impossible to clinically distinguish SD from TD in a given individual. Another possible explanation, not considered by this committee, is the diagnosis of edentulous dyskinesia. Major dental problems, including dentures are very common in psychiatric patients, especially from lower socio-economic backgrounds, and may account for some cases of SD. Since there is no biomarker for TD, clinicians can only stratify patients at risk and formulate a probability statement based on the age and the patient's conditions predisposing to SD, TD, or other movement disorder.

Risk factors for TD can be classified into modifiable and nonmodifiable.[25] The latter can be further subdivided into patient-related and illness-related. Nonmodifiable patient-related risk factors for TD include age (patients aged over 50 years are three to five times more likely to develop TD than younger patients, and patients over 65 are five to six times more likely), female sex, African or white descent (Asian descent appears to be protective), and genetic variations regarding drug metabolism (mainly abnormal CYP2D6 metabolizer status) or dopaminergic systems (such as the catechol-O-methyltransferase valine homozygous genotype—Val/Val COMT; the vesicular monoamine transporter 2—VMAT2—gene; or certain dopamine receptor 2—DRD2—polymorphisms). In the case of nonmodifiable illness-related risk factors, the main ones are longer illness duration, negative symptoms in schizophrenia, diagnosis of mood disorder, cognitive impairment, intellectual disability, and history of brain damage.

The modifiable risk factors can be divided into comorbidity-related and treatment-related. The former include comorbid conditions like diabetes, human immunodeficiency virus (HIV) infection, dementia, and substance use (e.g., smoking, alcohol, cocaine), which increase the risk of TD. Modifiable treatment-related risk factors comprise history of parkinsonian side effects, acute dystonic reactions, akathisia, WED, higher dose and/or longer duration of DRBA use, previous electroconvulsive therapy sessions, intermittent antipsychotic treatment (drug holidays and nonadherence), and anticholinergic cotreatment. It is still debatable whether anticholinergic drugs increase the risk of TD, but they seem to be detrimental once TD has developed. In addition to these, the main factor related to treatment involves the DRBAs themselves. Although many drugs have been associated with the development of TD, among all DRBAs, antipsychotics are the group of medications most related to this outcome. However, the risk does not appear to be the same for each antipsychotic individually.

The first reports of the era of FGA found a prevalence of TD in chronic users of these drugs from 24% to 56%, with an average prevalence of 20% in pooled heterogeneous studies.[26,27] The risk of TD after exposure to FGA for 5 years was estimated to be 32%; 57% for 15 years; and 68% after 25 years.[28] In 1977, Kane and colleagues started the Hillside Study including more than 900 patients who would be monitored prospectively for 20 years.[29] At the end of the follow-up, they observed that the cumulative incidence of TD was 5% in the first year, 27% in the fifth year, 43% in the tenth year, and 52% after 20 years of exposure.[30] This study suggested an overall annual incidence of 5% (including both transient as persistent TD) and about 3% for persistent TD, i.e., the presence of symptoms exceeding 3 months. In 1987, Morgenstern and colleagues investigated the prevalence of TD in a cross-sectional study involving 180 patients, finding a prevalence of 33%. With respect to individual drugs, the prevalence varied as follows: perphenazine (34.4%), fluphenazine decanoate (16.6%), thioridazine (15.6%), chlorpromazine (11.1%), trifluoperazine (8.3%), fluphenazine orally (6.7%), thiotixene (5.3%), and haloperidol (5.0%).[31] However, neither the equivalent dose of chlorpromazine nor the potency of antipsychotic had any significant effect on the prevalence of TD. The main predictive factors for TD in this study included age over 55 years, use of the depot (injectable) version of the antipsychotic, and more than six years of antipsychotic use. Another longitudinal study evaluating the use of FGA found results similar to the Hillside Study, estimating the annual incidence of persistent TD at 5.3% with a spontaneous remission rate of 2.5% per year.[28] Unlike the study conducted by Kane and colleagues, patients were, on average, 10 years older and the time of exposure to FGA was about 14 times longer, without significantly influencing the results. In the elderly population, however, the estimated annual incidence of TD was much higher: 26% after one year and about 60% after three years.

It was expected that, with the introduction of SGA, this scenario would be mitigated. Indeed, the first comparative studies attributed a lower risk of TD with the use of SGA.[32]

However, subsequent studies did not confirm these findings. Large prospective studies based in the United States (Intervention Antipsychotic Clinical Trials of Effectiveness—CATIE) and the United Kingdom (Cost Utility of the Latest Antipsychotic Drug Studies in Schizophrenia—CUtLASS-1) have failed to show a decrease in the onset of TD with SGA.[33,34] Conversely, a meta-analysis including 41 studies published since 2000, which assessed more than 11,000 patients, mostly with psychotic disorders, indicated that the prevalence of TD was significantly higher in patients who were using FGA than in those using SGA.[35] The overall mean TD prevalence found was 25.3%. The prevalence of probable TD was 30% in individuals treated with FGA and about 21% in those treated with SGA. The lowest prevalence (7.2%) was observed among patients receiving SGA who had never been exposed to FGA, suggesting that the simple previous exposure to FGA may also increase the risk of subsequent TD with the use of SGA. The estimated annual incidence rate of TD was reported at 3.9% with SGA and 5.5% with FGA in a systematic review of long-term studies involving patients with schizophrenia.[32] Table 5.2 summarizes the risk factors for TD.

Almost all studies are also affected by the paradox that the drugs that cause TD can also mask it. This can result in counterintuitive observation in which a group of patients chronically treated with an antipsychotic will manifest previously masked TD when the drug is discontinued. As an example of this phenomenon, we can mention a large meta-analysis in which a relatively high incidence of TD was observed when patients taking FGA had their prescription switched to clozapine, a drug associated with a very low risk of motor side effects.[36]

Another aspect that complicates the assessment of the epidemiology of TD is the fact that patients with chronic psychotic disorders must continue taking medication and cannot go untreated for long periods, even when they have TD as a side effect. Since patients often undergo drug switches from one class to another, the ability to identify a "causative" agent is difficult, as the long-term effects of several different DRBA are likely to be cumulative.

Finally, the data currently available shows that TD is still a significant problem, affecting a quarter to a third of patients chronically treated with antipsychotics—FGAs or SGAs—with the exception of clozapine, which presents a considerably lower risk. It is likely that, with the growth in the use of antipsychotics in other clinical conditions in addition to psychotic disorders, the number of people at risk of developing TD will continue to increase.

Table 5.2 Risk Factors Associated With Tardive Dyskinesia

Modifiable	Nonmodifiable
Comorbidity-related	**Patient-related**
• Diabetes	• Age
• HIV infection	• Female gender
• Dementia	• African/white descent
• Substance use (smoking, alcohol, cocaine)	• Genetic polymorphisms
Treatment-related	**Illness-related**
• Acute extrapyramidal reactions	• Longer illness duration
• Withdrawal-emergent dyskinesia	• Negative symptoms
• High doses of DRBA	• Mood disorders
• Long duration of DRBA use	• Cognitive impairment
• Electroconvulsive therapy	• Intellectual disability
• Intermittent DRBA use	• History of brain damage
• Anticholinergic cotreatment	

Neurobiology

The pathophysiology of TD remains to be fully understood, yet it is possible to assert that it is complex and multifactorial.[10] Several hypotheses have been suggested in order to clarify its mechanisms, such as upregulation and increased postsynaptic sensitivity of DRD2 due to chronic dopamine receptor blockage; imbalance of gamma-aminobutyric acid (GABA) neurotransmission; excitotoxicity of N-methyl-D-aspartate (NMDA) receptors; degeneration of cholinergic striatal interneurons; and free radicals related burden leading to oxidative stress that hampers the proper functioning of the basal ganglia.[7,25,37]

The most well-established hypothesis proposes that TD results from dopamine hypersensitivity in the nigrostriatal pathway following DRD2 upregulation with DRBA use. The frontalstriatal motor circuit is formed by the frontal cortex, basal ganglia, and thalamus. In short, this circuit is involved in the control of voluntary movements since it facilitates "desired" movements and inhibits "unwanted" ones or those in competition with the "desired" ones. Cortical activation leads to both activation of the "desired" motor plan through a direct pathway and inhibition of competing motor plans by an indirect pathway. Dopamine receptors D1 (DRD1) in the striatum control the activation of the direct pathway, while DRD2s regulate the indirect pathway, thus limiting competing motor behaviors. With chronic DRBA, the indirect pathway becomes dysfunctional due to hypersensitivity of DRD2, and the direct pathway works without brake, producing a variety of hyperkinetic movement disorders. This model would explain why increasing doses of antipsychotics can alleviate or mask TD symptoms at least initially. However, this model fails to explain why TD often persists for long periods even after the discontinuation of the offending DRBA. Theoretically, dopamine receptors without continuous blockade would be expected to downregulate, resetting the system, but this is not observed. Furthermore, up-regulation probably occurs in everyone within days of receptor blockade, yet TD typical manifests much later. Therefore, although hypersensitivity to the striatal DRD2 receptors may be the initial manifestation of exposure to DRD2 antagonists, this mechanism may be more associated with withdrawal dyskinesias, while persistent forms of TD in humans could have a different pathophysiology.

Another proposal states that DRBA can increase dopamine turnover and lead to increased free radical formation by monoamine oxidase and also by the auto-oxidation of dopamine molecules to free radicals and quinines. Chronic exposure to antipsychotic drugs could increase lipid peroxidation and the formation of free radicals, coupled with impairment of the antioxidant system leading to increased oxidative stress. Compared with individuals without TD using antipsychotics or with normal controls, patients with TD have elevated plasma activity of manganese superoxide dismutase, one of the main enzymes involved in the antioxidant defense mechanism. The level of enzyme activity in patients with TD correlated with the severity of dyskinetic symptoms. A polymorphism in the superoxide dismutase gene has also been associated with TD. Finally, oxidative stress could lead to neuronal damage and therefore degeneration of different neurotransmitter systems. Experimental animal studies and postmortem neuropathological analysis of the brains of patients with TD revealed structural changes, including neuronal loss and gliosis in the basal ganglia after prolonged exposure to antipsychotic drugs.[38]

Another proposition involves the idea that DRD2 hypersensitivity associated with degenerative changes in neurons caused by increased oxidative stress can result in side effects on synaptic plasticity. These effects would be mediated by the altered function of glutamatergic

NMDA receptors in striatal interneurons, causing an imbalance between the direct and indirect pathways of the basal ganglia and, therefore, producing an abnormal output to the sensorimotor cortex. Maladaptive cortical synaptic plasticity, coupled with abnormal basal ganglia output, may allow the miscoding of motor programs, imbalance between the direct and indirect pathways and, consequently, abnormal movements.

Beyond these assumptions, there is evidence involving other mechanisms, such as DRD3 upregulation in the nigrostriatal regions and hypofunction and/or degeneration of striatal cholinergic interneurons and fast-spiking GABA interneurons that regulate balance between direct and indirect basal ganglia pathways.

Treatment

The first-line approach for TD is prevention since it is an iatrogenic disorder. In this sense, long-term treatment with DRBA should be avoided whenever possible, through the choice of alternative therapeutic strategies or drugs with less potential to cause TD.

When a DRBA is required, particular care should be taken in the assessment of individual risk factors, especially in older adults, women, or individuals of African descent, with comorbidities such as diabetes or mood disorders, prolonged psychiatric disorders, and who have cognitive symptoms, intellectual disability, brain damage, prominent negative symptoms or a history of psychoactive substance use (smoking, alcohol, or other substance abuse). To minimize the risks of TD, SGA should be prioritized over FGA. In the case of patients with nonmodifiable risk factors for TD, SGA with lower D2-5HT$_{2A}$ affinity ratio or compounds with a partial D2 agonist activity should be preferred instead of agents with strong and predominant D2-blocking properties. Once a DRBA has been selected, efforts should be made to use the minimum therapeutic dose and to treat for only as long as necessary, to minimize the risk of acute motor syndromes and to reduce the cumulative dose of DRBA. However, it is known that lifelong treatment is often necessary for many patients with psychiatric disorders.

Before starting treatment, clinicians should document the presence or absence of any pre-existing movement disorder, both by history and by physical examination, which can be complemented by the AIMS. Frequent re-evaluation of treatment and monitoring of early signs of TD, ideally quantified by AIMS, are of paramount importance as this leads to earlier intervention and potentially better results. Acute extrapyramidal reactions, such as dystonia, akathisia, or parkinsonism, and specific symptom patterns, including negative and cognitive symptoms, should also be assessed, preferably with standardized scales, in order to identify patients at higher risk for TD and indicate intensified monitoring. Effective smoking cessation interventions should be offered to patients treated with DRBA.

Once TD manifests, suspension (or dose reduction) of antipsychotics is still the basis of treatment. Since most patients with psychotic disorders require chronic treatment with a DRBA, switching to a different agent with a lower risk of TD is recommended. The reduction of the offending agent should be gradual, since sudden discontinuation is more likely to exacerbate the TD. Both FGA and SGA present a risk for TD, but, despite the lack of more robust evidence, switching to SGA is regarded as the first step in the management of recently started TD. Clozapine is seen as the last resort of treatment when other regimens fail, and remains a potentially interesting option for patients who require continued use of antipsychotics.

The American Academy of Neurology published an evidence-based guideline for treatment of TD in 2013, which was updated in 2018.[39,40] Table 5.3 presents some pharmacological options for the treatment of TD, with the respective level of evidence. Numerous substances have been evaluated with the goal of treating TD, such as *Ginkgo biloba*, levetiracetam, buspirone, dehydrogenated ergot alkaloids, pemoline, promethazine, insulin, branched chain amino acids, isocarboxazid, ceruletine, phenylalanine, piracetam, melatonin, lithium, ritanserin, selegiline, oestrogen, gamma-linolenic acid, diltiazem, and GABA agonists as well as benzodiazepines and vitamin B6, in addition to methods like hypnosis or relaxation, all of which proved unconvincing for the use to be recommended.

Other than ceasing or switching antipsychotic medication, the strongest current evidence for TD treatment are the selective vesicular monoamine transporter 2 (VMAT2) inhibitors, deutetrabenazine and valbenazine.[41] The VMAT2 protein acts in the transport of monoamine neurotransmitters such as dopamine, serotonin, histamine, and norepinephrine to the presynaptic vesicles. The proposed mechanism of action is related to the depletion of presynaptic dopamine levels, without increasing the risk of oversensitization of postsynaptic receptors. Deutetrabenazine and valbenazine are the only medications with US Food and Drugs Administration (FDA) approval to treat TD. Tetrabenazine, an FDA-approved VMAT2 inhibitor for the treatment of Huntington's disease, has also long been used but has limited published data. Given the higher-quality evidence in support of valbenazine and deutetrabenazine with fewer adverse effects, they should be preferred over tetrabenazine.

The adverse events most commonly seen with valbenazine are drowsiness, headache, urinary retention, dry mouth, and akathisia. Valbenazine demonstrated efficacy and tolerability at one year of follow-up. The recommended starting dose is 40 mg once per day, which can then be increased to 60 mg or 80 mg once daily after one week, if needed. In the case of deutetrabenazine, headache, anxiety, and diarrhea are the most common adverse events. Initial dosing for deutetrabenazine is 6 mg twice daily, which can be increased by 6 mg weekly to a maximum dose of 24 mg twice daily, if indicated. It seems to be efficacious and well tolerated, with dosages up to 48 mg/day. Both VMAT2 inhibitors should not be prescribed in patients with congenital long QT syndrome or arrhythmias related to QT prolongation, in pregnant or breast-feeding women, or in patients taking monoamine oxidase inhibitors.

However, clinical experience with the new VMAT2 inhibitory agents, other than tetrabenazine is still incipient and these drugs need to confirm the results of clinical trials in the real world. If their value is confirmed, they may in fact represent a genuine advance in the

Table 5.3 Treatment Options for Tardive Dyskinesia

Drug	Mechanism of action	Dose	Grade of recommendation
Valbenazine	VMAT2 Inhibitor	40–80 mg/day	A
Deutetrabenazine	VMAT2 Inhibitor	6–48 mg/day	A
Clozapine	SGA	25–900 mg/day	B
Vitamin E	Antioxidant	400–1600 IU/day	B
Melatonin	Antioxidant	2–20 mg/day	C

pharmacological management of TD. Of note, it is important to mention that, with regard to the long-term data available from valbenazine, dyskinetic movements returned within four weeks after its discontinuation. Thus, at this point in time, indefinite duration of therapy is recommended for VMAT2 inhibitors.

Other pharmacological strategies lack more robust evidence. Among them, one can mention the use of vitamin E, which has antioxidant effect and does not seem to lead to clinically important improvements in TD once it is established but may protect against deterioration of dyskinetic symptoms; amantadine, which acts through different pharmacological mechanisms, including dopamine reuptake blockade, NMDA antagonism, or noradrenergic effects, and can be used as a second-line agent when other solutions fail; propranolol, which is a beta blocker and can be used with other agents, such as amantadine, as a part of a multidrug treatment strategy for resistant cases. It should be noted that anticholinergic agents, such as benztropine or trihexiphenidyl, which are routinely used in the management of acute motor side effects such as dystonia and parkinsonism, are not recommended for the treatment of TD. On the contrary, anticholinergic agents can potentially worsen the dyskinetic symptoms and cause cognitive impairment. If a patient is already using anticholinergic drugs to control parkinsonism and presents with TD, the clinician may consider discontinuing them, yet keeping in mind that there is very little evidence to support a positive effect on TD and that drug-induced parkinsonism may worsen.

Regarding nonpharmacological strategies, there is limited but impressive evidence for the use of deep brain stimulation (DBS) of the *globus pallidus internus* for TD. DBS should be considered an alternative treatment for select cases where TD symptoms are severe and distressing and pharmacological interventions are not effective or tolerated, as long as the psychiatric clinical status is stabilized.

For all these reasons, it is clear that there is still no single treatment strategy capable of dealing with the complexities of TD. Thus, this only highlights and reinforces to the clinician the fundamental importance of prevention strategies.

Natural history

The natural history of TD, as expected, is difficult to assess. The heterogeneity in the duration of the follow-up studies along with the variability in the characteristics of the evaluated populations contribute to a great diversity in the course reported for TD. In addition, the fact that most patients require continued use of DRBA interferes with the observed course of TD.

Several studies have already shown that TD can persist, improve, or have an unpredictable course depending on different characteristics of the studied population and the time of follow-up.[10,25] In long-term studies, the likelihood of clinical improvement in TD correlates with the duration of time without DRBA or, alternatively, the duration of follow-up. Studies that have monitored patients for more than five years are those that also show the highest rates of clinical improvement. Despite these optimistic views, some cases of TD persist indefinitely and may worsen over time.[42] Apparently, TD is irreversible in up to 50% of cases. The clinical course can negatively impact quality of life, leading to deficiency in food consumption, speech or ambulation, and generating social stigma. Consequently, TD has been associated with increased morbidity and mortality rates in psychiatric patients.

Conclusion

TD is still a common clinical condition that should not be overlooked. It is a very disabling iatrogenic disorder that is often difficult to manage and to treat. There is a real need to advance the pathophysiological understanding of TD, in addition to deepening the knowledge about its psychological, physical, social, and economic burden. Clinicians should be aware of the potential risk of developing TD in patients on long-term treatment with DRBAs. This approach requires an active attitude, which must go beyond protocol and disinterested evaluations. This would involve the investigation with patients and their caregivers about specific circumstances of daily life, such as situations of public exposure, where strange postures and movements can cause embarrassment, leading to shame, withdrawal, and stigma.

References

1. Rogers, D. (1985). The motor disorders of severe psychiatric illness: a conflict of paradigms. *Br J Psychiatry*, 147, 221–232.
2. Caroff, S.N., Ungvari, G.S., Cunningham Owens, D.G. (2018). Historical perspectives on tardive dyskinesia. *J Neurol Sci*, 389, 4–9.
3. Laborit, H., Huguenard, P., Alluaume, R. (1952). A new vegetative stabilizer; 4560 R.P. *Presse Med*, 60(10), 206–208.
4. Delay, J., Deniker, P., Harl, J.M. (1952). Therapeutic use in psychiatry of phenothiazine of central elective action (4560 RP). *Ann Med Psychol (Paris),* 110(2:1), 112–117.
5. Rifkin, A. (1987). Extrapyramidal side effects: a historical perspective. *J Clin Psychiatry*, 48(Suppl. 3), 6.
6. Schonecker, M. (1957). Beitrag zu der Mitteilung von Kulenkampff und Tarnow; Ein eigentümliches Syndrom im ovalen Bereich bei Megaphen applikation. *Nervenarzt*, 28, 35.
7. Macaluso, M., Flynn, A., Preskorn, S.H. (2017). Tardive dyskinesia: a historical perspective. *J Psychiatr Pract*, 23(2), 121–129.
8. Faurbye, A., Rasch, P.J., Petersen, P.B., Brandborg, G., Pakkenberg, H. (1964). Neurological symptoms in pharmacotherapy of psychoses. *Acta Psychiatr Scand*, 40, 10–27.
9. Freedman, D.X. (1973). Neurological syndromes associated with antipsychotic drug use: a special report. *Arch Gen Psychiatry*, 28(4), 463–467.
10. Salem, H., Pigott, T., Zhang, X.Y., Zeni, C.P., Teixeira, A.L. (2017). Antipsychotic-induced tardive dyskinesia: from biological basis to clinical management. *Expert Rev Neurother*, 17(9), 883–894.
11. Gureje, O. (1988). Topographic subtypes of tardive dyskinesia in schizophrenic patients aged less than 60 years: relationship to demographic, clinical, treatment, and neuropsychological variables. *J Neurol Neurosurg Psychiatry*, 51, 1525–1530.
12. Gureje, O. (1989). The significance of subtyping tardive dyskinesia: a study of prevalence and associated factors. *Psychol Med*, 19, 121–128.
13. Waddington, J.L., Youssef, H.A., Dolphin, C., Kinsella, A. (1987). Cognitive dysfunction, negative symptoms, and tardive dyskinesia in schizophrenia: their association in relation to topography of involuntary movements and criterion of their abnormality. *Arch Gen Psychiatry*, 44, 907–912.

14. American Psychiatric Association. (2013). *Diagnostic and statistical manual of mental disorders* (5th ed.). Washington, DC: American Psychiatric Association.

15. Guy, W. (1976). *ECDEU assessment manual for psychopharmacology*. Rockville, MD: U.S. Dept. of Health, Education, and Welfare.

16. Simpson, G.M., Lee, J.H., Zoubok, B., Gardos, G. (1979). A rating scale for tardive dyskinesia. *Psychopharmacology*, 64(2), 171–179.

17. Chouinard, G., Margolese, H.C. (2005). Manual for the extrapyramidal symptom rating scale (ESRS). *Schizophr Res*, 76(2–3), 247–265. Erratum in: (2006). *Schizophr Res*, 85(1–3), 305.

18. Touma, K., Scarff, J. R. (2018). Valbenazine and deutetrabenazine for tardive dyskinesia. *Innovations in clinical neuroscience*, 15(5–6), 13–16.

19. Schooler, N.R., Kane, J.M. (1982). Research diagnoses for tardive dyskinesia. *Arch Gen Psychiatry*, 39(4), 486–487.

20. Morgenstern, H., Glazer, W.M. (1993). Identifying risk factors for tardive dyskinesia among long-term outpatients maintained with neuroleptic medications: results of the Yale tardive dyskinesia study. *Arch Gen Psychiatry*, 50(9), 723–733.

21. American Psychiatric Association. (2021). *The American Psychiatric Association Practice Guideline for the Treatment of Patients with Schizophrenia*. Washington, DC: American Psychiatric Association.

22. Gervin, M., Browne, S., Lane, A., Clarke, M., Waddington, J.L., Larkin, C., O'Callaghan, E. (1998). Spontaneous abnormal involuntary movements in first-episode schizophrenia and schizophreniform disorder: baseline rate in a group of patients from an Irish catchment area. *Am J Psychiatry*, 155, 1202–1206.

23. McCreadie, R.G., Padmavati, R., Thara, R., Srinivasan, T.N. (2002). Spontaneous dyskinesia and parkinsonism in never-medicated, chronically ill patients with schizophrenia: 18-month follow-up. *Br J Psychiatry*, 181, 135–137.

24. American Psychiatric Association. (1980). Tardive dyskinesia: summary of a Task Force Report of the American Psychiatric Association; by the task force on late neurological effects of antipsychotic drugs. *Am J Psychiatry*, 137, 1163–1172.

25. Solmi, M., Pigato, G., Kane, J.M., Correll, C.U. (2018). Clinical risk factors for the development of tardive dyskinesia. *J Neurol Sci*, 389, 21–27.

26. Tepper, S.J., Haas, J. (1979). Prevalence of tardive dyskinesia. *J Clin Psychiatry*, 40(12), 508–516.

27. D'Abreu, A., Akbar, U., Friedman, J.H. (2018). Tardive dyskinesia: Epidemiology. *J Neurol Sci*, 389, 17–20.

28. Glazer, W.M., Morgenstern, H., Doucette, J.T. (1993). Predicting the long-term risk of tardive dyskinesia in outpatients maintained on neuroleptic medications. *J Clin Psychiatry*, 54(4), 133–139.

29. Kane, J., Woener, M., Weinhold, P., Wegner, J. (1982). Results from a prospective study of tardive dyskinesia development: preliminary findings over a 2-year period. *Psychopharmacol Bull*, 18, 82–83.

30. Tarsy, D., Baldessarini, R.J. (2006). Epidemiology of tardive dyskinesia: is risk declining with modern antipsychotics? *Mov Disord*, 21(5), 589–598.

31. Morgenstern, H., Glazer, W.M., Gibowski, L.D., Holmberg, S. (1987). Predictors of tardive dyskinesia: results of a cross-sectional study in an outpatient population. *J Chronic Dis*, 40(4), 319–327.

32. Correll, C.U., Schenk, E.M. (2008). Tardive dyskinesia and new antipsychotics. *Curr Opin Psychiatry*, 21(2), 151–156.

33. Peluso, M.J., Lewis, S.W., Barnes, T.R., Jones, P.B. (2012). Extrapyramidal motor side-effects of first-and second-generation antipsychotic drugs. *Br J Psychiatry*, 200(5), 387–392.

34. Miller, D.D., Caroff, S.N., Davis, S.M., et al. (2008). Extrapyramidal side-effects of antipsychotics in a randomised trial. *Br J Psychiatry*, 193(4), 279–288.

35. Carbon, M., Hsieh, C.-H., Kane, J.M., Correll, C.U. (2017). Tardive dyskinesia prevalence in the period of second-generation antipsychotic use: a meta-analysis. *J Clin Psychiatry*, 78(3), e264–e278.

36. Woods, S.W., Morgenstern, H., Saksa, J.R., et al. (2010). Incidence of tardive dyskinesia with atypical and conventional antipsychotic medications: prospective cohort study. *J Clin Psychiatry*, 71(4), 463–474.

37. Arya, D., Khan, T., Margolius, A.J., Fernandez, H.H. (2019). Tardive dyskinesia: treatment update. *Curr Neurol Neurosci Rep*, 19(9), 69.

38. Waln, O., Jankovic, J. (2013). An update on tardive dyskinesia: from phenomenology to treatment. *Tremor Other Hyperkinet Mov (NY)*, 3, tre-03-161-4138-1.

39. Bhidayasiri, R., Fahn, S., Weiner, W.J., Gronseth, G.S., Sullivan, K.L., Zesiewicz, T.A. (2013). American Academy of Neurology. Evidence-based guideline: treatment of tardive syndromes: report of the Guideline Development Subcommittee of the American Academy of Neurology. *Neurology*, 81(5), 463–469. Erratum in: (2013). *Neurology*, 81(22), 1968.

40. Bhidayasiri, R., Jitkritsadakul, O., Friedman, J.H., Fahn, S. (2018). Updating the recommendations for treatment of tardive syndromes: a systematic review of new evidence and practical treatment algorithm. *J Neurol Sci*, 389, 67–75.

41. Hauser, R.A., Truong, D. (2018). Tardive dyskinesia: out of the shadows. *J Neurol Sci*, 389, 1–3.

42. Miyawaki, E. (2003). Tardive dyskinesia and other drug-related movement disorders. In Samuels, M., Feske, S. (Eds.), *Office Practice of Neurology* (2nd ed., pp. 810–816). Philadelphia: Churchill Livingstone.

6

Serotonin Syndrome and Neuroleptic Malignant Syndrome

Haitham Salem, Brittany Finocchio, and Teresa Pigott

Introduction and Epidemiology

Serotonin, 5-hydroxytryptamine (5-HT), is an essential neurotransmitter produced within presynaptic nerve terminals via the metabolism (decarboxylation and hydroxylation) of L-tryptophan from dietary protein intake. 5-HT acts both peripherally and centrally. Centrally, serotonin arises from the midbrain raphe nuclei of the brainstem down to the medulla, where it is responsible for a wide array of functions from inhibiting excitatory neurotransmission to modulating wakefulness, attention, affective and sexual behavior, appetite, thermoregulation, motor tone, migraine propensity, emesis, nociception, and aggression. Peripheral serotonin is primarily a product of the enterochromaffin cells of the gastrointestinal tract and plays a critical role in stimulating vasoconstriction, uterine contraction, bronchoconstriction, gastrointestinal motility, and platelet aggregation.[1–4]

Serotonin syndrome (SS) is a potentially life-threatening condition due to excessive serotonin activity throughout the central nervous system (CNS) as a result of medication exposure. Although SS can manifest in a wide variety of clinical presentations, the clinical triad of mental status changes, autonomic instability, and neuromuscular hyperactivity (rigidity and clonus) are considered the classic SS symptoms (Figure 6.1). SS results from central and peripheral serotonin receptor overactivation. Medications that increase serotonin activity as monotherapy, in combination with other drugs, or even a withdrawal from a serotonergic medication can induce SS.[5,6,7]

Attempts to determine the actual incidence or prevalence of SS remain hindered not only by underrecognition but also by underreporting of milder cases. Nonetheless, cases of SS are increasing and likely reflect the widespread use of serotonergic enhancing agents in medical practice. SS can occur at any age and no significant sex difference appears to exist.[8,9] SS can be lethal, with mortality estimates ranging from 2% to 12%.[10] Apart from modest increased risk of SS associated with the presence of certain genetic polymorphisms, research has failed to show a consistent association between SS and any general risk factors.[3,11]

Manifestations, Diagnostic Criteria, and Differential Diagnosis

The diagnosis of SS remains a clinical one, based largely on the presence of key clinical features including mental status changes, autonomic instability, hyperthermia, and rigidity in the context of exposure to serotonergic medication(s) (Figure 6.2). Early and accurate identification of SS is essential, as severity ranges from mild cases presenting with subacute

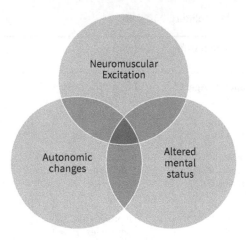

Figure 6.1 Serotonin syndrome: Critical symptom triad.

symptoms to severe cases that progress rapidly to death.[12] Although there is no definitive laboratory test to identify SS, specific criteria for diagnosing and assessing symptom severity have been proposed. Three of the most widely used criteria are the Sternbach, Radomski, and Hunter criteria.[13–15]

The differential diagnosis of SS includes neuroleptic malignant syndrome (NMS), anticholinergic toxicity, malignant hyperthermia, intoxication from sympathomimetic agents, sedative-hypnotic withdrawal, meningitis, and encephalitis. Although SS and NMS share some symptoms, they can be rapidly differentiated by history. For example, obtaining the suspected type of medication exposure (serotonergic enhancer vs. dopaminergic antagonist) as part of the patient's history is essential to making a rapid and accurate diagnosis. In addition, the neurological exam is critical. SS is characterized by neuromuscular hyperreactivity (tremors, hyperreflexia, myoclonus), whereas hyporeflexia often accompanies rigidity in NMS. Clinical course is also distinct between SS and NMS. SS develops over 24 hours and generally resolves within 24 hours of treatment. In contrast, NMS generally emerges after days to weeks and takes an average of 9 days to resolve. Unlike SS, NMS is

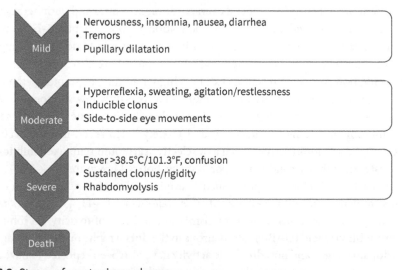

Figure 6.2 Stages of serotonin syndrome.

Table 6.1 SS vs. NMS vs. Anticholinergic Toxicity

	Serotonin Syndrome	NMS	Anticholinergic Toxicity
Causative Agent	Serotonergic Agent	Dopamine Antagonist or Withdrawal from Dopamine Agonist	Anticholinergic Agent
Onset	Within 24 hr.	Days to Weeks	Within 1-2 hr.
Similar Sx	Mental status changes Autonomic instability Hyperthermia Rigidity	Mental status changes Autonomic instability Hyperthermia Rigidity	Mental status changes Hyperthermia
Distinct Clinical Features	Hyperactivity Hyperreflexia Tremors Clonus Diarrhea Nausea or Vomiting	Hypoactivity Hyporeflexia Lead pipe rigidity Extrapyramidal fx	Dry skin & mucous membranes Urinary retention Reduced bowel sounds Normal muscle tone and reflexes
Resolution	Within 24 hr.	Average of 9 days	Within hours to days

also associated with a distinct profile of laboratory abnormalities including a low serum iron level coupled with elevations of creatine kinase, liver function tests (lactate dehydrogenase, aspartate transaminase), and the white blood cell count.[16-18] In contrast with SS, muscular tone and reflexes are normal in anticholinergic poisoning. Malignant hyperthermia is a rare genetic disorder that occurs in susceptible individuals exposed to halogenated volatile anesthetics and depolarizing muscle relaxants.[19,20] Table 6.1 summarizes the key differences between SS, NMS, and anticholinergic toxicity.

Pathophysiology and Pharmacology

While serotonin toxicity involves general overactivation of central and peripheral serotonin receptors, considerable evidence implicates activation of postsynaptic 5-HT$_{2A}$ receptors in the emergence of the most severe manifestations of serotonin toxicity including hyperthermia and hyperreflexia.[5,21] Postsynaptic 5-HT$_{1A}$ receptors have also been linked with serotonin toxicity; however, these receptors exhibit a higher affinity for serotonin than 5-HT$_{2A}$ receptors, i.e., 5-HT$_{2A}$ receptors are highly saturated at relatively low serotonergic medication doses.[21] As such, overstimulation of 5-HT$_{1A}$ likely only contributes to milder serotonin toxicity symptoms including hyperactivity and anxiety.[21] However, if a medication that increases synaptic serotonin activity, such as a selective serotonin reuptake inhibitor (SSRI) is coadministered with a second-generation antipsychotics known to block 5-HT$_{2A}$ receptors and also activate 5-HT$_{1A}$ receptors, such as aripiprazole, this could result in excessive serotonin stimulation and ultimately toxicity.[22] Antagonism of 5-HT$_{2A}$ receptors may also increase endogenous serotonergic neurotransmission and risk of toxicity via inhibition of gamma-aminobutyric acid (GABA) interneurons in the dorsal raphe nuclei.[21] Though glutamatergic, dopaminergic, and noradrenergic activity have also been reported to have a role in the emergence of serotonin toxicity, their specific contribution remains elusive at this time.[5]

Besides the SSRI antidepressants, serotonin norepinephrine reuptake inhibitors (SNRIs) and tricyclic antidepressants (TCAs) can increase serotonin. In addition, monoamine oxidase inhibitors (MAOIs) selective for MAO-A increase serotonin concentrations by delaying the degradation of serotonin.[22] Serotonin toxicity is possible with any of these therapeutic agents, yet it is relatively rare in monotherapy. In fact, only about 15% of patients receiving supratherapeutic SSRI dosages develop even a moderate level of serotonin toxicity.[21,22] Table 6.2 shows a list of many of the medications with primary serotonergic actions that have been associated with serotonin toxicity.

Severe serotonin toxicity is most likely to occur due to pharmacodynamic interactions from concomitant administration of more than one serotonergic agent.[21] The combination

Table 6.2 Medications and Illicit Drugs that Mediate Serotonergic Activity[22,23,59,79-90]

Mechanism of Action	Medication/Illicit Drug		
Increased 5-HT Synthesis	L-tryptophan		
Increased S-HT Release	Amphetamines Bromocriptine Buprenorphine Carbamazepine Cocaine	Dextromethorphan Ecstasy (3,4-MDMA) Fentanyl Lithium Levodopa	Meperidine Mirtazapine Phentermine Synthetic cathinones Tramadol
5-HT Reuptake Inhibition	Amphetamines Brompheniramine Chlorpheniramine Cocaine Cyclobenzaprine Dextromethorphan Ecstasy	Methadone Meperidine Metoclopramide Nefazodone Phentermine SNRIs SSRIs	St. John's Wort TCAs Tramadol Trazodone Vilazodone Vortioxetine
MAD Inhibition and Reduced 5-HT Metabolism	Isocarboxazid (irreversible, non-selective) Isoniazid (irreversible, non-selective) Linezolid (reversible, non-selective)	Phenelzine (irreversible, non-selective) Rasagillne (irreversible, selective MAO-B inhibitor at < 1 mg/day)	Selegiline (irreversible, selective MAD-EI inhibitor at < 10 mg/day) Tranylcypromine (Irreversible, non-selective)
S-HT₁ Receptor Activation	Bromocriptine Buspirone Carbamazepine Ergot derivatives Fentanyl	Lithium Lysergic acid diethylamide (LSD) Mirtazapine Trazodone	Triptans Valproats Vilazodone Vortioxetine
5-HT₂ Receptor Activation	LSD		
5-HT₂ₐ Receptor Antagonism	Mirtazapine Nefazodone	Second generation antipsychotics Trazodone	
Other	Bupropion (5-HT activity controversial; may upregulate VMATs) Lithium (may increase sensitivity of post-synaptic serotonin receptors.)		

Table 6.3 Pharmacokinetic Interactions That May Increase Risk of Serotonin Toxicity[1,3,23,58,82,84,91-95]

Metabolic Enzyme	Select Substrates			Select Notable Inhibitors	
CYPlA2	Amitriptyline Clomipramine Clozapine Cyclobenzaprine	Desipramine Doxepin Duloxetine Fluvoxamine	Imipramine Olanzapine Zolmitriptan	Ciprofloxacin Fluvoxamine	
CYP2C9	Fluoxetine Trimipramine Valproate	Venlafaxine Vortioxetine		Amiodarone Capecitabine Fluconazohe	Fluvoxamine Voriconazole
CYP2C19	Citalopram Clomipramine Escitalopram	Trimiprarmine Venlafaxine Valproate	Vortioxetine	Amiodarone Capecitabine Fluconazole	Fluvoxamine Voriconazole
CYP2D6	Amitriptyline Aripiprazole Brexpiprazole Clomipramine Cyclobenzaprine Desipramine Dextromethorphan Doxepin Duloxetine	Ecstasy Escitalopram Fluoxetine Fluwoxarmine Imipramine Mirtazapine Nortriptyline Paroxetine Phentermine	Pimavanserin Protriptyline Risperidone Serotonin Sertraline Tramadol Trimipramine Venlafaxine Vortioxetine	Bupropion Cinacalcet Duloxetine Ecstasy Fluoxetine Paroxetine Quinidine Terbinafine	
CYP3A4	Aripiprazole Bromocriptine Buprenorphine Buspirone Carbamazepine Citalopram Cocaine	Cyclobenzaprine Eletriptan Fentanyl Mirtazapine Nortriptyline Pantoprazole Pimavanserin Quetiapine	Risperidone Serotonin Trazodone Venlafaxine Vilazodone Vortioxetine Ziprasidone	Ciprofloxacin Clarithromycin Diltiazem Erythromycin Fluconazole Fluoxetine Fluoxetine Indinavir	Itraconazole Ketoconazole Nefazodone Nelfinavir Ritonavir Telithromycin Verapamil Voriconazole
P-Glycoprotein	Doxepin Paroxetine Venlafaxine			Cyclosporine Fluvoxamine Norfluoxetine	Paroxetine Tacrolimus

of an MAOI with an SSRI or SNRI has been associated with life-threatening cases of serotoninergic toxicity.[23] Pharmacokinetic interactions shown in Table 6.3 have been linked to serotonin toxicity as well. Metabolic enzymes may be inhibited by a given drug, causing serotonergic substrates for that metabolic enzyme to accumulate to toxic levels. The World Health Organization (WHO), Food and Drug Administration (FDA) and Health Canada have also reported that $5\text{-}HT_3$ antagonists (e.g., the antiemetic ondansetron) and triptans prescribed for migraines may also lead to serotonin toxicity; however, this remains controversial and the risk appears very low at this time.[24-26]

Management and Prognosis

Discontinuation of the serotonergic agent(s) and supportive management remain the primary management modality. With treatment, the syndrome usually resolves within one

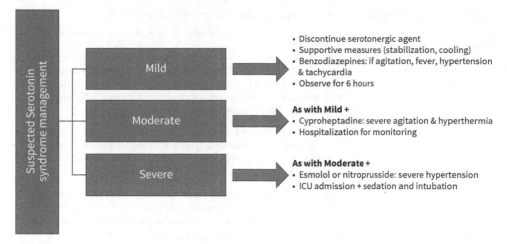

Figure 6.3 Serotonin syndrome management algorithm.

week. Treatment for mild cases includes discontinuation of the serotonergic agent, supportive care, sedation with benzodiazepines, and observation for at least 6 hours. Moderate cases can be similarly treated along with the addition of a serotonin antagonist (e.g., cyproheptadine) and admission to the hospital for cardiac monitoring and observation. In severe, life-threatening cases, the patient should also be treated with the addition of sedation, muscle paralysis, and intubation/ventilation in the intensive care unit (Figure 6.3).[5,21,22]

Common management pitfalls include failure to recognize serotonin syndrome, misdiagnosis, and failure to understand serotonin syndrome's potentially rapid rate of progression. A high degree of suspicion from the clinician is critical to ensure that serotonergic agents are withheld, and timely, aggressive supportive care is provided. The need for additional interventions must be anticipated before the patient's condition deteriorates. Prognosis is generally favorable, as long as the syndrome is promptly recognized and complications are appropriately treated.

Special Considerations

Medication-Specific Considerations

The potential role of a serotoninergic drug in causing serotonin toxicity cannot be discounted until the medication is expected to have been fully eliminated from the body based on its elimination half-life.[5] A general rule of thumb for the duration of a medication to be fully eliminated from the body is within 3–7 (an average of 5) elimination half-lives. Table 6.4 summarizes some additional considerations designed to limit the risk of serotonin toxicity with certain serotonergic medications and medication classes.

Although certain drug classes and combinations have a much higher risk of serotonin toxicity than others, caution is advised when prescribing any drug or combination of drugs that increase serotonergic activity. Moreover, patients should be educated about the signs and symptoms of serotonin toxicity, as well as potential interactions between their serotonergic medication(s) and other prescribed or over-the-counter medications along with herbal supplements and of course illicit drugs.

Table 6.4 Prescribing Considerations to Limit Risk of Serotonin Toxicity[5],[96-99]

Medication Class	Considerations
non-Selective, Irreversible MAOis or MAO-A Inhibitors	Do not prescribe with other serotonergic agents. A 2.week washout is recommended when transitioning to or from another serotonergic agent (5-weeks when transitioning from fluoxetine due to the long elimination half-life of this agent and its active metabolite)
MAO-B Inhibitors (e.g., selegiline or rasagiline)	May be prescribed with other serotonergic agents (e.g.,SSRIs) with caution. This practice should be limited, when possible. Titrate slowly to the lowest effective dosage of each agent prescribed. MAO-B inhibitors should be dosed within the appropriate dosage range for MAO-B selectivity.
Non-selective, Reversible, Weak MAOI Antibiotic (i.e. linezolid)	If an alternative antibiotic cannot be utilized, linezolid initiation should not he postponed due to a perceived need to washout SSRI or SNR I therapy. The decision to continue vs. temporarily discontinue antidepressant pharmacotherapy should be based on control of psychiatric sx. Patients should be monitored closely for serotonin toxicity.
Serotonin Reuptake Inhibitors (e.g., SSRIs and SNRIs)	Dose-optimized treatment with a single serotonin reuptake inhibitor should be considered to manage medical and mental health conditions, rather than use of an SSRI with an SNRI, for example. While older literature supported combining a TCA with an SSRI for treatment-resistant depression, this does not reflect current practice.
Opioids	Consider use of lower risk opioids when serotonergic agents are prescribed. Risk of serotonin toxicity among opioid agents is outlined below: • High risk opioids (avoid with MAOls or in patients with a history of serotonin toxicity): tramadol and meperidine • Moderate risk opioids (monitor closely for signs of serotonin toxicity): fentanyl, methadone, oxycodone • Low risk opioids (no restrictions): codeine, morphine, buprenorphine,, hydrornorphone, and oxymorphone
Triptans	May be given in combination with an SSRI or SNRI, with close monitoring for signs and symptoms of serotonin toxicity
5-HT, antagonists (e.g. ondansetron, granisetron)	May be prescribed with other serotonergic drugs, if necessary. Monitor for signs and symptoms of serotonin toxicity.

Pediatric Population

Serotonin syndrome in the pediatric population resembles that in the adult population. The same diagnostic criteria apply to the pediatric population. Hyperreflexia, clonus, and hyperthermia remain important findings. However, additional obstacles may make the diagnosis of SS more difficult in pediatric patients. Children often communicate vague symptoms and clinicians often do not consider the syndrome as a differential diagnosis in pediatric patients. Moreover, adolescents may be reluctant to disclose illicit drug use. Once identified, the basic tenants of management and treatment options for serotonin syndrome in pediatric patients remains the same as in adult patients. All serotonergic agents need to be stopped and supportive care provided with the goal being adequate patient sedation and normal vital signs.[27-30]

Neuroleptic Malignant syndrome (NMS)

Introduction and Epidemiology

Neuroleptic malignant syndrome (NMS) is a life-threatening emergency caused by adverse reaction to antipsychotic medication (or other antidopaminergic agent) and characterized by a distinctive clinical syndrome of mental status change, rigidity, fever, and dysautonomia (Figure 6.4). Dysautonomia and systemic complications are the main cause of death from the syndrome.[31] The first reported case of NMS appeared in 1956, shortly after the introduction of the antipsychotic drug chlorpromazine (Thorazine).[32] In 1960, a group of French clinicians reported an adverse event in association with haloperidol that they identified as "syndrome malin des neuroleptiques," that was subsequently translated to neuroleptic malignant syndrome.[33,34]

The incidence of NMS is estimated between 0.02%–3% among patients treated with antipsychotic antidopaminergic medication. Recent data suggest a decline in NMS rates to 0.01%–0.02% presumably due to increased awareness of the risk of NMS as well as a relatively reduced risk in patients prescribed second generation antipsychotic medication. There are also encouraging data suggesting that mortality rates in NMS have drastically declined from 20% to 6% in recent years.[35,36]

NMS can occur at any age, but males under 40 years of age demonstrated a two-times greater risk for development of NMS compared to female patients.[37] There are also data suggesting the possibility of a genetic risk for NMS in identical twins as well as a mother and two of her daughters as reported in one article.[38] However, the most consistent risk factors for the development of NMS remain high-potency for D2 receptor antipsychotic medication, rapid dose increases in antipsychotic medication, and the use of long-acting depot formulations of antipsychotics. It should be noted that patients with Lewy body dementia are not only extremely sensitive to adverse events with antipsychotic medication but also may have an increased risk of NMS like symptoms.[39,40]

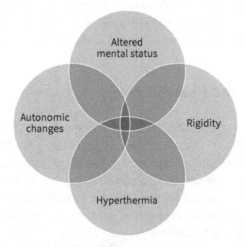

Figure 6.4 Neuroleptic malignant syndrome tetrad.

Manifestations, Diagnostic Criteria, and Differential Diagnosis

Typically, diagnosis is made in a patient taking antipsychotics who develops clinical symptoms consistent with NMS (Figure 6.4). In 2011, the International Multispecialty Consensus Group published diagnostic criteria for NMS using the Delphi method based on clinical symptoms and laboratory findings and specifying the "core symptoms."[41] Unfortunately, there are still no universally accepted criteria for NMS at this time.[41] DSM-5, published in 2013, lists NMS under "medication-induced movement disorders and other adverse effects of medication;" however no specific diagnostic criteria are listed.[42]

Given this complex scenario, NMS remains a diagnostic challenge. Although there is currently no specific diagnostic test that stablishes a diagnosis of NMS, lab testing does play a crucial role in the evaluation of patients with potential NMS. Serum creatine kinase (CK) levels are particularly essential and typically are more than 1,000 international units/L in NMS; and CK levels as high as 100,000 international units/L can occur. However, CK levels may be normal early in the onset of NMS especially if muscular rigidity has not yet developed.[43-46] Other lab findings commonly present but not specific to NMS include leukocytosis (10,000-400,000/mm^3), elevated lactate dehydrogenase, alkaline phosphatase and liver transaminase levels, low serum iron and electrolyte abnormalities.

Cases of atypical NMS have also been reported, in which milder forms were linked to the use of lower potency D2 antagonistic agents. In such cases, rigidity may be milder and perhaps even absent. While fever is considered an essential feature of NMS, mild cases without fever are reported. As a result, it may be reasonable to consider the diagnosis whenever any two of the tetrad of NMS symptoms emerge in the setting of a dopamine antagonist.[47-52]

The differential diagnosis of NMS includes SS (Table 6.1), malignant hyperthermia (rare genetic disorder with susceptible individuals exposed to halogenated volatile anesthetics and depolarizing muscle relaxants),[19,20] catatonia (prodrome of psychosis, agitation, and excitement as well as specific motor symptoms; posturing, waxy flexibility, stereotypic movements, and others),[53-55] drug induced parkinsonism, and CNS infections (prodrome of viral illness).

Pathophysiology and Pharmacology

The pathogenesis of NMS is generally considered to be secondary to dopamine blockade with subsequent disruption of the hypothalamus and corpus striatum resulting in temperature dysregulation and muscle contractions.[56] Since the dopamine pathway is crucial to hypothalamic function and temperature regulation, dopamine receptor antagonists (antipsychotics) can precipitate hyperthermia, arrhythmias, irregular blood pressure and respiratory dysfunction. Additionally, dopamine blockade in the corpus striatum can produce increased muscular rigidity that in turn may trigger rhabdomyolysis.[31] Blockage of the D2 has historically been recognized as the sine qua non of antipsychotic efficacy. Rapid antipsychotic dosage reduction was reported to predispose patients to a similar risk of NMS as that associated with rapid dose escalation.[57] Moreover, abrupt discontinuation of an antipsychotic medication may trigger NMS again as a secondary manifestation of dopaminergic dysregulation.

Although antipsychotic medications are most commonly associated with NMS, other medications with dopamine antagonist properties can also result in NMS. The tricyclic antidepressant amoxapine has low-potency D2 antagonism and is associated with an increased risk of NMS in comparison to other antidepressants.[58] Carbamazepine, deutetrabenazine, droperidol, metoclopramide, prochlorperazine, promethazine, tetrabenazine, and valbenazine also have antidopaminergic activity that may predispose to NMS, although not all of these have been clinically established.[58-61] Valproic acid has been associated with NMS; the mechanism is thought to be related to GABA-mediated modulation of dopaminergic activity.[62] Lithium is also associated with NMS presumably by promoting dopaminergic hypoactivity through its ability to block the accumulation of intracellular cyclic adenosine monophosphate.[63] Case reports have also reported NMS in association with lamotrigine; the purported mechanism remains unclear, although experimental studies with lamotrigine have implicated indirect effects on glutamatergic and GABAergic activity resulting in dopaminergic hypofunction.[64,65]

The reduction in dopaminergic activity associated with abrupt discontinuation of dopamine agonists, such as amantadine, baclofen, or levodopa, may also increase risk for an NMS like symptoms, although it is not clear that this represents the same entity.[66] NMS can also be seen with anticholinergic agents especially when they are prescribed in combination with an antipsychotic.[66] Chronic anticholinergic therapy leads to cholinergic receptor supersensitivity. Therefore, abrupt discontinuation results in an acute hypercholinergic state.[67] Since both clozapine and amitriptyline possess potent anticholinergic activity, they are also associated with an increased NMS risk. Use of more than one dopaminergic agent increases the risk of NMS.[36,18] NMS may occur through pharmacodynamic and pharmacokinetic interactions (Table 6.5).

Management and Prognosis

As with SS, discontinuation of the offending agents (dopaminergic drugs) or other potential contributing agents is the cornerstone of NMS management. If the syndrome occurs in the setting of abrupt withdrawal of a dopaminergic medication, then the medication should be reinstituted as soon as possible unless contraindications exist. Initiation of supportive medical therapy is paramount in achieving a favorable clinical outcome. This includes aggressive hydration if CK is elevated (to protect the kidneys from rhabdomyolysis and disseminated intravascular coagulation), treatment of hyperthermia through cooling or ice packs, or correction of metabolic disturbances (Figure 6.5).[68-70]

In more severe cases of NMS, empiric pharmacologic therapy is typically tried. The two most frequently used medications are bromocriptine, which is given to reverse the hypodopaminergic state,[46,71] and dantrolene sodium for muscle rigidity.[72-74] Amantadine and levodopa as well as benzodiazepines have also been used in the treatment of NMS (Figure 6.5).[75]

Based on its reported efficacy in malignant catatonia, electroconvulsive therapy (ECT) has also been proposed as a potential treatment in NMS. Though controlled data are not available, there are case reports indicating ECT was effective in select patients. However, ECT is generally reserved for patients that are refractory and/or poor candidates for standard

Table 6.5 Pharmacokinetic Interactions That May Increase Risk of NMS[5,58,94,95,100-102]

Metabolic Enzyme	Select Substrates			Select Notable Inhibitors	
CYP1A2	Asenapine	Loxapine	Thiothixene	Ciprofloxacin	
	Chlorpromazine	Olanzapine	Trifluoperazine	Flivoxamine	
	Clozapine	Pimozide	Ziprasidone		
	Haloperidol				
CYP2C9	Valproate			Amiodarone	Fluvoxamine
				Capecitabine	Voriconazole
CYP2C19	Loxapine			Esomeprazole	Oxcarbazepine
	Valproate			Omeprazole	Voriconazole
CYP2D6	Amoxapine	Haloperridol	Pimavanserin	Asenapine	Haloperidol
	Aripiprazole	lloperidone	Pimozide	Bupropion	Metoclopramide
	Brexpiprazole	Loxapine	Promethazine	Cinacalcet	Paroxetine
	Chloapromazine	Metociopramind	Risperidone	Duloxetine	Promethazine
	Deutetrabenazine	Olanzapine	Tetrabenazine	Ecstasy	Terbinafine
	Fluphenazine	Paliperidone	Thiroridazine	Fluoxetine	Thioridazine
		Perphenazine	Valbenazine	Fluphenazine	
CYP3A4	Aripiprazole		Paliperidone	Ciprofloxacin	Itraconazole
	Brexpiprazole		Pantoprazole	Clarithromycin	Ketoconazole
	Carbamazepine		Pimavanserin	Diltiazem	Nelfinavir
	Cariprazine		Pimozide	Erythromycin	Ritonavir
	Haloperidol		Quetiapine	Fluconazole	Telithromycin
	Iloperidone		Risperidone	Fluvoxamine	Verapamil
	Loxapine		Valbenazine	Haloperidol	Voriconazole
	Lurasidone		Ziprasidone	Indinavir	

treatment interventions for NMS. If pursued as a treatment in NMS, it is recommended that ECT be used early in refractory cases as a life-saving intervention.[76,77]

NMS is potentially lethal with reported mortality rates of 5%–20%. Fortunately, early intervention is associated with a favorable prognosis and NMS usually resolves within two

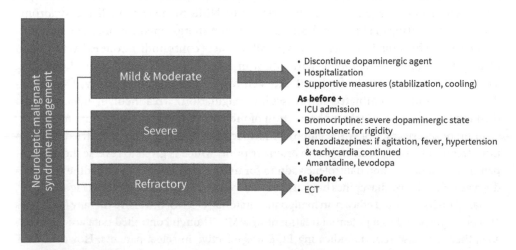

Figure 6.5 Neuroleptic malignant syndrome management algorithm.

weeks (mean recovery time of 7 to 11 days). Most patients recover without neurologic sequelae unless severe hypoxia or grossly elevated temperatures were present for a long duration. There are a few reports of residual NMS symptoms persisting for up to 6 months.[72,73]

Special Considerations: Restarting Antipsychotics

Patients restarted on antipsychotic agents after NMS are at an increased risk for recurrent NMS. Estimated relapse rates may be as high as 30%. However, risk of NMS recurrence can be reduced by waiting at least two weeks or longer before restarting antipsychotic medication after recovery as well as using lower-potency second-generation antipsychotic medication with gradual dose titration and lower overall dosage regimens. Careful monitoring of patients for early signs of NMS is also critical.[69,78]

Conclusion and Future Directions

SS and NMS are rare, but potentially life-threatening medication-induced emergencies. Whereas serotonergic excess appears to underlie the emergence of SS, dopaminergic deficits are essential to the development of NMS. Close attention to clinical symptoms, a detailed physical exam, and a high level of suspicion for potential offending agents is key in diagnosing the two syndromes. When multiple medications are present, consideration of potential pharmacokinetic and pharmacodynamic factors including drug interactions is absolutely critical. Laboratory abnormalities may aid in making the correct diagnosis of NMS, but SS lacks characteristic lab findings. Prompt recognition and discontinuation of the causative agents is imperative in preventing serious complications. Since SS and NMS are treated differently, clinicians must be able to rapidly and accurately differentiate between the two syndromes. Given their severity, raising awareness in patients about SS and NMS may also increase early recognition and prompt management. Both conditions require more research especially in terms of development of more universally accepted diagnostic criteria as well as further identification of risk factors and more effective treatment.

References

1. Kant, S., & Liebelt, E. (2012). Recognizing serotonin toxicity in the pediatric emergency department. *Pediatr Emer Care*. 28:817–824.
2. Foong, A.L., Grindrod, K.A., Patel, T., & Kellar, J. (2018). Demystifying serotonin syndrome (or serotonin toxicity). *Can Fam Physician*. 64:720–727.
3. Francescangeli, J., Karamchandani, K., Powell, M., & Bonavia, A. (2019). The serotonin syndrome: from molecular mechanisms to clinical practice. *Int J Mol Sci*. 20(9):2288. Published 2019 May 9. https://doi.org/10.3390/ijms20092288
4. Dvir, Y., & Smallwood, P. (2008). Serotonin syndrome: a complex but easily avoidable condition. *Gen Hosp Psychiatry*. 30(3):284–287. https://doi.org/10.1016/j.genhosppsych.2007.09.007
5. Volpi-Abadie, J., Kaye, A.M., & Kaye, A.D. (2013). Serotonin syndrome. *Ochsner J*. 13(4):533–540.

6. Katus, L.E., Frucht, S.J. (2016). Management of serotonin syndrome and neuroleptic malignant syndrome. *Curr Treat Options Neurol.* 18(9):39. https://doi.org/10.1007/s11940-016-0423-4

7. Foong, A.L., Patel, T., Kellar, J., & Grindrod, K.A. (2018). The scoop on serotonin syndrome. *Can Pharm J (Ott).* 151(4):233–239. Published 2018 May 30. https://doi.org/10.1177/1715163518779096

8. Bronstein, A.C., Spyker, D.A., Cantilena, L.R. Jr., Rumack, B.H., & Dart, R.C. (2012). 2011 Annual report of the American Association of Poison Control Centers' National Poison Data System (NPDS): 29th Annual Report [published correction appears in Clin Toxicol (Phila). Dec;52(10):1286–7]. Clin Toxicol (Phila). 2012;50(10):911–1164. https://doi.org/10.3109/15563650.2012.746424

9. Karkow, D.C., Kauer, J.F., & Ernst, E.J. (2017). Incidence of serotonin syndrome with combined use of linezolid and serotonin reuptake inhibitors compared with linezolid monotherapy. *J Clin Psychopharmacol* 37(5):518–523. https://doi.org/10.1097/JCP.0000000000000751

10. Gummin, D.D., Mowry, J.B., Spyker, D.A., et al. (2019) 2018 Annual Report of the American Association of Poison Control Centers' National Poison Data System (NPDS): 36th Annual Report. *Clin Toxicol.* 57(12):1220–1413. https://doi.org/10.1080/15563650.2019.1677022

11. Nguyen, C.T., Xie, L., Alley, S., McCarron, R.M., Baser, O., & Wang, Z. (2017). Epidemiology and economic burden of serotonin syndrome with concomitant use of serotonergic agents: a retrospective study utilizing two large US claims databases. *Prim Care Companion CNS Disord.* 19(6):17m02200. Published 2017 December 28. https://doi.org/10.4088/PCC.17m02200.

12. Uddin, M.F., Alweis, R., Shah, S.R., et al. (2017). Controversies in serotonin syndrome diagnosis and management: a review. *J Clin Diagn Res.* 11(9):OE05–OE07. https://doi.org/10.7860/JCDR/2017/29473.10696

13. Sternbach, H. (1991). The serotonin syndrome. *Am J Psychiatry.* 148:705–713.

14. Radomski, J.W., Dursun, S.M., Reveley, M.A., & Kutcher, S.P. (2000). An exploratory approach to the serotonin syndrome: an update of clinical phenomenology and revised diagnostic criteria. *Med Hypotheses.* 55:218–224. https://doi.org/10.1054/mehy.2000.1047

15. Dunkley E.J., Isbister G.K., Sibbritt D., Dawson A.H., & Whyte I.M. (2003). The hunter serotonin toxicity criteria: simple and accurate diagnostic decision rules for serotonin toxicity. *QJM.* 96:635–642. https://doi.org/10.1093/qjmed/hcg109

16. Greenberg, M.I. (2003). NMS versus serotonin syndrome: a clinical conundrum. *Emerg Med News.* 25(3):23–23.

17. Sokoro, A.A., Zivot, J., & Ariano, R.E. (2011). Neuroleptic malignant syndrome versus serotonin syndrome: the search for a diagnostic tool. *Ann Pharmacother.* 45:e50.

18. Perry, P.J., & Wilborn, C.A. (2012). Serotonin syndrome vs neuroleptic malignant syndrome: a contrast of causes, diagnoses, and management. *Ann Clin Psychiatry.* 24(2):155–162.

19. Rosenberg, H., Pollock, N., Schiemann, A., Bulger, T., & Stowell, K. (2015). Malignant hyperthermia: a review. *Orphanet J Rare Dis.* 10:93. https://doi.org/10.1186/s13023-015-0310-1

20. Litman, R.S., Griggs, S.M., Dowling, J.J., & Riazi, S. (2018). Malignant hyperthermia susceptibility and related diseases. *Anesthesiology.* 128(1):159–167. https://doi.org/ https://doi.org/10.1097/ALN.0000000000001877 .

21. Scotton, W.J., Hill, L.J., Williams, A.C., & Barnes, N.M. (2019). Serotonin syndrome: pathophysiology, clinical features, management, and potential future directions. *Int J Tryptophan Res.* 12:1178646919873925. https://doi.org/10.1177/1178646919873925

22. Frank, C. (2008). Recognition and treatment of serotonin syndrome. *Can Fam Physician.* 54;988–992.

23. Park, S.H., Wackernah, R.C., & Stimmel, G.L. (2014). Serotonin syndrome: is it a reason to avoid the use of tramadol with antidepressants? *J Pharm Pract.* 27(1):71–78.

24. Gillman, P.K. (2010). Triptans, serotonin agonists and serotonin syndrome (serotonin toxicity): a review. *Headache.* 50(2):264–272.

25. Gillman, P.K. (2014). Regulatory agencies (WHO, FDA) offer ill-conceived advice about serotonin toxicity (serotonin syndrome) with 5-HT3 antagonists: a worldwide problem. March 4, 2015. Health Canada. Summary safety review—serotonin blocking drugs (serotonin antagonists) ALOXI (palonosetron), ANZEMET (dolasetron), KYTRIP (granisetron) and generics and ZOFRAN (ondansetron) and generics—serotonin syndrome. May 14, 2014.

26. Gillman, P.K. (2009). Is there sufficient evidence to suggest cyclobenzaprine might be implicated in causing serotonin toxicity? *Am J Emerg Med.* 27(4):509–501.

27. Gill, M., LoVecchio, F., & Selden, B. (1999). Serotonin syndrome in a child after a single dose of fluvoxamine. *Ann Emerg Med.* 33(4):457–459. https://doi.org/10.1016/s0196-0644(99)70313-6

28. Pao, M., & Tipnis, T. (1997). Serotonin syndrome after sertraline overdose in a 5-year-old girl. *Arch Pediatr Adolesc Med.* 151(10):1064–1067. https://doi.org/10.1001/archpedi.1997.02170470098028

29. Godinho, E.M., Thompson, A.E., & Bramble, D.J. (2002). Neuroleptic withdrawal versus serotonergic syndrome in an 8-year-old child. *J Child Adolesc Psychopharmacol.* 12(3):265–270. https://doi.org/10.1089/104454602760386969

30. Laine, K., Heikkinen, T., Ekblad, U., & Kero, P.(2003). Effects of exposure to selective serotonin reuptake inhibitors during pregnancy on serotonergic symptoms in newborns and cord blood monoamine and prolactin concentrations. *Arch Gen Psychiatry.* 60(7):720–726. https://doi.org/10.1001/archpsyc.60.7.720

31. Modi, S., Dharaiya, D., Schultz, L., & Varelas, P. (2016). Neuroleptic malignant syndrome: complications, outcomes, and mortality. *Neurocrit Care.* 24(1):97–103. https://doi.org/10.1007/s12028-015-0162-5

32. Ayd, F.J., Jr. (1956). Fatal hyperpyrexia during chlorpromazine therapy. *J Clin Exp Psychopathol.* 17(2):189–192.

33. Buckley, P.F., & Hutchinson, M. (1995). Neuroleptic malignant syndrome. *J Neurol Neurosurg Psychiatry.* 58(3):271–273.

34. Khaldi, S., Kornreich, C., Choubani, Z., & Gourevitch, R. (2008). Antipsychotiques atypiques et syndrome malin des neuroleptiques: brève revue de la littérature [Neuroleptic malignant syndrome and atypical antipsychotics: A brief review] (pdf). *Encephale.* 34(6):618–624. https://doi.org/10.1016/j.encep.2007.11.007

35. Berman, B.D. (2011). Neuroleptic malignant syndrome: a review for neurohospitalists. *Neurohospitalist.* 1(1):41–47. https://doi.org/10.1177/1941875210386491

36. Tse, L., Barr, A.M., Scarapicchia, V., & Vila-Rodriguez, F. (2015). Neuroleptic malignant syndrome: a review from a clinically oriented perspective. *Curr Neuropharmacol.* 13(3):395–406. https://doi.org/10.2174/1570159x13999150424113345

37. Gupta, V., Magon, R., Mishra, B.P., Sidhu, G.B., & Mahajan, R. (2003). Risk factors in neuroleptic malignant syndrome. *Indian J Psychiatry.* 45(1):30–35.

38. Otani, K., Horiuchi, M., Kondo, T., Kaneko, S., & Fukushima, Y. (1991). Is the predisposition to neuroleptic malignant syndrome genetically transmitted? *Brit J Psychiatry.* 158(6):850–853. https://doi.org/10.1192/bjp.158.6.850

39. Zweig, Y.R., & Galvin, J.E. (2014). Lewy body dementia: the impact on patients and caregivers. *Alzheimers Res Ther.* 6(2):21. Published 2014 April 25. https://doi.org/10.1186/alzrt25

40. Oruch, R., Pryme, I.F., Engelsen, B.A., & Lund, A. (2017). Neuroleptic malignant syndrome: an easily overlooked neurologic emergency. *Neuropsychiatr Dis Treat.* 13:161–175. Published 2017 January 16. https://doi.org/10.2147/NDT.S118438.

41. Gurrera, R.J., Caroff, S.N., Cohen, A., et al. (2011). An international consensus study of neuroleptic malignant syndrome diagnostic criteria using the Delphi method. *J Clin Psychiatry.* 72(9):1222–1228.

42. American Psychiatric Association. (2013). *Diagnostic and Statistical Manual of Mental Disorders.* 5th ed. Arlington, VA: American Psychiatric Association Publishing.

43. Gurrera, R.J. (2002). Is neuroleptic malignant syndrome a neurogenic form of malignant hyperthermia? *Clin Neuropharmacol.* 25(4):183–193. https://doi.org/10.1097/00002826-200207000-00001

44. Hermesh, H., Manor, I., Shiloh, R., et al. (2002). High serum creatinine kinase level: possible risk factor for neuroleptic malignant syndrome. *J Clin Psychopharmacol.* 22(3):252–256. https://doi.org/10.1097/00004714-200206000-00004

45. Ambulkar, R.P., Patil, V.P., & Moiyadi, A.V. (2012). Neuroleptic malignant syndrome: a diagnostic challenge. *J Anaesthesiol Clin Pharmacol.* 28(4):517–519. https://doi.org/10.4103/0970-9185.101946

46. Al Danaf, J., Madara, J., & Dietsche, C. (2015). Neuroleptic malignant syndrome: a case aimed at raising clinical awareness. *Case Rep Med.* 2015:769576. https://doi.org/10.1155/2015/769576.

47. Reeves, R.R., Torres, R.A., Liberto, V., & Hart, H.H. (2002). Atypical neuroleptic malignant syndrome associated with olanzapine. *Pharmacotherapy.* 2(5):641–644. https://doi.org/10.1592/phco.22.8.641.33211

48. Picard, L.S., Lindsay, S., Strawn, J.R., Kaneria, R.M., Patel, N.C., & Keck, P.E., Jr. (2008). Atypical neuroleptic malignant syndrome: diagnostic controversies and considerations. *Pharmacotherapy.* 28(4):530–535. https://doi.org/10.1592/phco.22.8.641.33211

49. Carroll, B.T., & Surber, S.A. (2009). The problem of atypical neuroleptic malignant syndrome: a case report. *Psychiatry.* 6(7):45–47.

50. Collins, A., Davies, D., & Menon, S. (2016). Atypical neuroleptic malignant syndrome. *Case Reports BMJ.* 2016:bcr2016214901.

51. Leonardo, Q.F., Juliana, G.R., & Fernando, C.J. (2017). Atypical neuroleptic malignant syndrome associated with use of clozapine. *Case Rep Emerg Med.* 2017:2174379. https://doi.org/10.1155/2017/2174379

52. Özdemir, İ., Kuru, E., Safak, Y., & Tulacı, R.G. (2018). A neuroleptic malignant syndrome without rigidity. *Psychiatry Investig.* 15(2):226–229. https://doi.org/10.30773/pi.2017.06.05

53. Rasmussen, S.A., Mazurek, M.F., & Rosebush, P.I. (2016). Catatonia: our current understanding of its diagnosis, treatment and pathophysiology. *World J Psychiatry.* 6(4):391–398. Published 2016 December 22. https://doi.org/10.5498/wjp.v6.i4.39

54. Pelzer, A.C., van der Heijden, F.M., & den Boer. E. (2018). Systematic review of catatonia treatment. *Neuropsychiatr Dis Treat.* 14:317–326. Published 2018 January 17. https://doi.org/10.2147/NDT.S147897

55. Walther, S., Stegmayer, K., Wilson, J.E., & Heckers, S. (2019). Structure and neural mechanisms of catatonia. *Lancet Psychiatry.* 6(7):610–619. https://doi.org/10.1016/S2215-0366(18)30474-7

56. Bottoni, T.N. (2002). Neuroleptic malignant syndrome: a brief review. *Hosp Physician.* 38(3):58–63.

57. Amore, M., & Zazzeri, N. (1995). Neuroleptic malignant syndrome after neuroleptic discontinuation. *Prog Neuro-Psychopharmacol Biol Psychiatry.* 19:1323–1334.

58. Stahl, S. M., & Grady, M. M. (2017). *Stahl's Essential Psychopharmacology: The Prescriber's Guide* (6th ed.). Cambridge, UK; New York: Cambridge University Press.

59. Turner, A.H., Kim, J.J., McCarron, R.M., & Nguyen C.T. (2019). Differentiating serotonin syndrome and neuroleptic malignant syndrome. *Current Psychiatry.* 18(2):30–36.

60. Berman, B.D. (2011). Neuroleptic malignant syndrome: a review for neurohospitalists. *Neurohospitalist*. 1(1):41–47.
61. Teva Pharmaceuticals USA , Inc. Austedo˚ Package Insert. North Wales, PA: 2017, August.
62. Yildirim, V., Direk, M.C., Gunes, S., Okuyaz, Ç., & Toros, F. (2017). Neuroleptic malignant syndrome associated with valproate in an adolescent. *Clin Psychopharm Neurosci*. 15(1):76–78.
63. Patil, V., Gupta, R., Verma, R., & Balhara, Y.P.S. (2016). Neuroleptic malignant syndrome associated with lithium toxicity. *Oman Med*. 31(4):309–311.
64. Ishioka, M., Yasui-Furukori, N., Hashimoto, K., & Sugawara, N. (2013). Neuroleptic malignant syndrome induced by lamotrigine. *Clin Neuropharmacol*. 36:131–132.
65. Motomura, E., Tanii, H., Usami, A., Ohoyama, K., Nakagawa, M., & Okada, M. (2012). Lamotrigine-induced neuroleptic malignant syndrome under risperidone treatment: a case report. *J Neuropsychiatry Clin Neurosci*. 24(2):E38–E39.
66. Margetic, B., & Margetic, B.A. (2010). Neuroleptic malignant syndrome and its controversies. *Pharmacoepidemiol Drug Saf*. 19:429–435.
67. Alexander, P.J., Thomas, R.M., & Das, A. (1996). Occurrence of neuroleptic malignant syndrome on trihexyphenidyl discontinuation. *Indian J Psychiatry*. 38(4):250–253.
68. Strawn, J.R., & Keck, P.E Jr. (2006). Early bicarbonate loading and dantroline for ziprasidone/haloperidol-induced neuroleptic malignant syndrome. *J Clin Psychiatry*. 67(4):677. https://doi.org/10.4088/jcp. v67n0420e
69. Strawn, J.R., Keck, P.E., Jr., & Caroff, S.N. (2007). Neuroleptic malignant syndrome. *Am J Psychiatry*. 164(6):870–876. https://doi.org/10.1176/ajp.2007.164.6.870
70. Wijdicks, E.F. (2020). Neuroleptic malignant syndrome. [Accessed June 10, 2020]. https://www.uptodate.com/contents/neuroleptic-malignant-syndrome
71. Drews, J.D., Christopher, A., & Evans, D.C. (2017). Neuroleptic malignant syndrome in the trauma intensive care unit: diagnosis and management of a rare disease in a challenging population. *Int J Crit Illn Inj Sci*. 7(2):119–121. https://doi.org/10.4103/IJCIIS.IJCIIS_100_16
72. Reulbach, U., Dütsch, C., Biermann, T., et al. (2007). Managing an effective treatment for neuroleptic malignant syndrome. *Crit Care*. 11(1):R4. https://doi.org/10.1186/cc5148
73. Muehlschlegel, S., & Sims, J.R. (2009). Dantrolene: mechanisms of neuroprotection and possible clinical applications in the neurointensive care unit. *Neurocrit Care*. 10(1):103–115. https://doi.org/10.1007/s12028-008-9133-4
74. Whyte, C.J., & Rosini, J.M. (2018). Dantrolene for treatment of suspected neuroleptic malignant syndrome. *J Emerg Nurs*. 44(2):207–209. https://doi.org/10.1016/j.jen.2017.11.008
75. Ngo, V., Guerrero, A., Lanum, D., et al. (2019). Emergent treatment of neuroleptic malignant syndrome induced by antipsychotic monotherapy using dantrolene. *Clin Pract Cases Emerg Med*. 3(1):16–23. Published 2019 January 4. https://doi.org/10.5811/cpcem.2018.11.39667
76. Foguet-Boreu, Q., Coll-Negre, M., Serra-Millàs, M., & Cavalleria-Verdaguer, M. (2018). Neuroleptic malignant syndrome: a case responding to electroconvulsive therapy plus bupropion. *Clin Pract*. 8(1):1044. Published 2018 January 26. https://doi.org/10.4081/cp.2018.1044
77. Morcos, N., Rosinski, A., & Maixner, D.F. (2019). Electroconvulsive therapy for neuroleptic malignant syndrome. *Journal of ECT*. 35(4):225–230. https://doi.org/10.1097/YCT.0000000000000600
78. Simon, L.V., Hashmi, M.F., & Callahan, A,L. (2020). *Neuroleptic Malignant Syndrome*. StatPearls. Treasure Island (FL): StatPearls Publishing.

7

Movement Disorders Associated With SSRIs

Jennifer G. Goldman and Carlos Manuel Guerra Galicia

Introduction

Selective serotonin reuptake inhibitors (SSRIs) occupy a central place in today's neuropsychiatric therapeutic arsenal. These versatile agents are regularly used as first-line agents for treating depression, but are also useful for treating anxiety, panic, eating disorders, and obsessive-compulsive behaviors by potentiating the action of serotonin.[1,2] In general, SSRIs are easy to use and well tolerated, with reasonably good predictable clinical responses and usually few adverse effects. These attributes contribute to their widespread use in many medical specialties.[3,4]

Adverse effects, however, can occur with SSRIs, and movement disorders have been associated with SSRI use, which is the focus of this chapter. Adverse effects reported with SSRIs include gastrointestinal symptoms (nausea, vomiting, or diarrhea), sedation or stimulation, hyponatremia, seizures, sexual dysfunction, changes in appetite, alterations in platelet function, and the classic serotonin syndrome (serotonin toxicity).[5,6] Many of these adverse effects are typically mild, and for many people, the benefits of SSRIs overweigh their risk. SSRI toxicity, however, is a serious drug reaction, and dose augmentation or pharmacologic interactions, including with herbal supplements, can lead to severe reactions.[7–13] Table 7.1 shows drugs that enhance serotonin levels when used in combination. Classically, the Hunter Serotonin Toxicity Criteria include: spontaneous clonus, inducible clonus and agitation or diaphoresis, ocular clonus with agitation and diaphoresis, tremor and hyperreflexia, ocular clonus, hypertonicity, and temperature greater than 38°C in the context of serotonin medication exposure or overdose.[14] Serotonin toxicity usually resolves within 24 hours of discontinuation of serotonergic therapies and should be differentiated with neuroleptic malignant syndrome, which shares some features such as bradykinesia, rigidity, fever, and autonomic dysfunction, but with more insidious onset and slower resolution.[15] Of note, trazodone, fluoxetine, and sertraline were the most frequent antidepressants taken in excess in 2019, as reported in the American Association of Poison Control Centers' National Poison Data System Annual Report.[16]

SSRIs and Their Relationship to Neurochemistry

SSRIs were rationally designed in order to avoid the side effects associated with prior medications, namely tricyclic antidepressants (TCAs) and monoamine oxidase inhibitors (MAOIs), by targeting a specific site of action. Fluoxetine was the first SSRI introduced to the market in 1987, and after its approval by the US Food and Drug Administration (FDA), many others

Table 7.1 Drugs That Enhance Serotonin Levels in Combination With SSRIs

Mechanism	Drugs
Serotonin Reuptake Blocking	ondansetron, methadone, clomipramine, amitriptyline, dextromethorphan, fentanyl, meperidine, tramadol, trazodone, venlafaxine, pentazocine
Serotonin Metabolism Inhibition	linezoid, methylene blue, St. John's wort, phenelzine, selegiline, isocarboxazid
Serotonin Release Enhancers	methylenedioxymethamphatemine (mdma), mirtazapine
Serotonin Receptors Stimulation	buspirone, fentanyl, dihydroergotamine, lithium, metoclopramide, lysergic acid diethylamide (lsd)
Serotonin Precursor	tryptophan
Increase Serotonin Synthesis	cocaine
Serotonin Transporter (SERT) Inhibition	opioids

have been added to this pharmacological class.[17] These oral compounds share similarities regarding equivalent acute and maintenance antidepressant efficacy, a flat dose-response curve and ascending dose-response curve for antidepressant efficacy and good response rate for both depressive and anxiety disorders.[18] Table 7.2 shows currently available SSRIs, year of introduction, FDA-approved indications, receptor activity, and potential mechanism for movement disorders generation as adverse events.

The relationship between SSRIs and movement disorders involves understanding the concept that serotonin (5-HT) enhancement influences dopamine (DA) pathways in many brain regions, and has effects on other neurochemical systems. This enhancement may disrupt those neural networks and thereby manifest as a wide array of dopamine dysfunction symptoms. DA-containing neurons such as in the mesolimbic, mesocortical, and nigrostriatal systems receive rich innervation from 5-HT originating in the raphe nuclei of the brainstem, and both 5-HT and DA systems are closely related throughout the central nervous system.[19] Studies suggest that dysfunction of 5-HT and DA systems contributes to various neuropsychiatric disorders including depression, schizophrenia, drug abuse, and Parkinson's disease (PD).[20] Figure 7.1 depicts the dopaminergic pathways with serotonergic influence and effects.

The serotonergic system is complex with seven classes of 5-HT receptors, which are then subdivided into subclasses, resulting in at least 14 different receptors. The broad serotonergic system allows this neurotransmitter to exert many effects not only directly as a dopaminergic modulator, but also indirectly modifying GABAergic and glutamatergic input to the ventral tegmental area (VTA) and the substantia nigra pars compacta (SNc) and pars reticulata.[21] Experimental data demonstrated that 5-HT receptors 1A, 1B, 2A, 3, and 4 act to facilitate neuronal DA function and release, while the 5-HT receptor 2C mediates an inhibitory effect on the basal electrical activity of DA neurons and DA release.[19,22]

Serotonergic pathways and modulation remain a field of neuroscience research and discovery.[23] Interestingly, sigma-1 receptors have been proposed as potential therapeutic targets for neurodegenerative diseases such as Alzheimer's disease, PD, amyotrophic lateral

Table 7.2 Currently Available SSRIs, FDA Approved Indications, 5-HTA Receptor Activity, and Potential Mechanism of Movement Disorders Adverse Events Generation

SSRI (year of approval)	Indications (FDA)	Dose/day	Half life	5-HTA receptor activity	Potential mechanism for MD-AE
Fluoxetine (1987)	D (>8), PD, OCD (>7), BN, PMDD	20–80 mg 90 mg/week *(delayed release)*	2–4 days *metabolite Norfluoxetine:* 7–9 days	SERT inhibitor 5-HT$_{1A}$ agonist 5-HT$_{2A}$ mild antagonist 5-HT$_{2B}$ agonist 5-HT$_{2C}$ mild antagonist	5-HT enhanced effect, Facilitates neuronal DA release
Sertraline (1991)	D, PD, OCD, SAD, PTSD, PMDD	50–200 mg	22–36 hours	SERT potent inhibitor DAT inhibitor mild σ1 receptor antagonist	5-HT enhanced effect, Increases DA
Paroxetine (1992)	D, PD, OCD, SAD, GAD, PTSD, PMDD	20–60 mg	21 hours	SERT inhibitor NET inhibitor *(high doses)* M1 blockade	5-HT enhanced effect, NE enhanced effect, Muscarinic
Fluvoxamine (1994)	OCD (>8)	8–11 years 25–200 mg >11 years 25–300 mg	16 hours (26 hours in elderly, 58 hours in brain)	SERT inhibitor σ1 receptor agonist	5-HT enhanced effect
Citalopram (1998)	D	20–40 mg	35 hours	SERT inhibitor H1 mild antagonist	5-HT enhanced effect
Escitalopram (2002)	D (>12), GAD	10–20 mg	27–32 hours	SERT inhibitor	5-HT enhanced effect
Vilazodone (2011)	D	10–40 mg	25 hours	SERT inhibitor 5-HT$_{1A}$ partial agonist	5-HT enhanced effect, Increases Glut, Da, NA, HA, ACh
Vortioxetine (2013)	D	10–20 mg	66 hours	SERT inhibitor 5-HT$_{1A}$ agonist 5-HT$_{1B}$ partial agonist 5-HT$_{1D}$ antagonist 5-HT$_{7}$ antagonist 5-HT$_{3}$ antagonist	5-HT enhanced effect, Increases Glut, Da, NA, HA, Ach, Decreases GABA

(SSRI) Selective Serotonin receptor inhibitor; (FDA) Food and Drug Administration; (MD-AE) movement disorder adverse event; (D) Depression; (A) Anxiety; (PD) Panic Disorder; (OCD) obsessive-compulsive disorder; (BN) Bulimia nervosa; (PMDD) premenstrual dysphoric disorder; (SAD) Social anxiety disorder; (GAD) Generalized anxiety disorder; (PTSD) Posttraumatic stress disorder; (SERT) Serotonin transporter; (DAT) Dopamine Transporter; (NET) Norepinephrine Transporter

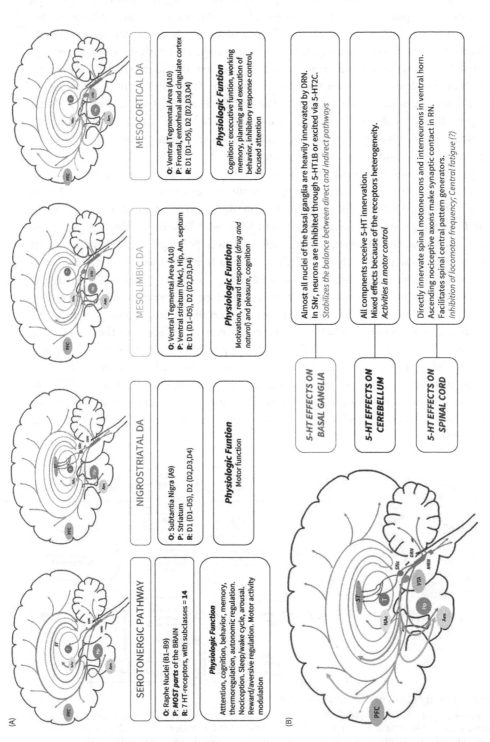

Figure 7.1 DA pathways with 5-HT influence and effects.

A) Diagrams of 5-HT and DA networks (O: origin; P: projections; R: receptors) with physiologic function. B) 5-HT-DA interactions PFC: prefrontal cortex; ST: striatum; T: thalamus; NAc: nucleus accumbens; SNc: substantia nigra pars compacta; SNr: substantia nigra pars reticulata; VTA: ventral tegmental area; DRN: dorsal raphe nucleus; MRN: midbrain raphe nucleus; Hp: hippocampus; Am: amygdala; DA: dopamine; 5-HT: serotonin.

sclerosis, and others, due to their action on calcium homeostasis, glutamate activity, NMDA inhibition, ion channel regulation, oxygen-reactive species production mitigation, glial cell anti-inflammatory properties, and mitochondrial/endoplasmic reticulum function modulation.[24–26] It is not clear, however, whether fluvoxamine's sigma-1 receptor agonist activity or sertraline's sigma-1 receptor antagonist activity are associated with the clinical development of movement disorders as adverse events SSRI use. Strong evidence of the serotonergic system's influence and involvement in motor control was demonstrated in the early 1960s, in the field of movement disorders research, when Dr. Barbeau demonstrated reduced levels of serotonin in the basal ganglia in postmortem studies of brains of people who died with PD.[27] Furthermore, basal ganglia serotonin modulation has been implicated in dystonia, Huntington's disease, and tremor in children and adults.[28]

During initial acute treatment with SSRIs, an increase in serotonergic transmission at the limbic system (nucleus accumbens, hippocampus, or cortex) and VTA/locus coeruleus induce a reduction in dopaminergic transmission, due to an antagonist 5-HT_{2C} receptor effect in GABA-ergic interneurons projecting to VTA, with little or no effect on noradrenergic activity.[29] Chronic treatment significantly enhances 5-HT pathways, resulting in an increase in dopaminergic activity with diminished noradrenergic transmission. This is partially explained because the persistent selective activation of 5-HT_{1A} and 5-HT_{1B} receptors diminishes the system's negative feedback, resulting in desensitization of both auto receptors, enhancing 5-HT liberation and effect.[28] Additionally, chronic serotonin transporter (SERT) inhibition activates microglia and alters regulation of tyrosine hydroxylase, the rate limiting enzyme for dopamine biosynthesis, and also offers a potential explanation for the various extrapyramidal adverse effects related to SSRIs.[30] The time needed to obtain sufficient serotonergic stimulation correlates well with timing that one usually anticipates for SSRIs to manifest their clinical effect, but this timing also correlates with the onset of movement disorders as adverse events. Figure 7.2 illustrates the acute and chronic changes with serotonin enhancement therapies.

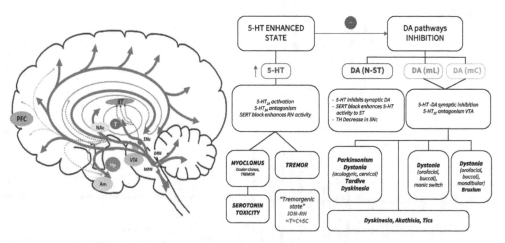

Figure 7.2 Changes in hyperserotonergic state.

Dopamine network dysfunction and the correspondent movement disorder evoked by each network dysfunction. See text for details. PFC: prefrontal cortex; st: striatum; T: thalamus; NAc: nucleus accumbens; SNc: substantia nigra pars compacta; VTA: ventral tegmental area; DRN: dorsal raphe nucleus; MRN: midbrain raphe nucleus; Hp: hippocampus; Am: amygdala; DA: dopamine; 5-HT: serotonin; N-ST: nigrostriatal; mL: mesolimbic; mC: mesocortical; iON: inferior olivary nucleus; RN: red nucleus; T + C+SC: thalamocorticosubcortical; TH: tyrosine hydroxylase.

Movement Disorders Associated With SSRIs

A first step when approaching a patient with a movement disorder is to define the phenomenology of the abnormal movement. Accurate clinical identification of the movement disorder phenomenology is crucial for the integration of clinical thinking and proper decision-making. Table 7.3 summarizes the definition and clinical characteristics of different drug-induced movement disorders.

With an estimated incidence of about 1 per 1,000 SSRI users, drug-induced movement disorders were not identified in early prerelease Phase III trials, and even currently, antidepressants are not routinely associated with extrapyramidal reactions.[31] Early reports linked fluoxetine, paroxetine, fluvoxamine, and sertraline as the most frequent causative agents of SSRI-related movement disorders, but evidence shows that movement disorders can occur with other SSRIs such as citalopram, escitalopram, and others.[32] Thus, it is recommended that this adverse effect should reflect a "drug class effect," taking into account the differences between the SSRI mechanisms of action and the fact that our current knowledge about the effect of potentiation of the serotonergic pathway has not been fully elucidated in motor or behavioral control.[33–35]

Table 7.3 Phenomenology and Clinical Findings of Drug-Induced Movement Disorders

Movement Disorder	Definition	Clinical Findings
Akathisia	State of agitation and restlessness, inability to be still	Restlessness, patient is unable to remain still, extremities crossing and uncrossing; pacing; anxiety
Dyskinesia	Abnormal, uncontrollable and involuntary movements, referring to acute or tardive dyskinesia here	Involuntary movements of the tongue, face (grimaces), limbs or trunk; chewing; lip smacking or puckering
Dystonia	Abnormal involuntary movements or postures, giving rise to sustained or intermittent muscle contractions	Twitching, muscular spasms, tongue protrusions, jaw tightening stiffening/opening, neck stiffness/deviation, conjugated eye deviation (oculogyric crisis), blepharospasm. Sensory trick, may have null point for the abnormal movement
Myoclonus	Quick involuntary and irregular muscle contraction	Nonrhythmic twitching or jerking of a muscle or a group of muscles
Parkinsonism	Bradykinesia Rigidity Parkinsonian Tremor Postural instability and gait disorder	Slowness, rigidity, rest tremor, diminished arm swing during walking, masked face, sialorrhea, micrographia, hypophonia.
Tics	Repetitive and patterned motor or vocal actions, preceded by uncomfortable sensory experiences (urge), suppressible	Simple brief movements or complex sequences, mostly head (ocular and facial), neck and upper body (rostrocaudal progression)
Tremor	Involuntary, rhythmic, oscillatory movement of a body part	Shaking of a body part, can be rest tremor or posture/action tremor

Various movement disorders have been reported with SSRI use. A report in 1996 included 71 cases of "SSRI-induced extrapyramidal symptoms," finding that akathisia was the most common (45.1%), followed by dystonia (28.2%), parkinsonism (14.1%), and tardive-dyskinesia-like states (11.3%); the latter three movement disorders were also related to older age.[36] In addition, the report included worsening of parkinsonism in 16 individuals with PD. Of note, 67.6% of all the affected patients were females. Agonism of serotonergic input to dopaminergic pathways within the CNS was proposed to explain the development of movement disorders with SSRI use.

Potential risk factors for extrapyramidal symptoms associated with SSRIs have been reported to include advanced age, female gender, and pharmacokinetic drug interaction through CYP2D6 inhibition.[37] Hawthorne et al. reported a follow-up review of extrapyramidal reactions and serotonergic antidepressants based on studies published between 1998 and 2015.[38] They reviewed 86 case reports for a total of 91 patients (57.1% female, age range of 15 months to 83 years), where SSRIs were thought to be implicated in 80.2% of the cases. Their findings differed from Leo's 1996 report in the rates of adverse effects and extrapyramidal reaction type, with dystonia as the most common (29.7%), followed by parkinsonism (21%), dyskinesia (19.7%), akathisia (18.6%), and then other mixed movement disorders (9.1%).[36] Movement disorder symptoms occurred within 30 days of either drug initiation or dose increase. Interestingly, the authors rated 55% of the cases as being "probably" related to a specific antidepressant, since there was not fully convincing evidence of a direct relation or causation. The most frequent SSRIs implicated were citalopram or escitalopram (22%), fluoxetine (20.9%) and sertraline (15.4%). The proposed mechanism for involuntary or abnormal movements is that serotonin reuptake blockade enhances raphe serotonin activity onto striatal or tegmental dopamine receptors, acting as a dopaminergic activity inhibitor, and thereby generating the extrapyramidal effects.

Dystonia

Dystonia is a condition characterized by abnormal involuntary movements or postures, giving rise to sustained or intermittent muscle contractions. Dystonia may involve impaired neural networks with aberrant input versus output plasticity of sensorimotor mismatch and involvement of the cerebellum as afferent limb of the dystonic pathway, with spinocerebellar and cerebellothalamostriatal projection abnormalities.[39]

SSRI-related dystonia is thought to occur due to dopaminergic inhibition secondary to 5-HT enhancement, particularly 5-HT2 to D2 receptor occupancy within basal ganglia circuits and a noradrenergic/cholinergic imbalance in the feedback loops. Table 7.4 illustrates case series of SSRI-related dystonia, clinical presentations, proposed mechanisms for specific types of dystonia, and therapeutic strategies that resolved the complication.[40-49]

Recently, Zoons et al. studied the effect of adding escitalopram 10 mg/day on dystonic jerks/tremor in patients with cervical dystonia.[50] This was a randomized, double-blind, placebo-controlled crossover trial of 53 primary dystonia patients treated with botulinum neurotoxin. Although there were no differences between add-on therapies, authors concluded that they found no reason to withhold treatment with SSRIs for depression and anxiety in a patient with dystonia, since there was no worsening of dystonia in the escitalopram group. Zandifar et al., however, reported a case series of five patients who

Table 7.4 Dystonia: Case Reports Associated With Different SSRIs

SSRI	Dystonia type	Case characteristics	Mechanisms
Paroxetine[49]	Severe orofacial and buccal	Case report 39-year-old female, PD-D. reversible with aripiprazole	Mesocorticolimbic DA-ergic 5-HT inhibition *Treatment: activation of 5-HTA$_{1A}$*
Fluvoxamine[46]	Oculogyric + Mania	Case report 21-year-old male, OCD-D	*Rapid dose hiking* a) Dystonia: - Imbalance on HTD$_2$:D$_2$ *toward* D$_2$ - σ1 agonism: reduces NMDA activity, abnormal GLU transmission in *C-St-T circuit (motor projections)* b) Mania: - Disturbance in 5-HT, DA, NA balance - σ1 agonism: Abnormal GLU transmission in C-St-T circuit (*limbic projections*) *Treatment: Promethazine IM injection, Fluvoxamine dose adjustment, plus lithium.*
Fluoxetine + Lurasidone[44]	Glosso-pharyngeal	Case report, 27-year-old male, SCZ-D	*Drug interaction* Fluoxetine inhibition of CYP-3A4, the metabolic route for lurasidone *Treatment: diphenhydramine IV*
Citalopram[42]	Acute dystonia	Retrospective case series, 9 patients (6 female), mean age 29 years	5-HT inhibitory input to DA on synaptic release and synthesis midB, St & C Decrease tyrosine hydroxylase, SNc *Treatment: Biperiden 5 mg IM*
Escitalopram[43]	Cervical dystonia (anterocollis)	Case report, 78-year-old male, D	5-HTT inhibition of the nigrostriatal pathways, and decrease of tyrosine hydroxylase cells in SNc in high risk subject (*postradiotherapy, previous use of antipsychotics*) *Treatment: diphenhydramine IV; escitalopram discontinuation.*
Sertraline[40,41,45,47]	Oromandibular Mandibular (+ bruxism)	Case reports a) 10-year-old boy, D+ PTSD; b) 29-year-old female, D; c) 25-year-old female, PD	a) 5-HT inhibition in DA-mesocortical circuits VTA; *Treatment: 2.5 biperiden, IM* b) *Treatment: SSRI switch to TCA* c) *Treatment: SSRI switch to TeCA.*
	Cervical	Case report 35-year-old male, OCD	5-HT inhibition in DA regulation *Treatment: lower dose SSRI*

(continued)

Table 7.4 Continued

SSRI	Dystonia type	Case characteristics	Mechanisms
Vortioxetine[48]	Meige Syndrome	Case report Two Sisters 35-year-old female, D 32-year-old female, D	Possible genetic predisposition, Central dopaminergic hyperactivity, Decreased inhibitory neurons (GABA) *Treatment: SSRI discontinuation*

(D) depression; (PD) panic disorder; (OCD) obsessive-compulsive disorder; (SCZ) schizophrenia; (C-St-T) cortico-subcortical-thalamic circuit; (DA) dopamine; (GLU) glutamate; (GABA) gamma-amino-butyric acid; (TCA) tricyclic antidepressant; (TeCA) tetracyclic antidepressant; (IM) intramuscular

developed bruxism and mandibular dystonia secondary to SSRIs (3 received sertraline, 1 fluoxetine and 1 citalopram), along with akathisia and insomnia.[51] These patients were treated with low-dose quetiapine, a medication with potent 5-HT2 receptor blocking activity, between 25 and 50 mg/day with improved bruxism and dystonia after 5–10 days of treatment.

Parkinsonism

Studies regarding the relationship between SSRI use and drug-induced parkinsonism in people without PD or worsened motor features in those with diagnosed PD have been conflicting. There are several case-reports of drug-induced parkinsonism in SSRIs users (without known PD). Escitalopram has been reported in several studies to cause drug-induced reversible parkinsonism.[52-55] There are also reports with sertraline and fluoxetine; in some cases however, the parkinsonian features were irreversible.[54,56] General treatment strategies include discontinuation of the SSRI, lowering of the SSRI dose, and in some cases, anticholinergic or antiparkinsonian drugs. One putative mechanism for the occurrence of parkinsonism in the setting of SSRIs is that tyrosine hydroxylase synthesis is significantly decreased in the substantia nigra due to microglia activation and downregulation of the enzyme, which is activated by SERT inhibition by the SSRIs such as citalopram and fluoxetine.[30] Movement disorders such as parkinsonism linked to SSRIs may be attributed to the effects that serotonin has on dopamine metabolism and resultant decreased production and release of dopamine. Animal studies suggest that SSRIs affect dopamine turnover, such that the SSRIs interference with dopamine reuptake, leads to increased synaptic dopamine levels, stimulation of striatal dopamine autoreceptors, and thereby, inhibition of dopamine release and metabolism.[57] It is important to keep in mind that SSRI-induced parkinsonism may actually unmask a underlying PD symptoms, in that case, parkinsonism would be expected to be irreversible.[58]

Regarding SSRIs and PD, these medications comprise an important and effective treatment option for depression and anxiety in PD.[59,60] Several cases and reports, however, describe worsened motor parkinsonian disability with increased tremor, rigidity, or bradykinesia in people with PD and depression treated with SSRIs, including fluvoxamine, fluoxetine, paroxetine, and sertraline.[36,61–63] Dell'Agnello et al. studied 62 consecutive depressed PD patients treated with citalopram (*n* = 15), fluoxetine (*n* = 16), fluvoxamine (n = 16), and sertraline (*n* = 15) and found that over 6 months, motor scores on the Unified PD Rating Scale were not significantly modified by the addition of SSRIs and thus, concluded that SSRIs do not significantly worsen motor features in PD.[64] SSRIs including paroxetine and citalopram have been studied in randomized, double-blind, placebo-controlled trials for depression in PD.[65–67] In all three of these randomized trials, adverse events in general were mild, and did not indicate worsened parkinsonian features, or to any degree greater than placebo or drug comparators. One participant in the citalopram group (*n* = 15) reported worsened tremor, compared to two individuals in the placebo group (*n* = 16) and one individual in the desipramine group (*n* = 17).[66] In the SAD-PD study, tremor was reported in 7 participants (16.7%) of the paroxetine group (*n* = 42), compared to 20.6% in the venlafaxine XR group (*n* = 34) and 7.7% in the placebo group (*n* = 39), and dyskinesia was reported in one participant (2.4%) in the paroxetine group, 11.8% in the venlafaxine XR group, and 7.7% of the placebo group.[67]

Acute and Tardive Dyskinesia

There are case reports of acute dyskinesia involving oral, lingual, facial, and limb regions and choreic dyskinesia with three reports with fluoxetine, two with sertraline, and one with paroxetine, citalopram, and escitalopram.[68–73] The basic mechanism for the development of dyskinetic movements seems to be similar to that proposed for dystonia after SSRI use. Some authors, however, have questioned the association of SSRIs with dyskinesia, since reported patients often receive concomitant medications (antipsychotics) that could also explain the dyskinetic movements themselves.[69,71] In addition, the phenomenological description of acute dyskinesia has been questioned with some arguing that those "dyskinesias" could be tremors, tics, or even dystonic movements.[74] Of note, these movement disorders were reported to resolve spontaneously or after dose lowering strategies in the reports.

Tardive dyskinesia or "TD" is defined in the DSM-5 as "involuntary athetoid or choreiform movements lasting at least a few weeks, developing in association with the use of a neuroleptic (dopamine antagonists) medication for at least a few months, and persisting beyond 4–8 weeks," making it almost a neuroleptic-exclusive side effect condition.[75] Nevertheless, the phenomenology of tardive dyskinesia has been reported with non-dopamine-receptor-blocking drugs such as the SSRIs fluoxetine, sertraline, and paroxetine, in much lower prevalence compared to neuroleptics, but associated with older age.[76–81] A bucco-lingual-masticatory pattern has been consistently reported, with symptom resolution after drug discontinuation, unlike typical TD. Older age, prior use of antipsychotics (neuroleptics), history of drug-induced extrapyramidal symptoms and PD are other identified risk factors for SSRI-related tardive dyskinesia.[80] D'Abreu and Friedman reviewed the literature of tardive dyskinesia not attributed to antipsychotics, termed "tardive dyskinesia–like" syndromes. They proposed that SSRIs and tricyclic antidepressants may exacerbate an underlying dyskinetic disorder, that was generated by a dopamine receptor blocking drug as in a number of the cases, people had previously or concurrently taken dopamine receptor blocking agents.[82] In other words, SSRIs antidepressants may unmask subclinical tardive dyskinesia in patients who have taken these drugs, even in the past. Their recommendation is that SSRIs and other non-dopamine-receptor-blocking drugs should be considered the cause of tardive dyskinesia only after excluding other causes and that tardive dyskinesia-like syndromes in people who have not taken dopamine blocking medications are extraordinarily rare. In follow up to this article, Walker also warned about the possibility of confusing late-onset primary dystonia (cranial segmental dystonia) with tardive dyskinesia, and that, in such cases, SSRIs could potentially exacerbate the dystonic disorder, rather than causing tardive dyskinesia.[83] A systematic phenomenology description and ideally, an expert opinion of a movement disorders specialist can help clarify those complex clinical manifestations.

Akathisia

Akathisia is represented by an inability to stay still and an intense sensation of restlessness that results in a compulsion to move.[84] Akathisia has variable presentations and may be misdiagnosed as panic attacks, anxiety, agitation, restless legs syndrome, tardive dyskinesias, and other conditions.[85] Akathisia is most frequently associated with use of antipsychotics with dopamine receptor blocking properties, neuropsychiatric syndromes, and has been linked to an increased risk of suicidal ideation/behavior in first-episode schizophrenia, which resolves rapidly after akathisia is treated.[86] Treatment for akathisia, most typically associated with antipsychotics, includes stopping or changing the antipsychotic, or considering beta blockers (e.g., propranolol 20 to 40 mg twice daily), or low-dose mirtazapine.[87]

Akathisia has also been associated with SSRIs, though it is frequently underrecognized, although the exact description is often a little different. The SSRIs fluvoxamine, fluoxetine, sertraline, citalopram, and escitalopram all have been reported to cause akathisia.[88–92] Deficiency of dopaminergic nigrostriatal pathway is thought to be the basic mechanism for akathisia, along with serotonergic enhancement in the mesocorticolimbic dopaminergic pathway.[93]

Tremor

Tremor is probably the most frequent movement disorder associated with SSRIs.[94] Approximately 20% of patients treated with SSRIs develop tremor.[95] Paroxetine, citalopram, and fluoxetine have been reported to cause this abnormal movement in several studies.[96–101] Tremor is typically mild and postural, although there are also reports of rest or kinetic/intention tremor in the extremities, jaw, chin, and mouth. Tremor development in the setting of SSRIs has been thought to relate to the presence of specific 5-HT receptors at the inferior olivary nucleus that are thought to cause an overexcitation of this structure, resulting in a stimulant effect by the SSRIs. The inferior olivary nucleus, in turn, stimulates the red nucleus, and both project to the thalamus, cortical neurons, and spinal cord and peripheral nervous system, generating an overexcited tremorgenic state. After SSRI discontinuation, it is anticipated that tremor will remit, with some suggesting tremor resolution within one month.[95] It is important to note that tremor present predominantly in the legs may also represent an early manifestation of serotonin toxicity syndrome.[102] Paradoxically, tremor is also a characteristic of SSRI withdrawal syndrome, along with anxiety, irritability, and paresthesia.[103]

A comprehensive evaluation with emphasis on timing and duration of medication use and clinical symptoms can guide the clinician to distinguish these complications.

Other Movement Disorders Induced by SSRIs

There are case reports of several other movement disorders induced by SSRI use, including myoclonus, hemichorea or hemiballism, sleep-related disorders, bruxism, and tics. Myoclonus, quick, involuntary muscle jerk movements, have been reported with SSRI use. The presence of myoclonus has been identified after the addition of fluoxetine to a trazodone-treated patient, and also in other SSRI treatments with concomitant use of metoclopramide, ondansetron plus HAART in a HIV positive patient, dextromethorphan, and alcohol intake.[104-108] Myoclonus can occur in patients with specific conditions such as schizophrenia and liver cirrhosis as well as those with metabolic derangments.[109,110] Myoclonus also can be a manifestation of serotonin toxicity syndrome and signify 5-HT hyperactivity. There is one case report of negative myoclonus in a 77-year-old man who mistakenly took paroxetine instead of fluoxetine. The explanatory mechanism is that hyperexcitability of the primary somatosensory cortex in turn, inhibits primary motor cortex output.[111] In a case-series report of 19 patients with isolated generalized polymyoclonus, seven patients were taking either opioids, SSRIs, or serotonin norepinephrine reuptake inhibitors (SNRIs).[112] Regarding phenomenology, it is important to distinguish myoclonus from tremor, tics, or other movement disorders.

Hemichorea and hemiballism are involuntary and nonpatterned movement disorders involving one side of the body that usually result from contralateral basal ganglia lesion or in the context of metabolic disturbances.[113] There has been a case report of sertraline-induced hemichorea in a 65-year-old woman, who developed this involuntary movement only one week after drug initiation; after an extensive diagnostic evaluation, hemichorea was determined to be associated to sertraline and disappeared after 7 days of drug discontinuation.[114]

SSRIs-induced or aggravation of pre-existing restless leg syndrome has been demonstrated in some case reports,[115] but this notion has been questioned in a Danish study of 10,875 restless leg syndrome patients followed for one year, where researchers found no association between the initiation of an SSRI and the development or worsening of restless leg syndrome.[116]

Periodic limb movements disorder has been consistently reported in the literature as a SSRIs adverse reaction. Up to 44% of adults treated with fluoxetine present this movement disorder, but it has been reported also with citalopram, paroxetine, and sertraline.[117,118] Children had a 5.4-fold higher risk to develop periodic limb movements of sleep with the use of SSRIs (OR of 5.45; 95% confidence interval 2.71–10.96 in SSRIs users vs. non-SSRIs-users).[75] The underlying mechanism is thought to relate to an abnormal function of spinal activity control of the dopaminergic system, secondary to 5-HT inhibitory action.

Bruxism and jaw spasm have been reported with SSRIs including fluoxetine, sertraline, and paroxetine occurring after 3 or 4 weeks of treatment, as well as with SNRIs.[119] These abnormal movements are often painful and are a frequent cause of dentist consultation, but their incidence is unknown. These symptoms tend to resolve spontaneously after 3–4 weeks of drug discontinuation or treatment with buspirone in some.[120] Given the potential occurrence of bruxism and jaw spasm related to SSRIs and SNRIs, a careful selection of antidepressants may be considered with some recommending starting with TCAs, atypical antidepressants, or MAO inhibitors.[121] The mechanism of SSRI-induced bruxism is not fully elucidated but is thought to be secondary to disruption of the dopamine mesocortical pathways.

Tics are sudden, involuntary, and intermittent movements or sounds that can be temporarily suppressible by the patient, but increase with stress and tension. There is a case report of sertraline-induced tics in an elderly woman who developed bursts of involuntary neck extension, eyebrow elevation, shoulder shrug, gasping, and throat clearing noises; these were suppressible voluntarily, aggravated by stress, and identified as tics after comprehensive diagnostic evaluation.[122] Other authors found worsening of pre-existing tic disorders such as Tourette's syndrome with the addition of sertraline.[123] Escitalopram-induced tics were reported in one patient, and switching to sertraline stopped the abnormal motor behavior.[124] Striatum disinhibition is the proposed mechanism for tics generation after SSRIs exposure. The intermittent, waxing and waning nature of tics, however, may make it challenging to establish relationships between medication timing and the development or resolution of tics.

Summary

SSRI-related movement disorders in general have been estimated to occur in about 1 per 1000 SSRI users, but may occur much more frequently, especially tremor and periodic limb movements. Multiple phenomenologies of movement disorders, however, have been reported in the context of SSRI use. Establishing cause and effect or relationships can often be challenging due to determining timing and relevance, concomitant use of other medications such as dopamine receptor blocking agents, or the intermittent nature of some involuntary movement disorders. Of the SSRIs reported to have association with movement disorders, fluoxetine, citalopram, escitalopram, and sertraline are the most frequently included in cases and reports. The majority of cases occur within 30 days of SSRI treatment initiation or augmentation and usually resolve after drug discontinuation or dose lowering. In some cases, the movement disorder symptoms require additional treatment such as with anticholinergic or dopaminergic medications, buspirone, propranolol, or mirtazapine, depending on the phenomenology of the hyper- or hypokinetic disorder. Treatment decisions require consideration of risks and benefits related to medication use, medication selection, and need for management of psychiatric symptoms such as depression and anxiety. Risk factors for SSRI-induced movement disorders include age, gender, genetics, previous drug-related movement disorder adverse effects, comorbidities, and concomitant medication use. In addition to individual-related risk factors, the vast presence and complexity of serotonin receptors within the brain, whose activity is not yet fully understood, and serotonin influences in other neurotransmitter pathways besides dopamine, opens the possibility to explain heterogeneous phenomenology of movement disorders within this drug class. The complex interaction between the monoaminergic systems highlights the complexity of neurochemical and cellular mechanisms that remain to be further elucidated.

Acknowledgments

We thank Andrea Hernandez and Julie Guerra for their assistance with research and illustrations in this chapter.

References

1. Cipriani A, Furukawa TA, Salanti G, et al. Comparative efficacy and acceptability of 21 antidepressant drugs for the acute treatment of adults with major depressive disorder: a systematic review and network meta-analysis. Lancet 2018;391:1357–1366.
2. Sangkuhl K, Klein TE, Altman RB. Selective serotonin reuptake inhibitors pathway. Pharmacogenet Genomics 2009;19:907–909.
3. Haller E, Watzke B, Blozik E, et al. Antidepressant prescription practice and related factors in Switzerland: a cross-sectional analysis of health claims data. BMC Psychiatry 2019;19:196.
4. Verhaak PFM, de Beurs D, Spreeuwenberg P. What proportion of initially prescribed antidepressants is still being prescribed chronically after 5 years in general practice? A longitudinal cohort analysis. BMJ Open 2019;9:e024051.
5. Bruggeman C, O'Day CS. Selective Serotonin Reuptake Inhibitor Toxicity. [Updated 2021 Jul 10]. In: StatPearls [Internet]. Treasure Island (FL): StatPearls Publishing; 2022 Jan-. Available from: https://www.ncbi.nlm.nih.gov/books/NBK534815/
6. Foong AL, Grindrod KA, Patel T, Kellar J. Demystifying serotonin syndrome (or serotonin toxicity). Can Fam Physician 2018;64:720–727.
7. Andrews PW , Bharwani A, Lee KR, Fox M, Thomson JA, Jr. Is serotonin an upper or a downer? The evolution of the serotonergic system and its role in depression and the antidepressant response. Neurosci Biobehav Rev 2015;51:164–188.
8. Baldo BA. Opioid analgesic drugs and serotonin toxicity (syndrome): mechanisms, animal models, and links to clinical effects. Arch Toxicol 2018;92:2457–2473.
9. Bartlett D. Drug-induced serotonin syndrome. Crit Care Nurse 2017;37:49–54.
10. de Leon J, Spina E. Possible pharmacodynamic and pharmacokinetic drug-drug interactions that are likely to be clinically relevant and/or frequent in bipolar disorder. Curr Psychiatry Rep 2018;20:17.
11. Ornoy A, Koren G. Selective serotonin reuptake inhibitor use in pregnant women; pharmacogenetics, drug-drug interactions and adverse effects. Expert Opin Drug Metab Toxicol 2018;14:247–259.
12. Schellander R, Donnerer J. Antidepressants: clinically relevant drug interactions to be considered. Pharmacology 2010;86:203–215.
13. Spoelhof B, Farrokh S, Rivera-Lara L. Drug interactions in neurocritical care. Neurocrit Care 2017;27:287–296.
14. Dunkley EJ, Isbister GK, Sibbritt D, Dawson AH, Whyte IM. The Hunter serotonin toxicity criteria: simple and accurate diagnostic decision rules for serotonin toxicity. QJM 2003;96:635–642.
15. Tormoehlen LM, Rusyniak DE. Neuroleptic malignant syndrome and serotonin syndrome. Handb Clin Neurol 2018;157:663–675.

16. Gummin DD, Mowry JB, Spyker DA, et al. 2018 Annual Report of the American Association of Poison Control Centers' National Poison Data System (NPDS): 36th Annual Report. Clin Toxicol (Phila) 2019;57:1220–1413.

17. Lochmann D, Richardson T. Selective serotonin reuptake inhibitors. Handb Exp Pharmacol 2019;250:135–144.

18. Jakubovski E, Varigonda AL, Freemantle N, Taylor MJ, Bloch MH. Systematic review and meta-analysis: dose-response relationship of selective serotonin reuptake inhibitors in major depressive disorder. Am J Psychiatry 2016;173:174–183.

19. Di Giovanni G, Esposito E, Di Matteo V. Role of serotonin in central dopamine dysfunction. CNS Neurosci Ther 2010;16:179–194.

20. Fischer AG, Ullsperger M. An update on the role of serotonin and its interplay with dopamine for reward. Front Hum Neurosci 2017;11:484.

21. Burke MV, Nocjar C, Sonneborn AJ, McCreary AC, Pehek EA. Striatal serotonin 2C receptors decrease nigrostriatal dopamine release by increasing GABA-A receptor tone in the substantia nigra. J Neurochem 2014;131:432–443.

22. Palacios JM. Serotonin receptors in brain revisited. Brain Res 2016;1645:46–49.

23. Li Y, Zhong W, Wang D, et al. Serotonin neurons in the dorsal raphe nucleus encode reward signals. Nat Commun 2016;7:10503.

24. Nguyen L, Lucke-Wold BP, Mookerjee SA, et al. Role of sigma-1 receptors in neurodegenerative diseases. J Pharmacol Sci 2015;127:17–29.

25. Ryskamp DA, Korban S, Zhemkov V, Kraskovskaya N, Bezprozvanny I. Neuronal sigma-1 receptors: signaling functions and protective roles in neurodegenerative diseases. Front Neurosci 2019;13:862.

26. Weng TY, Tsai SA, Su TP. Roles of sigma-1 receptors on mitochondrial functions relevant to neurodegenerative diseases. J Biomed Sci 2017;24:74.

27. Barbeau A. The pathogenesis of Parkinson's disease: a new hypothesis. Can Med Assoc J 1962;87:802–807.

28. Doummar D, Moussa F, Nougues MC, et al. Monoamine neurotransmitters and movement disorders in children and adults. Rev Neurol (Paris) 2018;174:581–588.

29. El Mansari M, Sanchez C, Chouvet G, Renaud B, Haddjeri N. Effects of acute and long-term administration of escitalopram and citalopram on serotonin neurotransmission: an in vivo electrophysiological study in rat brain. Neuropsychopharmacology 2005;30:1269–1277.

30. MacGillivray L, Reynolds KB, Sickand M, Rosebush PI, Mazurek MF. Inhibition of the serotonin transporter induces microglial activation and downregulation of dopaminergic neurons in the substantia nigra. Synapse 2011;65:1166–1172.

31. Coulter DM, Pillans PI. Fluoxetine and extrapyramidal side effects. Am J Psychiatry 1995;152:122–125.

32. Gerber PE, Lynd LD. Selective serotonin-reuptake inhibitor-induced movement disorders. Ann Pharmacother 1998;32:692–698.

33. Factor SA, Burkhard PR, Caroff S, et al. Recent developments in drug-induced movement disorders: a mixed picture. Lancet Neurol 2019;18:880–890.

34. Kawashima T. The role of the serotonergic system in motor control. Neurosci Res 2018;129:32–39.

35. Yohn CN, Gergues MM, Samuels BA. The role of 5-HT receptors in depression. Mol Brain 2017;10:28.

36. Leo RJ. Movement disorders associated with the serotonin selective reuptake inhibitors. J Clin Psychiatry 1996;57:449–454.

37. Madhusoodanan S, Alexeenko L, Sanders R, Brenner R. Extrapyramidal symptoms associated with antidepressants—a review of the literature and an analysis of spontaneous reports. Ann Clin Psychiatry 2010;22:148–156.

38. Hawthorne JM, Caley CF. Extrapyramidal reactions associated with serotonergic antidepressants. Ann Pharmacother 2015;49:1136–1152.

39. Kaji R, Bhatia K, Graybiel AM. Pathogenesis of dystonia: is it of cerebellar or basal ganglia origin? J Neurol Neurosurg Psychiatry 2018;89:488–492.

40. Gupta B, Ahmad J, Kar SK, Shrivastava A. Sertraline induced cervical dystonia in a patient of obsessive compulsive disorder. Asian J Psychiatr 2018;31:77–78.

41. Kutuk MO, Guler Aksu G, Tufan AE, Celik T. Oromandibular dystonia related to sertraline treatment in a child. J Child Adolesc Psychopharmacol 2019;29:164–165.

42. Moosavi SM, Ahmadi M, Monajemi MB. Acute dystonia due to citalopram treatment: a case series. Glob J Health Sci 2014;6:295–299.

43. Morgan RJ, Dolenc TJ. Escitalopram-induced progressive cervical dystonia. Psychosomatics 2015;56:572–575.

44. Paul S, Cooke BK, Nguyen M. Glossopharyngeal dystonia secondary to a lurasidone-fluoxetine CYP-3A4 interaction. Case Rep Psychiatry 2013;2013:136194.

45. Raveendranathan D, Rao SG. Sertraline induced acute mandibular dystonia. J Neurosci Rural Pract 2015;6:586–587.

46. Tikka SK, Garg S, Das B. Fluvoxamine induced oculogyric dystonia and manic switch in a patient with obsessive compulsive disorder. Indian J Pharmacol 2013;45:532–533.

47. Uvais NA, Sreeraj VS, Sathish Kumar SV. Sertraline induced mandibular dystonia and bruxism. J Family Med Prim Care 2016;5:882–884.

48. Kocamer Sahin S, Elboga G, Altindag A. Meige syndrome related to vortioxetine in 2 sisters: case reports. J Clin Psychopharmacol 2019;39:679–681.

49. Oulis P, Konstantakopoulos G, Nathanailidis E, Tsiamoura M, Kollias K. Low-dose aripiprazole in the treatment of selective serotonin reuptake inhibitors-induced orofacial and buccal dystonia. Psychiatry Clin Neurosci 2012;66:462–463.

50. Zoons E, Booij J, Delnooz CCS, et al. Randomised controlled trial of escitalopram for cervical dystonia with dystonic jerks/tremor. J Neurol Neurosurg Psychiatry 2018;89:579–585.

51. Zandifar A, Mohammadi MR, Badrfam R. Low-dose quetiapine in the treatment of SSRI-induced bruxism and mandibular dystonia: case series. Iran J Psychiatry 2018;13:227–229.

52. Ak S, Anil Yagcioglu AE. Escitalopram-induced parkinsonism. Gen Hosp Psychiatry 2014;36:126 e121–122.

53. Kumar PNS, Krishnan AG, Suresh R. Escitalopram-induced extrapyramidal symptoms. Indian J Psychiatry 2019;61:318–319.

54. Ozalp E, Soygur H, Cankurtaran ES, et al. Sertraline, escitalopram and tianeptine related abnormal movements but not with bupropion: a case report. Prog Neuropsychopharmacol Biol Psychiatry 2006;30:1337–1339.

55. Erdogan S, Demir S, Celikel F. The relationship of selective serotonin reuptake inhibitors with Parkinson's disease and parkinsonism: two case reports. Anadolu Psikiyatri Dergisi 2011;12:315–317.

56. Dixit S, Khan SA, Azad S. A case of SSRI induced irreversible parkinsonism. J Clin Diagn Res 2015;9:VD01–VD02.

57. Di Rocco A, Brannan T, Prikhojan A, Yahr MD. Sertraline induced parkinsonism: a case report and an in-vivo study of the effect of sertraline on dopamine metabolism. J Neural Transm (Vienna) 1998;105:247–251.

58. Gonul AS, Aksu M. SSRI-induced parkinsonism may be an early sign of future Parkinson's disease. J Clin Psychiatry 1999;60:410.

59. Goldman JG, Guerra CM. Treatment of nonmotor symptoms associated with Parkinson disease. Neurol Clin 2020;38:269–292.

60. Seppi K, Ray Chaudhuri K, Coelho M, et al. Update on treatments for nonmotor symptoms of Parkinson's disease-an evidence-based medicine review. Mov Disord 2019;34:180–198.

61. Steur EN. Increase of Parkinson disability after fluoxetine medication. Neurology 1993;43:211–213.

62. Simons JA. Fluoxetine in Parkinson's disease. Mov Disord 1996;11:581–582.

63. Richard IH, Maughn A, Kurlan R. Do serotonin reuptake inhibitor antidepressants worsen Parkinson's disease? A retrospective case series. Mov Disord 1999;14:155–157.

64. Dell'Agnello G, Ceravolo R, Nuti A, et al. SSRIs do not worsen Parkinson's disease: evidence from an open-label, prospective study. Clin Neuropharmacol 2001;24:221–227.

65. Devos D, Dujardin K, Poirot I, et al. Comparison of desipramine and citalopram treatments for depression in Parkinson's disease: a double-blind, randomized, placebo-controlled study. Mov Disord 2008;23:850–857.

66. Menza M, Dobkin RD, Marin H, et al. A controlled trial of antidepressants in patients with Parkinson disease and depression. Neurology 2009;72:886–892.

67. Richard IH, McDermott MP, Kurlan R, et al. A randomized, double-blind, placebo-controlled trial of antidepressants in Parkinson disease. Neurology 2012;78:1229–1236.

68. Albertini G, Majolini L, Di Gennaro G, et al. Oral dyskinesia induced by fluoxetine therapy for infantile autism. Pediatr Neurol 2004;31:76.

69. Allsbrook M, Fries BE, Szafara KL, Regal RE. Do SSRI antidepressants increase the risk of extrapyramidal side effects in patients taking antipsychotics? P T 2016;41:115–119.

70. Gaanderse M, Kliffen J, Linssen W. Citalopram-induced dyskinesia of the tongue: a video presentation. BMJ Case Rep 2016;2016:bcr2016216126.

71. Lauterbach EC, Meyer JM, Simpson GM. Clinical manifestations of dystonia and dyskinesia after SSRI administration. J Clin Psychiatry 1997;58:403–404.

72. Madhusoodanan S, Brenner R. Reversible choreiform dyskinesia and extrapyramidal symptoms associated with sertraline therapy. J Clin Psychopharmacol 1997;17:138–139.

73. Mander A, McCausland M, Workman B, Flamer H, Christophidis N. Fluoxetine induced dyskinesia. Aust N Z J Psychiatry 1994;28:328–330.

74. Muthusami S, Basu S, Kumar A, Dash A. Acute dyskinesia and extrapyramidal disorder in a child after ingestion of escitalopram. J Child Adolesc Psychopharmacol 2009;19:317–318.

75. Vendrame M, Zarowski M, Loddenkemper T, Steinborn B, Kothare SV. Selective serotonin reuptake inhibitors and periodic limb movements of sleep. Pediatr Neurol 2011;45:175–177.

76. Botsaris SD, Sypek JM. Paroxetine and tardive dyskinesia. J Clin Psychopharmacol 1996;16:258–259.

77. Cornett EM, Novitch M, Kaye AD, Kata V, Kaye AM. Medication-induced tardive dyskinesia: a review and update. Ochsner J 2017;17:162–174.

78. Dubovsky SL, Thomas M. Tardive dyskinesia associated with fluoxetine. Psychiatr Serv 1996;47:991–993.

79. Raidoo DM. Fluoxetine-induced tardive dyskinesia in a patient with Parkinson's disease. Acta Neuropsychiatr 2012;24:306–309.

80. Waln O, Jankovic J. An update on tardive dyskinesia: from phenomenology to treatment. Tremor Other Hyperkinet Mov (N Y) 2013;3:tre-03-161-4138-1.

81. Wang LF, Huang JW, Shan SY, et al. Possible sertraline-induced extrapyramidal adverse effects in an adolescent. Neuropsychiatr Dis Treat 2016;12:1127–1129.

82. D'Abreu A, Friedman JH. Tardive dyskinesia-like syndrome due to drugs that do not block dopamine receptors: rare or non-existent: literature review. Tremor Other Hyperkinet Mov (NY) 2018;8:570.

83. Walker RH. Reply to: Tardive dyskinesia-like syndrome due to drugs that do not block dopamine receptors: rare or non-existent: literature review. Tremor Other Hyperkinet Mov (N Y) 2019;9:626.

84. O'Brien H, Kiely F, Barry A, Meaney S. Cross-sectional examination of extrapyramidal side effects in a specialist palliative care inpatient unit. BMJ Support Palliat Care 2019;9:271–273.

85. Nepal H, Black E, Bhattarai M. Self-harm in sertraline-induced akathisia. Prim Care Companion CNS Disord 2016;18(6). doi: 10.4088/PCC.16l01952.

86. Seemuller F, Schennach R, Mayr A, et al. Akathisia and suicidal ideation in first-episode schizophrenia. J Clin Psychopharmacol 2012;32:694–698.

87. Poyurovsky M, Pashinian A, Weizman R, Fuchs C, Weizman A. Low-dose mirtazapine: a new option in the treatment of antipsychotic-induced akathisia. A randomized, double-blind, placebo- and propranolol-controlled trial. Biol Psychiatry 2006;59:1071–1077.

88. Hensley PL, Reeve A. A case of antidepressant-induced akathisia in a patient with traumatic brain injury. J Head Trauma Rehabil 2001;16:302–305.

89. Koliscak LP, Makela EH. Selective serotonin reuptake inhibitor-induced akathisia. J Am Pharm Assoc (2003) 2009;49:e28–36; quiz e37–28.

90. Albayrak Y, Hashimoto K. Beneficial effects of sigma-1 agonist fluvoxamine for tardive dyskinesia and tardive akathisia in patients with schizophrenia: report of three cases. Psychiatry Investig 2013;10:417–420.

91. Basu B, Gangopadhyay T, Dutta N, Mandal B, De S, Mondal S. A case of akathisia induced by escitalopram: case report & review of literature. Curr Drug Saf 2014;9:56–59.

92. Schillevoort I, van Puijenbroek EP, de Boer A, Roos RA, Jansen PA, Leufkens HG. Extrapyramidal syndromes associated with selective serotonin reuptake inhibitors: a case-control study using spontaneous reports. Int Clin Psychopharmacol 2002;17:75–79.

93. Lane RM. SSRI-induced extrapyramidal side-effects and akathisia: implications for treatment. J Psychopharmacol 1998;12:192–214.

94. Louis ED. Tremor. Continuum (Minneap Minn) 2019;25:959–975.

95. Morgan JC, Kurek JA, Davis JL, Sethi KD. Insights into pathophysiology from medication-induced tremor. Tremor Other Hyperkinet Mov (N Y) 2017;7:442.

96. Anand KS, Prasad A, Pradhan SC, Biswas A. Fluoxetine-induced tremors. J Assoc Physicians India 1999;47:651–652.

97. John P, McConnell K, Saif MW. Chin tremors associated with paroxetine in a patient with pancreatic adenocarcinoma. JOP 2013;14:661–663.

98. Lai H, Tolat R. Paroxetine-related tremor. Geriatrics 2005;60:18–20.

99. Serrano-Duenas M. Fluoxetine-induced tremor: clinical features in 21 patients. Parkinsonism Relat Disord 2002;8:325–327.

100. Tarlaci S. Citalopram-induced jaw tremor. Clin Neurol Neurosurg 2004;107:73–75.

101. Arshaduddin M, Al Kadasah S, Biary N, Al Deeb S, Al Moutaery K, Tariq M. Citalopram, a selective serotonin reuptake inhibitor augments harmaline-induced tremor in rats. Behav Brain Res 2004;153:15–20.

102. Hudd TR, Blake CS, Rimola-Dejesus Y, Nguyen TT, Zaiken K. A case report of serotonin syndrome in a patient on selective serotonin reuptake inhibitor (SSRI) monotherapy. J Pharm Pract 2020;33:206–212.

103. Massabki I, Abi-Jaoude E. Selective serotonin reuptake inhibitor "discontinuation syndrome" or withdrawal. Br J Psychiatry 2021: 218(3), 168–171.

104. Darko W, Guharoy R, Rose F, Lehman D, Pappas V. Myoclonus secondary to the concurrent use of trazodone and fluoxetine. Vet Hum Toxicol 2001;43:214–215.

105. Dy P, Arcega V, Ghali W, Wolfe W. Serotonin syndrome caused by drug to drug interaction between escitalopram and dextromethorphan. BMJ Case Rep 2017; 2017:bcr2017221486.

106. Harada T, Hirosawa T, Morinaga K, Shimizu T. Metoclopramide-induced serotonin syndrome. Intern Med 2017;56:737–739.

107. Kolli V, Addula M. Ondansetron-induced myoclonus with escitalopram and HAART: role of drug interactions. Prim Care Companion CNS Disord 2019; 21(4):18l02364..

108. Suzuki A, Otani K. Serotonin syndrome after an alcohol intake in a patient treated with escitalopram and clomipramine. Clin Neuropharmacol 2019;42:103–104.

109. Forsberg-Gillving M, Bode M, Sindrup SH. [Myoclonus as a side effect to citalopram treatment in a patient with liver cirrhosis]. Ugeskr Laeger 2015;177:V04150325.

110. Horga G, Horga A, Baeza I, Castro-Fornieles J, Lazaro L, Pons A. Drug-induced speech dysfluency and myoclonus preceding generalized tonic-clonic seizures in an adolescent male with schizophrenia. J Child Adolesc Psychopharmacol 2010;20:233–234.

111. Correia P, Ribeiro JA, Bento C, Sales F. Negative myoclonus secondary to paroxetine intake. BMJ Case Rep 2018; bcr201822458.

112. McKeon A, Pittock SJ, Glass GA, et al. Whole-body tremulousness: isolated generalized polymyoclonus. Arch Neurol 2007;64:1318–1322.

113. Laganiere S, Boes AD, Fox MD. Network localization of hemichorea-hemiballismus. Neurology 2016;86:2187–2195.

114. Gatto EM, Aldinio V, Parisi V, et al. Sertraline-induced hemichorea. Tremor Other Hyperkinet Mov (N Y) 2017;7:518.

115. Patatanian E, Claborn MK. Drug-induced restless legs syndrome. Ann Pharmacother 2018;52:662–672.

116. Dunvald AD, Henriksen DP, Hallas J, Christensen MMH, Lund LC. Selective serotonin reuptake inhibitors and the risk of restless legs syndrome: a symmetry analysis. Eur J Clin Pharmacol 2020;76:719–722.

117. Dorsey CM, Lukas SE, Cunningham SL. Fluoxetine-induced sleep disturbance in depressed patients. Neuropsychopharmacology 1996;14:437–442.

118. Hoque R, Chesson AL, Jr. Pharmacologically induced/exacerbated restless legs syndrome, periodic limb movements of sleep, and REM behavior disorder/REM sleep without atonia: literature review, qualitative scoring, and comparative analysis. J Clin Sleep Med 2010;6:79–83.

119. Uca AU, Uguz F, Kozak HH, et al. Antidepressant-induced sleep bruxism: prevalence, incidence, and related factors. Clin Neuropharmacol 2015;38:227–230.

120. Garrett AR, Hawley JS. SSRI-associated bruxism: a systematic review of published case reports. Neurol Clin Pract 2018;8:135–141.

121. Rajan R, Sun YM. Reevaluating antidepressant selection in patients with bruxism and temporomandibular joint disorder. J Psychiatr Pract 2017;23:173–179.

122. Rua A, Damasio J. Tics induced by sertraline: case report and literature review. Mov Disord Clin Pract 2014;1:243–244.

123. Hauser RA, Zesiewicz TA. Sertraline-induced exacerbation of tics in Tourette's syndrome. Mov Disord 1995;10:682–684.

124. Altindag A, Yanik M, Asoglu M. The emergence of tics during escitalopram and sertraline treatment. Int Clin Psychopharmacol 2005;20:177–178.

8

The Underrecognized Movement Disorders Associated With Mood Stabilizers

Melody Badii and William G. Ondo

Lithium-Induced Movement Disorders

Lithium, available in multiple salt preparations, is a complex, unique drug, employed since the 19th century, and now most commonly used to treat bipolar disorder. The precise mechanism of action is not well understood. Lithium was traditionally thought to alter cation transport across the nerve and muscle cell membranes, affect the reuptake of serotonin and norepinephrine, and inhibit second messenger systems.[1] Furthermore lithium may also have neuroprotective effects by increasing glutamate clearance,[2] inhibiting apoptotic glycogen synthase kinase activity,[3] increasing the levels of the antiapoptotic protein Bcl-2, and enhancing the expression of neurotropic factors, including brain-derived neurotrophic factor.[4]

Lithium has been reported to play a pathogenic role in multiple movement disorders including tremor, parkinsonism, chorea, dyskinesia, dystonia, ataxia, and somnambulism. However, there have also been studies assessing the effects of lithium in terms of treatment in movement disorders, which will be briefly discussed in each subsection.

Lithium-Induced Tremor

Action tremor is among the most common anticipated adverse effects of lithium, with an estimated prevalence of 4%–65% depending on assessment technique.[5] Action tremor may emerge anytime during treatment, but is mostly seen early in its course. Roughly 53% of patients develop tremor within the first week of treatment, and the number drops to 4% after 1–2 years of treatment.[6] Tremor is not necessarily correlated with serum lithium levels and is often seen with therapeutic levels, but can also be an early sign of lithium toxicity. Lithium-induced tremor in the early phase of treatment mainly manifests as postural and kinetic tremor, which is difficult to distinguish from mild essential tremor. It is mainly seen in hands, symmetrically. Certain risk factors such as increasing age, male sex, concurrent use of antidepressants and neuroleptics, anxiety, excessive caffeine intake, alcoholism, and a personal/family history of tremor increase the incidence of lithium-induced tremor in the acute phase of treatment.[7]

There is also a reported case of palatal tremor in a patient on chronic treatment with lithium and carbamazepine. Tremor was partially improved upon discontinuation of the medications.[8]

The mechanism of lithium-induced tremor is unclear. The most common postulated mechanism involves exaggerated physiologic tremor through central oscillation.[9] The two major components of physiologic tremor include: (1) peripheral reflex mechanical oscillation involving the monosynaptic reflex arch, and (2) normally occurring 8–12 Hz central oscillation. As lithium brain levels, and not the serum levels, are associated with tremor, an effect on central oscillation is postulated as the mechanism of enhancement. The olivocerebellar system, including inferior olive, climbing fibers, Purkinje cells, deep cerebellar nuclei, and eventually brainstem and spinal cord motoneurons are known to play a role in essential tremor. Inferior olive nuclei normally show rhythmic subthreshold oscillations that involve serial ion conductances. Harmaline used in animal models of tremor causes excitability in inferior olive neurons resulting in conversion of subthreshold oscillations to rhythmic burst firing.[10] Many drugs that are used to treat essential tremor, such as beta blockers, primidone, and GABA agonists, suppress harmaline-induced tremor in mice models. Interestingly, lithium actually suppresses harmaline tremor despite causing human tremor,[11] suggesting a different mechanism of tremor in humans.

Treatment of lithium tremor is based on symptom severity rather than lithium levels, as tremor is mostly seen with therapeutic serum levels. Gradually escalating the dose to therapeutic levels, once daily dosing, extended release forms of lithium, and avoidance of other trigger factors all decrease the probability of tremor development.[12] First-line management of lithium-induced tremor is conservative, including the avoidance of high serum levels of lithium and other trigger factors such as anxiety and caffeine. Action tremor usually does not require discontinuation of lithium, although it is reversible when lithium is stopped. If symptoms are bothersome, treatment is similar to essential tremor with noncardiac selective beta-adrenergic blockers. The mechanism of action of beta blockers is mostly via peripheral effect, as beta blockers with poor central nervous system penetration are still effective. Propranolol, metoprolol, and nadolol efficacy were established through multiple case series and two placebo-controlled cross over studies with total of 59 lithium tremor patients.[9,13–15] Other reported treatment options include primidone,[16] benzodiazepines, and vitamin B6.[17,18]

Lithium-Induced Parkinsonism

The characteristics of lithium-induced tremor can change from physiologic (high frequency, low amplitude, occurring with action) to parkinsonian tremor (low frequency, high amplitude, mostly occurring at rest) with chronic treatment, which indicates involvement of basal ganglia pathway.[19] Parkinsonism has been reported infrequently in case reports of patients on long-term lithium treatment, even with normal serum lithium levels.[20] The only published cross-sectional study of 110 subjects on lithium using the Extrapyramidal Symptoms Rating Scale (ESRS) reported a 7.7% prevalence of parkinsonism.[21]

DATscan—[^{123}I]N-ω-fluoropropyl-2β-carbomethoxy-3β-(4-iodophenyl)nortropane ([^{123}I]FP-CIT) SPECT—measures presynaptic dopamine transporter protein. This has been used off-label to differentiate idiopathic PD from dopamine receptor blocker drug-induced parkinsonism,[22] however lithium-induced parkinsonism can cause reversible abnormal DATscans that image dopamine transporter protein, which is normally thought to be a marker of true neurodegenerative parkinsonism. Cilia et al. presented a 71-year-old woman with an 8-year history of bipolar disorder who was being treated with lithium. She presented with bradykinesia, rigidity, bilateral hand postural and rest tremor, hypomimia, and hypophonia, and was initially diagnosed with idiopathic PD, based on clinical findings and supportive information from abnormal DATscan. As lithium was discontinued, parkinsonian symptoms improved over time with normalization of DATscan.[23] Of note, ^{18}F-dopa PET scan, which measures a precursor to dopamine, was normal. Based on these findings, it is postulated that lithium might cause functional downregulation of membrane DAT, despite normal dopamine levels in nerve terminals. Other medicines with known affinity to DAT such as bupropion or methylphenidate are known to impact DATscans, however lithium has no known affinity for DAT, and is not officially listed among medications that can artificially impact DaTscan results.

The authors have seen multiple cases of reversible lithium-induced parkinsonism, sometimes very severe. Typically these patients were on lithium for many years, thus were older, were no longer followed by a psychiatrist, and had normal lithium levels. One 69-year-old man had been on lithium for over 20 years before he developed parkinsonism, manifesting as severe rest tremor, bradykinesia, and hypophonia. Upon initial assessment, DATscan showed markedly decreased uptake consistent with idiopathic PD (Figure 8.1a). Lithium was gradually discontinued in addition to initiation of treatment with levodopa. Parkinsonian features greatly improved, although they persisted. A second DATscan was obtained 5 years later after complete discontinuation of lithium and L-dopa was normal (Figure 8.1b). These findings again support the hypothesis that lithium can potentially result in some form of

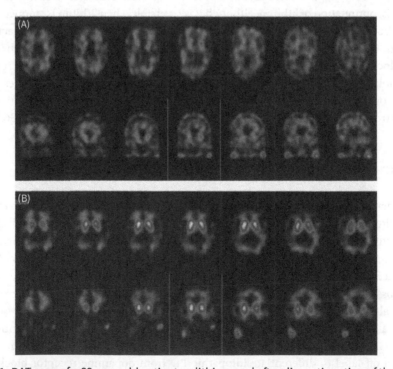

Figure 8.1 DAT scan of a 69-year-old patient on lithium and after discontinuation of therapy.

(A) Initial DAT scan when patient first presented with parkinsonism. Axial and coronal views demonstrate significantly reduced radioneurotransmitter reuptake in bilateral caudate and putamen regions. (B) Repeat DAT scan in the same patient 5 years after discontinuation of lithium. Radioneurotransmitter reuptake is increased to normal levels as evidenced on axial and coronal views. These findings were associated with improvement in parkinsonian symptoms.

downregulation or internalization of DAT receptors, causing abnormal DATscan in the absence of substantia nigra denervation. The exact mechanism still remains unclear, although Borre et al. postulated effects of lithium on DAT, as a dopamine sodium symporter.[24] This effect is reversible with discontinuation of lithium, but clinical improvement in parkinsonism may be very gradual over months. The exact rate of DATscan improvement after withdrawal is not established, but in our experience it can take months.

Lithium has been a drug of interest in neurodegenerative diseases because of its ability to decrease both alpha-synuclein and p-tau aggregation. It has also been shown to enhance the viability of dopaminergic cells in vitro and in vivo rodent models.[25–28] The low prevalence of Parkinson's disease (PD) in smokers has been attributed to tobacco's high lithium levels.[29,30] Lithium has been a promising drug in terms of progression of neurodegenerative disease in mice models, but the frequent anecdotal worsening in parkinsonism symptoms and signs in PD patients, makes lithium untenable in this population.

Lithium-Induced Chorea

Cases of reversible choreoathetosis secondary to lithium intoxication are reported, some in constellation with other typical lithium toxicity symptoms, including ataxia and encephalopathy.[31–34] Induced hypersensitivity of dopamine receptors in nigrostriatal pathways in the context of a patient's vulnerability has been postulated as a pathophysiology, but no mechanism of action is established. All cases were reversible and associated with high lithium levels.

In contrast, several case series report the efficacy of lithium in ameliorating hyperkinetic symptoms in Huntington's disease patients, in addition to its benefits in terms of mood improvement.[35] However, small placebo controlled trials failed to show any benefit.[36,37]

Lithium-Induced Ataxia

Reversible ataxia and cerebellar symptoms are common in lithium toxicity, however there are also reports of cerebellar degeneration associated with irreversible ataxia. Syndrome of irreversible lithium-effectuated neurotoxicity (SILENT) has been seen with both therapeutic serum lithium levels and post-lithium toxicity. Most of these cases were triggered by hyperthermia,[38–40] but there are reports of cerebellar atrophy in the absence of this trigger factor. Although patients presented with acute infection-induced hyperthermia, MRI findings show chronic cerebellar atrophy suggesting that the pathologic findings are chronic, despite the acute onset of symptoms. It is unclear whether fever acts as a trigger factor or is a component of the syndrome. One of the cases occurred in the context of Q fever, but no specific organisms were mentioned in the remainder of patients. Fever, hyperthermia, hyponatremia, and concurrent use of antipsychotics increase the risk of lithium cerebellar toxicity with normal serum levels.

Mangano et al. reported a case of incidental postmortem findings of chronic cerebellar atrophy after the patient died from acute lithium toxicity. The patient presented with acute lithium toxicity in the absence of prior similar episodes or any signs of chronic cerebellar atrophy.[41] There are several cases in the author's experience presenting with irreversible ataxia post-lithium intoxication. Figure 8.2 demonstrates MRI findings consistent with cerebellar atrophy after the patient presented with acute symptoms of lithium toxicity.

Lithium has a complex distribution in the body. Heurteaux et al. showed that in mice lithium levels in the thalamus, neocortex, and hippocampus were six times that in the plasma, and levels in the striatum and cerebellum were three times that in the plasma; therefore plasma concentration does not directly correlate with intracellular levels. Hyponatremia

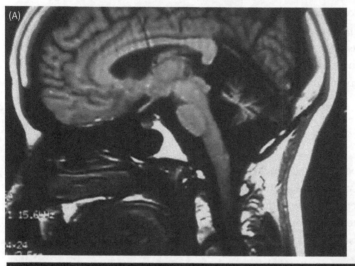

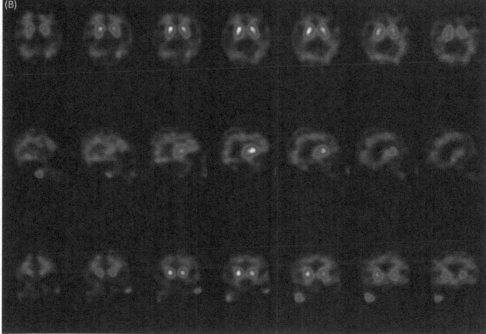

Figure 8.2 MRI findings of a patient presenting with acute onset irreversible ataxia post lithium intoxication.

Brain MRI shows chronic cerebellar atrophy in (A) sagittal and (B) axial/saggital/coronal views. Patient did not exhibit any signs or symptoms of cerebellar disease prior to acute lithium intoxication.

can result in the Na+/Li + transmembrane exchange rate increasing lithium influx into the cells and lithium toxicity symptoms.[38]

The pathologic findings in SILENT cases include significant loss of Purkinje cells with sparing of surrounding basket cells. This pathology is also found in patients with neuroleptic malignant syndrome (NMS).[42] However, neuropathological studies in NMS and heat stroke patients are few. Purkinje and deep cerebellar neuronal loss are striking findings in the case reports who had a longer course of disease.[43–45] Acute reversible lithium intoxication in rats has been associated with pathologic changes of vacuolization in the cerebellar white matter. Possible reasons for the selectivity of lithium for Purkinje cells are unknown, but might be attributed to excitotoxic effects secondary to lithium action on calcium channels.

Hemodialysis should be performed in cases of ataxia secondary to lithium toxicity, but it should be kept in mind that serum lithium levels do not necessarily correlate with intracellular levels and hemodialysis might need to be continued even after normalization of serum levels. There are no established treatments for the ataxia once it has presented.

Lithium-Induced Myoclonus

There are rare cases of cortical myoclonus reported in patients treated with lithium.[46,47] Carviness et al. noted that myoclonus was action induced in all five patients studied and rarely occurred at rest.[48] Facilitation of presynaptic serotonin release, serotonin augmentation, and cortical hyperexcitability have been postulated as mechanisms of these symptoms.[48] Certain factors might contribute to development of myoclonus including prolonged course of treatment, gluten sensitivity, alcoholism, concurrent treatment with other antidepressants, and possibly female sex. EEG/EMG polygraphy[47] is used to differentiate lithium-induced tremor and myoclonus in cases of debate. Based on a small sample, myoclonus is irreversible despite discontinuation of lithium. Treatment of myoclonus remains challenging in these patients, as no specific drug has been reported to help. Discontinuation of lithium and gluten free diet resulted in improvement of symptoms in some patients.[47]

Lithium-Induced Dystonia/Dyskinesia and Somnambulism

A few dystonia cases in the literature are associated with lithium treatment manifesting as acute or tardive adverse effects. Dystonia mentioned in these cases mostly involves the neck and trunk. They were observed in the combination therapy of lithium with other antipsychotics.[49,50] Dystonia improved with discontinuation of medications, but persisted to some extent. Although response of dystonia to clozapine is debatable, a trial of clozapine has been recommended.[50]

"Dyskinesia" is reported in rare cases with therapeutic or supratherapeutic serum lithium levels.[51,52] There have been reports of reversible orolingual dyskinesia in lithium intoxication. One case of "tardive dyskinesia" with lithium monotherapy at low doses and normal serum lithium levels was mentioned in 2019, which raised the concern of long term toxic effects of this commonly used medication.

Somnambulistic behavior is another movement disorder that has been attributed to lithium therapy.[53,54] As somnambulism occurs in the non-REM stage of sleep, increase in the non-REM sleep caused by lithium might contribute to this finding.

Valproate-Induced Movement Disorders

Valproate is a branched short-chain fatty acid used for treatment of seizures, bipolar disorder, anxiety disorder, and migraine prophylaxis. Valproate reduces metabolism of GABA and increases its synthesis, resulting in an increase of synaptic GABA levels. It may also cause direct suppression of sodium, potassium, and calcium channels.[55-57] Although antiepileptic effects are probably mainly secondary to GABA enhancement and sodium channel suppression, the exact mechanism through which valproate improves symptoms in bipolar disorder, anxiety disorder, and migraine, remains unknown.

Valproate-Induced Tremor and Parkinsonism

The prevalence of action tremor in patients on valproate is between 6%–45%.[58] Approximately 25% of patients develop tremor within 3–12 months after initiation of valproate, making it the most common neurologic adverse effect of this medication.[59] The objective presence of tremor measured by accelerometry seems to be as high as 80%.[60] The phenomenology of tremor resembles that of essential tremor, manifesting as kinetic and postural tremor, although it is sometimes associated with resting tremor and even parkinsonism.[61-64] Fine high-frequency tremor can be observed in the head, mouth, and extremities. The prevalence of tongue postural tremor is higher in valproate-induced tremor in comparison to essential tremor.[65] In a series of 125 patients on valproate for either epilepsy or migraine, 14 (11.2%) had upper limb rest tremor in at least one arm, among which two (1.6%) also had other parkinsonism features.[61] One of these patients was diagnosed with PD, and the other one was diagnosed with valproate-induced parkinsonism, as the symptoms resolved with discontinuation of valproate. Rest tremor in this series also correlated with greater action tremor. Only 1.6% of the total cohort had parkinsonism but their own meta-analysis of the literature describing 717 patients found a 3.0% prevalence of parkinsonism in subjects taking valproate. Armon et al. stopped valproate in 36 epilepsy patients for a variety of side effects and followed 32 prospectively to observe for improvement.[66] In this group, they reported 44% had tremor, which resolved in 14/16 subjects, and 75% had parkinsonism, which resolved in 23/24 subjects. They also reported high rates of cognitive, psychiatric, and audiometry problems. It should be noted that their abnormal findings were often subtle.

Galizia et al. described a patient who developed reversible parkinsonism after 20 years of treatment with valproate. The patient was on multiple antiepileptics, but akinetic rigid symptoms resolved only after discontinuation of valproate.[67] A recent review by Brugger et al., estimated the prevalence of valproate-associated parkinsonism between 1.4% and 75% of patients taking valproate. In the majority of patients, valproate concentrations were within or below therapeutic range when parkinsonism appeared.[68] There is also a case report of valproate toxicity mimicking multiple system atrophy.[69] Anecdotally, valproate induced parkinsonism correlates with older age and longer duration of use. A recent review by Muralidharan et al. in 2020 concluded that valproate-induced parkinsonism occurred in equal incidence in both genders and was higher in older populations. All patients were taking typical doses of valproate with therapeutic serum levels. Symptoms improved in most cases after discontinuation of the drug. In those cases who did not improve, parkinsonian symptoms responded well to levodopa treatment, supporting the hypothesis that valproate may have unmasked underlying PD.[70]

There are multiple possible mechanisms through which valproate may cause tremor and parkinsonism. Tremor may be caused by decrease in dopamine levels.[71,72] In one study, patients who developed tremor on valproate had lower serum dopamine levels in comparison to the control group and patients who did not develop tremor. However, further investigations with CSF dopamine measurement are required.[72] Parkinsonism could also be potentially explained by alterations in GABA metabolism in substantia nigra and striatum.[72] Interestingly, valproate, like lithium, actually improves the harmaline mouse model of essential tremor, so the pathophysiology likely is distinct from that of essential tremor.

Valproate is 90% protein bound in the plasma and is metabolized in the liver through glucuronidation, beta-oxidation and cytochrome P450 system.[12] Therefore any factor that can interfere with plasma protein binding or metabolization, can potentially increase the plasma free levels and result in adverse effects such as tremor. Karas et al. reported that tremor is more related with daily dose of valproate than actual plasma levels.[60] The tremorgenic effect of valproate also depends on the formulation. Tremor is less with controlled release preparations compared to conventional forms, presumably due to less peak-trough variation[73] although no data clearly correlates tremor with serum levels. In most studies serum levels are within normal ranges.

It has been estimated that tremor is severe enough in roughly 24% of patients to require intervention.[74] Tremor is reversible with discontinuation of valproate but if discontinuation is not feasible, few effective treatment options have been proposed in the literature. Karas et al. evaluated the therapeutic effects of propranolol, amantadine, benztropine, diphenhydramine, and cyproheptadine on 19 patients with valproate-induced tremor.[75] Tremor was assessed with serial accelerometric recordings. Results showed that propranolol was superior to other drugs. Amantadine was moderately effective, in contrast to benztropine, diphenhydramine, and cyproheptadine that gave little or no relief. There is also a case report of acetazolamide improving valproate-induced tremor.[76] There are no specific reports of treating valproate parkinsonism other than drug withdrawal.

Valproate-Induced Chorea

Chorea is a rare dose-dependent side effect of valproate.[77] Chorea was reversible upon cessation of valproate in all of the few reported cases. History of prior brain damage and concomitant use of other antiepileptic drugs increased the risk of chorea in these patients.[78] The pathophysiology of this phenomenon remains unclear and it contradicts valproate's known action on GABA. It is postulated that in these patients, possibly in the presence of other risk factors, different effects on GABA are seen in the basal ganglia–thalamocortical circuits, leading to activation rather than inhibition.[79] In contrast, valproate has also been used as treatment of chorea in patients with Sydenham's or rheumatic chorea.

Carbamazepine-Induced Movement Disorders

Carbamazepine was first discovered in 1953 and was marketed in 1963 as an antiepileptic drug. Since its marketing, various indications have been added to its profile, including treatment for trigeminal neuralgia, acute mania, and as a mood stabilizer. Carbamazepine achieves its effects through different mechanisms, predominately voltage-dependent sodium channel blockage/stabilization, but its metabolites may also increase serotonin release, antagonize adenosine receptors, increase dopamine release, inhibit glutamate release, and interact with GABA-B receptors.[80] The clinical relevance of these other mechanisms is unclear.[81] Efficacy for some indications, such as seizure control and trigeminal neuralgia are expected rapidly, in contrast to mood stabilizing effects, which take longer time to occur. Movement disorders caused by carbamazepine can possibly be explained by modulation of neurotransmitters as mentioned above.

Carbamazepine-Induced Myoclonus

Myoclonus is the most frequent movement disorder caused by carbamazepine. In general, anatomic origin of myoclonus can be cortical or subcortical based on EEG findings.[82] Most EEG studies performed on patients taking carbamazepine, were among epileptic patients. The presence of seizure among these patients might have biased the EEG findings, as the cortical locus can be secondary to seizure focus. Interestingly, EEG findings in patients with bipolar disorder being treated with carbamazepine showed subcortical origins for myoclonus, which might provide more accurate assessment in comparison to an epilepsy population. Carbamazepine can increase extracellular serotonin concentration, possibly resulting in subcortical myoclonus. Carbamazepine-induced myoclonus is not dose-dependent but is considered as a threshold side effect.

Of note, carbamazepine is also among treatment modalities tried for cortical, subcortical, supraspinal, spinal, and peripheral myoclonus, though there is little trial data supporting its use. Sanjari Moghaddam et al. reported a case of a 7-year-old patient with diagnosis of myoclonus-dystonia, in which the symptoms were significantly improved after treatment with carbamazepine. The myoclonus in this patient was subcortical based on normal EEG findings. The therapeutic effect of carbamazepine in this case was assumed to be due to changes in sodium channels, serotonin and dopamine levels at subcortical levels and basal ganglia.[83] Rahko et al. reported good response in three patients with objective myoclonus tinnitus to carbamazepine treatment.[84] Hirose et al. reported a patient with postanoxic myoclonus, where response to carbamazepine was noted.[85] Anecdotally, most patients with postanoxic myoclonus do not respond well.

Carbamazepine-Induced Dystonia

Carbamazepine has been associated with multiple dystonia phenotypes. The body regions involved in the order of prevalence include: focal/segmental limb, axial, cervical, oromandibular, blepharospasm, and dystonic tremor.[86] Dystonia is reversible upon drug withdrawal.

Although the benefits of continuing the medication should be compared to the degree of disability from dystonia. In particular cases where a patient has been refractory to other treatments other than carbamazepine, it can be continued with some chance of resolution of dystonia.[87]

The mechanism of dystonia is postulated to be the interaction of carbamazepine with GABA channels. This interaction causes elevation of GABA concentrations resulting in inactivation of the indirect pathway. Inactivation of indirect pathway results in more impact of the direct pathway, which manifests as sustained muscle contractions and dystonia.

Carbamazepine-Induced Hyperkinetic Dyskinesia

Different forms of dyskinesia including ballism, chorea, choreoathetosis, and orofacial dyskinesia are reported to be associated with carbamazepine. Patients with baseline structural brain abnormalities are at higher risk of developing dyskinesia. Treatment is similar to other adverse effects and includes discontinuation of the medication. Despite this approach, some reported cases continue to have irreversible dyskinesia.

Carbamazepine-Induced Tics

Both motor and phonic tics are reported with carbamazepine consumption. Neglia et al. reported three children who either developed or had exacerbation of Tourette's syndrome after initiation of carbamazepine. The tics in these children did not resolve despite discontinuation of carbamazepine.[88] Robertson et al. noted motor tics in three children after the start of treatment with carbamazepine, which were reversible with medication cessation.[89] Tics occur irrespective of serum carbamazepine levels, in contrast to most other abnormal movements, and can be seen with lower carbamazepine levels. Populations of patients with baseline tic predisposition may be more prone to develop this uncommon finding.

Tics in general may originate from increased dopamine sensitivity, as well as alterations in other monoamines, GABA, and glutamate neurotransmitters. Carbamazepine may modestly downregulate the dopaminergic system, so tic manifestation secondary to carbamazepine is attributed to alterations in glutamate concentration in striatum. Treatment is drug withdrawal or symptomatic treatment with tic medications, although maintenance was associated with spontaneous improvement or resolution in some patients.[89]

Carbamazepine Drug Interactions

There are no reports of parkinsonism resulting from carbamazepine monotherapy. However, carbamazepine can potentially increase 'parkinsonogenic' effects of other medications such as valproate, lithium, SSRIs, and antipsychotics through inhibition of their metabolism. Gernaat et al. described two patients who developed parkinsonism after addition of fluoxetine and thioridazine to carbamazepine.[90] Froomes et al. reported a case of reversible parkinsonism who developed after adding carbamazepine to preexisting valproate and confirmed the recurrence by rechallenging.[91] Carbamazepine has this effect partly by alterations in the other drugs' metabolism, increasing acetylcholine, increasing serotonin or decreasing the dopamine levels in striatum. The authors have seen idiosyncratic interactions with selegiline (used for PD and depression) and carbamazepine where levels of both drugs can be elevated resulting in marked ataxia and encephalopathy.

Lamotrigine-Induced Movement Disorders

Lamotrigine is a broad spectrum antiepileptic that is indicated for seizure disorders and bi-polar disorder. Like carbamazepine, its primary mechanism of action is inhibition of sodium channels. Lamotrigine is mostly associated with skin adverse effects, although there have been some reports of neurological side effects. It should also be noted that lamotrigine markedly increases levels of valproate, so concurrent use could markedly increase valproate toxicity.

Lamotrigine-Induced Tics and Blepharospasm

Tics and blepharospasm are reported to be rarely associated with lamotrigine.[92] Initially it was believed that lamotrigine only worsened tics in patients with remote history of tics, obsessive-compulsive disorder, or significant neurologic impairments. Recently, tics have been attributed to lamotrigine in the absence of such past medical history.[92–94] There is complete or partial resolution of tics after drug discontinuation.

Lamotrigine-Induced Dyskinesia

Dyskinesia and chorea were thought to be seen in combination therapy of lamotrigine and phenytoin,[95] although later two cases were reported with lamotrigine monotherapy.[96] Conversely, some physicians reported lamotrigine as effective treatment to reduce chorea in patients with paroxysmal kinesigenic choreoathetosis, which also responds well to other sodium channel blockers.[97,98]

Lamotrigine-Induced Dystonia

Marrero-Gonzalez et al. reported a case of acute dystonic reaction in a patient receiving lamotrigine as a mood stabilizer, in addition to other psychotherapeutic medications. The patient developed cervical dystonia, which resolved after discontinuation of lamotrigine and re-emerged upon a second introduction of lamotrigine.[99] Lamotrigine prodystonic effects were previously seen in a hamster model.[100]

Miscellaneous

Cinnarizine and flunarizine are calcium channel blockers, available in some countries, which are used off-label as mood stabilizers, and for other neurologic symptoms such as vertigo, migraine prophylaxis, epilepsy, and cerebrovascular blood flow insufficiency. These two medications have similar structures, pharmacodynamics and pharmacokinetics with flunarizine being 2.5–15 times more potent.[101] The primary mechanism of action is calcium channel blockade, although both have effects on other neurotransmitters, including histamine receptor-1 antagonism, anti-serotonergic, and a competitive dopamine type-2 antagonism.[102] Antidopaminergic effects may also result from presynaptic dopamine depletion (secondary to loss of tyrosine hydroxylase).[103] These drugs are strongly associated with movement disorders, including parkinsonism, tremor, dystonia, akathisia, and tardive dyskinesia.

In countries where these drugs are frequently prescribed (such as Brazil, Mexico, Taiwan, Japan, France, Spain), they constitute a higher percentage of drug-induced parkinsonism cases compared to antipsychotics.[104,105] The first case of flunarizine-induced parkinsonism was reported by De Melo-Souza in 1984.[106] Since then, numerous case reports and series discussed the extrapyramidal symptoms and signs.[107,108] The largest study to date was performed by Jhang et al. who conducted an epidemiologic study in Taiwan from 2005 to 2010 on more than 26,000 and 7,000 patients taking flunarizine and cinnarizine, respectively.[102] Both of these groups had higher cumulative incidence of extrapyramidal symptoms in comparison to the control group. The incidence risk may be overestimated, as patients on antipsychotics and metoclopramide were not excluded from the study. After adjustment for other factors, including antipsychotic exposure, hazard ratio for flunarizine and cinnarizine parkinsonism was estimated to be 8.03 and 3.41, respectively. Gimenez-Roldan et al. observed that older age and presence of essential tremor were risk factors for development of cinnarizine-induced parkinsonism.[109] Female sex is another risk factor.[107,108] In general, the course of motor symptoms after medication withdrawal is controversial. Negrotti et al. showed that prognosis is less benign, and associated with low remission after drug withdrawal.[110] In contrast, in another study, complete recovery rate was estimated to be 89%.[103]

Conclusion

Action tremor is a well-recognized movement disorder seen in the majority of patients on lithium and at least a large minority of those on valproate. Parkinsonism with both drugs, associated with reduced DAT binding, better established with lithium, is a less recognized side effect, probably associated with longer duration of use and older age. Drug-induced parkinsonism may persist for months after drug withdrawal or reduction, but most other movements, aside from permanent lithium toxicity-associated ataxia, typically resolve quickly. The sodium channel blockers carbamazepine and lamotrigine are less associated with movement disorders but are reported to cause tics, dystonia, and other hyperkinetic disorders. Recognition of these conditions is critical for optimal management of the patient.

References

1. Ward, M. E., Musa, M. N., & Bailey, L. (1994). Clinical pharmacokinetics of lithium. *Journal of Clinical Pharmacology*, 34(4), 280–285. https://doi.org/10.1002/j.1552-4604.1994.tb01994.x
2. Sanacora, G., Zarate, C. A., Krystal, J. H., & Manji, H. K. (2008). Targeting the glutamatergic system to develop novel, improved therapeutics for mood disorders. *Nature Reviews. Drug Discovery*, 7(5), 426–437. https://doi.org/10.1038/nrd2462

3. De Sarno, P., Li, X., & Jope, R. S. (2002). Regulation of Akt and glycogen synthase kinase-3 beta phosphorylation by sodium valproate and lithium. *Neuropharmacology, 43*(7), 1158–1164. https://doi.org/10.1016/s0028-3908(02)00215-0

4. de Sousa, R. T., van de Bilt, M. T., Diniz, B. S., et al. (2011). Lithium increases plasma brain-derived neurotrophic factor in acute bipolar mania: a preliminary 4-week study. *Neurosci Lett, 494*(1), 54–56. https://doi.org/10.1016/j.neulet.2011.02.054

5. Gelenberg, A. J., & Jefferson, J. W. (1995). Lithium tremor. *J Clin Psychiatry, 56*(7), 283–287. https://www.ncbi.nlm.nih.gov/pubmed/7615481

6. Carroll, J. A., Jefferson, J. W., & Greist, J. H. (1987). Treating tremor induced by lithium. *Hosp Community Psychiatry, 38*(12), 1280, 1288. https://doi.org/10.1176/ps.38.12.1280

7. Orleans, R. A., Dubin, M. J., & Kast, K. A. (2018). The effect of a therapeutic lithium level on a stroke-related cerebellar tremor. *BMJ Case Rep, 2018*, 2018:bcr-2017-222920. https://doi.org/10.1136/bcr-2017-222920

8. Mahasuar, R., Kuruvilla, A., & Jacob, K. (2010). Palatal tremor after lithium and carbamazepine use: a case report. *J Med Case Rep, 4*, 176. https://doi.org/10.1186/1752-1947-4-176

9. Baek, J. H., Kinrys, G., & Nierenberg, A. A. (2014). Lithium tremor revisited: pathophysiology and treatment. *Acta Psychiatr Scand, 129*(1), 17–23. https://doi.org/10.1111/acps.12171

10. Handforth, A. (2012). Harmaline tremor: underlying mechanisms in a potential animal model of essential tremor. *Tremor Other Hyperkinet Mov (N Y), 2*:02-92-769-1. https://doi.org/10.7916/d8td9w2p

11. Paterson, N. E., Malekiani, S. A., Foreman, M. M., Olivier, B., & Hanania, T. (2009). Pharmacological characterization of harmaline-induced tremor activity in mice. *Eur J Pharmacol, 616*(1–3), 73–80. https://doi.org/10.1016/j.ejphar.2009.05.031

12. Canning, J. E., Burton, S., & Hall, B. (2012). Lithium and valproate-induced tremors. *Ment Health Clin 1*(7), 174–176. https://doi.org/10.9740/mhc.n92093

13. Kellett, J. M., Metcalfe, M., Bailey, J., & Coppen, A. J. (1975). Beta blockade in lithium tremor. *J Neurol Neurosurg, Psychiatry, 38*(7), 719–721. doi:10.1136/jnnp.38.7.719

14. Zubenko, G. S., Cohen, B. M., & Lipinski, J. F., Jr. (1984). Comparison of metoprolol and propranolol in the treatment of lithium tremor. *Psychiatry Res, 11*(2), 163–164. doi:10.1016/0165-1781(84)90100-8

15. Kirk, L., Baastrup, P. C., & Schou, M. (1973). Letter: propranolol treatment of lithium-induced tremor. *Lancet, 2*(7837), 1086–1087. https://doi.org/10.1016/s0140-6736(73)92692-5

16. Goumentouk, A. D., Hurwitz, T. A., & Zis, A. P. (1989). Primidone in drug-induced tremor. *J Clin Psychopharmacol, 9*(6), 451. https://doi.org/10.1097/00004714-198912000-00024

17. Miodownik, C., Witztum, E., & Lerner, V. (2002). Lithium-induced tremor treated with vitamin B6: a preliminary case series. *Int J Psychiatry Med, 32*(1), 103–108. https://doi.org/10.2190/db1v-85m4-e65t-r3qa

18. Dias Alves, M., Varin, L., Fiori, L. M., Etain, B., Azorin, J. M., & Belzeaux, R. (2017). Efficacy of vitamin B6 in lithium-associated tremor: a case series. *J Clin Psychopharmacol, 37*(2), 267–269. https://doi.org/10.1097/jcp.0000000000000650

19. Tyrer, P., Lee, I., & Trotter, C. (1981). Physiological characteristics of tremor after chronic lithium therapy. *Br J Psychiatry, 139*, 59–61. https://doi.org/10.1192/bjp.139.1.59

20. Holroyd, S., & Smith, D. (1995). Disabling parkinsonism due to lithium: a case report. *J Geriatr Psychiatry Neurol, 8*(2), 118–119. https://doi.org/10.1177/089198879500800208

21. Ghadirian, A. M., Annable, L., Bélanger, M. C., & Chouinard, G. (1996). A cross-sectional study of parkinsonism and tardive dyskinesia in lithium-treated affective disordered patients. *J Clin Psychiatry*, *57*(1), 22–28.

22. Hermida, A. P., Janjua, A. U., Glass, O. M., *et al.* (2016). A case of lithium-induced parkinsonism presenting with typical motor symptoms of Parkinson's disease in a bipolar patient. *Int Psychogeriatr*, *28*(12), 2101–2104. https://doi.org/10.1017/S1041610216001101

23. Cilia, R., Marotta, G., Belletti, A., Siri, C., & Pezzoli, G. (2014). Reversible dopamine transporter reduction in drug-induced Parkinsonism. *Mov Disord*, *29*(4), 575–577. https://doi.org/10.1002/mds.25828

24. Borre, L., Andreassen, T. F., Shi, L., Weinstein, H., & Gether, U. (2014). The second sodium site in the dopamine transporter controls cation permeation and is regulated by chloride. *J Biol Chem*, *289*(37), 25764–25773. https://doi.org/10.1074/jbc.M114.574269

25. Kim, Y. H., Rane, A., Lussier, S., & Andersen, J. K. (2011). Lithium protects against oxidative stress-mediated cell death in α-synuclein-overexpressing in vitro and in vivo models of Parkinson's disease. *J Neurosci Res*, *89*(10), 1666–1675. https://doi.org/10.1002/jnr.22700

26. Lieu, C. A., Dewey, C. M., Chinta, S. J., et al. (2014). Lithium prevents parkinsonian behavioral and striatal phenotypes in an aged parkin mutant transgenic mouse model. *Brain Res, 1591*, 111–117. https://doi.org/10.1016/j.brainres.2014.10.032

27. Youdim, M. B., & Arraf, Z. (2004). Prevention of MPTP (N-methyl-4-phenyl-1,2,3,6-tetrahydropyridine) dopaminergic neurotoxicity in mice by chronic lithium: involvements of Bcl-2 and Bax. *Neuropharmacology*, *46*(8), 1130–1140. https://doi.org/10.1016/j.neuropharm.2004.02.005

28. MacDonald, B. T., Tamai, K., & He, X. (2009). Wnt/beta-catenin signaling: components, mechanisms, and diseases. *Dev Cell*, *17*(1), 9–26. https://doi.org/10.1016/j.devcel.2009.06.016

29. Guttuso, T., Jr., Russak, E., De Blanco, M. T., & Ramanathan, M. (2019). Could high lithium levels in tobacco contribute to reduced risk of Parkinson's disease in smokers? *J Neurol Sci, 397*, 179–180. https://doi.org/10.1016/j.jns.2019.01.009

30. Guttuso, T., Jr. (2019). High lithium levels in tobacco may account for reduced incidences of both Parkinson's disease and melanoma in smokers through enhanced β-catenin-mediated activity. *Med Hypotheses, 131*, 109302. https://doi.org/10.1016/j.mehy.2019.109302

31. Podskalny, G. D., & Factor, S. A. (1996). Chorea caused by lithium intoxication: a case report and literature review. *Mov Disord*, *11*(6), 733–737. https://doi.org/10.1002/mds.870110623

32. Wada, K., Sasaki, T., Yoshimura, Y., & Erabi, H. (2003). [Reversible choreoathetosis associated with lithium intoxication]. *Seishin Shinkeigaku Zasshi*, *105*(9), 1206–1212.

33. Reed, S. M., Wise, M. G., & Timmerman, I. (1989). Choreoathetosis: a sign of lithium toxicity. *J Neuropsychiatry Clin Neurosci, 1*(1), 57–60. https://doi.org/10.1176/jnp.1.1.57

34. Loyd, R. B., Perkins, R. E., & Schwartz, A. C. (2010). Choreoathetosis in the setting of lithium toxicity. *Psychosomatics*, *51*(6), 529–531. https://doi.org/10.1176/appi.psy.51.6.529

35. Andén, N. E., Dalén, P., & Johansson, B. (1973). Baclofen and lithium in Huntington's chorea. *Lancet*, *2*(7820), 93. https://doi.org/10.1016/s0140-6736(73)93285-6

36. Leonard, D. P., Kidson, M. A., Brown, J. G., Shannon, P. J., & Taryan, S. (1975). A double blind trial of lithium carbonate and haloperidol in Huntington's chorea. *Aust N Z J Psychiatry*, *9*(2), 115–118. https://doi.org/10.3109/00048677509159834

37. Vestergaard, P., Baastrup, P. C., & Petersson, H. (1977). Lithium treatment of Huntington's chorea. *Acta Psychiatr Scand*, *56*(3), 183–188. https://doi.org/10.1111/j.1600-0447.1977.tb03561.x

38. Ozsoy, S., Basturk, M., & Esel, E. (2006). Cerebellar syndrome in a patient with pneumonia under lithium treatment: a case report. *Prog Neuropsychopharmacol Biol Psychiatry, 30*(8), 1532–1534. https://doi.org/10.1016/j.pnpbp.2006.05.003

39. Rossi, F. H., Rossi, E. M., Hoffmann, M., et al. (2017). Permanent cerebellar degeneration after acute hyperthermia with non-toxic lithium levels: a case report and review of literature. *Cerebellum, 16*(5-6), 973–978. https://doi.org/10.1007/s12311-017-0868-3

40. Pfadenhauer, K., & Stapf, U. (1993). [Acute cerebellar syndrome in preventive lithium treatment and atypical pneumonia in Q fever]. *Nervenarzt, 64*(8), 545–547.

41. Mangano, W. E., Montine, T. J., & Hulette, C. M. (1997). Pathologic assessment of cerebellar atrophy following acute lithium intoxication. *Clin Neuropathol, 16*(1), 30–33.

42. Niethammer, M., & Ford, B. (2007). Permanent lithium-induced cerebellar toxicity: three cases and review of literature. *Mov Disord, 22*(4), 570–573. https://doi.org/10.1002/mds.21318

43. Lee, S., Merriam, A., Kim, T. S., Liebling, M., Dickson, D. W., & Moore, G. R. (1989). Cerebellar degeneration in neuroleptic malignant syndrome: neuropathologic findings and review of the literature concerning heat-related nervous system injury. *J Neurol Neurosurg Psychiatry, 52*(3), 387–391. https://doi.org/10.1136/jnnp.52.3.387

44. Delgado, G., Tuñón, T., Gállego, J., & Villanueva, J. A. (1985). Spinal cord lesions in heat stroke. *J Neurol Neurosurg Psychiatry, 48*(10), 1065–1067. https://doi.org/10.1136/jnnp.48.10.1065

45. Malamud, N., Haymaker, W., & Custer, R. P. (1946). Heat stroke: a clinico-pathologic study of 125 fatal cases. *Mil Surg, 99*(5), 397–449.

46. Kores, B., & Lader, M. H. (1997). Irreversible lithium neurotoxicity: an overview. *Clin Neuropharmacol, 20*(4), 283–299. https://doi.org/10.1097/00002826-199708000-00001

47. Sarrigiannis, P. G., Zis, P., Unwin, Z. C., et al. (2019). Tremor after long term lithium treatment; is it cortical myoclonus? *Cerebellum Ataxias, 6*(1), 5. https://doi.org/10.1186/s40673-019-0100-y

48. Caviness, J. N., & Evidente, V. G. H. (2003). Cortical myoclonus during lithium exposure. *Arch Neurol, 60*(3), 401–404. https://doi.org/10.1001/archneur.60.3.401

49. Hsieh, H. T., & Yeh, Y. W. (2020). Dose-dependent effects of lithium treatment on the aggravation of antipsychotic-induced pisa syndrome. *Clin Neuropharmacol, 43*(3), 90–91. https://doi.org/10.1097/wnf.0000000000000388

50. Chakrabarti, S., & Chand, P. (2002). Lithium—induced tardive dystonia. *Neurol India, 50*(4), 473–475. http://www.neurologyindia.com/article.asp?issn=0028-3886;year=2002;volume=50;issue=4;spage=473;epage=5;aulast=Chakrabarti

51. Chen, W. Y., Chen, A. C., Tsai, S. J., & Lin, J. J. (2013). Reversible oro-lingual dyskinesia related to lithium intoxication. *Acta Neurol Taiwan, 22*(1), 32–35.

52. Fountoulakis, K. N., Tegos, T., & Kimiskidis, V. (2019). Lithium monotherapy-induced tardive dyskinesia. *J Affect Disord, 244*, 78–79. https://doi.org/10.1016/j.jad.2018.10.094

53. Charney, D. S., Kales, A., Soldatos, C. R., & Nelson, J. C. (1979). Somnambulistic-like episodes secondary to combined lithium-neuroleptic treatment. *Br J Psychiatry, 135*, 418–424. https://doi.org/10.1192/bjp.135.5.418

54. Landry, P., Warnes, H., Nielsen, T., & Montplaisir, J. (1999). Somnambulistic-like behaviour in patients attending a lithium clinic. *Int Clin Psychopharmacol, 14*(3), 173–175.

55. Rosenberg, G. (2007). The mechanisms of action of valproate in neuropsychiatric disorders: can we see the forest for the trees? *Cell Mol Life Sci, 64*(16), 2090–2103. https://doi.org/10.1007/s00018-007-7079-x

56. VanDongen, A. M., VanErp, M. G., & Voskuyl, R. A. (1986). Valproate reduces excitability by blockage of sodium and potassium conductance. *Epilepsia, 27*(3), 177–182. https://doi.org/10.1111/j.1528-1157.1986.tb03525.x

57. Broicher, T., Seidenbecher, T., Meuth, P., et al. (2007). T-current related effects of antiepileptic drugs and a Ca2+ channel antagonist on thalamic relay and local circuit interneurons in a rat model of absence epilepsy. *Neuropharmacology, 53*(3), 431–446. https://doi.org/10.1016/j.neuropharm.2007.05.030

58. Perucca, E. (2002). Pharmacological and therapeutic properties of valproate: a summary after 35 years of clinical experience. *CNS Drugs, 16*(10), 695–714. https://doi.org/10.2165/00023210-200216100-00004

59. Smaga, S. (2003). Tremor. *Am Fam Physician, 68*(8), 1545–1552.

60. Karas, B. J., Wilder, B. J., Hammond, E. J., & Bauman, A. W. (1982). Valproate tremors. *Neurology, 32*(4), 428–432. https://doi.org/10.1212/wnl.32.4.428

61. Baizabal-Carvallo, J. F., & Alonso-Juarez, M. (2021). Valproate-induced rest tremor and parkinsonism. *Acta Neurol Belg, 121*(2), 515–519. https://doi.org/10.1007/s13760-019-01239-8

62. Arbaizar, B., Gómez-Acebo, I., & Llorca, J. (2008). Postural induced-tremor in psychiatry. *Psychiatry Clin Neurosci, 62*(6), 638–645. https://doi.org/10.1111/j.1440-1819.2008.01877.x

63. Silver, M., & Factor, S. A. (2013). Valproic acid-induced parkinsonism: levodopa responsiveness with dyskinesia. *Parkinsonism Relat Disord, 19*(8), 758–760. https://doi.org/10.1016/j.parkreldis.2013.03.016

64. Alvarez-Gomez, M. J., Vaamonde, J., Narbona, J., et al. (1993). Parkinsonian syndrome in childhood after sodium valproate administration. *Clin Neuropharmacol, 16*(5), 451–455. https://doi.org/10.1097/00002826-199310000-00009

65. Alonso-Juarez, M., & Baizabal-Carvallo, J. F. (2018). Distinguishing features between valproate-induced tremor and essential tremor. *Acta Neurol Scand, 138*(2), 177–181. https://doi.org/10.1111/ane.12953

66. Armon, C., Shin, C., Miller, P., et al. (1996). Reversible parkinsonism and cognitive impairment with chronic valproate use. *Neurology, 47*(3), 626–635. https://doi.org/10.1212/wnl.47.3.626

67. Caruana Galizia, E., Isaacs, J. D., & Cock, H. R. (2017). Non-hyperammonaemic valproate encephalopathy after 20 years of treatment. *Epilepsy Behav Case Rep, 8*, 9–11. https://doi.org/10.1016/j.ebcr.2017.04.002

68. Brugger, F., Bhatia, K. P., & Besag, F. M. (2016). Valproate-associated parkinsonism: a critical review of the literature. *CNS Drugs, 30*(6), 527–540. https://doi.org/10.1007/s40263-016-0341-8

69. Shill, H. A., & Fife, T. D. (2000). Valproic acid toxicity mimicking multiple system atrophy. *Neurology, 55*(12), 1936–1937. https://doi.org/10.1212/wnl.55.12.1936

70. Abilash Muralidharan, J. R., Banerjee, D., Mohammad, A. R. H., & Malik, B. H. (2020). *Parkinsonism: A Rare Adverse Effect of Valproic Acid.* https://doi.org/10.7759/cureus.8782

71. Morgan, J. C., & Sethi, K. D. (2005). Drug-induced tremors. *Lancet Neurol, 4*(12), 866–876. https://doi.org/10.1016/s1474-4422(05)70250-7

72. Hamed, S. A., & Abdellah, M. M. (2017). The relationship between valproate induced tremors and circulating neurotransmitters: a preliminary study. *Int J Neurosci, 127*(3), 236–242. https://doi.org/10.1080/00207454.2016.1181631

73. Rinnerthaler, M., Luef, G., Mueller, J., et al. (2005). Computerized tremor analysis of valproate-induced tremor: a comparative study of controlled-release versus conventional valproate. *Epilepsia, 46*(2), 320–323. https://doi.org/10.1111/j.0013-9580.2005.36204.x

74. Alonso-Juarez, M., Torres-Russotto, D., Crespo-Morfin, P., & Baizabal-Carvallo, J. F. (2017). The clinical features and functional impact of valproate-induced tremor. *Parkinsonism Relat Disord, 44*, 147–150. https://doi.org/10.1016/j.parkreldis.2017.09.011

75. Karas, B. J., Wilder, B. J., Hammond, E. J., & Bauman, A. W. (1983). Treatment of valproate tremors. *Neurology, 33*(10), 1380–1382. https://doi.org/10.1212/wnl.33.10.1380

76. Lancman, M. E., Asconapé, J. J., & Walker, F. (1994). Acetazolamide appears effective in the management of valproate-induced tremor. *Mov Disord, 9*(3), 369. https://doi.org/10.1002/mds.870090321

77. van de Velde, K., Cras, P., & Helsen, G. (2011). Acute chorea caused by valproate in an elderly. *Acta Neurol Belg, 111*(3), 220–221.

78. Lancman, M. E., Asconapé, J. J., & Penry, J. K. (1994). Choreiform movements associated with the use of valproate. *Arch Neurol, 51*(7), 702–704. https://doi.org/10.1001/archneur.1994.00540190086020

79. Srinivasan, S., & Lok, A. W. (2010). Valproate-induced reversible hemichorea. *Mov Disord, 25*(10), 1511–1512. https://doi.org/10.1002/mds.23119

80. Ambrosio, A. F., Soares-Da-Silva, P., Carvalho, C. M., & Carvalho, A. P. (2002). Mechanisms of action of carbamazepine and its derivatives, oxcarbazepine, BIA 2-093, and BIA 2-024. *Neurochem Res, 27*(1–2), 121–130. https://doi.org/10.1023/a:1014814924965

81. Post, R. M. (1988). Time course of clinical effects of carbamazepine: implications for mechanisms of action. *J Clin Psychiatry, 49*(Suppl), 35–48.

82. Caviness, J. N. (2003). The clinical neurophysiology of myoclonus. *Hand Clin Neurophysiol, 1*, 521–548. https://doi.org/10.1016/S1567-4231(09)70180-7

83. Sanjari Moghaddam, H., Tafakhori, A., Darvish, H., Mahmoudi-Gharaei, J., Jamali, F., & Aghamollaii, V. (2018). Treatment of myoclonus-dystonia with carbamazepine. *Parkinsonism Relat Disord, 53*, 116–117. https://doi.org/10.1016/j.parkreldis.2018.05.005

84. Rahko, T., & Hakkinen, V. (1979). Carbamazepine in the treatment of objective myoclonus tinnitus. *J Laryngol Otol, 93*(2), 123–127. https://doi.org/10.1017/s0022215100086849

85. Hirose, G., Singer, P., & Bass, N. H. (1971). Successful treatment of posthypoxic action myoclonus with carbamazepine. *JAMA, 218*(9), 1432–1433.

86. Rissardo, J. P., & Caprara, A. L. F. (2020). Carbamazepine-, oxcarbazepine-, eslicarbazepine-associated movement disorder: a literature review. *Clin Neuropharmacol, 43*(3), 66–80. https://doi.org/10.1097/wnf.0000000000000387

87. O'Neal, W., Jr., Whitten, K. M., Baumann, R. J., Blouin, R. A., & Piecoro, J. J., Jr. (1984). Lack of serious toxicity following carbamazepine overdosage. *Clin Pharm, 3*(5), 545–547.

88. Neglia, J. P., Glaze, D. G., & Zion, T. E. (1984). Tics and vocalizations in children treated with carbamazepine. *Pediatrics, 73*(6), 841–844.

89. Robertson, P. L., Garofalo, E. A., Silverstein, F. S., & Komarynski, M. A. (1993). Carbamazepine-induced tics. *Epilepsia, 34*(5), 965–968. https://doi.org/10.1111/j.1528-1157.1993.tb02119.x

90. Gernaat, H. B., Van de Woude, J., & Touw, D. J. (1991). Fluoxetine and parkinsonism in patients taking carbamazepine. *Am J Psychiatry, 148*(11), 1604–1605. https://doi.org/10.1176/ajp.148.11.1604b

91. Froomes, P. R., & Stewart, M. R. (1994). A reversible parkinsonian syndrome and hepatotoxicity following addition of carbamazepine to sodium valproate. *Aust N Z J Med, 24*(4), 413–414. https://doi.org/10.1111/j.1445-5994.1994.tb01479.x

92. Sotero de Menezes, M. A., Rho, J. M., Murphy, P., & Cheyette, S. (2000). Lamotrigine-induced tic disorder: report of five pediatric cases. *Epilepsia, 41*(7), 862–867. https://doi.org/10.1111/j.1528-1157.2000.tb00254.x

93. Musiek, E. S., Anderson, C. T., Dahodwala, N. A., & Pollard, J. R. (2010). Facial tic associated with lamotrigine in adults. *Mov Disord, 25*(10), 1512–1513. https://doi.org/10.1002/mds.23120

94. Verma, A., Miller, P., Carwile, S. T., Husain, A. M., & Radtke, R. A. (1999). Lamotrigine-induced blepharospasm. *Pharmacotherapy, 19*(7), 877–880. https://doi.org/10.1592/phco.19.10.877.31554

95. Zaatreh, M., Tennison, M., D'Cruz, O., & Beach, R. L. (2001). Anticonvulsants-induced chorea: a role for pharmacodynamic drug interaction? *Seizure, 10*(8), 596–599. https://doi.org/10.1053/seiz.2001.0555

96. Frost, M. D., Ritter, F. J., Hoskin, C., Mims, J. and Espo-Lillo, J. (1996). Movement disorder associated with lamotrigine treatment in children and adolescents. *Epilepsia, 37*, 112.

97. Uberall, M. A., & Wenzel, D. (2000). Effectiveness of lamotrigine in children with paroxysmal kinesigenic choreoathetosis. *Dev Med Child Neurol, 42*(10), 699–700. https://doi.org/10.1017/s0012162200001286

98. Pereira, A. C., Loo, W. J., Bamford, M., & Wroe, S. J. (2000). Use of lamotrigine to treat paroxysmal kinesigenic choreoathetosis. *J Neurol Neurosurg Psychiatry, 68*(6), 796–797. https://doi.org/10.1136/jnnp.68.6.796a

99. Marrero-Gonzalez, P. C., Ruano, O. L., Catalano, G., & Catalano, M. C. (2014). Dystonia associated with lamotrigine therapy: a case report and review of the literature. *Curr Drug Saf, 9*(1), 60-62. https://doi.org/10.2174/18715249113136660060

100. Richter, A., Löschmann, P. A., & Löscher, W. (1994). The novel antiepileptic drug, lamotrigine, exerts prodystonic effects in a mutant hamster model of generalized dystonia. *Eur J Pharmacol, 264*(3), 345–351. https://doi.org/10.1016/0014-2999(94)00493-5

101. Teive, H. A., Troiano, A. R., Germiniani, F. M., & Werneck, L. C. (2004). Flunarizine and cinnarizine-induced parkinsonism: a historical and clinical analysis. *Parkinsonism Relat Disord, 10*(4), 243–245. https://doi.org/10.1016/j.parkreldis.2003.12.004

102. Jhang, K.-M., Huang, J.-Y., Nfor, O. N., et al. (2017). Extrapyramidal symptoms after exposure to calcium channel blocker-flunarizine or cinnarizine. *European Journal of Clinical Pharmacology, 73*(7), 911–916. https://doi.org/10.1007/s00228-017-2247-x

103. Martí-Massó, J. F., & Poza, J. J. (1998). Cinnarizine-induced parkinsonism: ten years later. *Mov Disord, 13*(3), 453–456. https://doi.org/10.1002/mds.870130313

104. Llau, M. E., Nguyen, L., Senard, J. M., Rascol, O., & Montastruc, J. L. (1994). [Drug-induced parkinsonian syndromes: a 10-year experience at a regional center of pharmaco-vigilance]. *Rev Neurol (Paris), 150*(11), 757–762.

105. Errea-Abad, J. M., Ara-Callizo, J. R., & Aibar-Remón, C. (1998). [Drug-induced parkinsonism. Clinical aspects compared with Parkinson disease]. *Rev Neurol, 27*(155), 35–39.

106. MELO-SOUZA, SE. Flunarizina, parkinsonismo e depressão. XI Congresso Brasileiro de Neurologia. Tema livre. Resumo p. 39. Goiania, 1984.

107. Capellà, D., Laporte, J. R., Castel, J. M., Tristán, C., Cos, A., & Morales-Olivas, F. J. (1988). Parkinsonism, tremor, and depression induced by cinnarizine and flunarizine. *BMJ (Clinical research ed.), 297*(6650), 722–723. https://doi.org/10.1136/bmj.297.6650.722

108. Micheli, F., Pardal, M. F., Gatto, M., et al. (1987). Flunarizine- and cinnarizine-induced extrapyramidal reactions. *Neurology, 37*(5), 881–884. https://doi.org/10.1212/wnl.37.5.881

109. Giménez-Roldán, S., & Mateo, D. (1991). Cinnarizine-induced parkinsonism: susceptibility related to aging and essential tremor. *Clin Neuropharmacol*, *14*(2), 156–164. https://doi.org/10.1097/00002826-199104000-00005

110. Negrotti, A., Calzetti, S., & Sasso, E. (1992). Calcium-entry blockers-induced parkinsonism: possible role of inherited susceptibility. *Neurotoxicology*, *13*(1), 261–264.

9

Movement Disorders Associated With Stimulants and Other Drugs of Abuse

Luiz Paulo Vasconcelos, Jordi Gandini, Antonio L. Teixeira, and Mario Manto

Introduction

Substance use disorders (SUDs) are the consequence of abuse of and/or dependence on drugs that affect multiple brain circuits, including the ones involved in effortful decision-making, motivation, and hedonic experience.[1] The clinical effects of these drugs result from the recurrent activation and plastic changes of the reward system, notably the dopaminergic mesolimbic pathway and the nigrostriatal pathway.[2]

Cannabis, amphetamines, cocaine, and opioids are among the illicit and/or controlled prescribed drugs most commonly used. The clandestine use of these drugs underestimates the real burden of SUD, including the impact on health services and social and occupational functioning.[3] Nonetheless, the Global Burden of Disease 2017 report estimated a prevalence of 175,588,800 people under illicit drug use worldwide, representing a 34.3% increase in the rate of years lived with disability (YLDs) from 1990 to 2017.[4] SUDs represent an international public health problem, since they are currently the seventh cause of YLDs among males and the eighteenth among females worldwide.[4] Opioid use disorder is the most prevalent SUD, affecting an estimated 40,484,600 illicit users, followed by cannabis (17,857.3 million patients), amphetamine (7,382.6 million patients) and cocaine (5,017.2 million patients) use disorders.[4]

Cannabis effects include euphoria, increased self-confidence and relaxation.[1] Similarly, opioid use promotes euphoria, anxiolysis, feelings of relaxation and drowsiness.[5] Psychostimulants, such as amphetamines and cocaine, can cause increased alertness, euphoria, and increased energy as well as decreasing appetite and need for sleep. Interestingly, even experienced drug abusers cannot distinguish significant differences between cocaine and amphetamines, since their clinical effects are quite similar.[1,6]

The recurrent use of psychostimulants can cause several acute and chronic medical issues. Furthermore, chronic psychostimulant users suffer from nutritional deficiencies and expose themselves to risk behaviors, being prone to traumatic injuries and sexually transmitted diseases, particularly AIDS.[7] The most frequent acute consequences of psychostimulants are hypertensive crises, stroke, headache, movement disorders, seizures, and psychosis.[1,8,9] Some long-term complications include mood and psychotic disorders, neurocognitive impairment and frontobasal circuits damage, leading to persistent movement disorders.[1,8] The main neurocognitive symptoms include deficits in executive functions and short and long-term memory.[1,9] Among acute movement disorders, psychostimulants may induce chorea, tics, akathisia, tremor, dystonic reactions, and stereotypies.[1,10] Chronic use of

Table 9.1 Most Common Movement Disorders Associated With Substance Use Disorders

Drugs of Abuse	Movement Disorders
Amphetamines	Choreaoathetosis
	Exacerbation of tics
	Stereotypies
	Parkinsonism
Cocaine	Chorea ("crack dancing")
	Exacerbation of tics
	Dystonic reactions and orofacial dyskinesia ("boca torcida")
Cathinones	Choreaoathetosis
	Dystonic reactions
	Parkinsonism*
Opioids	Myoclonia
	Choreoathetosis
	Muscular rigidity

*Parkinsonism in cathinones is associated with methcatinone use by manganese intoxication

psychostimulants can lead to stereotypic motor behaviors, tics, dystonia, chorea, and myoclonus.[11,12] Parkinsonism has been also associated with psychostimulants.[13–15]

In this chapter, we will describe the involuntary movements associated with SUD, mainly psychostimulants, focusing on the manifestations of outside the intoxication phase. In Table 9.1, we summarize the most frequent movement disorders associated with SUD.

Movement Disorders Associated With Amphetamines

Humans have used natural stimulants for thousands of years by consuming amphetamine-producing plants such as the ones from the genus Ephedrae (family Ephedraceae).[6] Synthetic amphetamines have been used both therapeutically and recreationally since the 1930s and their illicit use has been rising in the last decades.[4,16] Methamphetamine, for instance, was synthesized from ephedrine, derived from the plant *Ephedra sinica* by Nagai Nagayoshi in 1893. Initially, the drug was commercialized as an over-the-counter (OTC) nasal decongestant and a bronchodilator. Since the early 1960s, illegal production of methamphetamine and other amphetamines in clandestine labs has increased in the United States. By using OTC ephedrine and pseudoephedrine as the main precursors, the illegal production of methamphetamine became quite simple. Subsequently, in the 1980s, a crystalline form of methamphetamine that could be smoked was developed and became very popular.[17,18] Its low cost, relatively easy access, and long duration of effects are contributing factors to methamphetamine abuse.[1]

Despite international efforts to control access to ingredients and precursors of synthetic amphetamine and its illicit commerce, amphetamine use disorder (AUD) is currently the third most frequent SUD and represents a major public health problem worldwide.[4]

Accordingly, amphetamines are classified as a schedule II drug by the Food and Drug Administration (FDA), and are only currently approved for attention-deficit/hyperactivity disorder (ADHD), extreme obesity, or to treat narcolepsy.[14,19,20]

Methamphetamine and 3,4-methylenedioxymethamphetamine (MDMA), also known as ecstasy, are the most used and studied amphetamines. Methamphetamine is taken by oral, intravenous, nasal, or smoking routes, whereas MDMA is usually ingested orally. They are psychoactive substances with stimulant, euphoric, anorectic, and, in some cases, empathogenic and hallucinogenic properties. The associated hyperadrenergic state leads to increase in pulse rate and blood pressure, with the risk of hypertensive crisis and stroke.[1] Among amphetamines, MDMA has greater hallucinogenic properties, probably associated with its enhanced serotonergic effects, which is more prominent than the dopamine-releasing effects.[7] Methamphetamine and its metabolite amphetamine act by promoting changes in monoaminergic neurotransmission. They bind to dopamine (DAT), norepinephrine (NAT), and, to a lesser extent, serotonin transporters (SERTs) located on neuronal cell membranes, reducing the reuptake of neurotransmitters. At higher concentrations, amphetamines can cross cell membranes independent of their binding to transporters and promote the release of dopamine (DA), serotonin (5-HT), and noradrenalin (NE) from storage vesicles, increasing their cytoplasmic concentrations and their subsequent extracellular release. Methamphetamine enters synaptic vesicles through the vesicular monoamine transporter 2 (vMAT-2) and causes DA release into the cytoplasm. Therefore, methamphetamine can cause a rapid and sustained increase in the extracellular concentrations of monoamines.[1,7,17,18] Increased DA levels in the cytoplasm also lead to accumulation of reactive oxygen species and severe oxidative stress, causing mitochondrial dysfunction and peroxidative damage to presynaptic membranes. These events are probably responsible for the degeneration of DA terminals observed in animal models.[1,10] MDMA is a substrate of the SERT, which reduces 5-HT neuronal reuptake. MDMA also inhibits the activity of tryptophan hydroxylase (TPH), the rate-limiting enzyme for serotonin synthesis, and inhibits serotonin degradation by monoamine oxidase B. DA-induced oxidative stress in 5-HT terminals, and 5-HT2A and dopamine D1 receptor-mediated hyperthermia are potential causative factors for MDMA neurotoxicity.[1]

Movement disorders have been described both during acute amphetamine intoxication and with the chronic use of the drug, as a long-term complication. Acute movement disorders manifest because of the greater availability of DA in the nigrostriatal pathway, whereas persistent movement disorders might be related to basal ganglia (mainly striatal) damage due to oxidative stress. In fact, experimental studies show methamphetamine-induced structural damage in DA neurons with long-term neurotransmitter depletion.[7,21,22]

Chorea, tics, and stereotypies are the most common hyperkinetic movements reported.[6,23] Choreoathetoid movements typically involve the limbs, neck, and face.[6,10,21] Rhee et al. reported three patients admitted to an emergency department with amphetamine-induced chorea. All patients manifested symptoms between 2 hours to 2 days after having the drug and their chorea resolved within hours to 1 day with haloperidol.[24] Typical neuroleptics, anticholinergic drugs, and benzodiazepines have been used to control chorea in these cases.[25] Some authors argue that the development of chorea from amphetamines may require an underlying striatum pathology, since amphetamines worsened choreic movements in patients with other known causes of chorea, such as Sydenham's chorea, Huntington's disease, and lupus.[17,18] In some patients, movement disorders can last years after they have stopped using amphetamines, suggesting that chorea may be persistent due to damage in the striatum. Choreoathetoid movements may resurge after amphetamine relapse, suggesting a permanent susceptibility to this movement disorder.[17,18]

Chorea has also been reported with methylphenidate use, an amphetamine typically used for ADHD.[10] Balazs et al. reported a 6½-year-old boy with ADHD and intellectual disability who developed orofacial and limb chorea immediately after methylphenidate administration, which lasted for 5 hours.[26] Similarly, Yilmaz et al. reported a 7-year-old boy with controlled seizures who also developed orofacial and limb dyskinesia after 5 hours of methylphenidate administration, which lasted 10 hours.[27] In both cases, the associated conditions (possibly indicating an affected brain, i.e., intellectual disability and epilepsy) may have contributed to the chorea emergence after drug administration. Morgan et al. reported a 22-year-old man initially treated with methylphenidate for ADHD who developed manic-like and choreiform movements after switching to mixed amphetamine salts. Symptoms resolved within 3 days after amphetamine withdrawal and the use of diphenhydramine and benzodiazepines. Prior to discharge, methylphenidate was restarted without recurrence of chorea.[28] This case suggests that methylphenidate might display a safer profile than mixed amphetamines regarding dyskinesia. It is worth mentioning that amphetamines, including methylphenidate, can uncover a pre-existing cause for chorea. Waugh et al. reported an 8-year-old boy treated for ADHD with methylphenidate who developed generalized chorea. Despite discontinuation of methylphenidate, chorea persisted. His father had the diagnosis of Huntington's disease and genetic testing of the child revealed 75 CAG repeats.[29]

Emergence or exacerbation of tics including Tourette's syndrome (TS) has been reported with amphetamines.[30] While most patients manifest tics right after amphetamine administration, tardive Tourette-like syndrome has already been described in patients using methylphenidate.[30] The emergence of tics is a major concern in patients taking amphetamines for ADHD. However, there is no robust evidence for an elevated risk of first-onset tics during stimulant medication in children and adolescents with ADHD without pre-existing tics.[31] Moreover, tic exacerbation may occur in a small minority of patients with the disorder.[20] Lipkin et al. (1994) conducted a chart review of 122 children with ADHD treated with stimulants. Tics and dyskinesias were reported in 9% of the children. Only one child developed movements and tics sufficient for a diagnosis of TS. Age, medication, dosage, and history of tics did not predict the manifestation of tics or dyskinesias.[32] Accordingly, tics are no longer a contraindication for amphetamines in patients with ADHD in the European Union, but clinicians must be cautious since stimulant drugs may exacerbate tics in individual cases.[20] For patients with ADHD who are displaying tics, other therapeutic alternatives should be considered, such as atomoxetine and guanfacine, with less propensity for exacerbating tics.[20]

Similar to other amphetamines, movement disorders have been observed in MDMA users. They tend to occur immediately after drug use, although they can be more enduring. Off-drug tremors or twitches attributed to ecstasy/MDMA were reported by 14% of novice users, 20% of moderate users, and 38% of experienced users.[8] MDMA use has also been associated with acute dystonic reaction involving the neck and coarse action tremor in the upper limb and postural tremor hours after ecstasy intake.[33]

Alongside acute movement disorders, dopaminergic-related neurotoxicity may cause permanent damage to basal ganglia and, therefore, persistent cognitive impairment and movement disorders. Todd et al. (2019) found that chronic motor effects, such as deficits in fine dexterity and timed gait tasks, exist in methamphetamine users. These effects were observed in users who had been abstinent for at least 12 months, suggesting that some psychomotor changes may be persistent. Whether these movement disorders are associated with increased risk of future development of Parkinson's disease is unclear.[34] A postmortem brain analysis study carried out in methamphetamine users showed marked dopamine loss in the caudate, whereas in PD the putamen is distinctly more affected.[35] Substantia nigra (SN) loss of dopamine-containing cell bodies is characteristic of PD, but similar neuropathological studies remain to be demonstrated in methamphetamine users.[22] Despite such differences, in Table 9.2 we list different levels of evidence that have been identified supporting the association between PD and methamphetamine.[1,6,14,16,36–40] Interestingly, the high rates of nicotine smoking among methamphetamine users—a putative protective factor against PD—may somewhat mask the risk conferred by methamphetamine. Furthermore, high mortality among methamphetamine users may prevent many from reaching an age at which PD might otherwise become diagnosable.[21] Significant and enduring dopamine toxicity caused by meth/amphetamine might only become clinically evident in susceptible users who have advanced to middle or older age.[16] Besides methamphetamine, MDMA may cause parkinsonism with anecdotal reports.[41]

Table 9.2 Different Levels of Evidence Supporting the Association Between Methamphetamine and Parkinsonism/Parkinson's Disease (PD)

Level of Evidence	Main Findings	Reference
Neuroimaging and Neuropathological studies	Decrease in striatal dopamine, dopamine transporter, tyrosine hydroxylase similar to PD.	[1, 6]
	Amphetamines are associated with hyperechogenicity of the substantia nigra on transcranial sonography and subtle clinical parkinsonian signs compared to cannabis, MDMA and non-drug-users.	[40]
Epidemiological studies	Two- to threefold increase in the risk of PD in methamphetamine/amphetamine users compared to cocaine users and nonexposed controls.	[14, 36]
	PD patients previously exposed to amphetamines had younger age compared to the nonexposed PD group.	[16]
In vitro studies	Methamphetamine can act similar to other environmental stressors associated with PD, such as paraquat and 1-methyl-4-phenyl-1, 2, 3, 6-tetrahydropyridine (MPTP), by eliciting senescence in the aging brain.	[37]
	The use of substances that block both VT and dopamine transporter and not only the latter, such as amphetamines, leads to higher cytosolic dopamine concentration and elevated oxidative stress, which can mediate neurodegeneration.	[38]
	Methamphetamine binds to the N-terminus of α-synuclein and causes conformational changes in the protein, which may influence the formation of Lewy bodies and increase the incidence of PD among users of the drug.	[39]

Persistent tremors have also been observed in MDMA abstinent users and in patients with both current and previous mixed psychostimulant addiction, including MDMA, amphetamines, cocaine and mephedrone.[42,43] Using an accelerometer attached to the patients' dominant index finger, Flavel et al. found that abstinent MDMA users exhibit an abnormally large tremor during movements compared to abstinent users of cannabis, amphetamines and control subjects.[42] This finding of persistent tremor in MDMA patients was surprising, as the majority of individuals had minimal to moderate exposure to the drug and an average abstinent period of three months. Abstinent amphetamine users did not display persistent tremors, which could be partially explained by a longer duration of abstinence compared to MDMA group.[42] Similarly, Downey et al. reported psychomotor symptoms, including tremors, in current and former recreational drug users when compared to non-drug-users.[43] In this study, abstinent psychostimulants users, including MDMA and amphetamines, exhibited persistent tremors detected by a wrist accelerometer, which could last for at least 18 months.[43] Future studies are required to determine whether persistent tremors represent a risk marker for movement disorders development in MDMA, amphetamines and other stimulant users.[42,43]

Alongside persistent movement disorders and chronic cognitive and behavioral impairment, another unique long-term manifestation associated with amphetamine users is the development of punding. The word "punding" is derived from the Swedish and means "blockhead." It is characterized by stereotyped and persistent behaviors, notably with non-goal-directed activity. Patients perform complex repetitive behaviors, such as endless collecting and arranging objects, shoe-shining, or nail polishing to the point of bleeding. There seems to be a predilection for activities usually performed by the drug user. For example, an artist may doodle, draw, or paint excessively.[6,17,18] According to Rylander et al., 26% of heavy users of amphetamine experience punding.[44] It is important to emphasize that punding syndrome should not be confused with stereotypies, which manifest as simpler repetitive movements like repetitive trunk flexions or flapping. Of note, punding has also been described in patients with PD using dopaminergics.[45]

Movement Disorders Associated With Cocaine

Cocaine is a natural alkaloid with potent psychostimulant activity. It was first extracted from the plant *Erythroxylum coca* in the mid-nineteenth century. Indigenous population of the Andes have used the plant for centuries before the European conquest and it played an important role in the Inca rites and customs. Chewed coca leaves are still used by Andean population to alleviate altitude sickness.[46] Despite its criminalization as a recreational drug since 1950s, cocaine use has steadily risen, becoming a public health problem. In the 1980s, the drug became available in a smokable form known as "crack." Crack has relatively lower in price and soon became popular among urban low-income Americans.[6,46] Cocaine causes intense euphoria, increased alertness, and energy that are linked to inhibition of DAT function and consequent increase of DA levels in the synaptic cleft. DAT levels and DA uptake are increased in the ventral striatum of chronic cocaine abusers, while SERTs are increased in the nucleus accumbens and striatum of victims of cocaine overdose.[1,10] Cocaine also influences the activity of medium-size GABA-containing spiny neurons that represent the main striatal neuronal population. Conversely, chronic use results in dopamine depletion.[10] One possible explanation is that cocaine may decrease both TH activity and postsynaptic DA receptor sites, indicating that DA depletion may be a compensatory mechanism triggered by dopaminergic overstimulation.[47]

Cocaine overdose may be associated with several neurological complications such as seizures, headaches, stroke (ischemic and hemorrhagic), and behavioral and movement disorders. Other acute adverse consequences include cardiovascular, thermoregulatory, and respiratory symptoms.[1,6,46] Some patients may present a cocaine-induced excited delirium, a syndrome similar to neuroleptic malignant syndrome characterized by hyperthermia, extrapyramidal signs, altered consciousness, and autonomic dysfunction.[1] Long-term effects of the drug include mood symptoms, drug craving, and cognitive impairment.[1,6] As with amphetamines, cocaine neurocognitive impairment includes decline in different domains including verbal memory, learning, and executive function.[1]

Several different movement disorders secondary to cocaine have been published, such as multifocal tics and Tourette-like symptoms, choreic movements, akathisia, and dystonia.[48] Punding and exacerbation of opsoclonus-myoclonus have also been reported.[11,49] Despite anecdotally reported, prolonged dyskinetic movements seem to occur only after chronic cocaine use.[1,50] Tardive dyskinesia and TS can be worsened by cocaine use.[23,51] For instance, a subject with TS and a patient with paranoid schizophrenia and neuroleptic-related tardive dystonia had marked exacerbations and/or recurrence of their pre-existing movement disorders with cocaine exposure.[52] In the same line, pre-existing dystonia and essential-like tremor can be exacerbated by cocaine.[7,52] Dystonia can occur secondary to cocaine withdrawal and may manifest after recreational use of cocaine in patients previously exposed to neuroleptics.[7,49,53] Cocaine can also cause dystonic reactions in the absence of other risk factors.[53,54]

Although there is limited clinical or literature evidence documenting cocaine-induced choreic movements, multiple references to "crack-dancing" suggest that it may be more common than physicians recognize.[10] Clinically, patients displaying "crack-dancing" exhibit hyperkinetic, random, and involuntary movements in the trunk and limbs. In young cocaine users with choreic movements, facial dyskinesias were also observed.[55] Hispanic cocaine users call the buccolingual dyskinesias "boca torcida" (literally, twisted mouth). Daras et al. reported seven patients with acute dyskinesias among 701 cocaine-related emergency room visits or admissions. The abnormal movements consisted of choreoathetoid movements involving the extremities in all cases. In addition, two patients had akathisia, one had buccolingual dyskinesias, and one had eye-blinking and lip-smacking. The onset of abnormal movements following cocaine use was nearly immediate in three patients, after two hours in one, and after one night in two. All movements lasted from 2 to 6 days and gradually disappeared with minimal or no treatment.[47] In such patients, duration of cocaine use prior to the onset of movements ranged from 8 months to 5 years. History of exposure to neuroleptics was obtained in two patients; one had used methylphenidate in childhood and one had also used heroin.[47] Although most patients display short-lasting dyskinesias, Weiner et al. described a woman with persistent movements for 20 months.[48]

As cocaine users often take other psychostimulants, defining the specific cause of the involuntary movement can be challenging.[47] Moreover, many patients have predisposing factors such as neuropsychiatric conditions, such as TS, or prior exposure to neuroleptics,[47] amphetamines,[55] or opioids.[56]

In contrast to amphetamines, epidemiological studies do not show increased risk for PD with cocaine use.[9,14] Despite chronic cocaine use results in dopamine depletion, there is no robust evidence of parkinsonism in cocaine users. One explanation for this may stem from the fact that amphetamines block both VMAT and DAT, while cocaine only blocks DAT resulting in lesser cytosolic dopamine levels and decreased neurodegeneration in the basal ganglia in the latter.[38] Once cocaine users also abuse amphetamines, this may explain why some patients developed parkinsonism.[57] Conversely, Illés et al. reported a patient with mutation in LRRK2 gene who developed a reversible parkinsonism associated with chronic cocaine use, raising the possibility of a gene-environment interaction.[58]

Movement Disorders Associated With Cathinones ("Bath Salts")

Cathinone is a potent natural amphetamine extracted from *Catha edulis* (khat), a plant that grows at high altitudes in East Africa and the Arabian Peninsula.[6] Synthetic cathinones are among the new psychoactive substances which are a complex and diverse group of substances often known as either designer or synthetic drugs, or by "legal highs." They are analogues of existing controlled drugs and pharmaceutical products or newly synthesized chemicals created to mimic the actions and psychoactive effects of other controlled substances.[5] The synthetic cathinones are becoming increasingly popular. These β-keto amphetamine analogues are also known as research chemicals, bath salts, plant food. or glass cleaner.[59] Common first-generation synthetic cathinones include methcathinone, mephedrone, methylone, and 3,4-methylenedioxypyrovalerone (MDPV).[1,5]

These chemicals act by releasing catecholamines from presynaptic storage sites, causing amphetamine and cocaine-like effects.[60,61] Cathinones release DA by inhibiting the VMAT2, reversing the transporter influx, thereby stimulating neurotransmitter release from the cytosolic pool or synaptic vesicles, while inhibiting the reuptake of neurotransmitters from the synaptic cleft.[5] They are most frequently used as white powder or crystalline mixtures by intravenous route but also taken orally as tablets. The intranasal, intramuscular, and rectal routes of administration have also been reported for mephedrone and methylone. The intravenous route for cathinones, including mephedrone, represents a major health concern.[59]

Primary effects sought by cathinone users are euphoria, talkativeness, increased alertness, empathy, intensification of sensory experiences, reduced appetite, insomnia, increased sexual performance, and increased sociability.[59] Acute motor effects of mephedrone are jaw clenching, and bruxism/teeth grinding, suggesting some dystonic and stereotyped reactions, similar to that observed in amphetamine and cocaine users. Tremors are observed during mephedrone withdrawal.[59] Methylone, in turn, has a structure similar to MDMA and, therefore, shares many of the risks generally associated to MDMA.[59]

Chronic methcathinone (ephedrone) use is associated with a severe neurological syndrome characterized by levodopa unresponsive bradykinesia, retropulsion with falls backward, hypophonic dysarthria, risus sardonicus, involuntary laughter, upright unsteady gait, limb dystonia, and apraxia of eyelid opening. This syndrome, also termed "ephedrone encephalopathy," resembles progressive supranuclear palsy (PSP), except for normal eye movements.[5,61] Methcathinone is synthesized by oxidation of ephedrine or pseudoephedrine (present in OTC nasal decongestants) with potassium permanganate. Manganese poisoning is the most accepted hypothesis for this severe parkinsonian manifestation in methcathinone users. The likelihood that this manganese poisoning causes parkinsonism is supported by findings of increased signal in the globus pallidus (GP) and the reticular part of SN on T1 MR imaging and elevated whole blood manganese levels. Moreover, the clinical syndrome of methcathinone toxicity is also similar to the earlier reports of chronic manganism. Besides, it is possible that a chronic increase in catecholamine release in the brain by methcathinone could further increase the risk of manganese neurotoxicity.[5,61] The prognosis of methcathinone neurotoxicity is poor, with significant residual or permanent deficits.[61]

Synthetic cathinones constitute an expanding group of substances, since there is an attempt to maintain a supply of new psychoactive substances whose structures lie within the legislation.[62] Despite its functional similarity with amphetamines, the understanding of its motor effects is still limited.

Movement Disorders Associated With Opioids

Opioid addiction is the current most prevalent SUD worldwide and is a severe public health problem, especially in the United States.[4] Opioids have their biochemical and physiological effects via stimulation of three types of opiate receptors, μ, κ, and δ, present on cell membranes. The classical opioids used for pain management act at the μ receptor, whereas the opioid antagonists naloxone and naltrexone bind to all receptor subtypes. There are mixed agonists-antagonists, such as pentatocine, butorphanol, and nalbuphine, and partial agonists such as buprenorphine. Acting on the central nervous system, opioids produce analgesia, a sense of relaxation, a decreased sense of apprehension, and suppression of ventilation. Administered by the oral route, opioids have a lower risk for the development of dependence compared with intravenous use.[7]

The stimulation of μ and κ opioid receptors are thought to, respectively, inhibit and amplify GABAergic inhibitory interneurons in various brain regions, modulating putative brain areas involved in the physiology of movements. For instance, methadone and heroin μ-agonism inhibit GABAergic inhibitory pathways, which can lead to amplification of dopamine and glutamate release in striatum and induce choreiform hyperkinesias.[63] Experimental models also show that endogenous opioids induce hyperkinetic movement disorders through sustained activation of opioid receptors in the globus pallidus.[64–66] Interestingly, the development of heroin drug-seeking behavior in rodents does not seem to be dopamine-dependent. Dopamine release is not increased following opioid administration, but opioids activate DA neurons indirectly, either resulting in limited increase in DA release or its fast uptake by terminals, therefore other sites seem to be responsible for addiction in opioid use.[10]

Heroin (diacetylmorphine) is a potent addictive opioid and represents the most commonly abused illicit opiate. It is a semisynthetic drug derived from opium. The drug is taken orally, via inhalation, or by intravenous injections. Heroin users may suffer from embolic strokes and chronic microvascular ischemia. Usually they show several cognitive deficits in neuropsychological tests, notably impairment of visual memory, working memory, processing speed, and executive function.[1] Heroin addiction is also associated with alterations in gray and white matters. Preclinical studies of opioid-induced effects on neural systems support the idea that clinical changes in brain function and structure are consequences of chronic heroin exposure.[1]

Opioids can produce a spectrum of movement abnormalities, including myoclonus, chorea, and rigidity. Myoclonus is the best documented hyperkinetic complication of opioid use.[11] It is normally associated with the rapid escalation of opioid doses or the use of relatively high opioid doses, usually in the setting of acute or cancer related pain.[67] The reported incidence of opioid-related myoclonus varies widely, ranging from 2.7% to 87%.[12] Many authors postulate that the neuroexcitatory metabolites of opioids, such as morphine and hydromorphone metabolites, may be responsible for the development of myoclonus in cancer pain patients treated with high doses of opioids, with M3G being the most potent metabolite. The development of myoclonus and hyperalgesia, as well as chronic nausea, have been attributed respectively to a M3G and M6G accumulation during chronic morphine therapy.[12] However, Hoffman et al. reported a 75-year-old man with multiple system atrophy (MSA) who presented severe generalized myoclonus, decreased level of arousal, and muscular rigidity just after the administration of a single dose of hydromorphone for pain control. Within seconds of naloxone administration, his condition improved dramatically, with a complete reversal of the myoclonus and a return to normal consciousness. Although naloxone would be incapable of reversing side effects in cases in which accumulation of opioid metabolites is responsible for neurotoxicity, the drug might be effective in acute-onset instances. In this report, the comorbid MSA might have led to a predisposition to this unusual presentation of opioid-induced myoclonus.[68]

There are numerous case reports of chorea secondary to opioids including heroin, methadone, oxycodone, fentanyl, propoxyphene, and hydromorphone.[66] In a clinic of legal supervised consumption of drugs in Canada, from 1,581 opioid overdoses seen between October 2016, and April 2017, 497 (31.4%) had atypical features such as muscle rigidity, dyskinesia, slow or irregular heart rate, confusion, and anisocoria. Among these patients, acute dyskinesia was the second most common atypical overdose presentation in 150 cases (30% of atypical cases).[69]

Methadone is associated with chorea and occasionally ballism. Several case reports have documented this association.[10] For example, Wasserman and Yahr reported a 25-year-old man who developed choreic movements of the upper limbs and torso and speech impairment after receiving methadone for heroin addiction. Movements were so severe that discontinuation of methadone was required, with no subsequent recurrence.[70] Bonnet et al. (1998) also described choreoathetoid movements following rapid increase in methadone dose, which resolved with a lower methadone dose.[63] Lussier and Cruciani reported a female patient with reported relapses of heroin use two months after diagnosis of small cell lung cancer who had acute choreoathetoid movements after a single dose of methadone for lumbar pain control.[71] When methadone was discontinued and replaced by a transdermal fentanyl patch, the movements resolved within three days. Supersensitivity of dopamine receptors has been postulated in chronic opioid users. In both cases, methadone use in conjunction with previous heroin addiction might result in chronic changes that lead to basal ganglia excitatory dysfunction.[10] Clark and Elliot reported a patient with choreoathetoid movements induced by methadone used for complex regional pain syndrome. In this case, methadone probably enhanced or amplified the underlying movement disorder (tremor) related primarily to the complex regional pain syndrome.[67]

Taken together, many patients with opioid-induced hyperkinetic movement disorders present an underlying condition such as use other psychostimulant drugs and other basal ganglia diseases, which can co-influence dopaminergic activity in nigrostriatal and fronto-striatal pathways.

Levodopa-responsive parkinsonism is associated with the synthetic opioid 1-methyl-4-phenyl-1, 2, 3, 6-tetrahydropyridine (MPTP) or "new heroin" through its metabolite 1-methyl-4-phenylpyridium (MPP+). The MPTP is transformed in MPP+ by monoaminoxidase-B (MAO-B) and transported by DAT into dopaminergic neurons where it inhibits mitochondrial complex I function.[15,72] The neurotoxicity of MPTP is well-known in the literature and the MPTP animal model is frequently used in preclinical studies for PD and other parkinsonism disorders.

Conclusion

There is limited information about the prevalence, pathophysiology, and treatment of SUD-related movement disorders. Movement disorders are not frequently reported in SUD, but their prevalence may be much higher than documented, since drug users frequently employ street terms like "crack dancing" and "boca torcida" to refer to diskynetic movements. Actually, subtle movement disorders are frequently observed, but overlooked by patients with SUD. Drug users usually do not keep close attention to their own health, avoiding clinical consultations. Further studies are needed in the field, especially giving the emergence of novel psychoactive substances.

References

1. Cadet, J.L., V. Bisagno, and C.M. Milroy, *Neuropathology of substance use disorders.* Acta Neuropathol, 2014. **127**(1): p. 91–107.
2. Volkow, N.D., et al., *Addiction circuitry in the human brain.* Annu Rev Pharmacol Toxicol, 2012. **52**: p. 321–336.
3. Degenhardt, L., and W. Hall, *Extent of illicit drug use and dependence, and their contribution to the global burden of disease.* Lancet, 2012. **379**(9810): p. 55–70.
4. *Global, regional, and national incidence, prevalence, and years lived with disability for 354 diseases and injuries for 195 countries and territories, 1990–2017: a systematic analysis for the Global Burden of Disease Study 2017.* Lancet, 2018. **392**(10159): p. 1789–1858.
5. Shafi, A., et al., *New psychoactive substances: a review and updates.* Ther Adv Psychopharmacol, 2020. 10: p. 2045125320967197.
6. Sanchez-Ramos, J., *Neurologic complications of psychomotor stimulant abuse.* Int Rev Neurobiol, 2015. **120**: p. 131–160.
7. Neiman, J., H.M. Haapaniemi, and M. Hillbom, *Neurological complications of drug abuse: pathophysiological mechanisms.* Eur J Neurol, 2000. **7**(6): p. 595–606.
8. Parrott, A.C., et al., *Parkinson's disorder, psychomotor problems and dopaminergic neurotoxicity in recreational ecstasy/MDMA users.* Psychopharmacology (Berl), 2003. **167**(4): p. 449–450.
9. Lappin, J.M., and G.E. Sara, *Psychostimulant use and the brain.* Addiction, 2019. **114**(11): p. 2065–2077.
10. Miyasaki, J.M., *Chorea caused by toxins.* Handb Clin Neurol, 2011. **100**: p. 335–346.

11. Robottom, B.J., L.M. Shulman, and W.J. Weiner, *Drug-induced movement disorders: emergencies and management.* Neurol Clin, 2012. **30**(1): p. 309–320, x.

12. Mercadante, S., *Pathophysiology and treatment of opioid-related myoclonus in cancer patients.* Pain, 1998. **74**(1): p. 5–9.

13. Sikk, K., et al., *Manganese-induced parkinsonism due to ephedrone abuse.* Parkinsons Dis, 2011. **2011**: p. 865319.

14. Callaghan, R.C., et al., *Increased risk of Parkinson's disease in individuals hospitalized with conditions related to the use of methamphetamine or other amphetamine-type drugs.* Drug Alcohol Depend, 2012. **120**(1–3): p. 35–40.

15. Langston, J.W., et al., *Chronic Parkinsonism in humans due to a product of meperidine-analog synthesis.* Science, 1983. **219**(4587): p. 979–980.

16. Christine, C.W., et al., *Parkinsonism in patients with a history of amphetamine exposure.* Mov Disord, 2010. **25**(2): p. 228–231.

17. Rusyniak, D.E., *Neurologic manifestations of chronic methamphetamine abuse.* Psychiatr Clin North Am, 2013. **36**(2): p. 261–275.

18. Rusyniak, D.E., *Neurologic manifestations of chronic methamphetamine abuse.* Neurol Clin, 2011. **29**(3): p. 641–655.

19. Christine, C.W., W.J. Marks, Jr., and J.L. Ostrem, *Development of Parkinson's disease in patients with Narcolepsy.* J Neural Transm (Vienna), 2012. **119**(6): p. 697–699.

20. Cortese, S., et al., *Practitioner review: current best practice in the management of adverse events during treatment with ADHD medications in children and adolescents.* J Child Psychol Psychiatry, 2013. **54**(3): p. 227–246.

21. Lappin, J.M., S. Darke, and M. Farrell, *Methamphetamine use and future risk for Parkinson's disease: Evidence and clinical implications.* Drug Alcohol Depend, 2018. **187**: p. 134–140.

22. Kish, S.J., et al., *Brain dopamine neurone "damage": methamphetamine users vs. Parkinson's disease—a critical assessment of the evidence.* Eur J Neurosci, 2017. **45**(1): p. 58–66.

23. Lopez, W., and D.V. Jeste, *Movement disorders and substance abuse.* Psychiatr Serv, 1997. **48**(5): p. 634–636.

24. Rhee, K.J., T.E. Albertson, and J.C. Douglas, *Choreoathetoid disorder associated with amphetamine-like drugs.* Am J Emerg Med, 1988. **6**(2): p. 131–133.

25. Downes, M.A., and I.M. Whyte, *Amphetamine-induced movement disorder.* Emerg Med Australas, 2005. **17**(3): p. 277–280.

26. Balázs, J., M. Besnyo, and J. Gádoros, *Methylphenidate-induced orofacial and extremity dyskinesia.* J Child Adolesc Psychopharmacol, 2007. **17**(3): p. 378–381.

27. Yilmaz, A.E., et al., *Methylphenidate-induced acute orofacial and extremity dyskinesia.* J Child Neurol, 2013. **28**(6): p. 781–783.

28. Morgan, J.C., W.C. Winter, and G.F. Wooten, *Amphetamine-induced chorea in attention deficit-hyperactivity disorder.* Mov Disord, 2004. **19**(7): p. 840–842.

29. Waugh, J.L., et al., *Juvenile Huntington disease exacerbated by methylphenidate: case report.* J Child Neurol, 2008. **23**(7): p. 807–809.

30. Fountoulakis, K.N., et al., *Tardive Tourette-like syndrome: a systematic review.* Int Clin Psychopharmacol, 2011. **26**(5): p. 237–242.

31. Roessner, V., et al., *First-onset tics in patients with attention-deficit-hyperactivity disorder: impact of stimulants.* Dev Med Child Neurol, 2006. **48**(7): p. 616–621.

32. Lipkin, P.H., I.J. Goldstein, and A.R. Adesman, *Tics and dyskinesias associated with stimulant treatment in attention-deficit hyperactivity disorder.* Arch Pediatr Adolesc Med, 1994. **148**(8): p. 859–861.

33. Priori, A., et al., *Acute dystonic reaction to ecstasy*. Mov Disord, 1995. **10**(3): p. 353.

34. Todd, G., et al., *Prevalence of self-reported movement dysfunction among young adults with a history of ecstasy and methamphetamine use*. Drug Alcohol Depend, 2019. **205**: p. 107595.

35. Moszczynska, A., et al., *Why is parkinsonism not a feature of human methamphetamine users?* Brain, 2004. **127**(Pt 2): p. 363–370.

36. Curtin, K., et al., *Methamphetamine/amphetamine abuse and risk of Parkinson's disease in Utah: a population-based assessment*. Drug Alcohol Depend, 2015. **146**: p. 30–38.

37. Ceccatelli, S., *Mechanisms of neurotoxicity and implications for neurological disorders*. J Intern Med, 2013. **273**(5): p. 426–428.

38. Pregeljc, D., et al., *How important is the use of cocaine and amphetamines in the development of Parkinson disease? A computational study*. Neurotox Res, 2020. **37**(3): p. 724–731.

39. Tavassoly, O., and J.S. Lee, *Methamphetamine binds to α-synuclein and causes a conformational change which can be detected by nanopore analysis*. FEBS Lett, 2012. **586**(19): p. 3222–3228.

40. Todd, G., et al., *Adults with a history of illicit amphetamine use exhibit abnormal substantia nigra morphology and parkinsonism*. Parkinsonism Relat Disord, 2016. **25**: p. 27–32.

41. Mintzer, S., S. Hickenbottom, and S. Gilman, *Parkinsonism after taking ecstasy*. N Engl J Med, 1999. **340**(18): p. 1443.

42. Flavel, S.C., et al., *Illicit stimulant use in humans is associated with a long-term increase in tremor*. PLoS One, 2012. **7**(12): p. e52025.

43. Downey, L.A., et al., *Psychomotor tremor and proprioceptive control problems in current and former stimulant drug users: an accelerometer study of heavy users of amphetamine, MDMA, and other recreational stimulants*. J Clin Pharmacol, 2017. **57**(10): p. 1330–1337.

44. Rylander, G., *Psychoses and the punding and choreiform syndromes in addiction to central stimulant drugs*. Psychiatr Neurol Neurochir, 1972. **75**(3): p. 203–212.

45. O'Sullivan, S.S., A.H. Evans, and A.J. Lees, *Dopamine dysregulation syndrome: an overview of its epidemiology, mechanisms and management*. CNS Drugs, 2009. **23**(2): p. 157–170.

46. Asser, A., and P. Taba, *Psychostimulants and movement disorders*. Front Neurol, 2015. **6**: p. 75.

47. Daras, M., B.S. Koppel, and E. Atos-Radzion, *Cocaine-induced choreoathetoid movements ("crack dancing")*. Neurology, 1994. **44**(4): p. 751–752.

48. Weiner, W.J., et al., *Cocaine-induced persistent dyskinesias*. Neurology, 2001. **56**(7): p. 964–965.

49. Habal, R., et al., *Cocaine and chorea*. Am J Emerg Med, 1991. **9**(6): p. 618–620.

50. Villalba, R.M., and Y. Smith, *Differential striatal spine pathology in Parkinson's disease and cocaine addiction: a key role of dopamine?* Neuroscience, 2013. **251**: p. 2–20.

51. Daniels, J., D.G. Baker, and A.B. Norman, *Cocaine-induced tics in untreated Tourette's syndrome*. Am J Psychiatry, 1996. **153**(7): p. 965.

52. Cardoso, F.E., and J. Jankovic, *Cocaine-related movement disorders*. Mov Disord, 1993. **8**(2): p. 175–178.

53. Pinto, J.M., K. Babu, and C. Jenny, *Cocaine-induced dystonic reaction: an unlikely presentation of child neglect*. Pediatr Emerg Care, 2013. **29**(9): p. 1006–1008.

54. Farrell, P.E., and A.K. Diehl, *Acute dystonic reaction to crack cocaine*. Ann Emerg Med, 1991. **20**(3): p. 322.

55. Bartzokis, G., et al., *Choreoathetoid movements in cocaine dependence*. Biol Psychiatry, 1999. **45**(12): p. 1630–1635.

56. Kamath, S., and N. Bajaj, *Crack dancing in the United Kingdom: apropos a video case presentation*. Mov Disord, 2007. **22**(8): p. 1190–1191.

57. Bauer, L.O., *Psychomotor and electroencephalographic sequelae of cocaine dependence*. NIDA Res Monogr, 1996. **163**: p. 66–93.

58. Illés, A., et al., *Dynamic interaction of genetic risk factors and cocaine abuse in the background of Parkinsonism—a case report.* BMC Neurol, 2019. **19**(1): p. 260.

59. Karila, L., et al., *The effects and risks associated to mephedrone and methylone in humans: a review of the preliminary evidences.* Brain Res Bull, 2016. **126**(Pt 1): p. 61–67.

60. Osterhoudt, K.C., and M.D. Cook, *Clean but not sober: a 16-year-old with restlessness.* Pediatr Emerg Care, 2011. **27**(9): p. 892–894.

61. Selikhova, M., et al., *Parkinsonism and dystonia caused by the illicit use of ephedrone—a longitudinal study.* Mov Disord, 2008. **23**(15): p. 2224–2231.

62. Roberts, L., et al., *11 analytically confirmed cases of mexedrone use among polydrug users.* Clin Toxicol (Phila), 2017. **55**(3): p. 181–186.

63. Bonnet, U., et al., *Choreoathetoid movements associated with rapid adjustment to methadone.* Pharmacopsychiatry, 1998. **31**(4): p. 143–145.

64. Sandyk, R., *The endogenous opioid system in neurological disorders of the basal ganglia.* Life Sci, 1985. **37**(18): p. 1655–1663.

65. Pan, J., and H. Cai, *Opioid system in L-DOPA-induced dyskinesia.* Transl Neurodegener, 2017. **6**: p. 1.

66. Martin, E.J., et al., *Hydromorphone-induced chorea as an atypical presentation of opioid neurotoxicity: a case report and review of the literature.* Palliat Med, 2018. **32**(9): p. 1529–1532.

67. Clark, J.D., and J. Elliott, *A case of a methadone-induced movement disorder.* Clin J Pain, 2001. **17**(4): p. 375–377.

68. Hofmann, A., et al., *Myoclonus as an acute complication of low-dose hydromorphone in multiple system atrophy.* J Neurol Neurosurg Psychiatry, 2006. **77**(8): p. 994–995.

69. Kinshella, M.W., T. Gauthier, and M. Lysyshyn, *Rigidity, dyskinesia and other atypical overdose presentations observed at a supervised injection site, Vancouver, Canada.* Harm Reduct J, 2018. **15**(1): p. 64.

70. Wasserman, S., and M.D. Yahr, *Choreic movements induced by the use of methadone.* Arch Neurol, 1980. **37**(11): p. 727–728.

71. Lussier, D., and R.A. Cruciani, *Choreiform movements after a single dose of methadone.* J Pain Symptom Manage, 2003. **26**(2): p. 688–691.

72. Mätzler, W., et al., *Acute parkinsonism with corresponding lesions in the basal ganglia after heroin abuse.* Neurology, 2007. **68**(6): p. 414.

PART III
MOVEMENT DISORDERS SEEN IN PRIMARY PSYCHIATRIC DISORDERS

10

Neurological Soft Signs in Schizophrenia Spectrum Disorders

Johannes Schröder and Christina J. Herold

Introduction

Neurological soft signs (NSS)—i.e., minor motor and sensory deficits—are among the best established neurobiological findings in schizophrenia,[1] and comprise subtle deficits in sensory integration, motor coordination, and sequencing of complex motor acts which can be reliable assessed by using ratings instruments such as the Heidelberg NSS-scale in any clinical examination.[1] As demonstrated in a wealth of studies, NSS are more prevalent in all stages of schizophrenia, including first-episode cases and subjects with an ultra-high risk of psychosis, than in healthy subjects.[2,3] However, NSS also arise in other severe neuropsychiatric conditions, in particular bipolar disorder,[4] HIV-associated neurocognitive decline,[5,6] or Alzheimer's disease.[7–9]

NSS in schizophrenia are associated with psychopathological symptoms and cognitive deficits typical for the condition. These include thought disorders, negative symptoms, apathy, and executive and declarative memory dysfunction, but also extend to changes in more distinct domains such as episodic autobiographical memory, logical memory, theory of mind,[10] and visuospatial functions.[4] It is notable that similar associations also apply to the other severe neuropsychiatric conditions mentioned above. These findings give rise to the hypothesis that NSS can be conceptualized as a transdiagnostic phenomenon.[11]

As these clinical correlates of NSS in schizophrenia vary during the course of the disorder, NSS share at least some state-related aspects too. High NSS-scores typically found during acute psychosis decrease in the course of illness with remission of psychopathological symptoms. This effect is more pronounced in patients with a remitting course than in patients with a chronic course, although even in the former NSS do not "normalize" to the low range typically found in healthy controls[1] (for review: Bachmann et al.[12]). Instead, after remission of acute psychosis NSS-scores remain elevated when compared to controls and are in the range reported in subjects with an increased genetic liability to schizophrenia spectrum disorders, such as nonaffected monozygotic twins of pairs discordant for schizophrenia.[2,13]

Neuroimaging studies in patients with schizophrenia spectrum disorders identified the sensorimotor cortex and other motor areas, such as the supplementary motor area, basal ganglia and thalamus, and cerebellum as important structural correlates of NSS.[14] Although the parallel between structural brain and NSS changes was longitudinally investigated

---

[1] Although the term "schizophrenia spectrum disorders" corresponds to Eugen Bleuler's (1911) original concept, which replaced "dementia praecox" by the "group of schizophrenias," the term "schizophrenia" is used in the following for its linguistic simplicity.

in a single study only,[15] the findings conform with the results of clinical follow-up studies demonstrating persistence of increased NSS-scores in patients with a chronic course of the condition. Hence, NSS can be considered as an unfavorable prognostic marker if not a risk factor for chronicity of the disease.[16,17]

In this chapter, we will discuss the assessment of NSS before reviewing their development in the clinical course and their clinical correlates. The hypotheses derived from these clinical findings on the nature and the underlying neurobiological basis of NSS will be discussed with reference to findings from neuroimaging studies. Little is known about aging in schizophrenia. Given the importance of this issue, NSS in aging will form a topic of its own right. While most studies focused on schizophrenia, key findings were referenced to other neuropsychiatric disorders wherever possible.

Clinical Assessment and Clinical Background

While motor and sensory deficits in schizophrenia were already mentioned by both Kraepelin[18] and Bleuler[19] in their masterly textbooks, systematic studies were not published until the advent of biological psychiatry in the 1970s and 1980s. This delay can be attributed to a variety of factors, in particular the assumption that motor or sensory deficits in schizophrenia were secondary to severe psychopathological symptoms and neuropsychological deficits, such as catatonic signs in a minority of schizophrenic patients or due to extrapyramidal motor side effects in the majority of them.

The way NSS were clinically perceived by physicians is described by the American psychologist Meehl who played an important role in fostering and stimulating clinical research. He quoted an "old-style 'neuro-psychiatrist'" who "warned the medical students that they should be careful not to jump to the conclusion, when somebody had a plus/minus dysdiadochokinesia, or past pointing, or even a positive Romberg sign, that there was neurologic disease in the cerebellum or dorsal columns. He said that for some unknown reason, a sizable minority of schizophrenes showed these kinds of phenomena."[20] This notion still holds true in contemporary practice, as NSS can suggest an organic brain disorder particularly when the diagnosis of schizophrenia was not established before. Conversely, NSS can facilitate the diagnosis when demonstrated in patients in whom a major neuropsychiatric condition was not yet considered. These observations formed the basis of our first NSS study in the late 1980s.[1]

NSS can be assessed by using ratings instruments, such as the Heidelberg NSS scale,[1] the Neurological Examination Scale (NES[21]), or the Cambridge Neurological Inventory (CNI).[22] While the Heidelberg NSS scale and the CNI share a similar definition of NSS and mainly comprise motor and sensory NSS, the NES also includes tests for cerebral dominance and declarative memory. The psychometric properties of the Heidelberg scale (Table 10.1), which were established in a number of studies, including its internal reliability (Cronbach's alpha = 0.85–0.89), retest reliability (r = 0.80), and interrater reliability (r = 0.88) are good.[1,13] It comprises 16 items on five factors (motor coordination, sensory integration, complex motor tasks, right/left and spatial orientation and hard signs); ratings are given on a 0–3 point scale (no/slight/moderate/marked abnormality) according to a detailed manual.[2]

---

[2] Manuals are available on request in English, German, and Spanish. A Chinese version is in preparation.

Table 10.1 The Heidelberg NSS Scale

NSS—subscale	Test
1. Motor Coordination	Ozeretzki's Test
	Diadochokinesis
	Pronation/supination
	Finger-thumb-opposition
	Articulation
2. Sensory integration	Gait
	Tandem gait
	2-point discrimination
3. Complex motor tasks	Finger-to-nose test
	Fist-edge-palm test
4. Right-left and spatial orientation	Right-left orientation
	Graphesthesia
	Face-hand sensory test
	Stereognosis
5. Hard signs	Arm-holding test
	Mirror movements

Motor and sensory deficits related to NSS can be further differentiated by analyzing distinct motor actions, such as handwriting, grip force stability and diadochokinesis, or an overarm throwing task.[23–26] The development of adequate devices for direct measurement and quantification of motor action started already in Kraepelin's days.[23] Studies demonstrated an increased variability of movements—clinically a loss of steadiness and rhythm—rather than changes in velocity or amplitude.

NSS in the Course of Schizophrenia

High NSS-scores typically mark acute psychosis decrease in the course of illness with remission of psychopathological symptoms. This decrease under treatment can be demonstrated in both the acute psychotic phase (Figure 10.1) and after remission of acute psychosis over the next months and years with further consolidation (Figure 10.2), and also applies to patients treated for a first episode.[1,12,27]

This effect is more evident in patients with a favorable course of the disorder, but does not lead to a complete "normalization" of NSS scores to the low range found in healthy controls. Instead, even months after an acute exacerbation NSS scores are still elevated when compared to controls and remain in the range reported in subjects with an increased genetic liability, such as nonaffected monozygotic twins of pairs discordant for schizophrenia.[2,13] In healthy controls, only minor NSS-scores which changed little over time periods of one year[13,28] were reported (Figure 10.3).

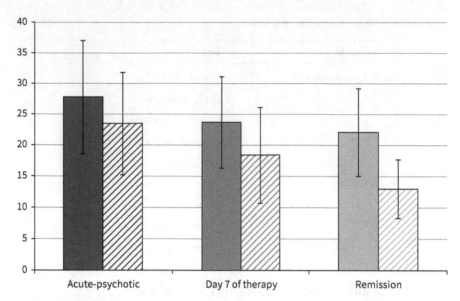

Figure 10.1 NSS in acute schizophrenia under treatment in patients with chronic (solid bars) vs. remitting schizophrenia.

Source: Data from Schröder et al., 1992.

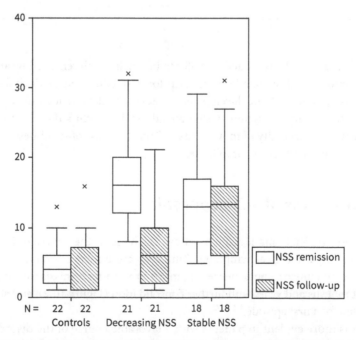

Figure 10.2 Neurological soft signs (NSS) in 22 healthy controls matched to 39 first-episode schizophrenic patients at remission of acute symptoms and at 14 months follow-up.

Although patients with decreasing NSS showed a better outcome than those with stable NSS, their NSS-scores (7.2 ± 5.8) did not remit to the level obtained in the controls, but stayed in the range of the level typically observed in subjects with a genetic liability.

Source: Data from Bachmann et al., 2005.

Based on our systematic review and meta-analysis of the literature,[12] we were able to identify 17 studies including between 10 to 93 patients with schizophrenia and yielding a total number of 858 patients who were followed for periods from 2 to 208 weeks. All but three studies found NSS to decrease with remission of psychopathological symptoms. While this effect was more pronounced in patients with a remitting than a chronic course (Cohen's d 0.81 vs. 0.28), even in the former NSS-scores did not decrease to the level typically observed in healthy controls. Since our meta-analysis was published, at least five additional studies confirmed these effects[16,28–31] of which Ferrucio and colleagues[16] established the long-term prognostic value of NSS in 233 patients with schizophrenia or affective disorder with psychotic features. On follow-up after 10 years, 147 patients had developed a chronic and 86 a remitting course of their disorder. NSS scores obtained at intake were significantly higher in patients who had a chronic course than in patients with a remitting disorder. Next to employment status, NSS were identified as predictors of functional outcome status. These findings confirm and extend results from earlier longitudinal studies with follow-up periods of up to 5 years and demonstrate that NSS are robust clinical predictors of the long-term course of schizophrenia and affective disorder. However, groups contrasted by Ferruccio et al.[16] differed significantly with respect to the proportion of patients with affective disorders, which was significantly higher in patients with a favorable course. When interpreting the results, this difference is of primary importance as affective disorders typically have a far better prognosis than schizophrenia. That the prognostic value of NSS applies to a mixed sample of patients with affective and schizophrenic psychoses conforms to their transdiagnostic nature.

These findings are pivotal for the clinical understanding of NSS since they demonstrate that NSS (a) are an essential part of clinical signs and symptoms characteristic for schizophrenia; (b) are both, state-related and a trait, and (c) can be used as a prognostic and a risk factor to monitor the disease progress and to identify subjects at risk to develop schizophrenia, respectively.

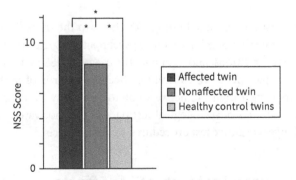

Figure 10.3 NSS-scores in affected and nonaffected monozygotic twins of pairs discordant for schizophrenia and healthy control twins.
*$p < 0.05$
Source: Data from Niethammer et al., 2000.

Clinical and Neuropsychological Correlates

The increase of NSS scores with clinical deterioration in chronic schizophrenia corresponds to the associations found between NSS and psychopathological symptoms, which were already described by Torrey[32] and Manschreck and Ames[33] in their pioneering studies. These associations especially involve formal thought disorder, increased activity and drive, and negative symptoms,[1] but also extend to apathy, which is also significantly correlated with NSS in Alzheimer's disease.[8,30]

Corresponding to these associations between NSS and psychopathological symptoms, earlier studies yielded significant correlations between NSS scores and poor reasoning, executive dysfunction, declarative memory, and attentional deficits.[27] or demonstrated pronounced cognitive impairments involving executive functioning, declarative memory, and attention in first-episode patients with high NSS scores when contrasted with low-NSS patients.[34] Similar associations were confirmed in patients with chronic schizophrenia,[10] in whom NSS scores were significantly correlated with deficits in a broad array of neuropsychological domains, including different memory functions (autobiographical, logical, and working memory), psychomotor speed, cognitive flexibility, and theory of mind. Except for autobiographic memory performance, these correlations also applied to healthy controls and did not appear to be accounted for by age, education, or severity of global cognitive deficits; a finding that paralleled an earlier study of Chan et al.[35] in elderly healthy adults. Taken together, associations between NSS and cognitive dysfunction in schizophrenia appear to be rather global than specific; a conclusion which corresponds to Chan et al.,[36] who suggested that NSS "capture more or less the same construct captured by conventional neurocognitive tests in patients with schizophrenia."

While longitudinal studies of NSS in organic brain diseases have not been published yet, cross-sectional studies yielded increasing NSS scores with deterioration of cognitive deficits from normal aging to mild neurocognitive disorder and manifest Alzheimer's disease or with manifestation of HIV-associated neurocognitive decline (HAND),[6,7,9] which corresponds to findings obtained in schizophrenia. In these conditions, similar patterns of associations between NSS and neuropsychological deficits were also reported.[5,9] That overall motor performance in Alzheimer's disease is related to executive functioning is further supported by the results of dual-task studies, which even yielded interactions between fall risk and executive dysfunctions.[37]

From a clinical perspective, these findings[1] conform to the transdiagnostic character of NSS as they demonstrate that NSS have similar psychopathological and neuropsychological correlates in different conditions, and[2] facilitate the usage of NSS as a screening instrument for neurocognitive impairments. In clinical practice, the latter is of particular importance as cognitive deficits have a high predictive value for everyday functioning, while human resources for thorough neuropsychological testing and the motivation and/or capacity of patients for such longer cognitive test procedures are often scarce.

NSS and Extrapyramidal Motor Side Effects

Extrapyramidal motor side effects, i.e., acute or tardive dyskinesia, parkinsonian symptoms, and akathisia, often arise under neuroleptic or antipsychotic treatment and have to be considered as a potential confounder, although contemporary atypical antipsychotics have a lower risk than conventional neuroleptics to provoke these side effects. The potential impact of extrapyramidal side effects is already counterbalanced by the decrease of NSS under neuroleptic treatment with remission of acute symptoms as described above. Moreover, several studies found only minor, nonsignificant differences between NSS-scores obtained in patients who received conventional neuroleptics or who were on clozapine.[38]

One multicenter trial[39] investigated motor NSS and extrapyramidal side effects in 82 patients with DSM-III-R schizophrenia who were examined twice in the subacute state at an interval average of 14 days. As discussed above, NSS correlated significantly with severity of illness, lower social functioning, and negative symptoms. Moderate, but significant correlations ($rs = .38; p = .001$) were found between NSS and parkinsonian side effects, while neither neuroleptic dose nor scores for tardive dyskinesia and akathisia correlated significantly with NSS. When compared between patients receiving clozapine monotherapy ($n = 33$) and those on conventional neuroleptics ($n = 45$), NSS scores obtained in both groups were almost identical (Figure 10.4), although patients taking clozapine displayed significantly fewer extrapyramidal symptoms.

Patients whose psychopathological symptoms remained stable or improved in the clinical course showed a significant reduction of NSS scores. This finding did not apply for those patients whose psychopathological symptoms deteriorated. These observations demonstrate that even motor NSS in schizophrenia are relatively independent of neuroleptic side effects, but are associated with severity and persistence of psychopathological symptoms and poor social functioning.

NSS have been already described in the "preneuroleptic era" long before antipsychotics became available. Later, studies in neuroleptic-naïve and/or first-episode patients or subjects with an increased liability, such as first-degree relatives, demonstrated increased NSS-scores before neuroleptic exposure.[1,27] Along with this, D2 dopamine receptor upregulation under treatment with (conventional) neuroleptics, which is often related to extrapyramidal side effects, was not correlated with NSS in a follow-up study under standardized neuroleptic treatment,[27] a finding that clearly argues against such a causative effect of neuroleptic therapy on NSS. On the contrary, the reverse may hold true, since NSS decrease under neuroleptic treatment.

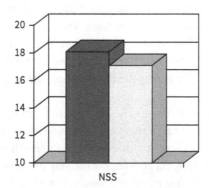

Figure 10.4 NSS under clozapine monotherapy (N = 33) (black) vs. NSS under conventional neuroleptics (N = 45) (gray)
Source: Data from Jahn et al., 2006.

The Potential Neurobiological Basis of NSS

Starting in the late 1970s with computerized tomography (CT), neuroimaging studies yielded associations between NSS and cerebral changes including global volume losses and regional abnormalities which particularly involved the thalamus and the caudate.[1] Despite numerous methodological limitations inherent to CT, these findings were confirmed in a wealth of magnetic resonance imaging (MRI) studies, which consistently found NSS to be associated with volumetric and gray matter changes in the frontal cortices including the pre- and postcentral gyrus, the inferior and middle frontal gyrus, the premotor area, the cerebellum, the caudate, and the thalamus.[15,40–43] As the respective sites are important nodes in cortico-cerebellar-thalamic-cortical circuit (CCTCC), which is hypothesized to play an important role in the development of symptoms such as motor dysfunction and cognitive deficits in schizophrenia,[44] these findings also correspond to the rather "global" associations between NSS, psychopathological symptoms, and cognitive deficits discussed above.

Extending beyond these gray matter morphometric studies, Kong et al.[14] sought to investigate the potential associations between NSS and gray matter networks in 101 first-episode patients with schizophrenia who were dichotomized into subgroups with high and low NSS scores according to a median split. Global analysis demonstrated that the subgroup with high NSS showed a weaker cliquishness or local interconnectivity and more diffuse patterns of connectivity. Further regional network analyses yielded subgroup differences that primarily affected the betweenness centrality mainly involving the orbital inferior frontal cortex, the middle temporal cortex, the supramarginal cortex, the amygdala, and the cerebellum. These changes especially involved regions in the sensorimotor system crucial for control and execution of motor acts and the integration of sensory functioning. In light of these findings, Kong et al.[14] suggested NSS may "represent a clinical proxy of the change in brain network architecture that putatively underlies psychotic disorders," a hypothesis that parallels the notion derived from psychopathological and neuropsychological studies that NSS reflect global rather than specific deficits. According to the results of a subsequent study, similar cerebral correlates refer to NSS in subjects with ultra-high risk for psychosis:[45] higher NSS scores were associated with decreased gray matter volumes of the superior and medial frontal cortex, the rectal cortex, the pre- and postcentral cortex, the insula, the caudate, and the cerebellum.

These cerebral sites may also be important for NSS in healthy controls although signs in this group are typically low and stable over time. This hypothesis was supported by using source-based morphometry for evaluating structural MRI obtained in 27 healthy adults (mean age 47.5 ± 14.9 a) by Wang et al.[44], who identified a cerebellar, a corticobasal ganglia-thalamic and a sensorimotor (including the motor strip) component as important correlates for NSS.

While demonstrated in a wealth of MRI-studies, these structural abnormalities do not prove that these structural cerebral changes are stable with time, as structural cerebral alterations may be changing in the clinical course of the disorder. The corresponding hypothesis that the cerebral changes underlying NSS are not entirely preformatted or static but increase or even develop in the course of psychosis is supported by a longitudinal MRI study[15] involving 20 patients with first-episode schizophrenia who were investigated after remission of the acute symptoms and at 1 year follow-up. At follow-up, patients were dichotomized into a subgroup with decreasing NSS scores and a subgroup with persistent NSS. While the former showed rather localized changes within the frontal lobe, cerebellum, and cingulate gyrus, patients with persistent NSS demonstrated pronounced changes of the sublobar claustrum, cingulate gyrus, cerebellum, and frontal lobe, including the middle frontal gyrus. These findings corroborate the results from longitudinal MRI studies that yielded progressive changes of the sensorimotor cortices and the supplementary motor area,[46] the thalamus[47] and the cerebellum[48] in patients with schizophrenia but did not examine NSS.

As demonstrated in the longitudinal studies, NSS in schizophrenia are not just the sequelae of a more vulnerable central nervous system, which predict or indicate schizophrenic psychopathology, but instead vary in the course of the disorder as they also appear de novo with manifestation of the disorder or develop in parallel with psychopathological symptoms in chronic courses. As the increased NSS scores in acute psychosis are partly reversible, this should also apply to the underlying cerebral changes. In addition, the putative cerebral changes may also be compensated for by cerebral mechanisms such as cognitive reserve. Therefore, functional rather than structural neuroimaging methods may be suitable to capture the underlying changes.

Findings obtained by functional magnetic resonance imaging (fMRI), among them the first fMRI study published in schizophrenia,[49] yielded associations between typical NSS (finger-to-thumb opposition;[26,49] fist-edge-palm test[3]) and a decreased activation of left frontal-parietal and frontal regions including the motor strip and the supplementary motor area. A lateralization effect with a greater activation of the right instead of the left sensorimotor cortices under ipsilateral movement, as first described by Kim et al.,[50] was confirmed in healthy controls but not in patients with schizophrenia.[49] The impact of task performance on sensorimotor cortex activation was investigated in each of 12 patients with schizophrenia and healthy controls during pronation/supination at three speed levels (low, medium, and high) with motor performance recorded simultaneously using a pronation/supination device.[26] Measures of motor retardation (i.e., repetition rate and amplitude of the movements) did not differ between patients and controls, while the variability of performance was significantly increased in the patient group. Sensorimotor cortex activation increased with speed, but was significantly lower in patients than controls.

With a special emphasis on task variability in schizophrenia, Dean and colleagues[24] investigated cerebral activation under a grip force stability task in 20 subjects with clinical high risk for psychosis and 21 healthy controls. Results confirmed a lower activation in motor regions including the caudate, putamen, cerebellum, and primary motor and somatosensory cortex in the risk than the control group. The coefficient of grip force variation was inversely associated with caudate activation in the high-risk group only.

During the palm-tapping task, Chan and colleagues[3] found activation of the left frontal-parietal region in fMRI to be lowest in patients with first-episode schizophrenia, intermediate in their nonpsychotic first-degree relatives, and highest in an independent group of healthy controls. Increased task complexity under the fist-edge-palm test led to a significant functional connectivity between the sensorimotor cortex and the right frontal gyrus in healthy controls only.

The effects of motor training on the performance of a sequential complex motor task executed with the right hand and cerebral activation was examined by Kodama and colleagues[51] by using fMRI in 9 patients with schizophrenia and 10 age-matched healthy controls. As described in the fMRI-studies cited above, patients showed a diminished activation in the premotor area before motor training than controls. Training led to activation increases in patients, but activation decreases in control subjects although training effects—i.e., the number of finger movement sequences achieved—did not differ between groups. Consistent effects of practice with a more efficient processing, requiring less neural engagement to perform the same task are described in literature. While an optimization of cerebral activation finds widespread support in healthy populations, in patient groups this effect has proven to be absent or reversed (for review: Schröder and Degen[52]). In a follow-up study, Bertolino et al.[53] confirmed a reduced activation of the left sensorimotor cortices while executing an n-back task with the right (dominant) hand in patients with schizophrenia, who had received a standardized treatment with olanzapine for four weeks, along with a diminished lateralization of left versus right sensorimotor cortex activation when compared with healthy controls. After continued olanzapine treatment for another four weeks, the activation of the left sensorimotor cortex had normalized while the diminished lateralization persisted. The authors referred their findings to state-related effects affecting the activation level and assigned the lateralization effects to persisting developmental abnormalities.

Excursus: NSS in Aging

Aging is a complex process that involves physical, psychological, and social changes. The consequences of the aging process differ between individuals and are modulated by preexisting conditions such as chronic schizophrenia leading to persisting psychopathological symptoms and cognitive deficits which, among other changes, hardly spare any aspect of life. Along with that, chronic schizophrenia is associated with an increased risk of physical conditions, such as metabolic syndrome compromising the general condition and—ultimately—leading to a highly reduced life-expectancy.[54]

Studies on NSS in elderly patients with chronic schizophrenia are scarce. In a large study including 3,105 participants from Beijing and Hong Kong, Chan and colleagues[55] demonstrated significantly higher NSS scores in 738 subjects with schizophrenia than 1,224 age-matched control subjects (age range: 14–82), which barely changed over the lifetime. In the control group, however, younger and older controls showed more NSS, resulting in a U-shaped relationship with age. However, potential effects of antipsychotic medication or psychopathological symptoms were not directly considered.

A cross-sectional comparison of NSS involving 90 patients with chronic schizophrenia (mean age: 43 ± 15; duration of illness: 19.5 ± 14.8) and 60 healthy controls (mean age: 43 ± 15), who were assigned to three age groups (18–29, 30–49, and + 50 years), also found NSS-scores to increase with age.[30] This effect was more pronounced in the patient group and paralleled the development of cognitive deficits, in particular executive dysfunctions, as indicated by diminished cognitive flexibility and decreased verbal fluency. This age effect was driven by a sharp increase of NSS-scores in the older patient group (Figure 10.5). Within the patient group, NSS-scores were significantly correlated with duration of illness, thought disorder, and positive symptoms, even when age and duration of illness were partialed out. Interestingly, apathy as a more "organic" psychopathological syndrome, but not negative symptoms, was significantly correlated with NSS.

A subsequent analysis of the same sample focused on the associations between NSS and neuropsychological deficits in patients with chronic schizophrenia.[10] In all neuropsychological domains but short-term memory patients performed significantly worse than controls.

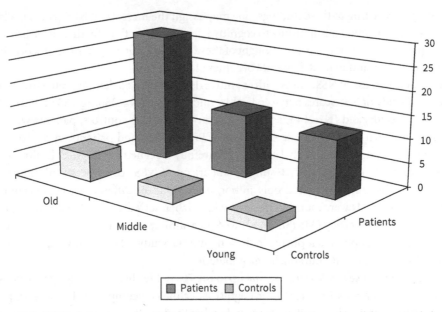

Figure 10.5 NSS total scores of patients with chronic schizophrenia and healthy controls by age group.
Source: Herold et al., 2018.

In both groups, NSS were significantly associated with deficits in a broad variety of neuro-psychological domains even when potential confounders, including the severity of global cognitive impairment, were controlled for. In healthy control subjects and patients with mild cognitive impairment and Alzheimer's disease, inverse correlations between NSS and executive and mnestic functions were also communicated by Chan et al.[35] and Urbanowitsch et al.[9]

A volumetric MRI-examination in a subgroup of 49 patients and 29 healthy controls identified the inferior and middle frontal gyri, the lingual, parahippocampal and superior temporal gyri, the thalamus and the cerebellum as important sites of NSS in chronic schizophrenia.[56,57] This pattern of cerebral changes corresponds with the associations between NSS and neuropsychological deficits demonstrated in the clinical study discussed above. Interestingly, these associations found in chronic schizophrenia also included mnestic deficits related to temporal lobe changes that were not frequently reported in other neuroimaging studies.

Twenty-one of the original 90 patients (initial mean duration of illness: 23±11; mean age: at intake 45±9; at follow-up 53±9) could be reexamined after 7 years.[57] NSS total scores and NSS subscales "motor coordination" and "integrative functions" increased in the follow-up period, although this effect failed to reach significance level ($p = 0.08$) for the total scores. While positive and negative symptoms, including apathy, remained rather stable on a high level, cognitive performance showed significant losses in verbal memory, verbal fluency and cognitive flexibility. Scores on the mini-mental status examination (MMSE) decreased significantly from 26±4 to 24±5 points at follow-up. That a further deterioration of psychopathological symptoms during the follow-up period was not demonstrated may well refer to ceiling effects of the rating scales applied as patients were in severe states requiring institutionalization already at intake. Seven patients were in need of nursing home care at follow-up. According to these findings, one may assign the increase of NSS scores in elderly patients with chronic schizophrenia to cognitive decline rather than further deterioration of psychopathological symptoms. In the light of these findings, the drop of MMSE scores into a range typically found in mild dementia becomes plausible.

A similar increase of NSS scores with cognitive decline was also demonstrated in a population based study of NSS scores between healthy middle-aged (N = 256, age: 55±1, born 1950–1952) and healthy old (N = 143, age: 74±1, born 1930–1932) controls, patients with mild cognitive impairment (N = 63, age: 74±1, born 1930–1932), and patients with Alzheimer's disease (N = 15, age: 75±1, born 1930–1932) carefully screened for physical health by clinical examination and laboratory testing. Comparison of NSS scores between middle-aged and old healthy controls yielded only minor, nonsignificant differences, while significant increased NSS levels were found in patients with Alzheimer's disease.[9] MMSE scores in the Alzheimer's disease group (MMSE: 24±2) were in a similar range as those from the patients with chronic schizophrenia reported in the longitudinal study.[57] Similar findings were documented by Seidl et al.[8] in a nursing home population.

Results from these studies suggest that up to the 70s of life "healthy aging" per se does not lead to increased NSS-scores. However, cognitive decline is accompanied by increasing NSS, as NSS were found to be significantly correlated with executive and mnestic dysfunctions. This effect also applied to cognitive decline from HIV infection[6] and could be demonstrated in elderly patients with chronic schizophrenia too. In addition, an impact of physical decline on NSS due to age-related conditions has to be considered.

Cognitive reserve—i.e., the ability to compensate for the cognitive consequences of cerebral changes—involves an ameliorating effect on NSS as demonstrated in the population-based study cited above[9] for both otherwise healthy controls and patients with mild cognitive impairment or Alzheimer's disease. A similar inverse correlation between educational levels as a proxy of cognitive reserve and NSS was communicated by Herold et al.[30], while Chan et al.[55] and Lizano et al.[28] reported a consisting negative association between NSS and intelligence coefficient. This observation conforms to the fact that the disease often prevents patients from achieving a higher school and/or professional education which involves a low cognitive reserve. Although still premature, these first findings suggest that the course of NSS in chronic schizophrenia during aging is driven not only by persistent psychopathological symptoms but also—to a perhaps even greater extent—by cognitive deficits. This is of particular clinical importance, as factors known to increase the risk of cognitive decline such as hypertension, hypercholesterinemia, obesity, or decreased physical and mental activity levels are typically more prevalent in patients with chronic schizophrenia and involve even a lower life expectancy than the general population enjoys.

Discussion

Evidence from the studies discussed above clearly confirm NSS as a characteristic feature of schizophrenia. Since NSS are closely related to psychopathological symptoms, neuropsychological deficits and cerebral changes, important traits such as genetic liability and clinical course of the disorder, they may even be considered to be inherent to schizophrenia. At the same time, NSS constitute a transdiagnostic phenomenon as they also arise in other severe neuropsychiatric conditions, such as bipolar disorder and Alzheimer's disease.

In schizophrenia, the highest NSS scores typically mark the acute psychotic state and decrease in the course of illness with remission of psychopathological symptoms. This effect is more pronounced in favorable courses, but does not lead to a complete "normalization" of, which remain in the range descripted in subjects with an increased genetic liability, such as nonaffected monozygotic twins of pairs discordant for schizophrenia. In contrast, NSS stay on rather stable levels or even increase with chronicity of psychopathological symptoms. While these effects do not correspond to potential confounders, specifically side effects of antipsychotic treatment, NSS are associated with psychopathological symptoms and a broad array of neuropsychological domains, in particular executive and declarative memory functions.

This clinical interpretation of NSS as an integral part of schizophrenia corresponds to the neuroimaging studies that identified broad cerebral changes affecting the frontal cortices, including pre- and postcentral gyrus, inferior and middle frontal gyrus, the premotor area, the cerebellum, the caudate, and the thalamus as correlates of NSS. This broad variety of sites reflects the clinical heterogeneity of NSS, which comprise both motor and sensory signs, and also corresponds to the diversity of neuropsychological deficits associated with NSS. In contrast, NSS do not seem to be caused by antipsychotic treatment, a finding clearly supported by the facts that signs were already noticed in the preneuroleptic era and decrease under therapy.

Chan and Gottesman[58] regard NSS as potential endophenotype for schizophrenia as they reflect the genetic liability toward the disease. On the other hand, the sharp increase of NSS scores in the acute psychotic state and their decrease with remission of acute symptoms clearly refers to an active disease process. Thus, NSS in schizophrenia seem to adopt characteristics of both state-like and trait-like features. While the state characteristics of NSS correspond to the acuity of the illness—the "process activity"—the trait-like features represent the genetic liability of the disease. That NSS refer to both trait- and state-related effects is further underlined by studies of identical twins discordant for schizophrenia,[2,59] which found the highest NSS-levels in affected twins from discordant pairs followed by their nonaffected co-twins and twins from healthy control pairs. However, the co-twins from affected pairs also presented significantly higher NSS-levels than the control twins. This differentiation between genetic and acquired risk factors was extended by Fountoulakis and colleagues[60] who reported lower NSS-scores in healthy controls carefully screened for a family history of any mental disorder than in previously published control samples. While the concept of process activity resembles both the trait and state characteristics of NSS, the worsening of cerebral changes with persisting NSS predicted hereby was only addressed and confirmed by Kong and coworkers.[15] If confirmed in further longitudinal studies involving patients in different stages of the disorder, NSS may provide reliable predictors of the clinical course, which may benefit the development of contemporary therapeutic concepts.

From a clinical perspective, the fluctuation of NSS in the course of the disorder may serve as a surrogate marker to monitor the underlying disease process and to identify subjects with an increased liability toward schizophrenia in general or more chronic courses in particular. NSS are inherent to schizophrenia and point at the involvement of motor and sensory sites within the cortico-cerebellar-thalamic-cortical circuits. These hypotheses warrant further longitudinal examinations of NSS and related clinical and neurobiological variables in first-episode schizophrenia, which should also imply special devices for direct measurement and quantification of motor action. Not only are results from these studies crucial to establish

NSS as prognostic signs but also they may help to further elucidate the interaction between genetic liability and state-related insults in schizophrenia.

References

1. Schröder, J., Niethammer, R., Geider, F.J. et al., (1992). Neurological soft signs in schizophrenia. *Schizophr Res*, 6, 25–30.
2. Niethammer, R., Weisbrod, M., Schiesser, S., et al. (2000). Genetic influence on laterality in schizophrenia? A twin study of neurological soft signs. *Am J Psychiatry*, 157: 272–274.
3. Chan, R.C.K., Huanga, J., Zhaob, Q., Wanga, Y., Laic, Y., Hong, N., Shumb, D.H.K., Cheung, E.F.C., Yu, X., Dazzan, P. (2015). Prefrontal cortex connectivity dysfunction in performing the Fist–Edge–Palm task in patients with first-episode schizophrenia and non-psychotic first-degree relatives. *NeuroImage: Clinical*, 9, 411–417.
4. Schröder, J., Richter, P., Geider, F.-J., Niethammer, R., Binkert, M., Reitz, C., Sauer, H. (1993). Diskrete motorische und sensorische Störungen (neurologische soft signs) im Akutverlauf endogener Psychosen. *Z Klin Psychol Psychopathol Psychotherap*, 41, 190–206.
5. Forno, G., Henriquez, F., Ceballos, M-E-, Gonzalez, M., Schröder, J., Toro, P (2020). Neurological soft signs (NSS) and cognitive deficits in HIV associated neurocognitive disorder. *Neuropsychologia*, 146:107545. https://doi.org/10.1016/j.neuropsychologia.2020.107545
6. Toro, P., Ceballos, M.E., Pesenti, J., Inostroza, M., Valenzuela, D., Henríquez, F., Forno, G., Herold, C., Schröder, J., Calderón, J. (2018). Neurological soft signs as a marker of cognitive impairment severity in people living with HIV. *Psychiatry Res*, 266, 138–142.
7. Kluger, A., Gianutsos, J.G., Golomb, J., et al. (1997) Patterns of motor impairment in normal aging, mild cognitive decline, and early Alzheimer's disease. *J Gerontology*, 528, P28–P39.
8. Seidl, U., Thomann, P.A., Schröder, J. (2009). Neurological soft signs in nursing home residents with Alzheimer's disease. *JAD*, 18, 525–530.
9. Urbanowitsch, N., Degen, C., Toro, P., Schröder, J. (2015). Neurological soft signs in aging, mild cognitive impairment, and Alzheimer's disease—the impact of cognitive decline and cognitive reserve. *Front Psychiatry*, 11(6), 12.
10. Herold, C.J., Duval, C.Z., Lässer, M.M., Schröder, J. (2019). Neurological soft signs (NSS) and cognitive impairment in chronic schizophrenia. *Schizophr Res Cogn*, 21(16), 17–24.
11. Toro, P., Schröder, J. (2018). Neurological soft signs in neuropsychiatric conditions. *Front Psychiatry*, 14(9), 736.
12. Bachmann, S., Degen, Ch., Geider, F.J., Schröder, J. (2014). Neurological soft signs in the clinical course of schizophrenia: results of a meta-analysis. *Front Psychiatry*, 5, 185.
13. Bachmann, S., Bottmer Ch., Schröder J. (2005). Neurological soft signs in first-episode schizophrenia—a follow-up study. *Am J Psychiatry*, 162, 1–7.
14. Kong, L., Herold, C.J., Cheung, E.F.C., Chan, R.C.K., Schröder, J. (2020). Neurological soft signs and brain network abnormalities in schizophrenia. *Schizophr Bull*, 46, 562–571.
15. Kong, L., Bachmann, S., Thomann, Ph. A., Essig, M., Schröder, J. (2012). Neurological soft signs and gray matter changes: a longitudinal analysis in first-episode schizophrenia. *Schizophr Res*, 134(1), 27–32.
16. Ferruccio, N.P., Tosato, S., Lappin, J.M., Heslin, M., Donoghue, K., Giordano, A., Lomas, B., Reininghaus, U., Onyejiaka, A., Chan, R.C.K., Croudace ,T., Jones, P.B., Murray, R.M., Fearon,

P., Doody, G.A., Morgan, C., Dazzan, P (2021). Neurological signs at the first psychotic episode as correlates of long-term outcome: results from the AESOP-10 Study. *Schizophr Bull*, 47(1), 118–127. https://doi.org/10.1093/schbul/sbaa089. Online ahead of print

17. Schröder, J., Toro, P. (2020) Neurological soft signs predict outcomes in schizophrenia. *Nat Rev Neurol.* 16(12), 659–660.https://doi.org/10.1038/s41582-020-0403-x. Online ahead of print.

18. Kraepelin, E. (1913). Psychiatrie. Barth, Leipzig.

19. Bleuler, E. (1911). Dementia praecox oder die Gruppe der Schizophrenien. In: Handbuch der Psychiatry (G. Aschaffenburg). Franz Deuticke Leipzig Wien.

20. Meehl, P.E. (1989). Schizotaxia revisited. *Arch Gen Psychiatry*, 46(10), 935–944.

21. Buchanan, R.W., Heinrichs, D.W. (1989). The Neurological Evaluation Scale (NES): a structured instrument for the assessment of neurological signs in schizophrenia. *Psychiatry Res*, 27(3), 335–350.

22. Chen, E.Y.H., Shapleske, J., Luque, R., McKenna, P.J., Hodges, J.R., Calloway, S.P., Hymas, N.F.S., Dening, T.R., Berrios, G.E. (1995). The Cambridge Neurological Inventory: a clinical instrument for assessment of soft neurological signs in psychiatric patients. *Psychiatry Research*, 56, 183–204.

23. Jahn T. (1999). Diskrete motorische Störungen bei Schizophrenie. Beltz Verlags Union, Weinheim.

24. Dean, D.J., Bernard, J.A., Damme, K.S.F., O'Reilly, R., Orr, J.M., Mittal ,V.A. (2020) Longitudinal assessment and functional neuroimaging of movement variability reveal novel insights into motor dysfunction in clinical high risk for psychosis. *Schizophr Bull.* 46(6), 1567–1576. https://doi.org/10.1093/schbul/sbaa072. Online ahead of print.

25. Sá, F., Marques, A., Rocha, N.B., Trigueiro, M.J., Campos, C., Schröder, J. (2015). Kinematic parameters of throwing performance in patients with schizophrenia using markerless motion capture system. *Somatosens Mot Res*, 32(2), 77–86.

26. Schröder, J., Essig, M., Baudendistel, K., Jahn, T., Gerdsen, I., Stockert, A., Schad, L.R., Knopp, M.V. (1999). Motor dysfunction and sensorimotor cortex activation changes in schizophrenia: a study with functional magnetic resonance imaging. *Neuroimage*, 9, 81–87.

27. Schröder, J., Silvestri, S., Bubeck, B., Karr, M., Demisch, S., Scherrer, S., Geider, F.J., Sauer, H. (1998). D2 dopamine receptor up-regulation, treatment response, neurological soft signs, and extrapyramidal side effects in schizophrenia: a follow-up study with 123I-iodobenzamid single photon emission computed tomography in the drug-naive state and after neuroleptic treatment. *Biol Psychiatry*, 43, 660–665.

28. Lizano, P., Dhaliwal, K., Lutz, O., et al. (2020). Trajectory of neurological examination abnormalities in antipsychotic-naïve first-episode psychosis population: a 1 year follow-up study. *Psychol Med*, 50(12), 2057–2065. https://doi.org/10.1017/S0033291719002162.

29. Emsley, R., Chiliza, B., Asmal, L., Kilian, S., Olivier, R.M., Phahladira, L., Ojagbemi, A., Scheffler, F., Carr, J., Kidd, M., Dazzan, P. (2017). Neurological soft signs in first-episode schizophrenia: State—and trait-related relationships to psychopathology, cognition and antipsychotic medication effects. *Schizophrenia Research,* 188 (2017) 144–150.

30. Herold, C.J., Lässer, M.M., Seidl, U.W., Hirjak, D., Thomann, P.A., Schröder, J. (2018). Neurological soft signs and psychopathology in chronic schizophrenia: a cross-sectional study in three age groups. *Front Psychiatry,* 9, 98.

31. Sambataro, F., Fritze, S., Rashidi, M., Topor, C.E., Kubera, K.M., Wolf, R.C., Hirjak, D. (2020). Moving forward: distinct sensorimotor abnormalities predict clinical outcome after 6 month in patients with schizophrenia. *Europ Neuropsychopharmacology*, 36, 72–82.

32. Torrey, E.F. (1980). Neurological abnormalities in schizophrenic patients. *Biol. Psychiatry,* 15(3), 381–388.

33. Manschreck, T.C., Ames, D. (1984). Neurological features and psychopathology. *Biol Psychiatry,* 19, 703–719.

34. Mohr F., Hubmann W., Albus M., et al. (2003). Neurological soft signs and neuropsychological performance in patients with first episode schizophrenia *Psychiatry Res,* 121(1), 21–30. https://doi.org/10.1016/s0165-1781(03)00203-8.

35. Chan, R.C., Xu, T., Li, H.J., Zhao, Q., Liu, H.H., Wang, Y., Yan, C., Cao, X.Y., Wang, Y.N., Shi, Y.F., Dazzan, P. (2011). Neurological abnormalities and neurocognitive functions in healthy elder people: a structural equation modeling analysis. *Behav Brain Funct,* 7, 32. https://doi.org/10.1186/1744-9081-7-32

36. Chan, R.C.K., Dai, S., Lui, S.S.Y., Ho, K.K.Y., Hung, K.S.Y., Wang, Y., Geng, F.-l., Li, Z., Cheung, E.F.C. (2015). Re-visiting the nature and relationships between neurological signs and neurocognitive functions in first-episode schizophrenia: an invariance model across time. *Sci Rep,* 5, 11850.

37. Sattler, C., Erickson, K.I., Toro, P., Schröder, J. (2011). Physical fitness as a protective factor for cognitive impairment in a prospective population-based study in Germany. *JAD,* 26 (4), 709–718.

38. Schröder, J. (2003). Neurological soft signs, neuroleptic side effects, and schizophrenia. *Psychiatr Annals,* 33, 215–220.

39. Jahn, Th., Hubmann, W., Karr, M., Mohr, F., Schlenker, R., Heidenreich, T., Cohen, R., Schröder J. (2006). Motoric neurological soft signs and psychopathological symptoms in schizophrenic psychoses. *Psych Res,* 142, 191–199.

40. Bottmer C, Bachmann S, Pantel J, Essig M, Amann M, Schad LR, Magnotta V, Schröder J. (2005). Reduced cerebellar volume and neurological soft signs in first-episode schizophrenia. *Psychiatry Res.* (2005 Dec 30), 140(3), 239–250.

41. Hirjak, D., Wolf, R.C., Stieltjes, B., Seidl, U., Schroder, J., Thomann, P.A. (2012). Neurological soft signs and subcortical brain morphology in recent onset schizophrenia. *J Psychiatr Res,* 46, 533–539.

42. Kong, L., Herold, C.J., Lässer, M.M., Schmid, L.A., Hirjak, D., Thomann, P.A., Essig, M. & Schröder, J. (2015). Association of cortical thickness and neurological soft signs in patients with chronic schizophrenia and healthy controls. *Neuropsychobiology,* 71, 225–233.

43. Thomann, P.A., Roebel, M., Dos Santos, V., Bachmann, S., Essig, M., Schröder, J. (2009). Cerebellar substructures and neurological soft signs in first-episode schizophrenia. *Psychiatry Res: Neuroimaging,* 173, 83–87.

44. Wang, X., Herold, C.J., Kong, L., Schröder. J. (2019). Associations between brain structural networks and neurological soft signs in healthy adults. *Psych Res: Neuroimaging,* 293, 1110989.

45. Kong, L., Cui, H., Zhang, T., Wang, Y., Huang, J., Zhu, Y., Tang, Y., Herold, C.J., Schröder, J., Cheung, E.F.C., Chan, R.C.K., Wang, J. (2019). Neurological soft signs and grey matter abnormalities in individuals with ultra-high risk for psychosis. *J Psych J,* 8(2), 252–260. https://doi.org/10.1002/pchj.258.

46. Thompson, P.M., Vidal, C., Giedd, J.N., et al. (2001). Mapping adolescent brain change reveals dynamic wave of accelerated gray matter loss in very early-onset schizophrenia. *Proc Natl Acad Sci USA,* 98, 11650–11655.

47. Rapoport, J.L., Kumra, J.G.S., Jacobsen, L., Smith, A., Lee, P., Nelson, J., Hamburger, S. (1997). Childhood-onset schizophrenia: progressive ventricular change during adolescence. *Arch Gen Psychiatry,* 54(10), 897–903. https://doi.org/10.1001/archpsyc.1997.01830220013002.

48. Pantelis, C., Velakoulis, D., McGorry, P.D., Wood, S.J., Suckling, J., Phillips, L.J., Yung, A.R. (2003). Neuroanatomical abnormalities before and after onset of psychosis: a cross-sectional and longitudinal MRI comparison. Lancet, 361, 281–288.

49. Schröder, J., Wenz, F., Schad, L.R., Baudendistel, K., Knopp, M.V. (1995). Senso-rimotor cortex and supplementary motor area changes in schizophrenia: a study with functional magnetic resonance imaging. *Br J Psychiatry,* 167, 197–201.

50. Kim, S.-G., Ashe, J., Hendrich, K., et al. (1993). Functional magnetic resonance imaging of motor cortex: hemispheric asymmetry and handedness. Science, 261, 615–618.

51. Schröder, J., Buchsbaum, M.S., Siegel, B.V., Haier, R.J., Lohr, J., Wu, J., Potkin, S.G. (1994). Patterns of cortical activation in schizophrenia. *Psychol Med,* 24, 947–955.

52. Kodama, S., Fukuzako, H., et al. (2001). Aberrant brain activation following motor skill learning in schizophrenic patients as shown by functional magnetic resonance imaging. *Psychological Medicine,* 31(6), 1079–1088. https://doi.org/10.1017/S0033291701004196

53. Schröder J, Degen C. Economization of cerebral activation under training: The inverse U-shaped function revisited. Psychiatry Res Neuroimaging. 2020 Dec 30;306:111177. doi: 10.1016/j.pscychresns.2020.111177.

54. Bertolino, A., Blasi, G., Caforio, G., et al. (2004). Functional lateralization of the sensomotor cortex in patients with schizophrenia: effects of treatments with olanzapine. *Biol Psychiatry,* 59, 190–197.

55. Laursen, T.M. (2011). Life expectancy among persons with schizophrenia or bipolar affective disorder. *Schizophr Res,* 131, 101–104.

56. Chan, R. C. K., Xie, W., Geng, F. L., Wang, Y., Lui, S. S., Wang, C. Y., Yu, X., Cheung, E. F., Rosenthal, R. (2016). Clinical utility and lifespan profiling of neurological soft signs in schizophrenia spectrum disorders. *Schizophr Bull,* 42, 560–570.

57. Herold, C.J., Essig, M., Schröder, J. (2020). Neurological soft signs (NSS) and brain morphology in patients with chronic schizophrenia and healthy controls. *PLoS One,* 15(4), e0231669.

58. Herold, C.J., Duval, C.Z., Schröder, J. (2021). Neurological soft signs and cognition in the late course of chronic schizophrenia: a longitudinal study. *Eur Arch Psychiatry Clin Neurosci,* 271(8), 1465–1473.

59. Chan, R.C.K.,Gottesman, I.I. (2008). Neurological sift signs as candidate endophenotypes for schizophrenia: a shooting star or a northern star? *Neuroscience Biohavioral Rev,* 32, 957–971.

60. Torrey E.F., Bowler A.E., Taylor E.H., Gottesman I.I. (1994). Schizophrenia and manic-depressive disorder: the biological roots of mental illness as revealed by the landmark study of identical twins. Naisc Books, New York, NY.

61. Fountoulakis, K.N., Panagiotidis, P., Kimiskidis, V., Nimatoudis, I., Gonga, X. (2018). Prevalence and correlates of neurological soft signs in healthy controls without family history of any mental disorder: a neurodevelopmental variation rather than a specific risk factor? *Int J Develop Neurosc,* 68, 59–65.

11

Stereotypies in Childhood Developmental Disorders and Neurodegenerative Diseases

Joohi Jimenez-Shahed

Introduction

A stereotypy is a repetitive, ritualistic, and patterned movement or behavior that occurs without an associated urge. While it can be confused with other hyperkinetic movement disorders such as tics, phenomenological characteristics and presenting manifestations can be used to differentiate it. Stereotypy can be seen in developmentally normal children or in neurodevelopmental disorders where it can form part of the diagnostic criteria for some conditions. In adults, stereotypy can occur in the context of concurrent psychiatric, cognitive, or neurologic conditions or drug therapy and drug abuse. This chapter reviews the definition and clinical features, classification, pathophysiology, work-up, and treatment of stereotypy in childhood developmental disorders and neurodegenerative diseases. Behavioral treatments, or pharmacologic treatment with dopamine receptor blocking agents or vesicular monoamine transporter type 2 inhibitors can be successful, with some evidence for the use of serotonin reuptake inhibitors in autistic patients.

Definition and Clinical Features

Stereotypies are coordinated, patterned, repetitive, rhythmic, purposeless but seemingly purposeful or ritualistic, movements, postures, or utterances that occur without an associated urge.[1] A recent recommendation to clarify the definition of this phenomenology proposes that stereotypy is a non-goal-directed movement pattern that is repeated continuously for a period of time in the same form and on multiple occasions, and that is typically distractible.[2] Stereotypies are common during periods of excitement, stress, fatigue, or boredom, and although they may seem purposeful, they serve no particular function. They tend to have a predictable pattern and location, can last seconds to minutes, and tend to occur in clusters several times per day.[1] Stereotypies are suppressible and notably can cease when the individual performing them is distracted. Stereotypies are also absent during sleep. Examples of stereotypic movements are provided in Table 11.1.

Stereotypies can be differentiated from other motor behaviors such as habits, mannerisms, and compulsions as well as other movement disorders based on a variety of features. Habits can be defined as repetitive, coordinated movements that are seen in otherwise normal individuals, commonly during times of boredom, fatigue, anxiety, or self-consciousness.[8,9] Habits may be socially inappropriate and tend to resolve with age. Mannerisms are defined

Table 11.1 Examples of Stereotypic Movements[3-7]

Anatomic Distribution	Examples
Face/Midline	Tongue twisting and protrusion; Lip smacking, pursing, and puckering; Chewing movements; Mouth/jaw opening; Blowing movements or sounds; Eyebrow movements; Facial grimacing; Bruxism (while awake); Head nodding, shaking, or tilting; Mouthing of the hands; Covering the ears; Tapping chin; Rocking, bending, or shaking of the trunk; Back arching; Shoulder shrugging
Upper extremities	Raising, lowering, or crossing of the arms; Internal and external twisting of the upper extremities; Flapping; Waving; Rotating of the wrists, hand-washing, or hand wringing; Rapid finger wiggling; Picking at fingertips; Banging arms against body
Lower extremities	Pacing; Leg elevation; Tapping or stomping the floor; Toe walking; Jumping; Feet twirling; Shifting weight from one leg to another or body swaying; Clapping thighs; Skipping; Spinning
Other	Punding; Rubbing face, arms, legs, or other body parts; Excoriations; Shaking, tapping, or twirling an object; Staring at an object or fingers out of the corner of the eyes

as an unusual or peculiar way of performing a normal activity, and may be considered odd, idiosyncratic, or bizarre variations of normal actions. Compulsions are purposeful behaviors that are carried out in response to an obsession, fear, or worry (as in obsessive-compulsive disorder) or according to certain rules (i.e., in a ritualistic manner).

Stereotypies can be differentiated from tics by their earlier age at onset (less than 3 years vs. over 3 years of age for tics), lack of premonitory urge, the characteristic suppression by external distraction (vs. suppression by the patient themselves), and the chance of more continuous and prolonged patterns of movement with a more constant and fixed pattern, whereas tics can wax and wane in frequency and the patterns of movement and noises can change frequently.[1,10] Although stereotypies may occur in paroxysms, they can clearly be differentiated from the diagnostic entity of kinesiogenic paroxysmal dyskinesias (which are precipitated by sudden movements) and nonkinesiogenic paroxysmal dyskinesias (not precipitated by movement)—each of these can be prolonged and while individual episodes can be quite similar to each other, they usually do not involve repeated, stereotyped movement patterns.[12] They also cannot be interrupted or suppressed. Chorea is a continuous nonpatterned movement that moves unpredictably from one body part to another and cannot be suppressed or interrupted.[13] Dystonia is characterized by a sustained contraction of a muscle or group of muscles producing an abnormal posture that recurs predictably with the same actions, though the movement pattern(s) do not repeat in the same form for a period of time.[14]

A classification scheme for stereotypies differentiates primary versus secondary types.[15] In this scheme, primary refers to "common," head nodding and complex hand/arm movement stereotypies, which can be present during normal development. The *Diagnostic and Statistical Manual of Mental Disorders* (DSM-5)[16] diagnostic criteria for such a stereotypic movement disorder is met when the repetitive, seemingly driven and apparently purposeless motor behaviors begin in the early developmental period and interfere with social, academic, or other activities, and may result in self-injury. Symptoms that are attributable to a physiologic effect of a substance or a neurologic condition, or that are better explained by a neurodevelopmental disorder or mental condition are excluded from this diagnosis. In secondary stereotypies,[14] the presence of an additional diagnosis with behavioral or neurologic signs is implied. Conditions included in this grouping are autistic spectrum disorders, intellectual impairment, sensory deprivation disorders, inborn errors of metabolism, neurodegenerative disorders, psychiatric conditions (e.g., schizophrenia), and drug-induced conditions (e.g., tardive dyskinesia).

Stereotypies are seen in a heterogeneous group of etiologies and likely result from differing pathophysiologies. For example, hand-flapping "stereotypy" commonly seen in children with autistic spectrum disorder is likely very different in physiology and certainly in etiology from orobuccal or finger-rubbing "stereotypies" seen in tardive dyskinesia. The published literature on stereotypy often focuses on a single etiology of stereotypy or single disease category associated with stereotypy, and conclusions from them therefore cannot be extrapolated to the entire scope of the phenomenology. This chapter will focus on secondary stereotypies in childhood developmental disorders and neurodegenerative diseases.

Pathophysiology of Stereotypies

In line with the fact that stereotypies can occur spontaneously as a part of normal development, or can be caused by a wide spectrum of genetic, developmental, toxic/metabolic, or other insults, there has been a wide variety of approaches to assessing their pathophysiology. It has long been postulated that, similar to other hyperkinetic movement disorders, stereotypies are a result of imbalance within basal ganglia motor pathways. The corticobasal ganglia-thalamocortical loops are well recognized to be organized in parallel circuits, where the motor loop is likely associated with continuous repetition of identical non-goal-directed movements, the associative loop is associated with inappropriate goal repetition, and the limbic loop is associated with motivational aspects of behavior control.[17] In order to localize whether the primary anatomic substrate is in the cortex or basal ganglia, a variety of imaging studies (e.g., assessing striatal volume, caudate-cortical connectivity, changes in activity of anterior cingulate and posterior parietal cortex, and structural changes of cortical white matter) have been performed in groups of patients with primary or secondary stereotypies, but have not consistently shown a uniform pattern of change. These discrepancies could be related to study design or inclusion of heterogeneous patient populations. Nonetheless, such investigations suggest that this movement disorder relates to dysfunction at the cortical or subcortical level, or by impaired connectivity or information exchange within the circuit.

Within the basal ganglia, increasing evidence suggests that reduced activity of the indirect pathway underlies stereotypy. Pharmacologic intervention in animal models with drugs whose basal ganglia manipulations end up disinhibiting thalamocortical projections (e.g., dopamine or dopamine agonist injection into the striatum, or GABA agonist injection into the substantia nigra) tend to induce stereotypy, while those whose end result is to increase inhibitory tone in the thalamus (e.g., serotonin antagonist injection into the subthalamic nucleus) tend to improve stereotypy.[18] Furthermore, it has been shown that following induction of stereotypy by bicuculline injection into the monkey limbic globus pallidus externa,[19] deep brain stimulation of the subthalamic nucleus (within the indirect pathway) reduced the abnormal movements.[20] In a series of experiments in deer mice, which express spontaneous stereotypy in the context of a restricted environment (such as when raised in laboratory cages), it has been shown that a low stereotypy condition is associated with high cytochrome oxidase activity in the motor context, striatum, nucleus accumbens, thalamus, and hippocampus, suggesting increased neuronal metabolic activity.[21] Following environmental enrichment in such animals, the low stereotypy condition yielded higher dendritic spine densities in the motor cortex and striatum, again implicating the corticobasal ganglia-thalamocortical loops in spontaneous stereotypy.[22] Stereotypies have been attenuated following intrastriatal injection or D1 dopamine receptor selective antagonists or an NMDA receptor-selective glutamate antagonist (involving disruption of the direct pathway).[23] When measuring dynorphin and enkephalin levels in medium spiny neurons of deer mice with stereotypies (as markers of the indirect and direct pathways, respectively), it was found that a significantly increased dynorphin: enkephalin concentration was associated with a high stereotypy condition and that enkephalin content negatively correlated with frequency of stereotypy.[24] These lines of evidence point to an important role of reduced indirect pathway activity in stereotypy generation.

In animal models of drug-induced stereotypy, repetitive behaviors in monkeys were found to associate with an immediate-early gene expression profile in striatal striosomes.[25] Furthermore, after chronic exposure to amphetamine and cocaine, this genetic profile predicted the presence of motor stereotypies and was more evident in the dorsal striatum, which contains the main corticostriatal connectivity of the motor loop.[26] An associated shift in metabolic activity from matrisomes to striosomes further supports this connectivity relationship from a functional standpoint.[27] Additional lines of investigation in cocaine-sensitized rats demonstrates the role of attenuated acetylcholine activity during repetitive behaviors (i.e., in striatal cholinergic interneurons), while restoration of cholinergic transmission is associated with arrest of stereotypy.[28] These findings may have additional implications for the recognized shift in early gene expression.

Studies assessing for pathophysiologic associations in humans with adult-onset stereotypies in frontotemporal dementia (FTD) are also revealing. These show that patients with FTD who have stereotypies have greater striatal volume loss compared to those without stereotypies.[29] Among genetic causes of FTD, patients with MAPT mutations were more likely to experience repetitive and stereotyped behaviors,[30] and stereotypy itself was associated with elevated default network connectivity in the right angular gyrus.[31] Patients with the behavioral variants of FTD also more commonly showed disrupted frontolimbic connectivity and elevated local connectivity within the prefrontal cortex. In an imaging study focusing on specific striatal subregions that used manual volumetric methods, panstriatal atrophy in the behavioral variant of FTD was found, whereas there was more selective putamen and nucleus accumbens atrophy in patients with the semantic dementia variant.[32] Such ventral striatal atrophy correlated with behavioral deficits but not parkinsonism; stereotypies were not specifically assessed. Regardless, these clinical data further support the pathophysiologic substrate of motor loop dysfunction within the corticobasal ganglia-thalamocortical circuitry, for which there may be different causes depending on the disease state in question.

Etiology of Stereotypies

From an etiologic standpoint, stereotypies are associated with a variety of clinical scenarios. The first is physiologic stereotypies that occur in developmentally normal children and often resolve spontaneously without sequelae,[33] or may continue through adolescence and the teenage years.[34] and are also recognized in a college-age population.[35] Although individuals with these young-onset stereotypies may also experience various psychiatric comorbidities[11] or family history, they are intellectually normal and symptoms do not progress; these stereotypies represent the group of primary stereotypies previously described and will not be reviewed further here.

Another clinical scenario is the group of childhood developmental disorders, in which stereotypies of various kinds can be a prominent and distinctive feature. These secondary stereotypies are characterized by more vocalizations, greater complexity and longer duration, and more frequent occurrence than primary stereotypies, which are predominantly motor, simple, and of shorter duration.[36] Among developmental disorders featuring prominent stereotypies, autism spectrum disorders and Rett syndrome are the most well recognized, though studies have described stereotypies in other conditions such as nonautistic developmental delay (e.g., developmental language disorder or those with nonautistic low IQ), Fragile X syndrome, Cornelia de Lange syndrome, Williams syndrome, Lesch-Nyhan syndrome, and Down syndrome, among others). Autism represents an etiologically diverse group of disorders with specific genetic causes only found in about 25%–35%.[37] Genetic abnormalities lead to disordered brain development. In addition to persistent deficits in social communication and social interaction, at least two types of restricted, repetitive patterns of behavior, interests, or activities must be present to satisfy DSM-5 diagnostic criteria for autism spectrum disorder,[16] and stereotypies represent one of the four types. Other types include insistence on sameness, restricted and fixated interests, and either hyper- or hypo-reactivity to sensory input. It is therefore possible that a child may meet diagnostic criteria for autism without evidence of stereotypies. Regardless, stereotypies are more prevalent in children with autism than in those with nonautistic developmental delay.[3] Those with gait and hand stereotypies are more likely to have a diagnosis of autism, and gazing at fingers or objects is a typical stereotypy seen in autism.

By contrast, Rett syndrome is a neurodevelopmental disorder that affects girls and is most commonly caused by loss of function mutations in the X-linked MECP2 gene.[38] Clinical diagnostic criteria include a period of regression followed by recovery or stabilization, partial or complete loss of purposeful hand skills, partial or complete loss of spoken language, gait abnormalities, and stereotypic hand movements. The stereotypic hand movements usually manifest after the onset of loss of purposeful hand movements.[4] Midline hand movements can be present in those with and without the MECP2 mutation, but those with known mutations had more varied stereotypies, and the number of stereotypies decreased significantly with age. Nonhand stereotypies were less common and tended to resolve over time. In comparison to children with autism spectrum disorder, the hand stereotypies in Rett syndrome are predominantly complex, more continuous, localized to the body midline, and involve mouthing, while in autism they are more simple, bilateral and intermittent, and often involve objects.[39]

Hand stereotypies (e.g., hand flapping, hand biting) are also the most common repetitive motor behavior in Fragile X syndrome, with onset most commonly before the age of 24 months, though they are not part of the diagnostic criteria for this condition.[40] Cornelia de Lange syndrome is a rare genetic neurodevelopmental disorder most often caused by mutations in the NIBPL gene, which impacts cell division and the regulation of developmental gene systems.[41] Intellectual disability and autistic features may be present, and repetitive behaviors including stereotypies and self-injurious behaviors are common (reported to occur in 42% and 70% of patients, respectively). Motor stereotypies are usually mild, including repetitive hand, body, or head movements and meaningless, recurring body movements (e.g., spinning, twirling, packing and rocking). Lesch-Nyhan syndrome is a disorder of purine metabolism caused by mutations in the HGPRT gene, with severity of the phenotype relating to the extent of HGPRT1 deficiency.[42] Stereotypies in this disorder typically take the form of self-injurious and self-mutilating behaviors, often associated with urges. This degree of self-injury is unique to this condition as opposed to other neurodevelopmental disorders. Among individuals with Down syndrome, caused by trisomy 21, those with an autistic phenotype are more likely to experience stereotypies, in particular involving the hands.[43]

In adult populations, secondary stereotypies are recognized in adults with onset of neurodegenerative disease. In a multicenter observational study, the frequency and type of stereotypies among patients with Alzheimer's disease, FTD, progressive supranuclear palsy, and Parkinson's disease dementia were evaluated.[44] Over 55% of subjects in each dementia category manifested at least one stereotypy, most often of the motor phenotype, though a diagnosis of FTD conferred a greater probability of manifesting stereotypies in general. Stereotypies were both more frequent and more severe in the FTD group compared to the other groups. Imaging studies have demonstrated that subjects with FTD with stereotypies had greater volume loss in the striatum, and those without stereotypy had more widespread pattern of cortical loss in the frontotemporal region.[29] Stereotypies in this form of dementia are more commonly motor, with both appendicular and craniocervical manifestations.[45]

Beyond the scope of this chapter, stereotypies can also be a motor feature in psychiatric disease such as catatonic schizophrenia.[46] Drug-induced stereotypies stemming from either dopamine receptor blockade (as in the case of tardive dyskinesia),[47] levodopa in Parkinson's disease (stereotypic levodopa-induced dyskinesias),[48] or drugs of abuse such as cocaine or amphetamines [49] are also common, but may represent a different pathophysiology. Central nervous system insults such as stroke or trauma have also been reported to lead to development of secondary stereotypies.[50,51] Additional rare causes of secondary stereotypies in adults and children have been summarized elsewhere.[8]

Diagnostic Testing

The recognition of the phenomenology of stereotypies is an important first step to pursuing diagnosis and management. An age-appropriate medical and psychiatric or behavioral history and a neurologic examination should be performed to determine if stereotypies are occurring as an isolated feature (primary stereotypy) or as a manifestation of a broader neurologic or medical condition (secondary stereotypy).[10] A history of comorbid behavioral changes should be sought, which in children may assist with distinguishing specific syndromes. Rating scales to assess severity of symptoms include the Motor Stereotypy Severity Scale, the Repetitive Behavior Scale, and the Behavior Problems Inventory; the latter two include subscales specifically directed to identification of stereotypic movements.[11] These and additional rating scales are described in Table 11.2. In adults, behavior changes should be considered alongside any history of exposure to psychoactive stimulants, serotonin reuptake inhibitors, neuroleptics or other dopamine antagonist medications, or drugs of abuse. Cognitive testing in adults should be considered, especially when other behavioral changes

Table 11.2 Scales Used to Assess Severity of Stereotypies

Scale	Reference	Description
Stereotypy Severity Scale	52	5-item caregiver questionnaire that rates the number, frequency, intensity, and interference of stereotypies (maximum, 18 points), and the global impairment (maximum, 50 points) during the past few days
Repetitive Behavior Scale—Revised	53	5 subscales addressing various symptoms of autism: Ritualistic/Sameness Behavior, *Stereotypic Behavior*, Self-injurious Behavior, Compulsive Behavior, and Restricted Interests
Behavior Problems Inventory	54	3 subscales assessing the three common types of troublesome behaviors in persons with intellectual and developmental disabilities: self-injurious behavior, *stereotyped behavior*, and aggressive/destructive behavior
Aberrant Behavior Checklist (ABC)	55	5 subscales: Irritability/Agitation/Crying, Lethargy and social withdrawal, *Stereotypic Behavior*, Hyperactivity/Noncompliance, and Inappropriate Speech
Nisonger Child Behaviour Rating Form	56	60 items subdivided among 6 scales: conduct problem, insecure/anxious, hyperactive, *self-injury/stereotypic*, self isolated/ritualistic, and overly sensitive
Ritvo-Freeman Real Life Rating Scale (RF-RLRS)	57	Video-based rating of pathologic behaviors on a Likert scale of observational measure for a variety of symptoms of autism. It comprises 5 subscales: Sensory-Motor scale (consists of 6 common motor stereoytpies and "other," each rated independently and averaged), Social-Relationship to People Scale, Affectual Response Scale, Sensory Response Scale, Language Scale

are present, to evaluate whether a more widespread and possibly neurodegenerative process is occurring. Brain imaging may also be considered to establish whether specific patterns of atrophy or other central nervous system insults (e.g., stroke) are present.

Treatment of Stereotypy

Primary stereotypies in children, adolescents or young adults may not require treatment, as affected individuals are often unaware of the frequency of the stereotypies and are generally not impaired by them. When treatment is required, habit reversal therapy may be successful in higher functioning individuals with little or no impairment in intellectual abilities.[52] Therapy delivered by the parents in the patient's home with guidance provided through an instructional DVD recording and from regular check-ins with a therapist has also been effective for management of primary and complex stereotypies.[9,58] Such behavioral approaches generally include consistent efforts at interruption of the stereotypic behavior and redirection.[60]

Pharmacologic interventions have been more extensively studied in the autistic population, though not exclusively for the management of stereotypies, as there are frequent coexisting psychiatric and behavioral features in autism that require management alongside the movement disorder. A Cochrane Database review[61] assessed evidence for the use of aripirazole in the treatment of behavioral aspects of autism. Short-term improvements in children and adolescents were found including reductions in irritability, hyperactivity, and stereotypies, but in the long-term these were counterbalanced by side effects such as weight gain, sedation, drooling, and tremor. In a discontinuation study,[62] there was no major difference in the relapse rate of those randomized to continue aripiprazole vs. those randomized to placebo. Risperidone treatment has also been found in a Cochrane Database review to confer significant improvements core features such as irritability, social withdrawal, hyperactivity and stereotypies, with the main side effect being weight gain.[63] Risperidone was also found to be more effective and better tolerated than haloperidol in this population.[64]

A meta-analysis of trials of serotonin reuptake inhibitors have suggested benefit in the treatment of repetitive behaviors in autism.[65] Amongst these, clomipramine, fluvoxamine, and fluoxetine were shown in double blind, placebo-controlled trials with small sample sizes to have efficacy in reducing repetitive behaviors.[66-69] In these trials, motor stereotypies were not specifically assessed by dedicated rating scales. In additional open label studies, sertraline and escitalopram were also found to have efficacy,[70-72] while a randomized controlled trial of citalopram failed to show benefit on repetitive behaviors,[73] as did a follow-up randomized trial of fluoxetine.[74] Furthermore, subsequent open label experiences found clomipramine to be less effective and tolerated than previously reported.[75]

Among adults with stereotypies in the context of neurodegenerative disorders, limited studies and reports exist. In a small case series, tetrabenazine, a vesicular monoamine transported type 2 inhibitor, was found to be effective in reducing stereotypy and well tolerated.[76] Case reports have noted positive effects with nonantidopaminergic medications such as buspirone and fluvoxamine.[8,77] Deep brain stimulation has been described in two cases with severe and refractory stereotypies associated with autism,[79] though with only robust and sustained results in one patient.

Conclusion

Stereotypies consist of non-goal-directed movement patterns that are repeated continuously for a period of time in the same form and on multiple occasions, and which are typically distractible and are not associated with an urge. They can be distinguished from other movement disorders based on their phenomenology and can be seen in normally developed children or in pathologic neurologic and psychiatric states, such as childhood developmental disorders and neurodegenerative diseases. Pathophysiology likely relates to reduced indirect pathway functioning within the motor loop of the corticobasal ganglia-thalamocortical circuit, with contributions from alterations in dopaminergic, cholinergic, and/or serotonergic signaling. When required, treatment can include behavioral therapy, dopamine receptor blocking or dopamine depleting agents, or serotonin reuptake inhibitors.

References

1. Hatcher-Martin JM SA, Factor SA. Stereotypies. In: Tolosa E, Jankovic J, editors. Parkinson's disease & movement disorders. Sixth edition. Philadelphia: Lippincott Williams & Wilkins; 2015. Pages 223–229.

2. Edwards MJ, Lang AE, Bhatia KP. Stereotypies: a critical appraisal and suggestion of a clinically useful definition. Mov Disord. 2012;27(2):179–185.

3. Goldman S, Wang C, Salgado MW, Greene PE, Kim M, Rapin I. Motor stereotypies in children with autism and other developmental disorders. Dev Med Child Neurol. 2009;51(1):30–38.

4. Temudo T, Oliveira P, Santos M, Dias K, Vieira J, Moreira A, et al. Stereotypies in Rett syndrome: analysis of 83 patients with and without detected MECP2 mutations. Neurology. 2007;68(15):1183–1187.

5. Mendez MF, Shapira JS, Miller BL. Stereotypical movements and frontotemporal dementia. Mov Disord. 2005;20(6):742–745.

6. O'Sullivan SS, Evans AH, Lees AJ. Punding in Parkinson's disease. Pract Neurol. 2007;7(6):397–399.

7. Fernandez HH, Friedman JH. Classification and treatment of tardive syndromes. Neurologist. 2003;9(1):16–27.

8. Barry S, Baird G, Lascelles K, Bunton P, Hedderly T. Neurodevelopmental movement disorders—an update on childhood motor stereotypies. Dev Med Child Neurol. 2011;53(11):979–985.

9. Kurlan RM. Habits, Mannerisms, Compulsions, and Steretoypies. In: Kurlan RM, Greene PE, Biglan KM, editors. Hyperkinetic movement disorders. Oxford: Oxford University Press; 2015. Page 99–105.

10. Martino D, Hedderly T. Tics and stereotypies: A comparative clinical review. Parkinsonism Relat Disord. 2019;59:117–124.

11. Katherine M. Stereotypic movement disorders. Semin Pediatr Neurol. 2018;25:19–24.

12. Zhang XJ, Xu ZY, Wu YC, Tan EK. Paroxysmal movement disorders: recent advances and proposal of a classification system. Parkinsonism Relat Disord. 2019;59:131–139.

13. Termsarasab P. Chorea. Continuum (Minneap Minn). 2019;25(4):1001–1035.

14. Singer HS. Motor stereotypies. Semin Pediatr Neurol. 2009;16(2):77–81.

15. Albanese A, Di Giovanni M, Lalli S. Dystonia: diagnosis and management. Eur J Neurol. 2019;26(1):5–17.

16. Diagnostic and statistical manual of mental disorders: DSM-5. Fifth edition. Arlington, VA: American Psychiatric Association; 2013. Page 947.

17. Langen M, Durston S, Kas MJ, van Engeland H, Staal WG. The neurobiology of repetitive behavior: . . . and men. Neurosci Biobehav Rev. 2011;35(3):356–365.

18. Muehlmann AM, Lewis MH. Abnormal repetitive behaviours: shared phenomenology and pathophysiology. J Intellect Disabil Res. 2012;56(5):427–440.

19. Grabli D, McCairn K, Hirsch EC, Agid Y, Feger J, Francois C, et al. Behavioural disorders induced by external globus pallidus dysfunction in primates: I. Behavioural study. Brain. 2004;127(Pt 9):2039–2054.

20. Baup N, Grabli D, Karachi C, Mounayar S, Francois C, Yelnik J, et al. High-frequency stimulation of the anterior subthalamic nucleus reduces stereotyped behaviors in primates. J Neurosci. 2008;28(35):8785–8788.

21. Turner CA, Yang MC, Lewis MH. Environmental enrichment: effects on stereotyped behavior and regional neuronal metabolic activity. Brain Res. 2002;938(1–2):15–21.

22. Turner CA, Lewis MH, King MA. Environmental enrichment: effects on stereotyped behavior and dendritic morphology. Dev Psychobiol. 2003;43(1):20–27.

23. Presti MF, Powell SB, Lewis MH. Dissociation between spontaneously emitted and apomorphine-induced stereotypy in Peromyscus maniculatus bairdii. Physiol Behav. 2002;75(3):347–353.

24. Presti MF, Lewis MH. Striatal opioid peptide content in an animal model of spontaneous stereotypic behavior. Behav Brain Res. 2005;157(2):363–368.

25. Saka E, Goodrich C, Harlan P, Madras BK, Graybiel AM. Repetitive behaviors in monkeys are linked to specific striatal activation patterns. J Neurosci. 2004;24(34):7557–7565.

26. Canales JJ, Graybiel AM. A measure of striatal function predicts motor stereotypy. Nat Neurosci. 2000;3(4):377–383.

27. Graybiel AM, Canales JJ, Capper-Loup C. Levodopa-induced dyskinesias and dopamine-dependent stereotypies: a new hypothesis. Trends Neurosci. 2000;23(10 Suppl):S71–S77.

28. Aliane V, Perez S, Bohren Y, Deniau JM, Kemel ML. Key role of striatal cholinergic interneurons in processes leading to arrest of motor stereotypies. Brain. 2011;134(Pt 1):110–118.

29. Josephs KA, Whitwell JL, Jack CR, Jr. Anatomic correlates of stereotypies in frontotemporal lobar degeneration. Neurobiol Aging. 2008;29(12):1859–1863.

30. Snowden JS, Adams J, Harris J, Thompson JC, Rollinson S, Richardson A, et al. Distinct clinical and pathological phenotypes in frontotemporal dementia associated with MAPT, PGRN and C9orf72 mutations. Amyotroph Lateral Scler Frontotemporal Degener. 2015;16(7–8):497–505.

31. Farb NA, Grady CL, Strother S, Tang-Wai DF, Masellis M, Black S, et al. Abnormal network connectivity in frontotemporal dementia: evidence for prefrontal isolation. Cortex. 2013;49(7):1856–1873.

32. Halabi C, Halabi A, Dean DL, Wang PN, Boxer AL, Trojanowski JQ, et al. Patterns of striatal degeneration in frontotemporal dementia. Alzheimer Dis Assoc Disord. 2013;27(1):74–83.

33. Harris KM, Mahone EM, Singer HS. Nonautistic motor stereotypies: clinical features and longitudinal follow-up. Pediatr Neurol. 2008;38(4):267–272.

34. Oakley C, Mahone EM, Morris-Berry C, Kline T, Singer HS. Primary complex motor stereotypies in older children and adolescents: clinical features and longitudinal follow-up. Pediatr Neurol. 2015;52(4):398–403 e1.

35. Niehaus DJ, Emsley RA, Brink P, Stein DJ. Stereotypies: prevalence and association with compulsive and impulsive symptoms in college students. Psychopathology. 2000;33(1):31–35.

36. Ghosh D, Rajan PV, Erenberg G. A comparative study of primary and secondary stereotypies. J Child Neurol. 2013;28(12):1562–1568.

37. Wisniowiecka-Kowalnik B, Nowakowska BA. Genetics and epigenetics of autism spectrum disorder: current evidence in the field. J Appl Genet. 2019;60(1):37–47.

38. Ehrhart F, Sangani NB, Curfs LMG. Current developments in the genetics of Rett and Rett-like syndrome. Curr Opin Psychiatry. 2018;31(2):103–108.

39. Goldman S, Temudo T. Hand stereotypies distinguish Rett syndrome from autism disorder. Mov Disord. 2012;27(8):1060–1062.

40. Zhang D, Poustka L, Marschik PB, Einspieler C. The onset of hand stereotypies in fragile X syndrome. Dev Med Child Neurol. 2018;60(10):1060–1061.

41. Srivastava S, Clark B, Landy-Schmitt C, Offermann EA, Kline AD, Wilkinson ST, et al. Repetitive and self-injurious behaviors in children with Cornelia de Lange syndrome. J Autism Dev Disord. 2021; 51(5):1748–1758.

42. Harris JC. Lesch-Nyhan syndrome and its variants: examining the behavioral and neurocognitive phenotype. Curr Opin Psychiatry. 2018;31(2):96–102.

43. Moss J, Richards C, Nelson L, Oliver C. Prevalence of autism spectrum disorder symptomatology and related behavioural characteristics in individuals with Down syndrome. Autism. 2013;17(4):390–404.

44. Prioni S, Fetoni V, Barocco F, Redaelli V, Falcone C, Soliveri P, et al. Stereotypic behaviors in degenerative dementias. J Neurol. 2012;259(11):2452–2459.

45. Mateen FJ, Josephs KA. The clinical spectrum of stereotypies in frontotemporal lobar degeneration. Mov Disord. 2009;24(8):1237–1240.

46. Ungvari GS, Gerevich J, Takacs R, Gazdag G. Schizophrenia with prominent catatonic features: a selective review. Schizophr Res. 2018;200:77–84.

47. Savitt D, Jankovic J. Tardive syndromes. J Neurol Sci. 2018;389:35–42.

48. Vijayakumar D, Jankovic J. Drug-induced dyskinesia, part 1: treatment of levodopa-induced dyskinesia. Drugs. 2016;76(7):759–777.

49. Maltete D. Adult-onset stereotypical motor behaviors. Rev Neurol (Paris). 2016;172(8–9):477–482.

50. Mehanna R, Jankovic J. Movement disorders in cerebrovascular disease. Lancet Neurol. 2013;12(6):597–608.

51. McGrath CM, Kennedy RE, Hoye W, Yablon SA. Stereotypic movement disorder after acquired brain injury. Brain Inj. 2002;16(5):447–451.

52. Miller JM, Singer HS, Bridges DD, Waranch HR. Behavioral therapy for treatment of stereotypic movements in nonautistic children. J Child Neurol. 2006;21(2):119–125.

53. Lam KS, Aman MG. The Repetitive Behavior Scale-Revised: independent validation in individuals with autism spectrum disorders. J Autism Dev Disord. 2007;37(5):855–866.

54. Rojahn J. Self-injurious and stereotypic behavior of noninstitutionalized mentally retarded people: prevalence and classification. Am J Ment Defic. 1986;91(3):268–276.

55. Aman MG, Singh NN, Stewart AW, Field CJ. The aberrant behavior checklist: a behavior rating scale for the assessment of treatment effects. Am J Ment Defic. 1985;89(5):485–491.

56. Aman MG, Tasse MJ, Rojahn J, Hammer D. The Nisonger CBRF: a child behavior rating form for children with developmental disabilities. Res Dev Disabil. 1996;17(1):41–57.

57. Freeman BJ, Ritvo ER, Yokota A, Ritvo A. A scale for rating symptoms of patients with the syndrome of autism in real life settings. J Am Acad Child Psychiatry. 1986;25(1):130–136.

58. Specht MW, Mahone EM, Kline T, Waranch R, Brabson L, Thompson CB, et al. Efficacy of parent-delivered behavioral therapy for primary complex motor stereotypies. Dev Med Child Neurol. 2017;59(2):168–173.

59. Singer HS, Rajendran S, Waranch HR, Mahone EM. Home-based, therapist-assisted, therapy for young children with primary complex motor stereotypies. Pediatr Neurol. 2018;85:51–57.

60. Miguel CF, Clark K, Tereshko L, Ahearn WH. The effects of response interruption and redirection and sertraline on vocal stereotypy. J Appl Behav Anal. 2009;42(4):883–888.

61. Hirsch LE, Pringsheim T. Aripiprazole for autism spectrum disorders (ASD). Cochrane Database Syst Rev. 2016(6):CD009043.

62. Findling RL, Mankoski R, Timko K, Lears K, McCartney T, McQuade RD, et al. A randomized controlled trial investigating the safety and efficacy of aripiprazole in the long-term maintenance treatment of pediatric patients with irritability associated with autistic disorder. J Clin Psychiatry. 2014;75(1):22–30.

63. Jesner OS, Aref-Adib M, Coren E. Risperidone for autism spectrum disorder. Cochrane Database Syst Rev. 2007(1):CD005040.

64. Miral S, Gencer O, Inal-Emiroglu FN, Baykara B, Baykara A, Dirik E. Risperidone versus haloperidol in children and adolescents with AD: a randomized, controlled, double-blind trial. Eur Child Adolesc Psychiatry. 2008;17(1):1–8.

65. Carrasco M, Volkmar FR, Bloch MH. Pharmacologic treatment of repetitive behaviors in autism spectrum disorders: evidence of publication bias. Pediatrics. 2012;129(5):e1301–1310.

66. Gordon CT, State RC, Nelson JE, Hamburger SD, Rapoport JL. A double-blind comparison of clomipramine, desipramine, and placebo in the treatment of autistic disorder. Arch Gen Psychiatry. 1993;50(6):441–447.

67. McDougle CJ, Naylor ST, Cohen DJ, Volkmar FR, Heninger GR, Price LH. A double-blind, placebo-controlled study of fluvoxamine in adults with autistic disorder. Arch Gen Psychiatry. 1996;53(11):1001–1008.

68. Hollander E, Phillips A, Chaplin W, Zagursky K, Novotny S, Wasserman S, et al. A placebo controlled crossover trial of liquid fluoxetine on repetitive behaviors in childhood and adolescent autism. Neuropsychopharmacology. 2005;30(3):582–589.

69. Hollander E, Soorya L, Chaplin W, Anagnostou E, Taylor BP, Ferretti CJ, et al. A double-blind placebo-controlled trial of fluoxetine for repetitive behaviors and global severity in adult autism spectrum disorders. Am J Psychiatry. 2012;169(3):292–299.

70. McDougle CJ, Brodkin ES, Naylor ST, Carlson DC, Cohen DJ, Price LH. Sertraline in adults with pervasive developmental disorders: a prospective open-label investigation. J Clin Psychopharmacol. 1998;18(1):62–66.

71. Steingard RJ, Zimnitzky B, DeMaso DR, Bauman ML, Bucci JP. Sertraline treatment of transition-associated anxiety and agitation in children with autistic disorder. J Child Adolesc Psychopharmacol. 1997;7(1):9–15.

72. Owley T, Walton L, Salt J, Guter SJ, Jr., Winnega M, Leventhal BL, et al. An open-label trial of escitalopram in pervasive developmental disorders. J Am Acad Child Adolesc Psychiatry. 2005;44(4):343–348.

73. King BH, Hollander E, Sikich L, McCracken JT, Scahill L, Bregman JD, et al. Lack of efficacy of citalopram in children with autism spectrum disorders and high levels of repetitive behavior: citalopram ineffective in children with autism. Arch Gen Psychiatry. 2009;66(6):583–590.

74. Herscu P, Handen BL, Arnold LE, Snape MF, Bregman JD, Ginsberg L, et al. The SOFIA study: negative multi-center study of low dose fluoxetine on repetitive behaviors in children and adolescents with autistic disorder. J Autism Dev Disord. 2020;50(9):3233–3244.

75. Soorya L, Kiarashi J, Hollander E. Psychopharmacologic interventions for repetitive behaviors in autism spectrum disorders. Child Adolesc Psychiatr Clin N Am. 2008;17(4):753–771, viii.

76. Ondo WG. Tetrabenazine treatment for stereotypies and tics associated with dementia. J Neuropsychiatry Clin Neurosci. 2012;24(2):208–214.

77. Helvink B, Holroyd S. Buspirone for stereotypic movements in elderly with cognitive impairment. J Neuropsychiatry Clin Neurosci. 2006;18(2):242–244.

78. Ishikawa H, Shimomura T, Shimizu T. [Stereotyped behaviors and compulsive complaints of pain improved by fluvoxamine in two cases of frontotemporal dementia]. Seishin Shinkeigaku Zasshi. 2006;108(10):1029–1035.

79. Stocco A, Baizabal-Carvallo JF. Deep brain stimulation for severe secondary stereotypies. Parkinsonism Relat Disord. 2014;20(9):1035–1036.

12
Catatonia and Hypokinetic Movement Disorders

Nidaullah Mian, Carla Bejjani, and Raja Mehanna

While dopamine blocking agents can cause drug-induced parkinsonism, and around half of patients with Parkinson's disease (PD) also complain of depression and other mood disorders,[1] patients with psychiatric disorders can present with noniatrogenic hypokinetic movement disorders, which are the topic of this chapter. We will first discuss catatonia as an individual entity, then review hypokinetic movement disorders in depression and schizophrenia.

Catatonia

Catatonia was first described by the German psychopathologist Karl Kahlbaum in 1874 as a complex syndrome of bizarre motor behavior, impaired volition, and vegetative abnormalities.[2,3] Subsequently, the psychopathologists Emil Kraepelin and Eugen Bleuler described catatonia within the spectrum of "dementia praecox" or premature dementia, later renamed schizophrenia.[4] A long-standing neglect of catatonia in clinical and scientific literature as well as underdiagnosis ensued due to debates about its nosology, operationalization, and suspected pathology.[5,6] While clinicians considered catatonia as part of schizophrenia,[7] the need to consider catatonia as an entity of its own was emphasized from the mid-1970s onward as it was seen in the setting of a variety of conditions such as psychiatric disorders other than schizophrenia, but also neurological, medical, and surgical conditions as well as the effect of certain drugs and toxins.[8]

Prevalence

The frequency of catatonia varies depending on the diagnostic criteria and duration of observation. In acute psychiatric admissions, the frequency is approximately 10%, with a range from 5% to 20% based on diagnostic criteria and duration of observation in inpatient psychiatric units, from 1 to 12 months.[9–12] Other surveys have reported a prevalence ranging between 7.6% and 38% of all psychiatric patients.[13–16] While patients with bipolar disorders probably constitute the largest subgroup of catatonic patients, around 43%,[17] and patients with schizophrenia represent around 30%,[17] 20%–39% of catatonia cases are due to a general medical condition.[18] In a minority of cases, no cause is found, but the prevalence of idiopathic catatonia is unknown.

Clinical Features

Catatonia usually presents acutely as a medical or psychiatric emergency.[19] However, it may also present insidiously, can be transient or chronic, and lasts for weeks, months, and even years. As such, patient may develop symptoms during hospitalization, such as in the intensive care unit (ICU).[20] Catatonia carries an excellent prognosis provided it is recognized early and treated appropriately.

Several prototypes of catatonic syndromes have been suggested for assisting with identification and clinical diagnosis.[21] For simplicity, catatonia can be divided into (a) withdrawn (or hypokinetic) form, and (b) excited (or hyperkinetic) form.[22] Occasionally, features of both types may appear in a patient during the course of their illness. The prototype of a hypokinetic or withdrawn presentation would be a patient manifesting features such as mutism, negativism, posturing, stupor, or obsessional slowness. On the other hand a hyperkinetic or excited prototype of catatonia would be a patient manifesting combativeness, agitation, stereotypies, grimacing, verbigeration, and echophenomena.

A brief description of the various clinical phenomena/terminology used in catatonic syndromes is presented in Table 12.1.

Diagnostic Criteria

The fifth *Diagnostic and Statistical Manual of Mental Disorders* (DSM-5) published the revised diagnostic criteria for catatonia in 2013, allowing application of these criteria across different clinical settings, whereas prior versions of the DSM used different sets of criteria for diagnosis of catatonia in schizophrenia and primary mood disorders versus neurological/medical conditions. The diagnosis of catatonia per the DSM-5 is based on clinical observation/examination of 12 clinical features, requiring the presence of at least 3 or more. These include: (1) catalepsy, (2) waxy flexibility, (3) posturing, (4) stupor, (5) agitation, (6) mutism, (7) negativism, (8) mannerisms, (9) stereotypies, (10) grimacing, (11) echolalia, or (12) echopraxia.

Of note, Kahlbaum originally reported 17 signs of catatonia.[2,3,24] Subsequent authors have expanded on those features and the list includes up to 40 clinical features across the different rating and screening scales.[24]

Rating Scales

Of the different scales in use to rate or screen for catatonia, the Bush-Francis Catatonia Rating Scale (BFCRS) is the most widely used.[17] This scale includes 23 items and up to 30 signs, including some that are not listed in the DSM-5 criteria. These include: staring, rigidity, withdrawal, automatic obedience, excitement, impulsivity, combativeness, perseveration, grasp reflex, ambitendency, verbigeration, mitgehen, and autonomic abnormality. Each item is scored on a 0–3 point scale, with the higher number indicating a more severe symptom. The BFCRS can be used to screen for catatonia and to rate its severity.

Table 12.1 Clinical Phenomena/Terminology Used in Catatonic Syndromes

Terminology	Description
Mutism	- minimal to no verbal communication in the absence of aphasia. - one of the most frequently observed signs of catatonia in the acute hospital setting.[23] - commonly seen in hypokinetic catatonia, but occasionally also seen in hyperkinetic catatonia.
Catatonic stupor	- lack of reaction or movement to stimuli including pain while patient is awake. - can be seen alone or in combination with mutism. - patient is extremely immobile or hypoactive. - normal awake EEG can help differentiate from sedation.
Posturing	- spontaneous and active maintenance of posture against gravity. - includes waxy flexibility, catalepsy, catatonic rigidity (see below).
Waxy flexibility	- ability of the extremities or body to assume certain postures for a long period of time when manipulated by an examiner. - "waxy" because of the slight and even resistance to movement as if bending a warm candle. - one of the characteristic motor signs of catatonia.
Catalepsy	- passive induction of posture held against gravity. - postures are fixed, unusual, and can be in the sitting or standing position for long periods of time. Can include statuesque postures, twisting of the body, standing on one leg like a stork, holding one arm outstretched for a long time, and squatting with extension of arms. - positions appear uncomfortable to the examiner and there is minimal movement regardless of external stimuli, including pain. - "psychological pillow": dramatic posturing where the patient lies in bed with the head and shoulder raised as if there is an imaginary pillow.
Catatonic Rigidity	- stiff position which the patient attempts to maintain despite efforts to be moved. - no cogwheeling or tremor (helps differentiate it from parkinsonian rigidity). - negativism is characterized by paratonia or gegenhalten. Paratonia is elicited by the examiner as increasing resistance to passive manipulation as if the patient were deliberately opposing the passive movement.
Stereotypies	- repetitive, rhythmic, involuntary, patterned, coordinated, seemingly purposeless movements or utterances (e.g., shoulder shrugging, repetitive mouth and jaw movements, or alternating eye opening and closing tightly . . .) - may be accompanied by self-injurious behavior. - catatonic patients can also have facial grimacing and exaggerated facial expressions. - can be phonic stereotypies (sniffing, snorting, moaning . . .)
Mannerism	- repetitive, idiosyncratic movements or gestures that are unique to the individual, such as using hands when talking.
Echopraxia	- mimicry of the examiner or other person's movements or gestures.
Echolalia	- mimicry or near simultaneous repetition of words or phrases spoken by others.
Verbigeration	- frequent repetition of meaningless words and phrases. - patient repeats themselves like a broken record.

Table 12.1 Continued

Terminology	Description
Motor Perseveration	- persistence of a particular movement long after the original command or intent.
Speech perseveration	- returning to the same topic again and again beyond its initial relevance.
Staring gaze	- eyes focused at a distance with little or no visual scanning of the environment.
	- decreased blinking with little eye contact.
Catatonic Excitement	- patient appears hyperactive with constant, apparently nonpurposeful, motor activity.
	- patient does not appear restless or uncomfortable (differentiates from akathisia).
	- may lead to autonomic changes including changes in cardiac and respiratory rate, blood pressure, temperature, and diaphoresis.
Catatonic Combativeness	- agitation and combativeness, generally undirected.
	- may lead to autonomic changes including changes in cardiac and respiratory rate, blood pressure, temperature, and diaphoresis.
Automatic Obedience	- patient automatically obeys every instruction from the examiner even if the task may be inappropriate or self-injurious.
	- Mitmachen and Mitgehen are forms of automatic obedience (see below).
Mitmachen	- a form of automatic obedience.
	- the body of the patient can be put into any posture, even if the patient is given instructions to resist.
Mitgehen	- examiner can move the patient's body with the slightest touch, with the body part immediately returning to the original position in an attempt to keep in physical contact with the examiner.
Grasp Reflex	- can be elicited by the examiner by offering a hand, which is forcibly and repeatedly grasped by the patient.
Ambitendency	- state of hesitant or indecisive movement.
	- manifested as alternating cooperation followed by resistance to examiner's instructions.
Impulsivity	- suddenly engaging in an inappropriate behavior such as running down hallway, screaming or taking off clothes without any provocation.

A different screening version of BFCRS, known as Bush-Francis Catatonia Rating Screening Instrument (BFCSI), can be used for screening. It contains the 14 most common catatonic signs, which are scored as "absent" or "present": rigidity, negativism, waxy flexibility and withdrawal, immobility/stupor, mutism, staring gaze, posturing/catalepsy, excitement, stereotypes, mannerisms, grimacing, echopraxia/echolalia, and verbigeration. If two or more of the BFCSI signs are present for 24 h or longer, catatonia should be considered as a possible diagnosis. To avoid overdiagnosis, impulsivity and combativeness are excluded from this screening instrument.

Pathophysiology

While the exact pathophysiology of catatonia is unclear, two hypotheses have been suggested: a dysfunction in neurotransmission or in brain circuitry.

Neurotransmission

Neurotransmitter disturbances involving dopamine, glutamate, and gamma-aminobutyric acid (GABA) have been considered as putative causes for catatonia. Among these, alterations in glutamatergic and GABAergic activity are felt to contribute to some but not all phenotypes of catatonia, while dopamine plays a less clear role.

Glutamate dysfunction is thought to contribute to some of the features of catatonia. Arguments in favor of this statement include appearance of catatonia-like signs in healthy patients upon administration of the N-methyl-D-aspartate (NMDA)-receptor antagonist ketamine.[25] Furthermore, many patients with anti-NMDA-receptor encephalitis mimic or present with acute catatonia with stereotypies, mutism, echophenomena, rigidity, and abnormal involuntary facial movements.[26] In fact, some acute catatonia cases may even be misdiagnosed as anti-NMDA-receptor encephalitis.[27] In addition, a mouse model of reduced NMDA-receptor expression indicated abnormal motor and social behavior.[28] In contrast, reports suggest some efficacy of the NMDA-antagonist amantadine in treating catatonia.[29–32]

Dysfunction of the GABAergic system may also contribute to catatonia. This idea is supported by GABAergic drugs (lorazepam, zolpidem, etc.) being most effective in treating acute catatonia in case reports and clinical trials.[17,33] Decreased GABA A-receptor density was also detected in the left sensorimotor cortex of catatonic patients, and was correlated with the severity of catatonia.[34] In addition, antibodies against GABA A-receptor subunits have been detected in patients with neuropsychiatric syndromes.[35]

Finally, dopamine has been thought to play an indirect role in the pathogenesis of catatonia. The argument is based on the role of dopamine D2 antagonists in worsening catatonia in some cases, as well as induction of immobility and rigor from dopamine antagonism.[17] However, dopamine antagonism alone cannot explain other signs of catatonia, and dopamine agonists fail to alleviate symptoms of chronic catatonia.[36] In addition, studies on dopamine metabolism or receptor occupancy in catatonia have been inconclusive.[37]

Brain Circuitry

Alterations of brain function or structure within the cerebral motor circuit have been suggested in catatonic syndromes. Studies utilizing regional cerebral blood flow (rCBF) revealed hypoperfusion in the frontal and parietal cortical motor areas in mixed groups of predominantly akinetic catatonia,[38,39] with other reporting increase in rCBF in these areas with improvement of catatonia by electroconvulsive therapy (ECT).[40,41] Studies utilizing cortical activity reported delayed onset of movement-related potentials in motor areas in akinetic catatonia.[42] Similarly, some studies reported reduced neural activation during motor tasks (finger-tapping or finger-opposition tasks) in cortical motor, premotor, and parietal areas in catatonic patients.[43–45] Impaired orbitofrontal function has also been reported during processing of negative emotions in catatonia.[46,47]

In contrast to the above, there have been reports of different patterns of frontal, striatal, and thalamic metabolism in chronic catatonia patients.[37,48–50] Thus, it is postulated that the patterns of altered cerebral metabolism or neural activity may correspond to specific symptoms.

Treatment

Most of the recommended treatments for catatonia are based on case series and reports and have not been subjected to randomized placebo-controlled trials.

Benzodiazepines are considered the first-line treatment for catatonia for their rapid onset of action and dramatic improvement in symptoms. They may also help in assisting with the diagnosis of unclear cases. Studies utilizing benzodiazepines have reported an overall response rate of 60%–80%.[51-53]

Lorazepam, oral or parenteral, is often selected as the drug of choice. Other benzodiazepines such as diazepam, clonazepam, or oxazepam have also been found effective.[17,54] One study involving 13 acute catatonic patients reported a 60% reduction in the BFCRS scale within 10 minutes of administration of 2 mg of intravenous lorazepam.[51,55] As such, a 1–2 mg intravenous dose of lorazepam (1–2 mg) can be used as a diagnostic test for catatonia with reduction or resolution of symptoms within minutes.[52,56] Since approximately 20% of the patients may not respond to such a challenge, the absence of response may not completely rule out catatonia.[51]

The typical starting dose of lorazepam in catatonia is 3 mg/day in divided doses, and can be titrated up as necessary. While oral route is preferred, in many cases the patient's mental status may warrant parenteral use (IM or IV), and studies have utilized a primary parenteral or even a combination of oral and parenteral administration.[54] Occasionally, 20–30 mg/day in divided doses may be needed. The vast majority of patients have complete resolution of their symptoms within 3 hours of receiving lorazepam 1–3 mg sublingually or intramuscularly. After resolution of the troublesome symptoms at the effective dose of lorazepam for a given patient, the patient should be maintained at that dose for several days until the underlying etiology is treated appropriately.[57] Side effects such as excessive sedation, hypoventilation in patients with sleep apnea or obesity, and falls in elderly patients should be considered when using benzodiazepines.

Zolpidem is another medication that is increasingly recognized as an efficient treatment of catatonia in case series and reports.[58-61] It acts by binding to GABA-A receptors at the same location as benzodiazepines, and potentiates the action of GABA. Zolpidem 10 mg PO is also suggested as a pharmacological test for catatonia with resolution of symptoms in 15 minutes.[59] Therapeutic effect is seen between plasma levels of 8–150 ng/l. Maintenance doses between 7.5–40 mg/day divided in three doses have been suggested.[61,62]

NMDA receptor antagonists can also be beneficial in catatonia. Amantadine in a single oral dose of 200 mg or single IV dose of 500 mg (or 200 mg TID in divided doses) has been reported to produce clinical improvement.[63] Similarly, maintenance doses of up to 600 mg/day in divided doses (three to four times per day) have been reported.[63] Memantine with doses from 10 mg/day to 20 mg/day have been shown to be effective in case series and case reports.[63,64]

Other medications with reported variable success include topiramate, amobarbital, tetrabenazine, corticosteroids and rituximab.[65]

Regarding neuroleptics, typical antipsychotics are generally not recommended as treatment for acute catatonia and should be avoided.[53] Clozapine was found to be beneficial in case reports and retrospective studies.[66] Olanzapine, quetiapine, and risperidone have shown benefit in some case reports.[66,67]

Electroconvulsive therapy (ECT) was reported effective for catatonia regardless of its etiology, including medication refractory catatonia, in retrospective studies, case reports, and case series,[53,68] with an improvement rate between 59% and 93%.[69,70] ECT factors associated with better outcomes include daily administration of ECT and longer duration of seizure activity at the final ECT session.[69] Daily treatments for 2–5 days may be required for lasting effect.[8] Patient factors associated with a faster response to ECT include shorter duration of illness, as well as waxy flexibility and gegenhalten, whereas patients with echophenomena have a slower response.[70] ECT should not be considered first-line therapy except for life-threatening malignant catatonia, in which case it should be used within 5 days of symptom onset to avoid an increase in mortality.[8,53] Some cases of catatonia may require maintenance ECT to prevent relapsing episodes.[71-73] Others, especially those with chronic catatonia might benefit from combination of ECT and clozapine.[74] A systemic review of patients with anti-NMDA receptor encephalitis who received ECT reported improvement in majority of cases, with some reporting improvement in the absence of immunomodulatory therapy.[75]

Finally, there have been case reports of benefits from 7 to 10 sessions of fast repetitive transcranial magnetic stimulation (10 Hz) of the left dorsolateral prefrontal cortex.[76-79]

Psychomotor Retardation in Depression

Psychomotor retardation (PMR) is recognized as one of the most fundamental and oldest features of major depressive disorder (MDD), as it was described by the earliest psychiatric authors. Indeed, Hippocrates and Aretaeus of Cappadocia both described PMR as a characteristic of depression.[80] In the late nineteenth century, Kraepelin further expanded on the phenomenon of PMR.[81] He reported it was more prominent than depressed mood and involved constrained speech, thought, and behavior. Other authors from the same era have reported disturbances in speech, ideation, facial expression, and fine and gross motor activity. Features mentioned in these accounts include slowness of movement and gait, motor stagnation, hesitant walking, and even nearly complete immobility.[82,83] More recently, the presence of PMR has been used to clinically delineate subtypes of depression (melancholic with and without psychotic features, bipolar and unipolar disorders).[84-86] Its presence has also been used to understand the underlying neurobiology and its relevance in therapeutic interventions.[82]

DSM-5 includes psychomotor retardation (or agitation) as one of criteria for diagnosing depression.

Prevalence

Exact definitions of psychomotor phenomena, as well as its strict incidence and prevalence remain unknown. Most of the mainstream rating tools either have not included components of motor phenomena or use one or two items focused on agitation or retardation. In this context, epidemiological studies on PMR in depression are lacking, and most of the studies aim at studying its pathophysiology, predicting treatment response or developing experimental tools for its assessment.

Clinical Features/Components of Psychomotor Retardation

PMR may involve changes in speech, facial expressions, eye movements, self-touching, posture, and speed and degree of movements. It is considered a prominent feature of major depression.[87]

Speech
Patients with depression and PMR may have alterations in paralinguistic aspects of speech, with changes in fluency and prosody. Based on audio tape recordings and computer-driven acoustic measuring systems of semistructured interviews and counting tasks, there is significant elongation of speech pause time in depressed patients. Reduced prosody is also seen. The phonation time may remain constant.[88-93]

Gross Motor Activity
Patients with a MDD and PMR may have alterations of gait, posture, or limb movement. These have been investigated by objective analysis of spatiotemporal gait parameters, actigraphy, cinematography, or ground reaction forces.[80] Depressed patients with PMR showed significantly slower gait velocity, reduced stride length, double limb support and cycle duration as compared to controls.[94,95] Nonverbal behavior is also altered in depression with increased brief repetitive body, hand-to-hand, and hand-to-head touching.[96] Circadian variations with reduction in activity levels in the late morning, early afternoon and early evening have also been reported.[97,98]

Fine Motor Activity
Fine motor system abnormalities that might not be clinically observed have also been reported in MDD. Kinematic analysis of handwriting or drawing movements, copying geometric figures allows precise objective recording of fine motor slowing that may not be noticed clinically. There is also a delay in initiation time and an increase in movement duration during simple and complex tasks.[99,100] The delay is increased in melancholic vs. nonmelancholic patients.[101] Internally cued movements are more severely affected than externally cued reactions, pointing toward impairments of visuospatial and attention processing cognitive aspects of psychomotor functioning.[87]

Eye Movements
Studies on eye movements in depression reveal intact reflexive and voluntary saccades, but increased duration with normal or slightly increased rates of response suppression errors.[102] There is reduced accuracy of memory-guided saccades.[103] Melancholic patients may have greater variability of latencies, lower peak saccade velocities, and reduced accuracy of the primary saccade.[103]

Facial Movements

Facial movements may also be reduced in patients with MDD. A study utilizing facial muscle electromyography (EMG) during affective imagery revealed depressed patients had significant reduction of EMG pattern for happiness, in the absence of any other obvious clinical signs of motor retardation.[104]

Cognitive Measures

Patients with PMR may complain of slow ideation. The components leading to slow ideation may include a central cognitive slowing and a peripheral motor slowing. There is slowing of the motor component in both melancholic and nonmelancholic depression patients, whereas the former have an additional central cognitive component.[105] A study in depressed bipolar patients also reported significant reduction in psychomotor speed.[106] The shifting of response from one side to the other as well as maximal response preparation are delayed in MDD compared to controls.[107-109]

Psychomotor Retardation Scales

Several rating scales have been used to quantify the severity of depression in clinical and research studies. However, most depression scales do not address the severity of PMR, with a minimal number of items to assess the overall psychomotor retardation.[110,111]

To address these shortcomings, rating scales have been devised to measure PMR, and can be used in both clinical practice and research.

Salpêtrière Retardation Rating Scale (SRRS)

The Salpêtrière Retardation Rating Scale (SRRS) is also known as the Widlocher Depressive Retardation Rating Scale or the Depressive Retardation Rating Scale. This scale measures both cognitive and motor aspects of PMR, and has a total of 15 items. Each item is scored from 0 (symptom absence) to 4 (severe) on a structured format, for a total score range of 0 to 60.[83] A score of 20 on the scale is used as a cutoff score for psychomotor retardation.

The scale measures 5 items related to movement. These include the quality of stride, and the slowness of limb, trunk, head, and neck movement. In regards to speech, the scale scores verbal flow, tone of voice, and length of response. It also has two items designed to objectively measure the patient's cognitive function. Five items are subjective and assess the level

---

Box 12.1 Components of Psychomotor Retardation

1. Decrease in fluency and prosody of speech.
2. Slowness and decrease in gross motor activity.
3. Slowness and delay in fine motor activity on kinematic analysis.
4. Abnormal ocular saccadic responses on specific analyses
5. Decreased facial expression
6. Cognitive slowing

of interest, fatigue, memory, perception of time, and concentration. The scale also includes an item for an overall assessment of the patient's PMR.

The SRSS has been found to correlate with both cognitive and motor aspects PMR in MDD. In addition to patients with MDD, the SRRS has been used to assess patients with dysthymic disorder. A study found high scores on SRSS inpatients with dysthymia, but only half of the patients scored above the threshold for psychomotor retardation.[112]

Short Version of Retardation Rating Scale for Elderly Patients (RRS-4)

A shorter version of the Salpêtrière Retardation Rating Scale (RRS-4) is available to evaluate psychomotor retardation in geriatric patients. It consists of 14 items scored on a 5-point scale from 0 (normal) to 4 (severe), with a total score range from 0 to 56. Compared to the SRRS, the modified scale has the same number of cognitive and subjective experience items, adds one additional item rating motility, and has one less item rating speech. It also lacks the item for overall impression.[113]

The CORE measure

The CORE measure was originally designed to classify melancholic and nonmelancholic subtypes of depression. Since the scale is constructed on rating certain clinical features of PMR to diagnose melancholic depression, it can be utilized to score PMR.

There are a total of 18 items on the CORE measure, divided into three subscales. These consist of 6 noninteractiveness scale items, 7 retardation scale items, and 5 agitation scale items. The noninteractiveness subscale items include attentiveness, reactivity, richness of associations, level of interactiveness, length of responses, and willingness to converse. The retardation subscale includes posture, level of facial and body immobility, speed of movement, amount of delay in motor movement and verbal responses, and speech rate. The items on the agitation subscale include repetitive speech, facial expression and movement. Each item is scored based on severity from 0 (absence of symptom) to 3 (severe) with a total score of 54. A patient score of 21 or higher is considered to have melancholic depression.[86] A cutoff score of 8 has been used to classify as psychomotor depression.[86]

It is recommended that the interview be conducted in the morning since psychomotor disturbances are more profound early in the day. To avoid the influence of anxiety on body movements, the scale should be used at least twenty minutes into the interview to allow the patient to get comfortable. The CORE measure was found to have high reliability and validity.[86]

Motor Agitation and Retardation Scale (MARS)

The Motor Agitation and Retardation Scale (MARS) was designed to assess only the motor features in depressed patients, without taking into account the cognitive effects of depression. There are a total of 19 items on the scale divided into five major body categories (eyes, face, voice, limbs, and trunk). In the eyes, the scale rates direction of gaze, eye movement, amount of blinking, and staring. In the face, the scale rates facial expression and facial expressivity. In the voice, the scale rates tone, volume, time for onset and slurring. Items under the limbs category include movement of the foot, leg and hand; tension in hand; motor slowness and stride. The trunk category items include posture, axial movement and immobility. Each item is scored from 1 to 4, with 4 being the most severe. In addition, the scale utilizes different scoring for discrete and comprehensive items. For discrete items such as erratic eye movement, the severity is scaled by: none, rare, periodic, and continual. For comprehensive items such as monotone speech, the severity is scaled by: none, mild, moderate, and severe.[114]

Each of the retardation scales mentioned here has different strengths and weaknesses, providing flexibility in the choice of the scale to adapt to different situations. The SRSS is the scale most commonly used by researchers.[115] Its modified version, RSS-4 can be used on elderly patients.[113] The CORE scale is primarily used for diagnosis of melancholia in clinic, or for research purposes.[86] The MARS scale is a quick and easy tool to use in clinical setting.[114]

Pathophysiology

Similar to catatonia, two hypotheses have been suggested for the pathophysiology of PMR: a dysfunction in neurotransmission or in brain circuitry.

Neurotransmission

Dysfunctional dopaminergic neurotransmission is postulated as an underlying feature of psychomotor changes in patients with melancholic depression. This theory is supported by studies on plasma dopamine precursors and cerebrospinal fluid levels of dopamine metabolites.[115,116] In addition, one study showed that reduced regional uptake in the left and right striatum was associated with psychomotor retardation in subjects with depression compared to healthy volunteers.[117] However, these findings could not be replicated in another study.[118]

Serotonin is also hypothesized to play a role in depression and cognitive slowing in PMR. One study utilizing 5-HT receptor agonist administration to healthy volunteers revealed cognitive slowing, but not motor slowing during reaction time and copying psychomotor tasks.[119]

Brain Circuitry

The basal ganglia is hypothesized to play a role in the pathophysiology of psychomotor changes in mood disorders. This hypothesis is based on the premise of high incidences of depressive symptomatology seen in other neuropsychiatric disorders where psychomotor changes are seen, such as Parkinson's disease, Huntington's disease and schizophrenia. In addition, the striatum receives cortical input via the thalamus and has projections to the prefrontal, premotor, and supplementary motor area that play a key role in motor planning.[115,120] Investigators have correlated specific neurocircuitry in the prefrontal cortex and basal ganglia with psychomotor changes in depression.[80] Structural imaging studies have suggested frontostriatal abnormalities including white matter changes in the basal ganglia and atrophy of the prefrontal cortex, caudate, and putamen in patients with depression; and these were more prominent in those with PMR.[121,122] Another study associated PMR with white matter hyperintensities on structural brain MRI in patients with depression after age 50, the authors were also able to predict poor response to ECT and pharmacotherapy in these patients.[122-124] Some authors have also hypothesized that decreased regional blood flow in the left neostriatum or activity in the left caudate may contribute to PMR.[125]

Involvement of areas beyond the basal ganglia especially the paralimbic regions of the frontal lobes have also been hypothesized to contribute to PMR in depression. Indeed, several studies utilizing functional neuroimaging have suggested decreased blood flow in the dorsolateral prefrontal cortex, left prefrontal cortex, angular gyrus, and the anterior cingulate region in patients with PMR in depression.[126-130] A positron emission tomography (PET) study also revealed hypometabolism of the orbital frontal-inferior prefrontal cortex in subjects with both MDD and Huntington's as compared to those with HD alone or healthy subjects.[131] Another single photon emission computed tomography (SPECT) study negatively correlated the severity of psychomotor retardation with prefrontal, frontal and temporal perfusion in severe depression.[127]

Finally, studies have shown an association of the hypothalamic–pituitary–adrenal (HPA) axis overactivity with PMR.[132-134] Arginine vasopressin (AVP), produced by hypothalamic neurons, is known to activate the HPA axis and studies have revealed elevated AVP levels in MDD patients with PMR.[135,136]

Treatment

Selective serotonin reuptake inhibitors (SSRIs) are the most frequently used medications for the treatment of depression. As such, they are the most studied class in patients with PMR with particular interest in determining if the presence of PMR could predict the response of depression to a specific agent. Given its greatest dopaminergic activity, two studies hypothesized sertraline as the optimal choice for patients with PMR.[137,138] However, the results of the studies are mixed. Studies have reported melancholia as a predictor of good response to sertraline[138] and fluoxetine[139] but not to citalopram.[140] Similarly, PMR was linked to nonresponse to fluoxetine,[141] or sertraline.[142] However, another study reported PMR had no predictive value for the response to SSRIs.[143]

Some authors have hypothesized that pharmacological agents with broader actions may be more efficacious for patients with PMR due to deficiencies in both the norepinephrine and dopamine systems. One study indeed demonstrated that PMR predicted response to selective serotonin-norepinephrine reuptake inhibitors (SNRIs) more so than to SSRIs.[144]

Tricyclic antidepressants (TCAs) may be considered in patients with PMR and resistance to SSRI or SNRI's. Multiple studies have compared SSRIs to TCAs in patients with PMR. Some studies found in PMR a better predictor of response to TCAs.[145,146] Another study reported TCAs as predictor of response if the definition of PMR in the study were changed.[147] To our knowledge, no study has reported a lack of response of PMR to TCAs.

Studies on MAOIs have reported mixed results with PMR predicting response, nonresponse or neither.[142,148,149]

There is a lack of evidence regarding other classes of antidepressants studied for depressed patients with PMR. These include norepinephrine-dopamine reuptake inhibitors (NDRIs), tetracyclics (TeCAs), and mood stabilizers. One study on NDRIs (bupropion) in psychomotor retardation predicted response,[142] while another predicted nonresponse.[150]

Regarding nonpharmacological interventions, PMR was found to be predictive of good response to ECT,[123,151,152] while repetitive transcranial magnetic stimulation (rTMS) was reported to help decrease the severity of PMR.[153,154]

Movement Disorders in Drug-Naïve Schizophrenic Patients

Movement disorders have been described as an intrinsic component of the disease process in schizophrenic patients before the advent of neuroleptic drugs.[4,155,156] After the discovery of the first-generation antipsychotics in the 1950s, focus shifted to the presumption that movement disorders in schizophrenia, including parkinsonism, constitute an antido-paminergic side effect of such medication.[157–159] However, recent studies on drug-naïve schizophrenic patients have shown that spontaneous movement disorders (SMDs), both parkinsonism and spontaneous dyskinesia, can be detected in schizophrenia at the first presentation and for several years thereafter.[160–163]

Prevalence

SMDs have been reported in 4% to 11% of schizophrenic patients with no prior exposure to antipsychotic medications.[160–163] Spontaneous parkinsonism is the most common SMD followed by abnormal involuntary movements in a tardive dyskinesia-like syndrome. A review comprising 13 studies reported a median rate of 17% for spontaneous parkinsonism followed by 9% for spontaneous dyskinesia.[160] In this section, we will focus on parkinsonism as spontaneous dyskinesias are hyperkinetic movement disorder and beyond the scope of this chapter.

Clinical Features

Parkinsonism in drug naïve schizophrenic patients is most often of the akinetic-rigid type, with bradykinesia and rigidity dominating the picture, while tremor is rarer.[155,160–164] Nonakinetic parkinsonian features (such as tremor) worsen following treatment with antipsychotics as compared to the akinetic type leading to the hypothesis that the former might primarily be a drug-induced phenomenon.[161,162]

The most common dyskinetic symptoms reported in drug naïve patients are involuntary stereotypies in the orofacial region,[165] that resemble those in antipsychotic-induced tardive dyskinesia and levodopa induced dyskinesias in Parkinson's disease patients.[166]

Parkinsonism and stereotypies can occasionally present together in patients with drug-naïve schizophrenia, with stereotypies in the orofacial region and parkinsonism in the limbs. In addition, patients with schizophrenia may have increased postural sway.[167,168]

SMDs have also been reported in subjects with schizotypal personality disorder,[167] as well as in relatives of patients with schizophrenia.[161]

Factors associated with an increased risk of stereotypies reported in a meta-analysis included age and increased duration of untreated schizophrenia. No such correlation could be found with parkinsonism.[161]

Pathogenesis

The pathobiological concepts behind these entities are not entirely clear and the concepts have evolved over the years. Similar to catatonia and PMR, these concepts include a dysfunction in neurotransmission or in brain circuitry.

Neurotransmission

The dopaminergic system is hypothesized to be involved. In schizophrenia, the nigrostriatal dopaminergic neurons are hyperactive and intact based on neuroimaging as well as postmortem neurochemical measure. The D2 receptor is hyperactive in the caudate and putamen, with a large increase in the dorsal (associative and sensorimotor) regions of the striatum, while the ventral (limbic) subdivision of the striatum is less involved.[169–172] This could explain the spontaneous stereotypies in drug naïve patients, as well as the propensity for neuroleptic induced tardive syndromes. However, it does not explain the spontaneous parkinsonism seen in schizophrenia.

Brain Circuitry

An alternative explanation utilizing an overlapping network/loop based dysfunction for both Parkinson's disease and schizophrenia has been proposed. There is involvement of the cortical-striatal-thalamocortical loop in Parkinson's disease. The dysfunctional cortical-subcortical neuronal network (including the putamen) mediates motor dysfunction; and the dysfunctional cortico-striato-thalamocortical neuronal network (including the caudate, frontal association cortex, limbic system and other neocortical areas) mediates both motor and non-motor features of Parkinson's disease, such as psychosis.[173,174] The loop may overlap with dysfunction in the prefrontal/anterior cingulate cortical-striatal-hippocampal neuronal network that is seen in psychosis and antipsychotic drug action in schizophrenia[175–177] Hence, it has been proposed that the hypokinetic movement disorders (such as parkinsonism) in schizophrenia involve dysfunction in the cingulate motor cortex/supplementary motor area/motor cortical-striatal-thalamocortical neuronal network.[178] It is also hypothesized that dopaminergic hypofunction (as in Parkinson's disease) and dopaminergic hyperfunction (as in schizophrenia) may have a common functional effect on an element of the cortico-striato-thalamocortical neuronal network.[179]

Finally, an involvement of the cerebellum (in addition to the basal ganglia) leading to the increased postural sway in schizophrenia spectrum disorders patients has been suggested. These cerebellar abnormalities include impairments in functional activation, connectivity, metabolism, gyrification and alteration in Purkinje cell morphology and protein expression.[180–183]

Treatment of Parkinsonism in Neuroleptic-Naïve Schizophrenia

There are limited data on treatment of parkinsonism in patients with schizophrenia and other psychotic conditions. Theoretically, the treatment poses a challenge as dopamine blockade from treating schizophrenia carries the potential risk of worsening parkinsonism and vice versa.[184]

A wise choice of the patient's antipsychotic regimen might be prudent to lessen the risk of worsening parkinsonism. Two antipsychotic medications shown not to exacerbate parkinsonism in idiopathic Parkinson's disease in double blind, placebo-controlled trials are quetiapine and clozapine.[185] The effect of quetiapine is hypothesized to be due to its faster dopamine receptor dissociation, whereas clozapine has poor dopamine selectivity.[186,187] If possible, preferring these two agents over other neuroleptics would be a first step in preventing worsening of parkinsonism in neuroleptic naïve schizophrenia. This choice of neuroleptics may not be possible in some patients, and parkinsonism may otherwise require direct symptomatic treatment because of its impact of quality of life and function. These patients may thus require dopaminergic therapy. Because of the higher risk of hallucinations and psychosis with amantadine and dopamine agonists, levodopa therapy remains the drug of choice. Indeed, while worsening of psychosis from levodopa therapy has been reported in individual cases,[188-190] several reports of a favorable outcome without worsening of psychosis can be found in literature. One study showed no worsening of psychosis in patients with drug induced parkinsonism after chronic levodopa therapy.[191] A meta-analysis of five studies of concomitant levodopa with antipsychotic drugs revealed an overall improvement. Sixteen other studies in which levodopa was added to antipsychotic drugs, but did not meet inclusion criteria for the meta-analysis, also reported a favorable improvement profile with worsening occurring in less than 20% of patients.[192] A case series of nine patients with parkinsonism and schizophrenia showed improvement of motor symptoms without worsening of psychosis with addition of carbidopa/levodopa to their regimen in 8 patients. One patient who was not on an antipsychotic had an initial worsening of psychosis that resolved with quetiapine.[193] To avoid a potential worsening of psychosis from levodopa, we recommend using the smallest amount that satisfactorily improves the parkinsonism.

Conclusion

Noniatrogenic hypokinetic movement disorders may be seen in patients with psychiatric disorders in the absence of a diagnosis of a primary movement disorder. Hypokinetic catatonia, psychomotor retardation in depression, and spontaneous parkinsonism in drug naïve schizophrenia patients are an example. It is important for clinicians and other healthcare providers to be cognizant of these features and entities in order to improve their diagnosis and management. The quality of life of patients afflicted with noniatrogenic hypokinetic movement disorders can be meaningfully improved with symptomatic therapies tailored to their specific needs.

References

1. Anguenot, A., Loll, P. Y., Neau, J. P., Ingrand, P., & Gil, R. (2002). Depression et maladie de Parkinson: étude d'une série de 135 parkinsoniens [Depression and Parkinson's disease: study of a series of 135 Parkinson's patients]. *Canadian journal of neurological sciences. Le journal canadien des sciences neurologiques, 29*(2), 139–146.
2. Kahlbaum, K. L., (1874). Die Katatonie oder das Spannungsirresein. Eineklinische Form psychischer Krankheit. Vol Erstdruck Berlin: A. Hirschwald.
3. Kahlbaum, K. L., (1973). Catatonia. Translated by Levi Y, Pridon T. Baltimore: Johns Hopkins University Press.
4. Kraepelin, E. (1919). Dementia praecox and paraphrenia. Translated by Barclay RM. Edinburgh: Livingstone.
5. Pfuhlmann, B., & Stöber, G. (2001). The different conceptions of catatonia: historical overview and critical discussion. *European archives of psychiatry and clinical neuroscience, 251*(Suppl 1), I4–I7.
6. van der Heijden, F. M., Tuinier, S., Arts, N. J., Hoogendoorn, M. L., Kahn, R. S., & Verhoeven, W. M. (2005). Catatonia: disappeared or under-diagnosed? *Psychopathology, 38*(1), 3–8.

7. Fink, M., Shorter, E., & Taylor, M. A. (2010). Catatonia is not schizophrenia: Kraepelin's error and the need to recognize catatonia as an independent syndrome in medical nomenclature. *Schizophrenia bulletin*, 36(2), 314–320.

8. Fink, M., & Taylor, M. A. (2009). The catatonia syndrome: forgotten but not gone. *Archives of general psychiatry*, 66(11), 1173–1177.

9. Rosebush, P. I., Hildebrand, A. M., Furlong, B. G., & Mazurek, M. F. (1990). Catatonic syndrome in a general psychiatric inpatient population: frequency, clinical presentation, and response to lorazepam. *Journal of clinical psychiatry*, 51(9), 357–362.

10. Chalasani, P., Healy, D., & Morriss, R. (2005). Presentation and frequency of catatonia in new admissions to two acute psychiatric admission units in India and Wales. *Psychological medicine*, 35(11), 1667–1675.

11. Stuivenga, M., & Morrens, M. (2014). Prevalence of the catatonic syndrome in an acute inpatient sample. *Frontiers in psychiatry*, 5, 17.

12. Grover, S., Chakrabarti, S., Ghormode, D., Agarwal, M., Sharma, A., & Avasthi, A. (2015). Catatonia in inpatients with psychiatric disorders: a comparison of schizophrenia and mood disorders. *Psychiatry research*, 229(3), 919–925.

13. Docx, L., Morrens, M., Bervoets, C., Hulstijn, W., Fransen, E., De Hert, M., et al. (2012). Parsing the components of the psychomotor syndrome in schizophrenia. *Acta psychiatrica Scandinavica*, 126(4), 256–265

14. Peralta, V., Campos, M. S., de Jalon, E. G., & Cuesta, M. J. (2010). DSM-IV catatonia signs and criteria in first-episode, drug-naive, psychotic patients: psychometric validity and response to antipsychotic medication. *Schizophrenia research*, 118(1–3), 168–175.

15. Ungvari, G. S., Leung, S. K., Ng, F. S., Cheung, H. K., & Leung, T. (2005). Schizophrenia with prominent catatonic features ("catatonic schizophrenia"): I. Demographic and clinical correlates in the chronic phase. *Progress in neuro-psychopharmacology & biological psychiatry*, 29(1), 27–38.

16. Kleinhaus, K., Harlap, S., Perrin, M. C., Manor, O., Weiser, M., Harkavy-Friedman, J. M., et al. (2012). Catatonic schizophrenia: a cohort prospective study. *Schizophrenia bulletin*, 38(2), 331–337.

17. Sienaert, P., Dhossche, D. M., Vancampfort, D., De Hert, M., & Gazdag, G. (2014). A clinical review of the treatment of catatonia. *Frontiers in psychiatry*, 5, 181.

18. Smith, J. H., Smith, V. D., Philbrick, K. L., & Kumar, N. (2012). Catatonic disorder due to a general medical or psychiatric condition. *Journal of neuropsychiatry and clinical neurosciences*, 24(2), 198–207.

19. Jaimes-Albornoz, W., & Serra-Mestres, J. (2012). Catatonia in the emergency department. *Emergency medicine journal: EMJ*, 29(11), 863–867.

20. Saddawi-Konefka, D., Berg, S. M., Nejad, S. H., & Bittner, E. A. (2014). Catatonia in the ICU: an important and underdiagnosed cause of altered mental status. a case series and review of the literature. *Critical care medicine*, 42(3), e234–e241.

21. Azzam, P. N., & Gopalan, P. (2013). Prototypes of catatonia: diagnostic and therapeutic challenges in the general hospital. *Psychosomatics*, 54(1), 88–93.

22. Taylor, M. A., & Fink, M. (2003). Catatonia in psychiatric classification: a home of its own. *American journal of psychiatry*, 160(7), 1233–1241.

23. Bush, G., Petrides, G., & Francis, A. (1997). Catatonia and other motor syndromes in a chronically hospitalized psychiatric population. *Schizophrenia research*, 27(1), 83–92.

24. Fink, M., Taylor, M.A. (2003). Catatonia: a clinician's guide to diagnosis and treatment. Cambridge, UK: Cambridge University Press; p. 276.

25. Gouzoulis-Mayfrank, E., Heekeren, K., Neukirch, A., Stoll, M., Stock, C., Obradovic, M., et al. (2005). Psychological effects of (S)-ketamine and N,N-dimethyltryptamine (DMT): a double-blind, cross-over study in healthy volunteers. *Pharmacopsychiatry*, *38*(6), 301–311.

26. Dalmau, J., Lancaster, E., Martinez-Hernandez, E., Rosenfeld, M. R., & Balice-Gordon, R. (2011). Clinical experience and laboratory investigations in patients with anti-NMDAR encephalitis. *Lancet. Neurology*, *10*(1), 63–74.

27. Steiner, J., Walter, M., Glanz, W., Sarnyai, Z., Bernstein, H. G., Vielhaber, S. et al., (2013). Increased prevalence of diverse N-methyl-D-aspartate glutamate receptor antibodies in patients with an initial diagnosis of schizophrenia: specific relevance of IgG NR1a antibodies for distinction from N-methyl-D-aspartate glutamate receptor encephalitis. *JAMA psychiatry*, *70*(3), 271–278.

28. Mohn, A. R., Gainetdinov, R. R., Caron, M. G., & Koller, B. H. (1999). Mice with reduced NMDA receptor expression display behaviors related to schizophrenia. *Cell*, *98*(4), 427–436.

29. Northoff, G., Eckert, J., & Fritze, J. (1997). Glutamatergic dysfunction in catatonia? Successful treatment of three acute akinetic catatonic patients with the NMDA antagonist amantadine. *Journal of neurology, neurosurgery, and psychiatry*, *62*(4), 404–406.

30. Babington, P. W., & Spiegel, D. R. (2007). Treatment of catatonia with olanzapine and amantadine. *Psychosomatics*, *48*(6), 534–536.

31. Muneoka, K., Shirayama, Y., Kon, K., Kawabe, M., Goto, M., & Kimura, S. (2010). Improvement of mutism in a catatonic schizophrenia case by add-on treatment with amantadine. *Pharmacopsychiatry*, *43*(4), 151–152.

32. Hervey, W. M., Stewart, J. T., & Catalano, G. (2012). Treatment of catatonia with amantadine. *Clinical neuropharmacology*, *35*(2), 86–87.

33. Northoff G. (2002). Catatonia and neuroleptic malignant syndrome: psychopathology and pathophysiology. *Journal of neural transmission (Vienna, Austria: 1996)*, *109*(12), 1453–1467.

34. Northoff, G., Steinke, R., Czcervenka, C., Krause, R., Ulrich, S., Danos, P., et al. (1999). Decreased density of GABA-A receptors in the left sensorimotor cortex in akinetic catatonia: investigation of in vivo benzodiazepine receptor binding. *Journal of neurology, neurosurgery, and psychiatry*, *67*(4), 445–450.

35. Pettingill, P., Kramer, H. B., Coebergh, J. A., Pettingill, R., Maxwell, S., Nibber, A., et al. (2015). Antibodies to GABAA receptor α1 and γ2 subunits: clinical and serologic characterization. *Neurology*, *84*(12), 1233–1241.

36. Ungvari G. S. (2010). Amineptine treatment of persistent catatonic symptoms in schizophrenia: a controlled study. *Neuropsychopharmacologia Hungarica: a Magyar Pszichofarmakologiai Egyesulet lapja = official journal of the Hungarian Association of Psychopharmacology*, *12*(4), 463–467.

37. Lauer, M., Schirrmeister, H., Gerhard, A., Ellitok, E., Beckmann, H., Reske, S. N., et al. (2001). Disturbed neural circuits in a subtype of chronic catatonic schizophrenia demonstrated by F-18-FDG-PET and F-18-DOPA-PET. *Journal of neural transmission (Vienna, Austria: 1996)*, *108*(6), 661–670.

38. Northoff, G., Steinke, R., Nagel D, Czerwenka, C., Grosser, O., Danos, P., Genz, A., et al. (2000). Right lower prefronto-parietal cortical dysfunction in akinetic catatonia: a combined study of neuropsychology and regional cerebral blood flow. *Psychological medicine*, *30*(3), 583–596.

39. Satoh, K., Suzuki, T., Narita, M., Ishikura, S., Shibasaki, M., Kato, T., et al. (1993). Regional cerebral blood flow in catatonic schizophrenia. *Psychiatry research*, *50*(4), 203–216.

40. Galynker, I. I., Weiss, J., Ongseng, F., & Finestone, H. (1997). ECT treatment and cerebral perfusion in Catatonia. *Journal of nuclear medicine: official publication, Society of Nuclear Medicine, 38*(2), 251–254.

41. Escobar, R., Rios, A., Montoya, I. D., Lopera, F., Ramos, D., Carvajal, C., et al. (2000). Clinical and cerebral blood flow changes in catatonic patients treated with ECT. *Journal of psychosomatic research, 49*(6), 423–429.

42. Northoff, G., Pfennig, A., Krug, M., Danos, P., Leschinger, A., Schwarz, A., et al. (2000). Delayed onset of late movement-related cortical potentials and abnormal response to lorazepam in catatonia. *Schizophrenia research, 44*(3), 193–211.

43. Northoff, G., Braus, D. F., Sartorius, A., Khoram-Sefat, D., Russ, M., Eckert, J., et al. (1999). Reduced activation and altered laterality in two neuroleptic-naive catatonic patients during a motor task in functional MRI. *Psychological medicine, 29*(4), 997–1002.

44. Payoux, P., Boulanouar, K., Sarramon, C., Fabre, N., Descombes, S., Galitsky, M., et al. (2004). Cortical motor activation in akinetic schizophrenic patients: a pilot functional MRI study. *Movement disorders: official journal of the Movement Disorder Society, 19*(1), 83–90.

45. Scheuerecker, J., Ufer, S., Käpernick, M., Wiesmann, M., Brückmann, H., Kraft, E., et al. (2009). Cerebral network deficits in post-acute catatonic schizophrenic patients measured by fMRI. *Journal of psychiatric research, 43*(6), 607–614.

46. Northoff, G., Kötter, R., Baumgart, F., Danos, P., Boeker, H., Kaulisch, T., et al. (2004). Orbitofrontal cortical dysfunction in akinetic catatonia: a functional magnetic resonance imaging study during negative emotional stimulation. *Schizophrenia bulletin, 30*(2), 405–427.

47. Richter, A., Grimm, S., & Northoff, G. (2010). Lorazepam modulates orbitofrontal signal changes during emotional processing in catatonia. *Human psychopharmacology, 25*(1), 55–62.

48. Tsujino, N., Nemoto, T., Yamaguchi, T., Katagiri, N., Tohgi, N., Ikeda, R., et al. (2011). Cerebral blood flow changes in very-late-onset schizophrenia-like psychosis with catatonia before and after successful treatment. *Psychiatry and clinical neurosciences, 65*(6), 600–603.

49. De Tiége, X., Bier, J. C., Massat, I., Laureys, S., Lotstra, F., Berré, J., et al. (2003). Regional cerebral glucose metabolism in akinetic catatonia and after remission. *Journal of neurology, neurosurgery, and psychiatry, 74*(7), 1003–1004.

50. Grignon, S., Forget, K., Durand, M., & Huppert, T. (2008). Increased left prefrontal activation during staring/mutism episodes in a patient with resistant catatonic schizophrenia: a near infrared spectroscopy study. *Cognitive and behavioral neurology: official journal of the Society for Behavioral and Cognitive Neurology, 21*(1), 41–45.

51. Bush, G., Fink, M., Petrides, G., Dowling, F., & Francis, A. (1996). Catatonia. II. Treatment with lorazepam and electroconvulsive therapy. *Acta psychiatrica Scandinavica, 93*(2), 137–143.

52. Daniels J. (2009). Catatonia: clinical aspects and neurobiological correlates. *Journal of neuropsychiatry and clinical neurosciences, 21*(4), 371–380.

53. Francis A. (2010). Catatonia: diagnosis, classification, and treatment. *Current psychiatry reports, 12*(3), 180–185.

54. Pelzer, A. C., van der Heijden, F. M., & den Boer, E. (2018). Systematic review of catatonia treatment. *Neuropsychiatric disease and treatment, 14,* 317–326.

55. Bush, G., Fink, M., Petrides, G., Dowling, F., & Francis, A. (1996). Catatonia. I. Rating scale and standardized examination. *Acta psychiatrica Scandinavica, 93*(2), 129–136.

56. Tibrewal, P., Narayanaswamy, J., Zutshi, A., Srinivasaraju, R., & Math, S. B. (2010). Response rate of lorazepam in catatonia: a developing country's perspective. *Progress in neuro-psychopharmacology & biological psychiatry, 34*(8), 1520–1522.

57. Rosebush, P. I., & Mazurek, M. F. (2010). Catatonia and its treatment. *Schizophrenia bulletin, 36*(2), 239–242.

58. Mastain, B., Vaiva, G., Guerouaou, D., Pommery, J., & Thomas, P. (1995). Effet favorable du zolpidem sur un état catatonique [Favorable effect of zolpidem on catatonia]. *Revue neurologique, 151*(1), 52–56.

59. Thomas, P., Rascle, C., Mastain, B., Maron, M., & Vaiva, G. (1997). Test for catatonia with zolpidem. *Lancet (London, England), 349*(9053), 702.

60. Zaw, Z. F., & Bates, G. D. (1997). Replication of zolpidem test for catatonia in an adolescent. *Lancet (London, England), 349*(9069), 1914.

61. Peglow, S., Prem, V., & McDaniel, W. (2013). Treatment of catatonia with zolpidem. *Journal of neuropsychiatry and clinical neurosciences, 25*(3), E13.

62. Hlal, H., Kettani, N., Berhili, N., Rammouz, I., & Aalouane, R. (2014). Place du zolpidem dans le traitement des catatonies résistantes aux benzodiazépines. À propos d'un cas [The role of zolpidem in improving catatonic schizophrenia. Case report]. *Presse medicale (Paris, France: 1983), 43*(9), 1018–1020.

63. Carroll, B. T., Goforth, H. W., Thomas, C., Ahuja, N., McDaniel, W. W., Kraus, M. F., et al. (2007). Review of adjunctive glutamate antagonist therapy in the treatment of catatonic syndromes. *Journal of neuropsychiatry and clinical neurosciences, 19*(4), 406–412.

64. Obregon, D. F., Velasco, R. M., Wuerz, T. P., Catalano, M. C., Catalano, G., & Kahn, D. (2011). Memantine and catatonia: a case report and literature review. *Journal of psychiatric practice, 17*(4), 292–299.

65. Wijemanne, S., & Jankovic, J. (2015). Movement disorders in catatonia. *Journal of neurology, neurosurgery, and psychiatry, 86*(8), 825–832.

66. Van Den Eede, F., Van Hecke, J., Van Dalfsen, A., Van den Bossche, B., Cosyns, P., & Sabbe, B. G. (2005). The use of atypical antipsychotics in the treatment of catatonia. *European psychiatry: the journal of the Association of European Psychiatrists, 20*(5–6), 422–429.

67. Hesslinger, B., Walden, J., & Normann, C. (2001). Acute and long-term treatment of catatonia with risperidone. *Pharmacopsychiatry, 34*(1), 25–26.

68. Zisselman, M. H., & Jaffe, R. L. (2010). ECT in the treatment of a patient with catatonia: consent and complications. *American journal of psychiatry, 167*(2), 127–132.

69. van Waarde, J. A., Tuerlings, J. H., Verwey, B., & van der Mast, R. C. (2010). Electroconvulsive therapy for catatonia: treatment characteristics and outcomes in 27 patients. *Journal of ECT, 26*(4), 248–252.

70. Raveendranathan, D., Narayanaswamy, J. C., & Reddi, S. V. (2012). Response rate of catatonia to electroconvulsive therapy and its clinical correlates. *European archives of psychiatry and clinical neuroscience, 262*(5), 425–430.

71. Suzuki, K., Awata, S., & Matsuoka, H. (2004). One-year outcome after response to ECT in middle-aged and elderly patients with intractable catatonic schizophrenia. *Journal of ECT, 20*(2), 99–106.

72. Suzuki, K., Awata, S., Takano, T., Ebina, Y., Iwasaki, H., & Matsuoka, H. (2005). Continuation electroconvulsive therapy for relapse prevention in middle-aged and elderly patients with intractable catatonic schizophrenia. *Psychiatry and clinical neurosciences, 59*(4), 481–489.

73. Suzuki, K., Awata, S., Takano, T., Ebina, Y., Shindo, T., Harada, N., et al. (2006). Adjusting the frequency of continuation and maintenance electroconvulsive therapy to prevent relapse of catatonic schizophrenia in middle-aged and elderly patients who are relapse-prone. *Psychiatry and clinical neurosciences, 60*(4), 486–492.

74. Gazdag, G., Kocsis-Ficzere, N., & Tolna, J. (2006). The augmentation of clozapine treatment with electroconvulsive therapy. *Ideggyogyaszati szemle, 59*(7–8), 261–267.

75. Warren, N., Grote, V., O'Gorman, C., & Siskind, D. (2019). Electroconvulsive therapy for anti-N-methyl-d-aspartate (NMDA) receptor encephalitis: a systematic review of cases. *Brain stimulation, 12*(2), 329–334.

76. Grisaru, N., Chudakov, B., Yaroslavsky, Y., & Belmaker, R. H. (1998). Catatonia treated with transcranial magnetic stimulation. *American journal of psychiatry, 155*(11), 1630.

77. Saba, G., Rocamora, J. F., Kalalou, K., Benadhira, R., Plaze, M., Aubriot-Delmas, B., & Januel, D. (2002). Catatonia and transcranial magnetic stimulation. *American journal of psychiatry, 159*(10), 1794.

78. Kate, M. P., Raju, D., Vishwanathan, V., Khan, F. R., Nair, & Thomas, S. V. (2011). Successful treatment of refractory organic catatonic disorder with repetitive transcranial magnetic stimulation (rTMS) therapy. *Journal of neuropsychiatry and clinical neurosciences, 23*(3), E2–E3

79. Trojak, B., Meille, V., Bonin, B., & Chauvet-Geliner, J. C. (2014). Repetitive transcranial magnetic stimulation for the treatment of catatonia: an alternative treatment to electroconvulsive therapy? *Journal of neuropsychiatry and clinical neurosciences, 26*(2), E42–E43.

80. Sobin, C., & Sackeim, H. A. (1997). Psychomotor symptoms of depression. *American journal of psychiatry, 154*(1), 4–17.

81. Kraepelin, E. (1993) La folie maniaque-dépressive. Grenoble: Editions Jérôme Millon; p. 160.

82. Greden, J. F., & Carroll, B. J. (1981). Psychomotor function in affective disorders: an overview of new monitoring techniques. *American journal of psychiatry, 138*(11), 1441–1448.

83. Dantchev, N., & Widlöcher, D. J. (1998). The measurement of retardation in depression. *Journal of clinical psychiatry, 59*(Suppl 14), 19–25.

84. Nelson, J. C., & Charney, D. S. (1981). The symptoms of major depressive illness. *American journal of psychiatry, 138*(1), 1–13.

85. Goodwin, F., & Jamison, K. R. (1990). Manic depressive illness. Oxford, UK: Oxford University Press.

86. Parker, G., & Hadzi-Pavlovic, D. (1996). Melancholia: a disorder of movement and mood: a phenomenological and neurobiological review. Cambridge, UK: Cambridge University Press.

87. Hoffstaedter, F., Sarlon, J., Grefkes, C., & Eickhoff, S. B. (2012). Internally vs. externally triggered movements in patients with major depression. *Behavioural brain research, 228*(1), 125–132.

88. Greden, J. F., Albala, A. A., Smokler, I. A., Gardner, R., & Carroll, B. J. (1981). Speech pause time: a marker of psychomotor retardation among endogenous depressives. *Biological psychiatry, 16*(9), 851–859.

89. Nilsonne, A. (1987). Acoustic analysis of speech variables during depression and after improvement. *Acta psychiatrica Scandinavica, 76*(3), 235–245.

90. Nilsonne, A. (1988). Speech characteristics as indicators of depressive illness. *Acta psychiatrica Scandinavica, 77*(3), 253–263.

91. Kuny, S., & Stassen, H. H. (1993). Speaking behavior and voice sound characteristics in depressive patients during recovery. *Journal of psychiatric research, 27*(3), 289–307.

92. Flint, A. J., Black, S. E., Campbell-Taylor, I., Gailey, G. F., & Levinton, C. (1993). Abnormal speech articulation, psychomotor retardation, and subcortical dysfunction in major depression. *Journal of psychiatric research, 27*(3), 309–319.

93. Alpert, M., Pouget, E. R., & Silva, R. R. (2001). Reflections of depression in acoustic measures of the patient's speech. *Journal of affective disorders, 66*(1), 59–69.

94. Hergueta, T., Delgado, F., & Lecrubier Y., (1996). Quantitative video analysis of gait in depressed inpatients. *European Neuropsychopharmacology, 6*(4) S4–S100.

95. Lemke, M. R., Wendorff, T., Mieth, B., Buhl, K., & Linnemann, M. (2000). Spatiotemporal gait patterns during over ground locomotion in major depression compared with healthy controls. *Journal of psychiatric research, 34*(4–5), 277–283.

96. Lemke, M. R., & Schleidt, M. (1999). Temporal segmentation of human short-term behavior in everyday activities and interview sessions. *Die Naturwissenschaften, 86*(6), 289–292.

97. Raoux, N., Benoit, O., Dantchev, N., Denise, P., Franc, B., Allilaire, J. F., & Widlöcher, D. (1994). Circadian pattern of motor activity in major depressed patients undergoing antidepressant therapy: relationship between actigraphic measures and clinical course. *Psychiatry research, 52*(1), 85–98.

98. Lemke, M. R., Broderick, A., Zeitelberger, M., & Hartmann, W. (1997). Motor activity and daily variation of symptom intensity in depressed patients. *Neuropsychobiology, 36*(2), 57–61.

99. Sabbe, B., Hulstijn, W., Van Hoof, J., & Zitman, F. (1996). Fine motor retardation and depression. *Journal of psychiatric research, 30*(4), 295–306.

100. Sabbe, B., Hulstijn, W., van Hoof, J., Tuynman-Qua, H. G., & Zitman, F. (1999). Retardation in depression: assessment by means of simple motor tasks. *Journal of affective disorders, 55*(1), 39–44.

101. Pier, M. P., Hulstijn, W., & Sabbe, B. G. (2004). Differential patterns of psychomotor functioning in unmedicated melancholic and nonmelancholic depressed patients. *Journal of psychiatric research, 38*(4), 425–435.

102. Sweeney, J. A., Strojwas, M. H., Mann, J. J., & Thase, M. E. (1998). Prefrontal and cerebellar abnormalities in major depression: evidence from oculomotor studies. *Biological psychiatry, 43*(8), 584–594.

103. Mahlberg, R., Steinacher, B., Mackert, A., & Flechtner, K. M. (2001). Basic parameters of saccadic eye movements—differences between unmedicated schizophrenia and affective disorder patients. *European archives of psychiatry and clinical neuroscience, 251*(5), 205–210.

104. Schwartz, G. E., Fair, P. L., Salt, P., Mandel, M. R., & Klerman, G. L. (1976). Facial expression and imagery in depression: an electromyographic study. *Psychosomatic medicine, 38*(5), 337–347.

105. Cornell, D. G., Suarez, R., & Berent, S. (1984). Psychomotor retardation in melancholic and nonmelancholic depression: cognitive and motor components. *Journal of abnormal psychology, 93*(2), 150–157.

106. Blackburn I. M. (1975). Mental and psychomotor speed in depression and mania. *British journal of psychiatry: the journal of mental science, 126*, 329–335.

107. Bonin-Guillaume, S., Hasbroucq, T., & Blin, O. (2008). Mise en évidence d'un ralentissement psychomoteur spécifique à la dépression chez le sujet âgé [Psychomotor retardation associated to depression differs from that of normal aging]. *Psychologie & neuropsychiatrie du vieillissement, 6*(2), 137–144.

108. Brébion, G., Smith, M. J., & Allilaire, J. F. (1995). Psychometric characteristics of ideational retardation in depressives. *British journal of clinical psychology, 34*(3), 371–381.

109. Smith, M. J., Brébion, G., Banquet, J. P., & Allilaire, J. F. (1994). Experimental evidence for two dimensions of cognitive disorders in depressives. *Journal of psychiatric research, 28*(4), 401–411.

110. Snaith R. P. (1977). Hamilton rating scale for depression. *British journal of psychiatry: the journal of mental science, 131,* 431–432.

111. Fantino, B., & Moore, N. (2009). The self-reported Montgomery-Asberg Depression Rating Scale is a useful evaluative tool in major depressive disorder. *BMC psychiatry, 9,* 26.

112. Pier, M. P., Hulstijn, W., & Sabbe, B. G. (2004). No psychomotor slowing in fine motor tasks in dysthymia. *Journal of affective disorders, 83*(2–3), 109–120.

113. Bonin-Guillaume, S., Jouve, E., Sautel, L., Fakra, E., & Blin, O. (2008). RRS-4: short version of the Retardation Rating Scale to screen for depression in elderly inpatients. *American journal of geriatric psychiatry: official journal of the American Association for Geriatric Psychiatry, 16*(4), 331–335.

114. Sobin, C., Mayer, L., & Endicott, J. (1998). The motor agitation and retardation scale: a scale for the assessment of motor abnormalities in depressed patients. *Journal of neuropsychiatry and clinical neurosciences, 10*(1), 85–92.

115. Schrijvers, D., Hulstijn, W., & Sabbe, B. G. (2008). Psychomotor symptoms in depression: a diagnostic, pathophysiological and therapeutic tool. *Journal of affective disorders, 109*(1–2), 1–20.

116. Kapur, S., & Mann, J. J. (1992). Role of the dopaminergic system in depression. *Biological psychiatry, 32*(1), 1–17.

117. Shah, P. J., Ogilvie, A. D., Goodwin, G. M., & Ebmeier, K. P. (1997). Clinical and psychometric correlates of dopamine D2 binding in depression. *Psychological medicine, 27*(6), 1247–1256.

118. Austin, M. P., Mitchell, P., Hadzi-Pavlovic, D., Hickie, I., Parker, G., Chan, J., et al. (2000). Effect of apomorphine on motor and cognitive function in melancholic patients: a preliminary report. *Psychiatry research, 97*(2–3), 207–215.

119. Sabbe, B., Hulstijn, W., Maes, M., Pier, M., Scharpé, S., & Zitman, F. (2001). Psychomotor slowing, neuroendocrine responses, and behavioral changes after oral administration of meta-chlorophenylpiperazine in normal volunteers. *Psychiatry research, 105*(3), 151–163.

120. Herrero, M. T., Barcia, C., & Navarro, J. M. (2002). Functional anatomy of thalamus and basal ganglia. *Child's nervous system: ChNS: official journal of the International Society for Pediatric Neurosurgery, 18*(8), 386–404.

121. Hickie, I., Scott, E., Mitchell, P., Wilhelm, K., Austin, M. P., & Bennett, B. (1995). Subcortical hyperintensities on magnetic resonance imaging: clinical correlates and prognostic significance in patients with severe depression. *Biological psychiatry, 37*(3), 151–160.

122. Naismith, S., Hickie, I., Ward, P. B., Turner, K., Scott, E., Little, C., et al. (2002). Caudate nucleus volumes and genetic determinants of homocysteine metabolism in the prediction of psychomotor speed in older persons with depression. *American journal of psychiatry, 159*(12), 2096–2098.

123. Hickie, I., Mason, C., Parker, G., & Brodaty, H. (1996). Prediction of ECT response: validation of a refined sign-based (CORE) system for defining melancholia. *British journal of psychiatry: the journal of mental science, 169*(1), 68–74.

124. Steffens, D. C., & Krishnan, K. R. (1998). Structural neuroimaging and mood disorders: recent findings, implications for classification, and future directions. *Biological psychiatry, 43*(10), 705–712.

125. Hickie, I., Ward, P., Scott, E., Haindl, W., Walker, B., Dixon, J., & Turner, K. (1999). Neostriatal rCBF correlates of psychomotor slowing in patients with major depression. *Psychiatry research*, *92*(2–3), 75–81.

126. Bench, C. J., Friston, K. J., Brown, R. G., Frackowiak, R. S., & Dolan, R. J. (1993). Regional cerebral blood flow in depression measured by positron emission tomography: the relationship with clinical dimensions. *Psychological medicine*, *23*(3), 579–590.

127. Mayberg, H. S., Lewis, P. J., Regenold, W., & Wagner, H. N., Jr (1994). Paralimbic hypoperfusion in unipolar depression. *Journal of nuclear medicine: official publication, Society of Nuclear Medicine*, *35*(6), 929–934.

128. Brody, A. L., Barsom, M. W., Bota, R. G., & Saxena, S. (2001). Prefrontal-subcortical and limbic circuit mediation of major depressive disorder. *Seminars in clinical neuropsychiatry*, *6*(2), 102–112.

129. Videbech, P., Ravnkilde, B., Pedersen, T. H., Hartvig, H., Egander, A., Clemmensen, K., et al. (2002). The Danish PET/depression project: clinical symptoms and cerebral blood flow: a regions-of-interest analysis. *Acta psychiatrica Scandinavica*, *106*(1), 35–44.

130. Narita, H., Odawara, T., Iseki, E., Kosaka, K., & Hirayasu, Y. (2004). Psychomotor retardation correlates with frontal hypoperfusion and the Modified Stroop Test in patients under 60-years-old with major depression. *Psychiatry and clinical neurosciences*, *58*(4), 389–395.

131. Mayberg, H. S., Starkstein, S. E., Peyser, C. E., Brandt, J., Dannals, R. F., & Folstein, S. E. (1992). Paralimbic frontal lobe hypometabolism in depression associated with Huntington's disease. *Neurology*, *42*(9), 1791–1797.

132. Klein, H. E., Bender, W., Mayr, H., Niederschweiberer, A., & Schmauss, M. (1984). The DST and its relationship to psychiatric diagnosis, symptoms and treatment outcome. *British journal of psychiatry: the journal of mental science*, *145*, 591–599.

133. Mitchell, P., Hadzi-Pavlovic, D., Parker, G., Hickie, I., Wilhelm, K., Brodaty, H., et al. (1996). Depressive psychomotor disturbance, cortisol, and dexamethasone. *Biological psychiatry*, *40*(10), 941–950.

134. Smith, J., Carr, V., Morris, H., & Gilliland, J. (1988). The dexamethasone suppression test in relation to symptomatology: preliminary findings controlling for serum dexamethasone concentrations. *Psychiatry research*, *25*(2), 123–133.

135. van Londen, L., Kerkhof, G. A., van den Berg, F., Goekoop, J. G., Zwinderman, K. H., Frankhuijzen-Sierevogel, A. C., et al. (1998). Plasma arginine vasopressin and motor activity in major depression. *Biological psychiatry*, *43*(3), 196–204.

136. de Winter, R. F., van Hemert, A. M., DeRijk, R. H., Zwinderman, K. H., Frankhuijzen-Sierevogel, A. C., Wiegant, V. M., et al. (2003). Anxious-retarded depression: relation with plasma vasopressin and cortisol. *Neuropsychopharmacology: official publication of the American College of Neuropsychopharmacology*, *28*(1), 140–147.

137. Amsterdam J. D. (1998). Selective serotonin reuptake inhibitor efficacy in severe and melancholic depression. *Journal of psychopharmacology (Oxford, England)*, *12*(3 Suppl B), S99–S111.

138. Flament, M. F., Lane, R. M., Zhu, R., & Ying, Z. (1999). Predictors of an acute antidepressant response to fluoxetine and sertraline. *International clinical psychopharmacology*, *14*(5), 259–275.

139. Heiligenstein, J. H., Tollefson, G. D., & Faries, D. E. (1994). Response patterns of depressed outpatients with and without melancholia: a double-blind, placebo-controlled trial of fluoxetine versus placebo. *Journal of affective disorders*, *30*(3), 163–173.

140. McGrath, P. J., Khan, A. Y., Trivedi, M. H., Stewart, J. W., Morris, D. W., Wisniewski, S. R., et al. (2008). Response to a selective serotonin reuptake inhibitor (citalopram) in major depressive disorder with melancholic features: a STAR*D report. *Journal of clinical psychiatry*, *69*(12), 1847–1855.

141. Burns, R. A., Lock, T., Edwards, D. R., Katona, C. L., Harrison, D. A., Robertson, M. M., et al. (1995). Predictors of response to amine-specific antidepressants. *Journal of affective disorders*, *35*(3), 97–106.

142. Caligiuri, M. P., Gentili, V., Eberson, S., Kelsoe, J., Rapaport, M., & Gillin, J. C. (2003). A quantitative neuromotor predictor of antidepressant non-response in patients with major depression. *Journal of affective disorders*, *77*(2), 135–141.

143. Sabbe, B., van Hoof, J., Hulstijn, W., & Zitman, F. (1997). Depressive retardation and treatment with fluoxetine: assessment of the motor component. *Journal of affective disorders*, *43*(1), 53–61.

144. Mallinckrodt, C. H., Prakash, A., Houston, J. P., Swindle, R., Detke, M. J., & Fava, M. (2007). Differential antidepressant symptom efficacy: placebo-controlled comparisons of duloxetine and SSRIs (fluoxetine, paroxetine, escitalopram). *Neuropsychobiology*, *56*(2–3), 73–85.

145. Laakmann, G., Blaschke, D., Engel, R., & Schwarz, A. (1988). Fluoxetine vs amitriptyline in the treatment of depressed out-patients. *British journal of psychiatry. Supplement*, (3), 64–68.

146. Roose, S. P., Glassman, A. H., Attia, E., & Woodring, S. (1994). Comparative efficacy of selective serotonin reuptake inhibitors and tricyclics in the treatment of melancholia. *American journal of psychiatry*, *151*(12), 1735–1739.

147. Joyce, P. R., Mulder, R. T., Luty, S. E., McKenzie, J. M., Sullivan, P. F., Abbott, R. M., et al. (2002). Melancholia: definitions, risk factors, personality, neuroendocrine markers and differential antidepressant response. *Australian and New Zealand journal of psychiatry*, *36*(3), 376–383.

148. White, K., & White, J. (1986). Tranylcypromine: patterns and predictors of response. *Journal of clinical psychiatry*, *47*(7), 380–382.

149. Del Zompo, M., Bernardi, F., Burrai, C., & Bocchetta, A. (1990). A double-blind study of minaprine versus amitriptyline in major depression. *Neuropsychobiology*, *24*(2), 79–83.

150. Herrera-Guzmán, I., Gudayol-Ferré, E., Lira-Mandujano, J., Herrera-Abarca, J., Herrera-Guzmán, D., Montoya-Pérez, K., et al. (2008). Cognitive predictors of treatment response to bupropion and cognitive effects of bupropion in patients with major depressive disorder. *Psychiatry research*, *160*(1), 72–82.

151. Mendels, J. (1965). Electroconvulsive therapy and depression. I. The prognostic significance of clinical factors. *British Journal of Psychiatry*, *111*(477), 675–681.

152. Gill, D., & Lambourn, J. (1979). Indications for electric convulsion therapy and its use by senior psychiatrists. *British medical journal*, *1*(6172), 1169–1171.

153. Baeken, C., De Raedt, R., Santermans, L., Zeeuws, D., Vanderhasselt, M. A., Meers, M., et al. (2010). HF-rTMS treatment decreases psychomotor retardation in medication-resistant melancholic depression. *Progress in neuro-psychopharmacology & biological psychiatry*, *34*(4), 684–687.

154. Hoeppner, J., Padberg, F., Domes, G., Zinke, A., Herpertz, S. C., Grossheinrich, N., et al. (2010). Influence of repetitive transcranial magnetic stimulation on psychomotor symptoms in major depression. *European archives of psychiatry and clinical neuroscience*, *260*(3), 197–202.

155. Waddington, J. L., & Crow, T. J. (1988). Abnormal involuntary movements and psychosis in the preneuroleptic era and in unmedicated patients: implications for the concept of tardive dyskinesia. In: Wolf M, Mosnaim AD, editors. Tardive dyskinesia: biological mechanisms and clinical aspects. Washington, DC: American Psychiatric Press;1988. p. 51–66.13.

156. Lader, M. H. (1970). Drug-induced extrapyramidal syndromes. *Journal of the Royal College of Physicians of London*, 5(1), 87–98.

157. Marsden, C. D., & Jenner, P. The pathophysiology of extrapyramidal side-effects of neuroleptic drugs. *Psychological Medicine*. 1980;10(1):55–72.

158. Casey D. E. (1991). Neuroleptic drug-induced extrapyramidal syndromes and tardive dyskinesia. *Schizophrenia research*, 4(2), 109–120.

159. Leucht, S., Corves, C., Arbter, D., Engel, R. R., Li, C., & Davis, J. M. (2009). Second-generation versus first-generation antipsychotic drugs for schizophrenia: a meta-analysis. *Lancet (London, England)*, 373(9657), 31–41.

160. Pappa, S., & Dazzan, P. (2009). Spontaneous movement disorders in antipsychotic-naive patients with first-episode psychoses: a systematic review. *Psychological medicine*, 39(7), 1065–1076.

161. Koning, J. P., Tenback, D. E., van Os, J., Aleman, A., Kahn, R. S., & van Harten, P. N. (2010). Dyskinesia and parkinsonism in antipsychotic-naive patients with schizophrenia, first-degree relatives and healthy controls: a meta-analysis. *Schizophrenia bulletin*, 36(4), 723–731.

162. Peralta, V., Campos, M. S., De Jalón, E. G., & Cuesta, M. J. (2010). Motor behavior abnormalities in drug-naïve patients with schizophrenia spectrum disorders. *Movement disorders: official journal of the Movement Disorder Society*, 25(8), 1068–1076.

163. Ayehu, M., Shibre, T., Milkias, B., & Fekadu, A. (2014). Movement disorders in neuroleptic-naïve patients with schizophrenia spectrum disorders. *BMC psychiatry*, 14, 280.

164. Whitty, P. F., Owoeye, O., & Waddington, J. L. (2009). Neurological signs and involuntary movements in schizophrenia: intrinsic to and informative on systems pathobiology. *Schizophrenia bulletin*, 35(2), 415–424.

165. Fenton W. S. (2000). Prevalence of spontaneous dyskinesia in schizophrenia. *Journal of clinical psychiatry*, 61(Suppl 4), 10–14.

166. Cortese, L., Caligiuri, M. P., Malla, A. K., Manchanda, R., Takhar, J., & Haricharan, R. (2005). Relationship of neuromotor disturbances to psychosis symptoms in first-episode neuroleptic-naive schizophrenia patients. *Schizophrenia research*, 75(1), 65–75.

167. Cassady, S. L., Adami, H., Moran, M., Kunkel, R., & Thaker, G. K. (1998). Spontaneous dyskinesia in subjects with schizophrenia spectrum personality. *American journal of psychiatry*, 155(1), 70–75.

168. Apthorp, D., Bolbecker, A. R., Bartolomeo, L. A., O'Donnell, B. F., & Hetrick, W. P. (2019). Postural sway abnormalities in schizotypal personality disorder. *Schizophrenia bulletin*, 45(3), 512–521.

169. Meltzer, H. Y., & Stahl, S. M. (1976). The dopamine hypothesis of schizophrenia: a review. *Schizophrenia bulletin*, 2(1), 19–76.

170. Fusar-Poli, P., & Meyer-Lindenberg, A. (2013). Striatal presynaptic dopamine in schizophrenia, part I: meta-analysis of dopamine active transporter (DAT) density. *Schizophrenia bulletin*, 39(1), 22–32.

171. Obeso, J. A., Rodríguez-Oroz, M. C., Benitez-Temino, B., Blesa, F. J., Guridi, J., Marin, C., et al. (2008). Functional organization of the basal ganglia: therapeutic implications for

Parkinson's disease. *Movement disorders: official journal of the Movement Disorder Society*, *23*(Suppl 3), S548–S559.

172. McCutcheon, R., Beck, K., Jauhar, S., & Howes, O. D. (2018). Defining the locus of dopaminergic dysfunction in schizophrenia: a meta-analysis and test of the mesolimbic hypothesis. *Schizophrenia bulletin*, *44*(6), 1301–1311.

173. Liu, S. Y., Wu, J. J., Zhao, J., Huang, S. F., Wang, Y. X., Ge, J. J., et al. (2015). Onset-related subtypes of Parkinson's disease differ in the patterns of striatal dopaminergic dysfunction: a positron emission tomography study. *Parkinsonism & related disorders*, *21*(12), 1448–1453.

174. Ffytche, D. H., Creese, B., Politis, M., Chaudhuri, K. R., Weintraub, D., Ballard, C., et al. (2017). The psychosis spectrum in Parkinson disease. *Nature reviews. Neurology*, *13*(2), 81–95.

175. Goodkind, M., Eickhoff, S. B., Oathes, D. J., Jiang, Y., Chang, A., Jones-Hagata, L. B., et al. (2015). Identification of a common neurobiological substrate for mental illness. *JAMA psychiatry*, *72*(4), 305–315.

176. Sarpal, D. K., Robinson, D. G., Lencz, T., Argyelan, M., Ikuta, T., Karlsgodt, K., et al. (2015). Antipsychotic treatment and functional connectivity of the striatum in first-episode schizophrenia. *JAMA psychiatry*, *72*(1), 5–13.

177. Kraguljac, N. V., White, D. M., Hadley, N., Hadley, J. A., Ver Hoef, L., Davis, E., et al. (2016). Aberrant hippocampal connectivity in unmedicated patients with schizophrenia and effects of antipsychotic medication: a longitudinal resting state functional MRI study. *Schizophrenia bulletin*, *42*(4), 1046–1055.

178. Walther S. (2015). Psychomotor symptoms of schizophrenia map on the cerebral motor circuit. *Psychiatry research*, *233*(3), 293–298.

179. Seamans, J. K., & Yang, C. R. (2004). The principal features and mechanisms of dopamine modulation in the prefrontal cortex. *Progress in neurobiology*, *74*(1), 1–58.

180. Andreasen, N. C., & Pierson, R. (2008). The role of the cerebellum in schizophrenia. *Biological psychiatry*, *64*(2), 81–88.

181. Picard, H., Amado, I., Mouchet-Mages, S., Olié, J. P., & Krebs, M. O. (2008). The role of the cerebellum in schizophrenia: an update of clinical, cognitive, and functional evidences. *Schizophrenia bulletin*, *34*(1), 155–172.

182. Kim, T., Lee, K. H., Oh, H., Lee, T. Y., Cho, K., Lee, J., et al. (2018). Cerebellar structural abnormalities associated with cognitive function in patients with first-episode psychosis. *Frontiers in psychiatry*, *9*, 286.

183. Moberget, T., Doan, N. T., Alnæs, D., Kaufmann, T., Córdova-Palomera, A., Lagerberg, T. V., et al. (2018). Cerebellar volume and cerebellocerebral structural covariance in schizophrenia: a multisite mega-analysis of 983 patients and 1349 healthy controls. *Molecular psychiatry*, *23*(6), 1512–1520.

184. Lan, C. C., Su, T. P., Chen, Y. S., & Bai, Y. M. (2011). Treatment dilemma in comorbidity of schizophrenia and idiopathic Parkinson's disease. *General hospital psychiatry*, *33*(4), 411.e3–411.e411005.

185. Chou, K. L., Borek, L. L., & Friedman, J. H. (2007). The management of psychosis in movement disorder patients. *Expert opinion on pharmacotherapy*, *8*(7), 935–943.

186. Menza, M. M., Palermo, B., & Mark, M. (1999). Quetiapine as an alternative to clozapine in the treatment of dopamimetic psychosis in patients with Parkinson's disease. *Annals of clinical psychiatry: official journal of the American Academy of Clinical Psychiatrists*, *11*(3), 141–144.

187. Ruggieri, S., De Pandis, M. F., Bonamartini, A., Vacca, L., & Stocchi, F. (1997). Low dose of clozapine in the treatment of dopaminergic psychosis in Parkinson's disease. *Clinical neuropharmacology, 20*(3), 204–209.

188. Lam R. W. (1993). Chronic schizophrenia and idiopathic Parkinson's disease. *Canadian journal of psychiatry. Revue canadienne de psychiatrie, 38*(2), 75–77.

189. Gadit A. (2011). Schizophrenia and Parkinson's disease: challenges in management. *BMJ case reports,* 2011, bcr1120115108.

190. Habermeyer, B., Kneifel, S., Lotz-Bläuer, I., & Müller-Spahn, F. (2008). Psychosis in a case of schizophrenia and Parkinson's disease. *Journal of neuropsychiatry and clinical neurosciences, 20*(3), 373–375.

191. Tinazzi, M., Antonini, A., Bovi, T., Pasquin, I., Steinmayr, M., Moretto, G., et al. (2009). Clinical and [123I]FP-CIT SPET imaging follow-up in patients with drug-induced parkinsonism. *Journal of neurology, 256*(6), 910–915.

192. Jaskiw, G. E., & Popli, A. P. (2004). A meta-analysis of the response to chronic L-dopa in patients with schizophrenia: therapeutic and heuristic implications. *Psychopharmacology, 171*(4), 365–374.

193. Friedman J. H. (2011). Managing idiopathic Parkinson's disease in patients with schizophrenic disorders. *Parkinsonism & related disorders, 17*(3), 198–200.

13

Functional Movement Disorders

Jennifer S. Sharma and Alberto J. Espay

Functional movement disorder (FMD) applies to abnormal movements that are determined to be inconsistent over time and incongruent with the broad spectrum of "organic" phenotypes. The impact on the individual, family, and society is hefty among the functional neurological disorders.[1] A British study from 2010 estimated that functional somatic symptoms involving multiple organ systems (a disorder within which FMD belongs) cost the economy £18 billion (almost US $28 billion at the 2021 exchange rate) per year.[2] Hospitalizations and emergency care are an important part of that expenditure, equivalent to costs incurred by anterior horn cell disorders in adults or in demyelinating or neuroinflammatory diseases in children.[3] Overall, there is at least a doubling of the outpatient and inpatient medical care utilization as well as annual medical care costs compared to comparable nonsomatizing patients.[4]

In one report, functional neurological disorders (FNDs) represented the second most common diagnosis in the outpatient neurology setting,[5] with FMD, a subset of FND, accounting for 2%–20% of patients seen in movement disorder clinics.[6,7] Prevalence varies between 2%–4%,[8] but these estimates differ per center and specialization of the clinic being sampled. Women outnumber men at almost a 3:1 ratio. Tremor is usually the most common (with one study showing dystonia being the most common presentation in women),[9] followed by dystonia, myoclonus, and parkinsonism.[6]

A Brief History of Functional Neurological Disorders

The concept of "hysteria" was proposed by the ancient Egyptians as far back as 1900 BC and rediscovered more than two thousand years later by Hippocrates, who named this phenomenon "hysterion." Both differentiated this entity from its "organic" counterpart and believed that it was caused by the "upward dislocation of the uterus and displacement of other organs."[10] In the first century BC, the Roman encyclopedist Aulus Celsus described functional epilepsy: "it so completely destroys the senses that on occasions the patient falls, as if in epilepsy. This case, however, differs in that the eyes are not turned, nor does froth issue forth, nor are there any convulsions: there is only a deep sleep."[11] The mid-1900s saw the advent of the culpable mind, with Pierre Janet proposing that hysteria is "the patient's own idea of pathology is translated into a physical disability."[12] "Conversion disorder" was coined by Freud and refers to the substitution of somatic symptoms for a repressed idea.[13] The term "psychogenic disorders" was introduced in the mid-1980s with Drs. Fahn and Williams creating diagnostic criteria in 1988. Both theories implied that this disorder is secondary to an abnormal psychological state rather than an organic process.

In neurology, the global transition to the term "functional" has taken place recently, truly starting in the early 2010s. However, this term has been debated about and used even as far back as the mid-1500s. Some early adopters of this term recognized that the previous iterations attributed a specific etiology to this disorder, in that this disorder was secondary to psychiatric causes. For example, "conversion disorder" implies that repression is the root of an individual's malady. When given the label of a "psychogenic" disorder, one can be sure that the cause of the symptoms are "born of the mind."[14] While "medically unexplained" disorders do not confer a psychiatric cause, this label conveys diagnostic uncertainty, implying that one only needs to do further testing and to look for the "real" disease.[15] These labels also impede a therapeutic relationship between a physician and their patient. Among patients in a general neurology clinic, the previously mentioned terms were considered equivalent to "putting it on," "being mad," or "imagining symptoms." These negative connotations were most associated with the terms "hysteria" (52%), "medically unexplained" (42%), and "psychosomatic" (35%), with "functional" (12%) being the least likely.[16] The recent push to adopt this term is not simply due to the its lack of a negative association but rather, it conveys our current understanding of the neurobiology without assigning etiology.

Pathophysiology from a Psychosocial Perspective

We are still in the midst of untangling the complex biopsychosocial factors underlying FMD (Figure 13.1). The historical context above provides the groundwork in which psychological factors have been thought to play a role. Multiple studies have shown higher rates of total childhood trauma (primarily emotional abuse and physical neglect), greater fear of traumatic events, and greater number of traumatic episodes than controls after controlling for depression and gender.[17,18] Interestingly, emotional neglect appears to confer higher risk compared to previously emphasized sexual and physical abuse, which seem more associated with psychogenic nonepileptic seizures.[10] Patients do have a higher risk of both lifetime trauma and stress directly preceding onset of symptoms. Various studies have used different definitions of "prior trauma." Importantly, there is a large proportion of patients (14%–77%) who do not have any known prior traumatic history.[18] Although not considered etiologic, psychiatric comorbidity is common: 61.9% of patients have a lifetime history of anxiety disorders, 42.9% have major depression, and 45% have personality disorders.

While the biological underpinning for phenotypic specificity of FMD expression in individuals is unknown, a role for "disease modeling," or exposure to the illness through family members or friends, has been argued as a possibility. Some small studies have noted that FMD occurs more in those with a family history of neurological or with reported exposure to neurological disease.[19,20] However, a larger retrospective study of 874 patients found that a first-degree relative with a movement disorder is present in only 9.7% of FMD patients compared with 29.6% of those with other neurological disorders.[21] It is currently difficult to assign it either as a risk factor for FMD or organic disorder.

Finally, psychiatric history and psychological evaluations as well as personality tests provide a relevant context for the psychosocial framework within which FMD arises and inform therapeutic considerations. It is important to emphasize that psychological stressors or

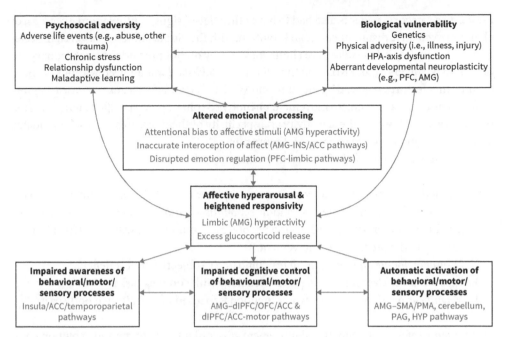

Figure 13.1 A summary of the possible role of emotional processing in generating (and perpetuating) functional neurological symptoms.

Key emotional processing differences include an attentional bias to affective stimuli, inaccurate interoception, and suboptimal emotional regulation. Affective hyperarousal and hyperreactivity are linked to elevated limbic (amygdalar, HPA-axis, PAG) activity, which exerts a disruptive influence on neurocircuits crucial for cognitive control, initiation of behavioral/motor responses, and awareness. Key: ACC = anterior cingulate gyrus; AMG = amygdala; dlPFC = dorsolateral prefrontal cortex; HPA = hypothalamic-pituitary-adrenal; HYP = hypothalamus; INS = insula; OFC = orbitofrontal cortex; PAG = periaqueductal gray; PFC = prefrontal cortex; PMA = premotor area; SMA = supplementary motor area.

Source: Reproduced with permission from Pick, S., Goldstein, L. H., Perez, D. L., & Nicholson, T. R. (2019). Emotional processing in functional neurological disorder: a review, biopsychosocial model and research agenda. *Journal of Neurology, Neurosurgery, & Psychiatry*, 90(6), 704–711. https://doi.org/10.1136/jnnp-2018-319201.

psychiatric comorbidities are neither necessary nor sufficient for making a diagnosis, which should rely exclusively on phenotypic rather than historical clues (see phenomenology section below). Subjects with FMD may have no suggestion on somatization or malingering on personality assessments.

The Central Role of Inconsistency and Incongruence in Diagnosis

The Fahn and William criteria from 1988 had four levels of diagnostic certainty, including *Documented* (remission with suggestion, physiotherapy, psychotherapy, placebo, and/or while unobserved), *Clinically Established*, *Probable*, and *Possible* ("obvious emotional disturbance").[22] The pillars of *incongruence* and *inconsistence* were only mandatory for the *Clinically*

Established category; patients also had to have other "false" signs, multiple somatizations, or obvious psychiatric disturbance. As an evolution, with the Gupta and Lang criteria, the categories of *Probable* and *Possible* were eliminated, as they do not preclude an exclusionary approach to the diagnosis of FMD, and the *Clinically Established* was allowed without the need for the other features required by the Fahn and Williams criteria.[23] Because *inconsistency and incongruence* vary according to movement phenotype, a phenotype-specific diagnostic criteria was created. However, the sensitivity and specificity of these features cannot be validated as there is no gold standard to compare them against.[24,25]

Inconsistency is composed of four components:

1. *Variability* of phenomenology and/or severity over time: This specifically refers to the change in *frequency, amplitude*, and *direction/distribution of movement.* Of these, the key differentiator between FMD and its "organic" counterpart will vary depending according to the predominant movement.
2. *Disproportionate amount of disability* compared to objective motor deficits.
3. *Suppression or clear changes* in phenomenology with complex tasks.
4. *Magnification of the disability* when attention is focused on the affected body part.

Incongruence refers to the functional movement's discordant phenotype and evolution compared to the presentation, progression, and disability of its known organic counterpart. This key feature demands extensive experience in organic movement disorders and is the main reason the diagnosis of FMD can only be confidently made by neurologists with expertise in movement disorders. Supportive features are incongruent (nonanatomical, nonphysiological) signs such as the Hoover's sign, lack of pronator drift, tubular vision defect, give-away weakness, and nonanatomical sensory loss.

Suggestibility refers to the amelioration or worsening of the movement with application of nonphysiological interventions, e.g., somatic trigger points, tuning fork, electrotherapy, and/ or placebo. This is an optional requirement for establishing the clinically definite diagnosis of FMD. This feature particularly, requires adequate rapport with the patient and nonjudgment sharing of the outcome.

Phenomenology

Historical clues such as abrupt onset, maximum deficit at onset, or spontaneous remission, and psychopathology features, such as multiple somatizations or history of psychiatric disorders, are neither necessary nor sufficient for the diagnosis of FMD.[24] The diagnosis of FMD is predominately dependent on the assessment of the phenomenology because FMDs are distinguished from other movement disorders by "rule violations" of their phenotypic spectrum, which defines *incongruence*, the major pillar required for its clinical ascertainment. This is also an acknowledgment that "bizarre presentations," which are not uncommonly confused with FMDs, are not internally inconsistent, and therefore *not incongruent.* We here present selected phenotype-specific considerations to aid in their recognition.

Functional Parkinsonism

Careful observation during both the neurological exam and casual manual tasks such as buttoning their shirt, tying shoelaces, reaching out for a glass of water, or gesticulating while talking reveal discordant speeds between voluntary and tasked movements. The finger-tapping and finger-to-nose task will show excessive slowness of movements without the sequence effect (progressive reduction in amplitude). The key element on examination is the variability of resistance against passive movements when assessing for muscle tone. The "huffing and puffing" sign (disproportionate demonstration of labored breathing) is a common supportive sign.[26]

Functional Tremor

The following features are required for the clinically definite diagnosis of functional tremor:

1. Entrainment or full suppressibility: By asking the patient to perform a rhythmic but complex task, a functional tremor will be suppressed or match the frequency of the complex task, a phenomenon called *entrainment*. While amplitude can vary in organic tremor disorders, changes in *frequency* are only seen in functional tremor.
2. Distractibility: The tremor worsens on attention to the affected limb and attenuates or ceases when the attention is driven away, as when the patient listens attentively to instructions or thinks of a response to an unrelated question.
3. Tonic coactivation at tremor onset: Approximately 300 ms before the onset of a tremor, electrophysiology shows tonic coactivation of both the agonist and antagonist muscles, as this can contribute to a state of clonus.[27] This electrophysiological feature can be appreciated by palpation of the forearm muscles when tremors pause intermittently.
4. Pause of tremor during ballistic movements: A sudden ballistic movement in the contralateral hand or limb should result in a pause in the functional tremor.
5. Variability in frequency, axis, and distribution: Spontaneous changes in frequency are a manifestation of definite functional tremor. A change in axis can sometimes be seen in a dystonic tremor, but the movement then demands that it follow the rules set out for a dystonic tremor (e.g., position-sensitive, action-induced, task-specific, weight-enhanced, and response to sensory tricks).[28]

Functional Myoclonus

Similar to functional tremor, functional myoclonus is ascertained by its variability in duration, topographical distribution and/or latency (if stimulus sensitive), and entrainability or full suppressibility. While not sufficient for a diagnosis, one can also see variability in amplitude.

Functional Dystonia

The key features (Figure 13.2) that need to be documented for a diagnosis of clinically definite functional dystonia are:[29]

1. Fixed dystonia at rest: Organic dystonia tends to evolve over months to years (this can occur *gradually* in some organic disorders).
2. Rapid onset: Tends to appear suddenly or rapidly (this is the only exception to the "history is neither necessary nor sufficient"; fixed dystonia is otherwise possible as a later occurrence of neurodegenerative or post-stroke dystonias).
3. Variable resistance to manipulation: There should be little to no active resistance to passive movements in organic dystonia. Variable resistance can also be seen in paratonia but tends to be proportional to the force applied and speed of movement.[30]

Some supportive features include associated pain (except for the cervical region, organic dystonia is often painless) and complex regional pain syndrome (CRPS). The latter feature has been hotly debated as to whether it falls under the "functional" category. While some

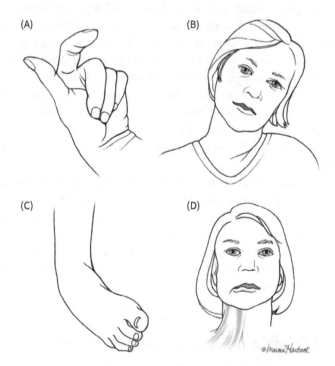

Figure 13.2 Classic functional dystonia phenotypes.

(A) Functional hand dystonia with preserved pincer function. (B) "Post-traumatic painful torticollis," with fixed laterocollis, ipsilateral shoulder elevation, and contralateral shoulder depression. (C) Foot dystonia with fixed foot plantar flexion and inversion. (D) Functional facial dystonia with unilateral tonic jaw and lip deviation, often with ipsilateral platysma involvement.

Source: Reproduced with permission from Schmerler, D. A., & Espay, A. J. (2016). Functional dystonia. *Handbook of Clinical Neurology*, 139, 235–245. Figure 20.1. https://doi.org/10.1016/B978-0-12-801 772-2.00020-5.

studies have proposed mechanisms for movement disorders in CRPS,[31] other studies have demonstrated mechanistic underpinnings, imaging and neurophysiology of CRPS consistent with FMD.[32]

Functional Gait

Pure functional gait disorders constitute 6%–8.5% of FMDs and are part of the phenotype in about 42% of all functional patients.[33] While many bizarre gait disorders can be mistaken as functional (e.g., diphasic dyskinetic gait in Parkinson's disease or the gait of chorea acanthocytosis patients) the ascertainment of inconsistency is critical even if incongruence may be difficult. As noted above, bizarre gait disorders, if internally consistent, are unlikely to be functional.[33] Common denominators are excessive slowness with prolonged single-leg stance, dragging gait with forefoot in contact with the ground, and application of inconsistent or uneconomic postures.[24] Knee buckling is a common manifestation when walking straight. The more common sideway-walking with variable base of support is typically associated with other features. Patients often demonstrate excessive arm movements, veering wildly from one side to another with improvement during complex dual tasks or eye closure; exaggerated sway without falling during Romberg's without sensory/vestibular findings; and astasia-abasia, which is exaggerated performance without side-steps during tandem gait, and can include scissoring and prolonged standing on one leg.[33]

Treatment

In the past, treatment of FND had been focused solely on treatment of underlying depression, anxiety, and/or posttraumatic stress disorder, if these psychiatric comorbidities were present. The past two decades have seen functional disorders legitimized as true neurological/cognitive disorders, due in no small part to evolving neuroimaging and electrophysiological advances reflecting subtle neurobiological changes that had eluded prior generations.

Treatment begins in the office at the time of the diagnostic debriefing. This multipart process includes acknowledging that while their movements are currently not under voluntary control, it is possible to fully reverse them. While subsequent therapies such as physical/occupational therapy (PT/OT) and cognitive-behavioral therapy (CBT) are infinitely useful, success hinges on the patient's ability to truly accept and understand the diagnosis, and thus it is worthwhile to spend time navigating and addressing their fears. The therapeutic alliance that is established during the interview and examination can help incur trust on which one can properly disclose the diagnosis and thus serve as the first stage of treatment.[34]

A general framework for diagnosis debriefing is summarized here:

1. Clearly state the diagnosis. We use "FND," which stands for functional neurological disorder as the overarching label for all FMD. Provide a brief explanation of what this diagnosis means.
2. Explain that the diagnosis is made definitively based on the neurological examination alone. It may be helpful to revisit selected aspects of the examination, such as how entrainment was elicited, in order to demonstrate expertise, begin to reveal the

movement's reversibility, and emphasize the lack of need for further laboratory or imaging investigations.

3. We have found it beneficial to add, "You are not crazy" and "You are not faking this" to allay very common subconscious fears that patients may be "making up" the movements and dispel perceptions arising from prior clinical encounters that the movements are "in the head." Eliminating these false perceptions can strengthen the therapeutic alliance with the patient and enhance his/her commitment to the therapeutic program.

4. Whether it be through encouraging questions or reviewing the diagnosis, the patient should have confidence in the diagnosis, which will lower the odds of seeking alternative medical opinions and muster the commitment and effort required of therapy.

While research continues in this field, current best practices suggest a multidisciplinary approach to patient care.[35] In addition to the clinician (neurologist and psychiatrist), it is beneficial to involve PT, OT, speech therapy, clinical social work, and both cognitive-behavioral talk therapy and CBT-informed psychotherapy.[36,26] Proper multidisciplinary care is contingent on communication and consensus among all providers, as hesitation or inconsistences across practitioners will hinder a patient's trust in the diagnosis, the fulcrum on which treatment success depends. Indeed, the major predictor in symptom improvement is acceptance of the diagnosis prior to further treatment.[24,37,38] If the patient continues to seek alternative medical explanations, it is useful to reassess their understanding of the diagnosis and reiterate the rationale behind it. Encourage open dialogue regarding their fears and in a non-judgmental manner.[36] If there is still concern regarding alternative diagnoses, a practitioner may continue to see them in follow-up or invite the patient to return to clinic when they are ready to revisit the diagnosis of FND.[36]

Physical therapy is a key treatment modality in patients with severe motor disability. In cases where psychological treatment is indicated, it may actually be more beneficial to undergo treatment *after* or *alongside* PT. In addition to continuing patient education, PT has an important role in demonstrating that normal movement can occur and retraining movement with attentional diverting maneuvers.[39] Occupational therapy works alongside PT in creating strategies and practicing movements that allow the patient to be functional in their everyday life, i.e., tying shoelaces, showering, and dressing. By integrating specific treatment techniques into their everyday functioning, and focusing on activity-based (functional) rather than impairment-based goals and intervention, OT encourages independence and reinforces an internal locus of control.[40] Both specialties use motor retraining techniques by establishing basic movements (e.g., weight-shifting) followed by more complex movements. Treadmill training, electrical stimulation, EMG and auditory biofeedback, and transcranial magnetic stimulation have all been used with varying success.[24]

Cognitive-behavioral therapy is a structured, time-limited therapy that helps identify conscious, or in many cases subconscious, maladaptive thought patterns and emotional states and their subsequent connection to the ensuing movements. By identifying the particular trigger, patients can learn to modulate their thought patterns and movements accordingly.[24,41] In a small prospective study, CBT led to remission or near remission in 12/15 patients with reduced functional MRI activity in the anterior cingulate and paracingulate regions (magnitude of change being highest in those with more severe baseline depression) without any functional changes in motor regions. Dysfunction within these regions has been associated with alexithymia, the exact deficit that CBT aims to address.[42] CBT can be concurrently used with treatment of psychiatric illnesses when appropriate: psychoeducation, acceptance commitment therapy, dialectical behavior therapy, psychodynamic, and narrative therapy to address current stressors, past trauma, and relational issues.[41] Expert consensus also suggests that involvement of family in treatment, addressing relationships and work life and encouraging social connectedness are all important for treatment success. Continued follow-up is important in renewing the above concepts and preventing relapses.

Currently, the prognosis of FND remains relatively poor partly due to the underrecognition of this condition, poorly delivered diagnoses, archaic understanding of this condition by clinicians, the public, and patients themselves, and by a dearth of medical and ancillary personnel who specialize in this field. Length of disease process with accumulated disability before diagnosis, litigation and disability proceedings, and personality disorders are associated with poor prognosis, whereas short disease duration prior to diagnosis and underlying depression are associated with favorable outcomes.[24]

Conclusion

Greater understanding and appreciation of the complex biopsychosocial factors that lead to functional disorders have evolved. Layered genetic, epigenetic, psychosocial, and traumatic vulnerabilities create the scaffolding and dysfunctional connections on which deficits in attention, emotional processing, sensorimotor function, and awareness can flourish to generate FMD. The diagnosis is always based on positive clinical findings rather than being treated as a diagnosis of exclusion; it requires the presence of both *inconsistency* and *incongruence*, which can only be established by a practitioner experienced in the full breadth and depth of neurological disorders. While there may not be a singular mechanism or etiology to address, a nonjudgmental and transparent delivery of the diagnosis serves as the first step in recovery. Adjunct physical and psychotherapy can considerably improve outcomes but are predicated foremost on the unequivocal acceptance of the diagnosis by the patient. The past two decades have seen considerable advances in the field, and while there continue to be many unknowns, destigmatization and education will serve to address the needs of this oft-forgotten population.

References

1. Carson, A., Stone, J., Hibberd, C., Murray, G., Duncan, R., Coleman, R., Warlow, C., Roberts, R., Pelosi, A., Cavanagh, J., Matthews, K., Goldbeck, R., Hansen, C., & Sharpe, M. (2011). Disability, distress and unemployment in neurology outpatients with symptoms "unexplained by organic disease." *Journal of Neurology, Neurosurgery & Psychiatry, 82*(7), 810–813. https://doi.org/10.1136/jnnp.2010.220640

2. Bermingham, S. L., Cohen, A., Hague, J., & Parsonage, M. (2010). The cost of somatisation among the working-age population in England for the year 2008–2009. *Mental Health in Family Medicine, 7*(2), 71–84.

3. Stephen, C. D., Fung, V., Lungu, C. I., & Espay, A. J. (2021). Assessment of emergency department and inpatient use and costs in adult and pediatric functional neurological disorders. *JAMA Neurology, 78*(1), 88. https://doi.org/10.1001/jamaneurol.2020.3753

4. Barsky, A. J., Orav, E. J., & Bates, D. W. (2005). Somatization increases medical utilization and costs independent of psychiatric and medical comorbidity. *Archives of General Psychiatry*, *62*(8), 903–910. https://doi.org/10.1001/archpsyc.62.8.903

5. Stone, J., Carson, A., Duncan, R., Roberts, R., Warlow, C., Hibberd, C., Coleman, R., Cull, R., Murray, G., Pelosi, A., Cavanagh, J., Matthews, K., Goldbeck, R., Smyth, R., Walker, J., & Sharpe, M. (2010). Who is referred to neurology clinics?—The diagnoses made in 3781 new patients. *Clinical Neurology and Neurosurgery*, *112*(9), 747–751. https://doi.org/10.1016/j.clineuro.2010.05.011

6. Factor, S. A., Podskalny, G. D., & Molho, E. S. (1995). Psychogenic movement disorders: Frequency, clinical profile, and characteristics. *Journal of Neurology, Neurosurgery & Psychiatry*, *59*(4), 406–412. https://doi.org/10.1136/jnnp.59.4.406

7. Williams, D. T., Ford, B., & Fahn, S. (1995). Phenomenology and psychopathology related to psychogenic movement disorders. *Phenomenology and Psychopathology Related to Psychogenic Movement Disorders*, *65*, 231–257.

8. Miyasaki, J., Hurtig, H. (2021) Functional neurological disorders. In A. F. Eichler (Ed.), *UpToDate*. Retrieved April 10, 2021, from https://www.uptodate.com/contents/functional-movement-disorders

9. Baizabal-Carvallo, J. F., & Jankovic, J. (2020). Gender differences in functional movement disorders. *Movement Disorders Clinical Practice*, *7*(2), 182–187. https://doi.org/10.1002/mdc3.12864

10. Erro, R., Brigo, F., Trinka, E., Turri, G., Edwards, M. J., & Tinazzi, M. (2016). Psychogenic nonepileptic seizures and movement disorders: A comparative review. *Neurology. Clinical Practice*, *6*(2), 138–149. https://doi.org/10.1212/CPJ.0000000000000235

11. Tasca, C., Rapetti, M., Carta, M. G., & Fadda, B. (2012). Women and hysteria in the history of mental health. *Clinical Practice and Epidemiology in Mental Health: CP & EMH*, *8*, 110–119. https://doi.org/10.2174/1745017901208010110

12. Haule, J. R. (1986). Pierre Janet and dissociation: The first transference theory and its origins in hypnosis. *American Journal of Clinical Hypnosis*, *29*(2), 86–94. https://doi.org/10.1080/00029157.1986.10402690

13. Ali, S., Jabeen, S., Pate, R. J., Shahid, M., Chinala, S., Nathani, M., & Shah, R. (2015). Conversion disorder—Mind versus body: A review. *Innovations in Clinical Neuroscience*, *12*(5–6), 27–33.

14. Trimble, M. R. (1982). Functional diseases. *British Medical Journal (Clinical Research Ed.)*, *285*(6357), 1768–1770. https://doi.org/10.1136/bmj.285.6357.1768

15. Edwards, M. J., Stone, J., & Lang, A. E. (2014). From psychogenic movement disorder to functional movement disorder: It's time to change the name. *Movement Disorders*, *29*(7), 849–852. https://doi.org/10.1002/mds.25562

16. Stone, J., Wojcik, W., Durrance, D., Carson, A., Lewis, S., MacKenzie, L., Warlow, C. P., & Sharpe, M. (2002). What should we say to patients with symptoms unexplained by disease? The "number needed to offend." *BMJ (Clinical Research Ed.)*, *325*(7378), 1449–1450. https://doi.org/10.1136/bmj.325.7378.1449

17. Epstein, S. A., Maurer, C. W., LaFaver, K., Ameli, R., Sinclair, S., & Hallett, M. (2016). Insights into chronic functional movement disorders: The value of qualitative psychiatric interviews. *Psychosomatics*, *57*(6), 566–575. https://doi.org/10.1016/j.psym.2016.04.005

18. Ludwig, L., Pasman, J. A., Nicholson, T., Aybek, S., David, A. S., Tuck, S., Kanaan, R. A., Roelofs, K., Carson, A., & Stone, J. (2018). Stressful life events and maltreatment in conversion

(functional neurological) disorder: Systematic review and meta-analysis of case-control studies. *Lancet. Psychiatry*, *5*(4), 307–320. https://doi.org/10.1016/S2215-0366(18)30051-8

19. Miyasaki, J. M., Sa, D. S., Galvez-Jimenez, N., & Lang, A. E. (2003). Psychogenic movement disorders. *Canadian journal of neurological sciences. Le journal canadien des sciences neurologiques*, *30*(Suppl 1), S94–S100. https://doi.org/10.1017/s0317167100003292

20. Shill, H., & Gerber, P. (2006). Evaluation of clinical diagnostic criteria for psychogenic movement disorders. *Movement Disorders: Official Journal of the Movement Disorder Society*, *21*(8), 1163–1168. https://doi.org/10.1002/mds.20921

21. Lagrand, T., Tuitert, I., Klamer, M., van der Meulen, A., van der Palen, J., Kramer, G., & Tijssen, M. (2021). Functional or not functional; that's the question: Can we predict the diagnosis functional movement disorder based on associated features?. *European Journal of Neurology*, *28*(1), 33–39. https://doi.org/10.1111/ene.14488

22. Fahn, S., & Williams, D. T. (1988). Psychogenic dystonia. *Advances in Neurology*, *50*, 431–455.

23. Gupta, A., & Lang, A. E. (2009). Psychogenic movement disorders. *Current Opinion in Neurology*, *22*(4), 430–436. https://doi.org/10.1097/WCO.0b013e32832dc169

24. Espay, A. J., Aybek, S., Carson, A., Edwards, M. J., Goldstein, L. H., Hallett, M., LaFaver, K., LaFrance, W. C., Lang, A. E., Nicholson, T., Nielsen, G., Reuber, M., Voon, V., Stone, J., & Morgante, F. (2018). Current concepts in diagnosis and treatment of functional neurological disorders. *JAMA Neurology*, *75*(9), 1132–1141. https://doi.org/10.1001/jamaneurol.2018.1264

25. Espay, A. J., Edwards, M. J., Oggioni, G. D., Phielipp, N., Cox, B., Gonzalez-Usigli, H., Pecina, C., Heldman, D. A., Mishra, J., & Lang, A. E. (2014). Tremor retrainment as therapeutic strategy in psychogenic (functional) tremor. *Parkinsonism & Related Disorders*, *20*(6), 647–650. https://doi.org/10.1016/j.parkreldis.2014.02.029

26. Laub, H. N., Dwivedi, A. K., Revilla, F. J., Duker, A. P., Pecina-Jacob, C., & Espay, A. J. (2015). Diagnostic performance of the "huffing and puffing" sign in psychogenic (functional) movement disorders. *Movement Disorders Clinical Practice*, *2*(1), 29–32. https://doi.org/10.1002/mdc3.12102

27. Chen, K.-H. S., & Chen, R. (2020). Principles of electrophysiological assessments for movement disorders. *Journal of Movement Disorders*, *13*(1), 27–38. https://doi.org/10.14802/jmd.19064

28. Sharma, J., Macias-Garcia, D., Zaidi, A., & Espay, A. J. (2018). Teaching video NeuroImages: The signs of dystonic tremor: Tremulous "escanciador." *Neurology*, *91*(12), e1204–e1205. https://doi.org/10.1212/WNL.0000000000006215

29. Schmerler, D. A., & Espay, A. J. (2016). Functional dystonia. *Handbook of Clinical Neurology*, *139*, 235–245. https://doi.org/10.1016/B978-0-12-801772-2.00020-5

30. Drenth, H., Zuidema, S., Bautmans, I., Marinelli, L., Kleiner, G., & Hobbelen, H. (2020). Paratonia in dementia: A systematic review. *Journal of Alzheimer's Disease*, *78*(4), 1615–1637. https://doi.org/10.3233/JAD-200691

31. Munts, A. G., van der Plas, A. A., Ferrari, M. D., Teepe-Twiss, I. M., Marinus, J., & van Hilten, J. J. (2010). Efficacy and safety of a single intrathecal methylprednisolone bolus in chronic complex regional pain syndrome. *European Journal of Pain (London, England)*, *14*(5), 523–528. https://doi.org/10.1016/j.ejpain.2009.11.004

32. Popkirov, S., Hoeritzauer, I., Colvin, L., Carson, A. J., & Stone, J. (2019). Complex regional pain syndrome and functional neurological disorders—time for reconciliation. *Journal of Neurology, Neurosurgery & Psychiatry*, *90*(5), 608–614. https://doi.org/10.1136/jnnp-2018-318298

33. Nonnekes, J., Růžička, E., Serranová, T., Reich, S. G., Bloem, B. R., & Hallett, M. (2020). Functional gait disorders. *Neurology*, *94*(24), 1093–1099. https://doi.org/10.1212/WNL.00000 00000009649

34. Stone, J. (2016). Functional neurological disorders: The neurological assessment as treatment. *Practical Neurology*, *16*(1), 7–17. https://doi.org/10.1136/practneurol-2015-001241

35. Jimenez, X. F., Aboussouan, A., & Johnson, J. (2019). Functional neurological disorder responds favorably to interdisciplinary rehabilitation models. *Psychosomatics*, *60*(6), 556–562. https://doi.org/10.1016/j.psym.2019.07.002

36. Adams, C., Anderson, J., Madva, E. N., Jr, W. C. L., & Perez, D. L. (2018). You've made the diagnosis of functional neurological disorder: Now what? *Practical Neurology*, *18*(4), 323–330. https://doi.org/10.1136/practneurol-2017-001835

37. LaFaver, K., Lang, A. E., Stone, J., Morgante, F., Edwards, M., Lidstone, S., Maurer, C. W., Hallett, M., Dwivedi, A. K., & Espay, A. J. (2020). Opinions and clinical practices related to diagnosing and managing functional (psychogenic) movement disorders: Changes in the last decade. *European Journal of Neurology*, *27*(6), 975–984. https://doi.org/10.1111/ene.14200

38. O'Connell, N., Watson, G., Grey, C., Pastena, R., McKeown, K., & David, A. S. (2020). Outpatient CBT for motor functional neurological disorder and other neuropsychiatric conditions: A retrospective case comparison. *Journal of Neuropsychiatry and Clinical Neurosciences*, *32*(1), 58–66. https://doi.org/10.1176/appi.neuropsych.19030067

39. Nielsen, G., Stone, J., Matthews, A., Brown, M., Sparkes, C., Farmer, R., Masterton, L., Duncan, L., Winters, A., Daniell, L., Lumsden, C., Carson, A., David, A. S., & Edwards, M. (2015). Physiotherapy for functional motor disorders: A consensus recommendation. *Journal of Neurology, Neurosurgery & Psychiatry*, *86*(10), 1113–1119. https://doi.org/10.1136/jnnp-2014-309255

40. Nicholson, C., Edwards, M. J., Carson, A. J., Gardiner, P., Golder, D., Hayward, K., Humblestone, S., Jinadu, H., Lumsden, C., MacLean, J., Main, L., Macgregor, L., Nielsen, G., Oakley, L., Price, J., Ranford, J., Ranu, J., Sum, E., & Stone, J. (2020). Occupational therapy consensus recommendations for functional neurological disorder. *Journal of Neurology, Neurosurgery & Psychiatry*, *91*(10), 1037–1045.

41. LaFaver, Kathrin, LaFrance, W. C., Price, M. E., Rosen, P. B., & Rapaport, M. (2021). Treatment of functional neurological disorder: Current state, future directions, and a research agenda. *CNS Spectrums*, *26*(6), 607–613. https://doi.org/10.1017/S1092852920002138

42. Espay, A. J., Ries, S., Maloney, T., Vannest, J., Neefus, E., Dwivedi, A. K., Allendorfer, J. B., Wulsin, L. R., LaFrance, W. C., Lang, A. E., & Szaflarski, J. P. (2019). Clinical and neural responses to cognitive behavioral therapy for functional tremor. *Neurology*, *93*(19), e1787–e1798. https://doi.org/10.1212/WNL.0000000000008442

PART IV

DISEASES WITH CONCURRENT PSYCHIATRIC AND MOVEMENT DISORDERS SYMPTOMS

14

Tics and Tourette's Syndrome

Abhishek Lenka and Joseph Jankovic

Introduction

Tourette's syndrome (TS), also known as Gilles de la Tourette syndrome, is a complex childhood-onset neurobehavioral disorder. The cardinal symptom of TS is a tic, which is defined as sudden-onset, recurrent, brief-lasting, irregular, involuntary movement (motor tic) or sound (phonic tics).[1] Besides motor and phonic tics, patients with TS often develop a variety of psychiatric comorbidities such as obsessive-compulsive disorder (OCD), attention deficit hyperactivity disorder (ADHD), anxiety, mood disorders, self-injurious behaviors, and impulse control disorder.[2] Prior studies have reported a wide range of prevalence of TS, partly attributed to the differences in the diagnostic criteria, study methodologies, and demographic distributions. A meta-analysis of 26 published studies estimated the population prevalence of TS in children to be 0.52% (0.3% to 0.9%).[3] Nearly all studies of TS report male preponderance with male:female ratio ranging from 3:1 to 4:1. The symptoms usually start manifesting between the 4th to 8th year of life and the peak in severity during the adolescent period just prior to onset of puberty. A prospective study revealed an annual decline in tic severity after adolescence, with 17.7% of adolescents >16 years having no tics and 59.5% having minimal or mild tics 6 years after the initial evaluation.[4] Severity of tics, OCD, and ADHD during childhood are strong predictors of the severity of these symptoms in adulthood.[5] Furthermore, female gender and severe childhood ADHD were reported to be the predictors of future emotional abnormalities in TS.[5]

Historical Background

This syndrome is named after the French neurologist Georges Gilles de la Tourette, protégé of Jean-Martin Charcot, the French neurologist considered by some as the "father of neurology." Although the first comprehensive description of this syndrome dates back to 1885, when Tourette elaborated on the clinical features of nine patients with motor and phonic tics ("maladies of tics"),[6] certain features were also highlighted by another French neurologist, Armand Trousseau, in 1873.[7] Tourette noticed a remarkable overlap of features in those nine patients with a group of disorders characterized by exaggerated startle reflex ("the jumping Frenchmen of Maine"). Although described in the 19th century, there were not many significant advances in the field of this disease until the second half of the 20th century. For several years, TS was thought to have a psychogenic (functional) basis. However, the observation in the 1960s that certain neuroleptic agents (by blocking the dopamine receptor blockers) were effective in ameliorating the tics diverted the attention toward potential organic etiologies of TS. Since the 1970s, there has been an exponential growth in the number of clinical and scientific publications on TS, attesting to the enormous growth in knowledge about clinical, epidemiological, pathophysiological, and therapeutic aspects.

Clinical Characteristics of TS

Phenomenology of Tics

The two categories of tics (motor and phonic) are further classified as simple tics (simple motor or simple phonic) and complex tics (complex motor or complex phonic).[8] Motor tics typically first appear in the face, manifested by frequent blinking and facial grimacing, but multiple parts of the body can be involved later in the course, usually in a rostrocaudal pattern. Phonic tics are typically manifested as sniffing, throat clearing, coughing, and other noises that are often wrongly attributed to allergies or some respiratory problems. Since the sounds made by patients with TS do not always involve vocal cords, it can be argued that these phenomena are fundamentally motor tics involving the nose, mouth, tongue, palate, pharynx, and larynx. Hence, we prefer the term "phonic" instead of "vocal" tics.

While simple motor tic refers to the abrupt, rapid, jerky, nonrhythmic involuntary movements of a single muscle or localized group of muscles (examples: repetitive blinking, head jerks, shoulder shrugs), the complex motor tics refer to either a cluster of simple actions or more coordinated, sequential movements which may be nonpurposeful or semipurposeful (sometimes referred to as "unvoluntary"). Examples of complex motor tics include touching, hitting, jumping, imitating observed movements (echopraxia), and making obscene gestures (copropraxia). From the phenomenology standpoint, the motor tics may be rhythmic clonic (resembling tremor), arrhythmic clonic (simple irregular jerks), tonic (staring, immobility, prolonged tensing of abdominal muscles), and dystonic (oculogyric movements, torticollis, blepharospasm). Patients with TS may also exhibit brief, recurrent cessation of motor output, which has been termed a "blocking phenomenon."[9]

Several sounds or noises, which are language nonspecific, fall under the spectrum of simple phonic tics. On the contrary, complex phonic tics include linguistically meaningful vocalizations. This may include repeating other people's words (echolalia), own words (palilalia), or utterance of obscene words (coprolalia). A study aimed at exploring the coprophenomena in 597 TS patients documented coprolalia in 19.3% of the male patients and 14.6% of the female patients.[10] In 11% of the patients, coprolalia was the initial manifestation of TS.[10] Patients may have pauses and hesitations in speech, word interjections, changes in tone/pitch, and prolongations of words.

The spectrum of severity of the tics in TS is wide and may vary from mild, barely perceptible movements or noises to very severe, even life-threatening, tics. The term "malignant TS" was coined by one of the authors (JJ) to draw attention to a small group of TS patients with dangerously self-injurious tics.[11] In the original series only 5.1% of all TS patients followed in a movement disorders clinic satisfied the criteria for malignant TS.[11] The severe tics in these patients have resulted in marked disability as a result of complex tics such as repetitive forceful whiplash tics that resulted in compression of cervical spinal cord and quadriparesis. Other examples included hitting oneself resulting in hematomas or persistent eye-poking leading to blindness. Patients with "malignant" TS are more likely to experience severe motor symptoms, complex phonic tics, OCD symptoms, suicidal ideations, and poor response to medication.[11]

One important characteristic of TS is that the tic phenomenology evolves and may wax and wane from day to day, week to week, or month to month. The fluctuations are not always predictable and do not always correlate with stress, although the latter does often exacerbate tics.

Premonitory Sensations and Urges

Patients with TS often report an uncomfortable sensation that precedes or accompanies the onset of the tics. This sensation, recognized as a premonitory sensation, encompasses the feeling of a wide array of discrete sensations (tingling, tightness, pressure, distress, etc.).[12,13] There seems to be a difference in the predilection of body parts associated with premonitory urges, as tics involving the head, neck, shoulders, or the midline abdomen tend to be commonly preceded by urges, whereas simple motor tics manifesting with eye blinking and mouth movement are less likely to be preceded by urges. Although the precise mechanism remains elusive, it has been speculated that the premonitory sensations precipitate an "urge" to tic (premonitory urge). It is, however, unclear why only a subset of patients develop the premonitory sensations and urges before the tics. While >90% of the older children and adolescents report experiencing these complex symptoms, it is rather uncommon in children. A questionnaire-based study on 50 TS patients reported the presence of premonitory urges in 92% of the participants and two-third of those had their urges disappeared with tic expression.[14]

It is essential to ask about and document the premonitory sensations/urges as these symptoms have diagnostic, prognostic, and therapeutic implications. Premonitory urges could be useful to distinguish organic tics from functional (psychogenic) tics, as patients with the latter usually do not report the premonitory urges.[15,16] Several studies have observed an association between the premonitory urges and greater severity of tics, OCD, and poor quality of life in patients with TS, more so in older children.[17–19]

Better understanding of the premonitory phenomenon is crucial for counseling the patients and their parents and potentially for formulating customized treatment approach. The presence of premonitory urges may aid in more targeted behavioral therapies that expose premonitory sensory expressions during therapy. Indeed, comprehensive behavioral therapy in tics (CBIT), which uses habit reversal training, relaxation training, and functional intervention, may be employed to teach the patients how to recognize the urge and gradually implement a substitutive behavior and response prevention to strengthen tic-suppression abilities.[20]

Distinguishing the Organic Tics From the Functional Tics

Rarely, functional (psychogenic) movement disorders (FMDs) may present with tic-like movements. In a series of 184 patients with FMD, 4.9% had movements resembling tics.[15] The clues to distinguish the functional tics from its organic counterpart are lack of clear premonitory urge, lack of suppressibility, the coexistence of other FMD, and lack of response to the tic-suppressing medications. In addition to these clues, another case series suggested that the absence of pali-, echo- and copro-phenomena, presence of blocking tics, and the lack of the typical rostrocaudal tic distribution are indicators of functional tics.[21] However, it is important to emphasize that functional and organic tics may coexist.[16]

Comorbid Psychiatric Symptoms

Patients with TS have a higher risk of developing ADHD, OCD, anxiety, and mood disorders.[2] A study estimated that the lifetime prevalence of having one psychiatric comorbidity in patients with TS is 85.7% and that of having two or more comorbidities is 57.7%.[2]

The prevalence of ADHD in TS is 30-%–50%.[2,22] Identifying ADHD has important implications in TS. As comorbid ADHD is associated with disruptive behavior and functional impairment in children with TS, adequate treatment of ADHD is essential. The presence of ADHD may guide in choosing medications that are effective for ameliorating both ADHD and tics. These include alpha-2 agonists such as clonidine and guanfacine (described in detail in the management section). When ADHD is particularly troublesome CNS stimulants may be required. Since these drugs may trigger or exacerbate tics, adequate control of tics with anti-tic medications is prudent before instituting CNS stimulants (see below).

Obsessive-compulsive behaviors may become apparent in up to one-third of the patients with TS.[8,23] Given the overlap in certain phenomenological characteristics, distinguishing tics from the obsession/compulsion may be challenging. From the phenomenology standpoint, in tic-free OCD, the commonly observed features are fear of contamination and repetitive washing and checking rituals. On the contrary, OC-like behaviors associated with TS are often characterized by repetitive touching, echophenomena, or self-injurious behaviors.[24,25] Thorough assessment and adequate treatment of OC symptoms in patients with TS are crucial as TS patients with OCD have a significantly higher risk of developing other comorbid disorders than those without OC symptoms.[26]

Diagnostic Criteria for TS

The fifth edition of the *Diagnostic and Statistical Manual* (DSM-5) includes the following criteria for the diagnosis of TS.[27]

1. The patient should have multiple motor tics and at least one vocal tic at some time during the illness, although not necessarily concurrently.
2. Tics have been present for >1 year since first tic onset (if persists for <1year, it is labeled as "provisional tic disorder")
3. Age at tic onset <18 years.
4. Symptoms are not attributable to the physiological effects of a substance (e.g., cocaine) or a general medical condition (e.g., Huntington's disease, postviral encephalitis).

The term "provisional tic disorder" is reserved for the tics present for less than 1 year, whereas the term "chronic motor/vocal tics" is used to describe the presence of either motor tics or phonic tics (not both) for >1 year.[28]

Table 14.1 Differential Diagnoses for the Tic Disorders [27]

Tic disorders	Tic characteristics (criterion A)	Duration (criterion B)	Age at tic onset (criterion C)
Tourette's syndrome	>1 motor **AND** ≥1 vocal tics (not necessarily concurrent)	> 1 year since onset	<18 years
Chronic motor/vocal tic disorder	≥1 motor **OR** vocal tics (not both)	> 1 year since onset	<18 years
Provisional tic disorder	≥1 motor **AND/OR** vocal tics	<1 year since onset	<18 years
Other tic disorders	Other specified tic disorder	The clinician records the specific reason that the presentation does not meet the criteria for a tic disorder or any other neurodevelopmental disorder.	
	Unspecified tic disorder	The clinician chooses not to communicate the specific reason that the presentation does not meet the criteria for a tic disorder or any other neurodevelopmental disorder, and/or there is insufficient information to make a more specific diagnosis.	

Criterion D: None of the disturbances attributable to the physiological effect of a substance (e.g., cocaine) or another medical condition (e.g., Huntington's disease, postviral encephalitis).

Etiology of TS

The exact underlying etiology of TS remains elusive. However, several lines of evidence suggest that TS has a genetic substrate as described below.

Genetics of TS

TS has been described as a polygenic disorder with a strong interaction with environmental factors.[1] Multiple lines of evidence suggest the potential role of heritability in TS. Studies have shown that there is a 15-fold risk of having TS or chronic motor/phonic tics in siblings of patients with TS and almost half of the patients with TS provided a history of tics. Besides, a high concordance rate of developing chronic motor/vocal tics (86%) in monozygotic twins further strengthens the argument in favor of the underlying genetic substrates.[29] Offsprings of the TS patients also carry a higher risk of developing the classic comorbidities associated with TS, such as OCD and ADHD.[30] Furthermore, while at least one parent is affected in over 80% of patients, bilineal transmission (inheritance from both parents) has been observed in at least 25% of families,[31] but this frequency is probably much higher.

Several potential susceptibility genes have been identified, but not yet confirmed. These include the *SLITRK1* located in 13q31.1[32] and mutation in the gene encoding L-histidine decarboxylase (HDC).[33] Several other studies have explored the genetic substrates of TS without identifying any specific causative gene mutation.[34,35]

Autoimmunity and TS

Although highly controversial, some evidence suggests the potential role of an underlying autoimmune process in the pathogenesis of TS. The association with pediatric autoimmune neuropsychiatric disorders associated with streptococcal infection (PANDAS) and pediatric acute-onset neuropsychiatric syndrome (PANS) has garnered attention from the autoimmune standpoint.[36] Some studies have provided evidence that striatal cholinergic neurons are a critical cellular target for antibodies in patients with PANDAS,[37] but the relationship between TS and PANDAS continues to be a controversial topic. In a case series involving 42 patients with streptococcal infections, 5 patients subsequently developed TS.[38] A study by Church and colleagues revealed elevated antistreptolysin O titer (ASO) and the presence of anti-basal-ganglia antibodies in patients with TS.[39] This raises the possibility that some individuals with Sydenham chorea may exhibit tics (and OCD) which overlap with known clinical manifestations of TS. Some animal models of TS developed oral stereotypies after injection of the antineuronal antibodies, which further suggests the role of an autoimmune etiology, but additional research is needed before the link between TS and immune system can be established.[40]

Pathogenesis of Tics

The pathogenesis and pathophysiology of tics is complex and remains to be fully understood. Although a multitude of studies based on structural and functional neuroimaging and electrophysiology have provided considerable insights, the precise pathophysiology remains elusive.[13]

There are debates over the nature of the movement or sound that is clinically diagnosed as "tic." One of the most fundamental questions is whether a tic is involuntary, unvoluntary, or voluntary.[13] There is some evidence in favor of a continuum from "involuntary" to "voluntary" nature of the tics with an overlap "unvoluntary" (i.e., in response to an inner urge) component in most patients. For example, the repetitive and persistent nature, presence of tics during sleep, and lack of a clear goal or benefit provides evidence that tics are "involuntary." The presence of premonitory urge before the tics, sense of "feeling better" after the tics associated with the premonitory urges, argues for "unvoluntary" component of tics. The frequently observed voluntary suppressibility, and reduction in tics while performing other voluntary activities argues for evidence of "voluntary" construct. One of the commonly used neurophysiological tools to objectively distinguish voluntary from the involuntary movements is the demonstration of the Bereitschaft potential (BP) in the former. It is also known as premotor potential or readiness potential, which usually precedes the voluntary movements. Unfortunately, the results of the studies based on the BP have yielded nonuniform results, i.e., in a few patients, BP preceded the tic onset[41] whereas it was absent in others.[42] Another study that explored BP in patients with psychogenic jerks, TS, and myoclonus revealed that 6 out of 14 (43%) TS patients had BP.[43] However, the characteristic of BP in TS was different from that in psychogenic jerks or healthy controls as the BP in the former was late-onset and had a shorter duration.[43] A recent study investigated the local field potential (LFP) from the centromedian (CM) thalamus and motor cortex in TS patients after deep brain stimulation and revealed an association of increase in low frequency power (3–10 hz) in CM thalamus with the tic onset.[44] As the increase in the low frequency power was independent of the voluntary movements, LFP monitoring could turn out to be a useful tool in future to guide neuromodulation-based therapeutics.

This conundrum about the nature of the tics has led to the speculation that involuntary activation of the neural networks associated with the voluntary motor pathways is associated with tic generation.[45] Besides, the role of an abnormal voluntary inhibitory control over the tic output has also been posited.[46] The cortico-striato-thalamo-cortical (CSTC) loop is considered the fundamental neural network for the voluntary motor functions. Previous structural and functional neuroimaging studies have found abnormalities in different components of the CSTC,[47] indicating the potential role of these structures in tic generation. A resting state functional MRI study demonstrated a temporal pattern of tic generation following the CSTC loop and activation of the cortical structures precede that of the subcortical structures.[48]

There is a growing body of evidence that supports a voluntary component of tics that might be triggered by a failure of compensatory motor inhibitory mechanisms.[49] Furthermore, in addition to the CSTC circuit, the insula has been shown to play a role in the severity of tics and premonitory phenomenon.[50] However, based on studies using voxel-based morphometry and "seed-to-voxel" structural covariance network mapping techniques, there is evidence that tics and the premonitory urges are generated in different parts of the brain and have distinct anatomical correlates.[51] Thus, while tic severity seems to be negatively associated with the gray matter volume values in a posterior region of the right insular cortex the severity of premonitory urge correlates positively with gray matter volume values in anterior-dorsal region of the right insula.[51]

As the neural networks are modulated by several neurotransmitters, it is possible that an imbalanced neurotransmission (excitatory vs. inhibitory) could be playing a key role in the genesis of tics. Two postmortem studies on patients with TS revealed an imbalance in the inhibitory neuron distribution in the striatum and globus pallidus interna (GPi)[52] and a selective deficit of cholinergic and GABAergic interneurons in the striatum.[53] The role of aberrant striatal cholinergic transmission in the pathogenesis of TS received support from a study by Xu et al., wherein targeted ablation of the cholinergic interneurons in the dorsolateral striatum in mice (corresponds to putamen in humans) resulted in tic-like stereotypies.[54] Abnormal GABA transmission in TS was further suggested by findings from several functional and other neuroimaging studies. A magnetic resonance spectroscopy (MRS) study revealed lower GABA concentration in the primary sensorimotor cortex in children with TS compared to controls.[55] The finding which further reinforced the role of GABA in TS pathogenesis was the negative correlation between GABA concentration and motor tic severity.[55] A positron emission tomography (PET) study using [11C]flumazenil as a GABA-ligand revealed widespread alterations in GABA transmission in TS patients compared to the controls (decreased—ventral striatum, globus pallidus, thalamus, amygdala, and right insula; increased—bilateral substantia nigra, left periaqueductal grey, right posterior cingulate cortex, and bilateral cerebellum).[56]

In addition to abnormal GABAergic and cholinergic transmission, multiple lines of evidence indicate the potential role of a hyperdopaminergic state in the TS pathogenesis. Clinical observations that support the hypothesis of the hyperdopaminergic state include suppression of tics by centrally acting dopamine depleting agents such as tetrabenazine (and its isomer deutetrabenazine).[57,58] Also, psychostimulants, such as amphetamine, which has dopaminergic properties has been observed to worsen tics.[59,60] Previous studies using molecular neuroimaging have observed high pre-and intrasynaptic dopaminergic activity (assessed through PET studies) and increased binding of the dopamine transporter in the striatum (assessed through SPECT-ligand studies).[61–64] However, functional PET scan utilizing presynaptic dopaminergic markers found no evidence of increased striatal dopaminergic innervation.[65] The same group also found no evidence of cholinergic abnormalities in TS.[66] However, a PET study on 12 drug-naïve TS patients with additional symptoms of OCD revealed two distinct abnormal brain networks, i.e., the existence of separate TS-related patterns and OCD-related patterns.[67] Postmortem studies have provided useful insights into the potential underlying pathophysiology of TS. These studies observed increased density of presynaptic nerve terminals,[68] elevated D2 receptor protein in the prefrontal cortex,[69] and a higher density of dopamine transporter and D1 receptors.[70]

In summary, the pathogenesis of TS is enigmatic, and yet to be fully understood. The available information from the structural, functional, and molecular neuroimaging and postmortem studies indicate the potential role of neurotransmitter imbalance, particularly involving the GABAergic system and abnormalities in the connectivity, predominantly in the CSTC loop as playing a pathophysiological role in "disinhibition" as the general underpinning mechanism in tic generation.

Screening Instruments and Severity Scales for Tics

A subcommittee of the Movement Disorders Society performed a systematic review of the currently available screening instruments and severity rating scales.[71] The subcommittee recommended 5 of the 16 rating scales reviewed for the assessment of the severity of tics and 2 of the 13 screening instruments for tics. The 5 recommended scales for severity assessment were the Yale Global Tic Severity Scale (YGTSS), Schapiro TS Severity Scale (STSS), TS Clinical Global Impression (TS-CGI), Tourette's Disorder Scale (TODS), and Premonitory Urges for Tics Scale (PUTS). Of these scales, the YGTCC is the most comprehensive and reliable. The PUTS has good psychometric properties for assessment of the severity of the premonitory urges, however, its use is limited to patients older than 10 years. A recent study has suggested additional revisions to the PUTS scale to make it more comprehensive.[72] The two screening instruments recommended by the subcommittee were Autism-Tics ADHD and other Comorbidities inventory (A-TAC) and Motor tic, Obsessions and compulsions, Vocal tics Evaluation Survey (MOVES).

Management of TS

Management of TS is challenging, and it requires a multidisciplinary approach.[73] The most crucial component of the management of TS is counseling the patients and caregivers and to provide them with appropriate resources for information regarding TS (e.g., the Tourette Association of America; https://tourette.org/). It is important to address the features leading toward overall functional impairment. Based on the nature and severity of the symptoms, nonpharmacological (behavioral treatment), pharmacological, and surgical treatment options may be provided.

Nonpharmacological Management

Patient and Caregiver Education

The education of the patients and the caregivers is the foremost step in the management of TS. Education should be aimed toward providing a clear picture of the spectrum, severity, and natural course of tics as well as the comorbid behavioral symptoms. As described earlier, tic severity reaches the peak just before puberty (10–12 years), and parents should closely monitor the worsening of tics or behavioral symptoms that would prompt initiation of treatment. It is essential to educate the patients and caregivers about the wide spectrum of tics, especially those associated with coprophenomena, which may be socially embarrassing. Although rare, patients with TS may develop self-injurious behaviors, the neurobiology of which is poorly understood, but protective devices, behavioral therapy, and pharmacological and neurosurgical interventions may be helpful in preventing serious self-harm.[74,75] The parents, teachers, and friends should be informed that affected individuals have limited ability to suppress this behavior, and a stressful environment may trigger or exacerbates tics. Providing educational information to teachers and peers enhances knowledge, positive attitudes, and behaviors toward TS patients.[76] Determining when and if pharmacologic therapy should be initiated for tic suppression is important as there is no predetermined threshold for symptom severity that warrants treatment. The decision is often fostered by the physical, emotional, and social disabilities associated with TS. Appropriate treatment expectations must be conveyed to patients and their caregivers, ensuring that they understand the treatments, while effective at reducing the tic burden, are purely symptomatic and are not disease modifying or curative.

Comprehensive Behavioral Intervention for Tics

Comprehensive behavioral intervention for tics (CBIT) is a form of cognitive-behavioral intervention that encompasses several strategies such as habit reversal training, relaxation training, and functional interventions to address the factors that may worsen tics. A multitude of studies has reported the efficacy of behavioral therapy in patients with TS.[77] Wilhelm and colleagues, in a study on 110 TS patients, reported a significant reduction in the YGTSS score in patients who had received 8 sessions of CBIT over 10 weeks compared to those who received conservative treatment.[78] A recent study on 110 patients with TS comparing CBIT, pharmacotherapy, and psychoeducation revealed that both behavioral and pharmacotherapy were comparable in terms of reducing the tic severity, whereas pharmacotherapy is superior in controlling the OCD symptoms.[79] As per the recently published guideline of the American Academy of Neurology (AAN),[80] there is the confidence that CBIT is more likely than psychoeducation and supportive therapy to reduce tics.

There are several barriers to CBIT which include unavailability of an adequate number of trained professionals, poor or no insurance coverage, and time and compliance demands on family and patients to adhere to the therapy, as well as patient age, self-motivation, and other factors.[81,82] Given the similarity in the effect size for CBIT and that of most of anti-tic medications, the former is recommended as first-line therapy for mild tics.[81,82] There is an ongoing clinical trial titled "Internet-Based CBIT for Children With Chronic Tics" (Clinical Trials ID NCT04087616) directed at evaluating the efficacy of CBIT when delivered via the Internet, in efforts to expand access.[83]

Pharmacological Treatment

Several classes of medications can partially ameliorate the tics. These include alpha-2 agonists, dopamine receptor blockers, dopamine-depleting drugs, antiepileptic drugs, serotonergic drugs, cannabinoids, and botulinum neurotoxin (BoNT). In the following section, we succinctly describe the role of the aforementioned classes of drugs and their adverse effects.

Alpha-2 Agonists

Clonidine and guanfacine are the two alpha-2 agonists that have been used as the tier-1 medications for the treatment of mild tics in newly diagnosed TS. The added advantage with these agents is the amelioration of ADHD symptoms along with tics. Previous studies have observed higher efficacy of the oral formulation,[22] as well as the transdermal patches of clonidine compared to the placebo in reducing tics in TS.[84] An open-label study[85] and a randomized double-blinded placebo-controlled study (RDBPCS) reported significant improvement in tic severity after treatment with guanfacine.[86] However, a recent RDBPCS did not find any significant improvement in tics with the use of extended-release guanfacine over eight weeks.[87] Although clonidine and guanfacine were reported to be effective in TS patients with coexisting ADHD, there appears to be only a small, nonsignificant benefit on tics in studies that excluded coexisting ADHD.[88] This suggests a possible moderator effect of ADHD.

The common side effects associated with the alpha-2 agonists include drowsiness, fatigue, irritability, bradycardia, and orthostatic hypotension. Sudden withdrawal of medication should be discouraged as the alpha-2 agonists often precipitate rebound hypertension. Given the small effect of this class of medication, the alpha-2 agonists are usually recommended for patients with mild tics and coexisting ADHD. As per the practice guideline recommendations from the American Academy of Neurology (AAN), physicians should counsel individuals with tics and comorbid ADHD that alpha-2 agonists may improve both conditions (Level B).[80]

Dopamine Receptor Blockers

Antipsychotics are the commonly used dopamine receptor blockers for the management of tics. The Food and Drug Administration (FDA) has approved three antipsychotics for the treatment of tics and these are haloperidol, pimozide, and aripiprazole. Haloperidol and pimozide are among the old typical antipsychotics which were noted to have efficacy in reducing tics. However, these two medications are associated with a range of side effects which often limit their long-term use. The neurological adverse effects include a full spectrum of drug-induced movement disorders (acute dystonic reaction, parkinsonism, tardive dyskinesias)[89] whereas many patients also develop several cardiovascular and metabolic side effects.[90] This warrants higher surveillance for cardiovascular side effects in TS patients who are otherwise at a higher risk of developing metabolic syndrome and cardiovascular diseases.[91] A baseline EKG is strongly recommended as these medications have the potential to prolong the QT-interval. Hence, a "start low–go slow" approach should be followed and other drugs that are associated with QT-prolongation should be avoided as much as possible. Aripiprazole was the third and the latest FDA-approved antipsychotics for the treatment of tics. A phase-3 RDBPCT of aripiprazole on 133 patients with TS resulted in a significant improvement in tics after eight weeks.[92] The treatment difference in YGTSS-TTS vs placebo was -6.3 ($p = 0.0020$) in the low (5–10 mg/day) dose group and -9.9 ($p = <0.0001$) in the high (10–20 mg/day) dose group.[92] Aripiprazole is pharmacodynamically different from haloperidol and pimozide as it acts as a partial agonist of the D2-receptor, resulting in relatively fewer extrapyramidal side effects. Risperidone and fluphenazine (in Europe) are the other antipsychotics (not FDA approved) that have undergone clinical trials for the treatment of tics. In a RDBPCS on 48 patients with TS, 60.8% of patients in the treatment group had improvement in the TS severity score (TSSS) compared to 26.1% in the placebo group, significantly favoring risperidone.[93] Later, another RDBPCS on 34 patients with TS, 8 weeks of treatment with risperidone resulted in a significant reduction in tics in the treatment group compared to the placebo group (32% vs. 7%, $p = 0.004$).[94] A comparative double-blinded parallel group study that compared the efficacy of risperidone and pimozide in reducing tics reported that both the antipsychotics were comparable in terms of efficacy.[95] The risperidone group had a greater improvement in comorbid OCD symptoms and had a higher number of extrapyramidal symptoms. Fluphenazine has not undergone any RDBPCS; however, several open-label studies have documented improvement in tics after treatment with fluphenazine.[96,97] Tiapride, a D2/D3 receptor blocker, has been used primarily in Europe for the treatment of tics. A placebo-controlled study found tiapride beneficial for tic suppression without any significant side effects.[98] Although there is scarcity of RDBPCS on tiapride, it is frequently prescribed outside the United States).[99]

The AAN practice guidelines recommend that physicians may prescribe antipsychotics for the treatment of tics when the benefits of treatment outweigh the risks (Level C).[80] Besides, the guidelines also highlight that there is insufficient evidence to determine the relative efficacy of the dopamine receptor blockers for the treatment of tics in TS. The prescribers should be aware of the fact that tics may become refractory to the highest tolerated dose of the antipsychotics in some patients necessitating a switch to other classes of medications. Among the FDA-approved agents, aripiprazole may be preferred over haloperidol and pimozide based on the relatively favorable adverse effect profile of the former. Given the metabolic and cardiac adverse effects and potential risk of tardive dyskinesia, antipsychotics should be considered second-line therapy after first-line agents have failed (Figure 14.1).

Dopamine-Depleting Drugs
The dopamine depleting agents work by inhibiting the vesicular monoamine transporter 2 (VMAT2). The currently available VMAT2 inhibitors are tetrabenazine (FDA-approved for chorea in Huntington's disease), deutetrabenazine (FDA-approved for tardive dyskinesia and Huntington's disease), and valbenazine (FDA-approved for tardive dyskinesia).[101] Tetrabenazine has also been shown to have some efficacy in reducing the tic severity and frequency.[102] It is one of the first-line agents for the treatment of severe tics in TS. However, tetrabenazine carries a black box warning about the potential association with depression and suicidal ideations. Besides, it is also associated with several other adverse effects such as drowsiness, parkinsonism, and akathisia.[58] One of the practical issues with the use of tetrabenazine is the short half-life (approximately 10 hours) resulting in the requirement of at least 3 times/day administration. To overcome this, longer-acting agents with a better side

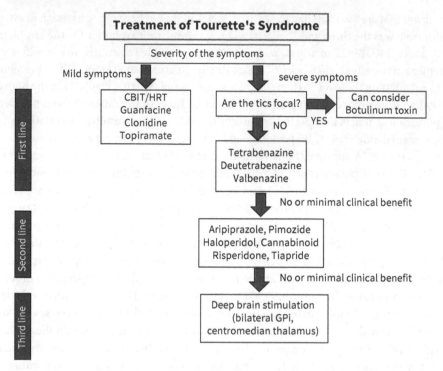

Figure 14.1 Treatment of Tourette's Syndrome.

effect profile i.e., deutetrabenazine and valbenazine have been investigated for the treatment of tics. Deutetrabenazine resulted in a 37.6% reduction in the tic severity (YGTSS score) in an open-label eight-week study.[57] A retrospective chart review that explored the use and efficacy of the VMAT2 inhibitors in hyperkinetic disorders revealed subjective improvement in tics in the majority of the responder.[103]

Unfortunately, the improvement observed in the open-label studies of deutetrabenazine could not be replicated in two recent RDBPCTs: ClinicalTrials.gov Identifier: NCT03452943: ARTISTS 1 (flexible-dose titration) and clinicalTrials.gov Identifier: NCT03571256: ARTISTS 2 (fixed dose). In the ARTIST 1 trial, 119 patients were enrolled and after initial dose titration study were followed for a total of 12 weeks, while in the ARTIST 2 trial 158 patients were recruited in a fixed-dose design and followed for 8 weeks. Although neither of the studies reached the primary endpoint,[104] there was clear evidence of improvement compared to placebo during early titration period, and there were some positive signals in the secondary endpoint analyses. There are many possible explanations for the unexpected results, including difficulties in assessing a highly variable disorder, and subtherapeutic dosing. The latter explanation is supported by the observation of a very low frequency of adverse effects, including depression.

Given the benefits observed by many clinicians around the world in many TS patients, along with good tolerability and favorable adverse effect profile, VMAT2 inhibitors should be considered viable alternative therapy to antipsychotic medications, and despite the disappointing results because of failure to meet the primary endpoint in above-cited RDBPCS, we still consider the VMAT2 inhibitors as the first line of therapy in patients with troublesome tics (Figure 14.1).

Antiepileptic Medications

Topiramate and levetiracetam have been investigated for the treatment of tics in TS. In a multicenter placebo-controlled study on 29 patients with TS, topiramate resulted in significant improvement not only in the tic severity but also in the clinical global impression and premonitory urge compared to that by the placebo.[105] Subsequently, a meta-analysis revealed a significant decrease in the YGTSS score in children with TS who were on topiramate than those on placebo.[106] Topiramate can be used as a frontline agent for the treatment of mild tics, more so for TS patients with other comorbidities such as epilepsy, migraine, and obesity for which topiramate is widely used. The AAN practice guidelines have given a level-B recommendation (should prescribe when the benefits of treatment outweigh the risks) for use of topiramate for treatment of tics in TS. The prescribers should be vigilant about the common side effects of topiramate which include drowsiness, weight loss, and nephrolithiasis. Levetiracetam is the other antiepileptic medication that was investigated in TS. Although it showed some effect in open-label studies, small controlled trials have yielded conflicting results.[107,108]

Cannabinoids

Cannabinoids have surged a lot of public interest in their utility in many chronic diseases. Several studies have investigated the efficacy of cannabinoid in ameliorating tics in TS. Although patients report overall subjective improvement after starting cannabinoid, it is challenging to interpret the effects of the medication based on the nonspecific subjective improvement.[109] Although a RDBPCS on 24 patients with TS demonstrated the efficacy of cannabinoids in controlling tics, subsequently[110] a Cochrane review concluded that definite conclusions about the safety and efficacy of cannabinoids in the treatment of TS cannot be drawn.[111] A recently published meta-analysis on the use of cannabinoids for mental disorders suggested that there is little evidence for the effectiveness of pharmaceutical cannabinoids or medicinal cannabis for the treatment of various disorders, including TS.[112] Several studies are currently investigating a compound named ABX-1431, an enzyme that regulates 2-arachidonoylglycerol, which is an endogenous agonist of cannabinoid CB1 and CB2 receptors. A double-blind study on 19 patients assessing the efficacy of a single dose of this compound resulted in a significant reduction in YGTSS score 8 hours after the intake.[113] Additional trials are needed to confirm the findings of the study.

As per the AAN practice guidelines, where regional legislation allows, physicians may consider treatment with cannabis-based medication in otherwise treatment-resistant adults with clinically relevant tics (Level C).

Botulinum Neurotoxin Injection

Several studies have assessed the utility of botulinum neurotoxin (BoNT) for medication-refractory motor and phonic tics.[114] A RDBPCS on 18 TS patients documented improvement in the tic frequency and urge after BoNT therapy compared to the placebo group.[115] However, there was no effect of BoNT on the tic severity and the patients did not report an overall benefit from the treatment. In an open-label study on 35 TS patients, BoNT resulted

Table 14.2 Oral Pharmacotherapy for the Treatment of Tics in Tourette's Syndrome

Pharmacological class	Medications	Initial dose (mg)	Dose range (mg/d)	Side effects
Dopamine receptor blockers	Typical neuroleptics:			Sedation, DIMD
	Haloperidol	0.25–0.5	1–4	Sedation, DIMD, QT prolongation
	Pimozide	0.5–1	2–8	
	Atypical neuroleptics:			Sedation, DIMD, weight gain
	Aripiprazole	2.5–5	10–20	
	Risperidone	1–3	1–3	Sedation, DIMD, weight gain
	Fluphenazine	0.5–1	1.5–10	Sedation, DIMD
	Tiapride (in Europe)	50–100	50–500	Sedation, increased appetite
Dopamine depleting agents	Tetrabenazine	25	37.5–100	Parkinsonism, suicidal ideations, sedation
	Deutetrabenazine	6	under study	Sedation, tiredness, dry mouth
Alpha-2 agonists	Clonidine	0.025–0.05	0.1–0.3	Orthostasis, bradycardia, sedation
	Guanfacine	0.5–1	1–3	Orthostasis, bradycardia, sedation
Benzodiazepines	Clonazepam	0.5	0.5–5	Drowsiness
Antiepileptics	Topiramate	25	25–150	Sedation, weight loss, kidney stones cognitive dysfunction

DIMD: Drug-induced movement disorders.

in significant improvement in the motor component of tic and the premonitory sensations.[116] Importantly, the effect of BoNT lasted for a median duration of 14.4 weeks.

Considering the lack of systemic adverse effects and long-term effects, BoNT can be considered in TS patients with medication-refractory focal motor and phonic tics. This can be especially beneficial in severe motor tics with repetitive cervical extension, often referred to as whiplash tics or malignant tics[11] BoNT was reported to reverse cervical myelopathy secondary to severe tics.[117]

Surgical Management of Tics

Deep Brain Stimulation for Medication-Refractory Tics
Deep brain stimulation (DBS) has been revolutionary for the treatment of medication refractory movement disorders and there is a growing interest in the use of DBS for the treatment

of severe tics.[118] There is a limited number of studies with a controlled design that have investigated the role of DBS in TS. In a randomized, double-blind, crossover trial on medication refractory TS patients, DBS of the GPi resulted in a significant decrease in YGTSS scores during the stimulation-ON period compared to the stimulation-OFF period.[119] A systematic review and meta-analysis (57 studies, 156 patients) also suggested that irrespective of the stimulation targets (GPi, centromedian thalamus, internal capsule) there was a significant improvement in the tic severity after DB.[120] In an international registry of patients who had undergone DBS for TS, the mean total YGTSS score of 157 patients improved by 45% at 1-year follow-up compared to the baseline score. When the data was stratified based on the site of stimulation, improvement in the mean total YGTSS at 1-year follow-up was greatest in those with anterior GPi stimulation (50.5% improvement), followed by centromedian thalamic stimulation (46.3% improvement), and posterior GPi stimulation (27.7% improvement).[118] A meta-analysis comparing several studies of efficacy and safety of DBS, pharmacotherapy, and psychotherapy concluded that DBS results in a greater reduction of YGTSS compared with relatively fewer adverse effects compared to psychotherapy and pharmacotherapy.[121]

The AAN guideline report, which is weighted toward controlled trials and evidence-based data, found low confidence that GPi DBS results in significant improvement in tics compared to placebo. However, because the number of trials is limited, the conclusions of the AAN guideline report should be balanced against and coupled with a more practical approach, based on long-term experience and expert opinion. At present, the practice guidelines give a level C recommendation for DBS in TS (Physicians may consider DBS for severe, self-injurious tics, such as severe cervical tics that result in spinal injury).

Conclusion

TS is a complex childhood-onset neurobehavioral disorder with marked clinical heterogeneity. In addition to tics, which are the defining symptoms of TS, patients may develop several comorbid psychiatric issues (ADHD, OCD, anxiety, mood disorders). The etiology and pathogenesis of TS remain elusive. Educating the patients, caregivers, and school officials in detail about the spectrum, severity, and natural course of the symptoms of TS is the cornerstone of the management of TS. CBIT should be offered to all the patients as the initial step of management, if available. Comorbid medical and behavioral abnormalities should be kept in mind and individualized when choosing the most appropriate pharmacotherapy for tics (Figure 14.1). While BoNT should be considered for severe focal tics, DBS should be considered as an option for drug-resistant disabling tics and OCD. A multidisciplinary approach along with appropriate utilization of the aforementioned therapeutic options should lead to optimal functional outcome in TS patients.

References

1. Robertson MM, Eapen V, Singer HS, et al. Gilles de la Tourette syndrome. *Nat Rev Dis Prim*. 2017;3:1–20. https://doi.org/10.1038/nrdp.2016.97

2. Hirschtritt ME, Lee PC, Pauls DL, et al. Lifetime prevalence, age of risk, and genetic relationships of comorbid psychiatric disorders in Tourette syndrome. *JAMA Psychiatry*. 2015;72(4):325. https://doi.org/10.1001/jamapsychiatry.2014.2650

3. Scharf JM, Miller LL, Gauvin CA, Alabiso J, Mathews CA, Ben-Shlomo Y. Population prevalence of Tourette syndrome: a systematic review and meta-analysis. *Mov Disord*. 2015;30(2):221–228. https://doi.org/10.1002/mds.26089

4. Groth C, Mol Debes N, Rask CU, Lange T, Skov L. Course of Tourette syndrome and comorbidities in a large prospective clinical study. *Journal of the American Academy of Child and Adolescent Psychiatry*. 2017;56(4):304–312. https://doi.org/10.1016/j.jaac.2017.01.010

5. Groth C, Skov L, Lange T, Debes NM. Predictors of the clinical course of Tourette syndrome: a longitudinal study. *J Child Neurol*. 2019;34(12):913–921. https://doi.org/10.1177/0883073819867245

6. Lajonchere C. Gilles de la Tourette and the discovery of Tourette syndrome. *Arch Neurol*. 1996;53(6):567–574. https://doi.org/10.1001/archneur.1996.00550060111024

7. Rickards H, Woolf I, Cavanna AE. "Trousseau's disease": a description of the Gilles de la Tourette syndrome 12 years before 1885. *Mov Disord*. 2010; 25(14):2285–2289. https://doi.org/10.1002/mds.23202

8. Ganos C, Münchau A, Bhatia KP. The semiology of tics, Tourette's, and their associations. *Mov Disord Clin Pract*. 2014;1(3):145–153. https://doi.org/10.1002/mdc3.12043

9. Ganos C, Müller-Vahl K, Bhatia KP. Blocking phenomena in Gilles de la Tourette syndrome. *Mov Disord Clin Pract*. 2015;2(4):438–439. https://doi.org/10.1002/mdc3.12199

10. Freeman RD, Zinner SH, Müller-Vahl KR, et al. Coprophenomena in Tourette syndrome. *Dev Med Child Neurol*. 2009;51(3):218–227. https://doi.org/10.1111/j.1469-8749.2008.03135.x

11. Cheung MYC, Shahed J, Jankovic J. Malignant Tourette syndrome. *Mov Disord*. 2007;22(12):1743–1750. https://doi.org/10.1002/mds.21599

12. Cavanna AE, Black KJ, Hallett M, Voon V. Neurobiology of the premonitory urge in Tourette's syndrome: pathophysiology and treatment implications. *J Neuropsychiatry Clin Neurosci*. 2017;29(2):95–104. https://doi.org/10.1176/appi.neuropsych.16070141

13. Singer HS, Augustine F. Controversies surrounding the pathophysiology of tics. *J Child Neurol*. 2019; 34(13):851–862. https://doi.org/10.1177/0883073819862121

14. Kwak C, Dat Vuong K, Jankovic J. Premonitory sensory phenomenon in Tourette's syndrome. *Mov Disord*. 2003;18(12):1530–1533. https://doi.org/10.1002/mds.10618

15. Baizabal-Carvallo JF, Jankovic J. The clinical features of psychogenic movement disorders resembling tics. *J Neurol Neurosurg Psychiatry*. 2014;85(5):573–575. https://doi.org/10.1136/jnnp-2013-305594

16. Ganos C, Martino D, Espay AJ, Lang AE, Bhatia KP, Edwards MJ. Tics and functional tic-like movements: can we tell them apart? *Neurology*. 2019;93(17):750–758. https://doi.org/10.1212/WNL.0000000000008372

17. Eddy CM, Cavanna AE. Premonitory urges in adults with complicated and uncomplicated Tourette syndrome. *Behav Modif*. 2014;38(2):264–275. https://doi.org/10.1177/0145445513504432

18. Kyriazi M, Kalyva E, Vargiami E, Krikonis K, Zafeiriou D. Premonitory urges and their link with tic severity in children and adolescents with tic disorders. *Front Psychiatry*. 2019;10(569):1–5. https://doi.org/10.3389/fpsyt.2019.00569

19. Li Y, Wang F, Liu J, et al. The correlation between the severity of premonitory urges and tic symptoms: a meta-analysis. *J Child Adolesc Psychopharmacol*. 2019;29(9):652–658. https://doi.org/10.1089/cap.2019.0048

20. Verdellen CWJ, Keijsers GPJ, Cath DC, Hoogduin CAL. Exposure with response prevention versus habit reversal in Tourettes's syndrome: a controlled study. *Behav Res Ther*. 2004;42(5):501–511. https://doi.org/10.1016/S0005-7967(03)00154-2

21. Demartini B, Ricciardi L, Parees I, Ganos C, Bhatia KP, Edwards MJ. A positive diagnosis of functional (psychogenic) tics. *Eur J Neurol*. 2015;22(3):1–7. https://doi.org/10.1111/ene.12609

22. Kurlan R, Goetz CG, McDermott MP, et al. Treatment of ADHD in children with tics: a randomized controlled trial. *Neurology*. 2002;58(4):527–536. https://doi.org/10.1212/WNL.58.4.527

23. Freeman RD, Fast DK, Burd L, Kerbeshian J, Robertson MM, Sandor P. An international perspective on Tourette syndrome: selected findings from 3500 individuals in 22 countries. *Dev Med Child Neurol*. 2000;42(7):436–447. https://doi.org/10.1017/S0012162200000839

24. Cath DC, Spinhoven P, Hoogduin CAL, et al. Repetitive behaviors in Tourette's syndrome and OCD with and without tics: what are the differences? *Psychiatry Res*. 2001;101(2):171–185. https://doi.org/10.1016/S0165-1781(01)00219-0

25. Stafford M, Cavanna AE. Prevalence and clinical correlates of self-injurious behavior in Tourette syndrome. *Neurosci Biobehav Rev*. 2020;113:299–307. https://doi.org/10.1016/j.neubiorev.2020.03.022

26. Wanderer S, Roessner V, Freeman R, Bock N, Rothenberger A, Becker A. Relationship of obsessive-compulsive disorder to age-related comorbidity in children and adolescents with Tourette syndrome. *J Dev Behav Pediatr*. 2012;33(2):124–133. https://doi.org/10.1097/DBP.0b013e31823f6933

27. American Psychiatric Association. *American Psychiatric Association: Diagnostic and Statistical Manual of Mental Disorders*, fifth edition. 2013. https://doi.org/10.1176/appi.books.9780890425596.744053

28. Singer HS. Tics and Tourette syndrome. *Continuum (Minneap Minn)*. 2019;25(4):936–958. https://doi.org/10.1212/CON.0000000000000752

29. Mataix-Cols D, Isomura K, Pérez-Vigil A, et al. Familial risks of Tourette syndrome and chronic tic disorders a population-based cohort study. *JAMA Psychiatry*. 2015;72(8):787–793. https://doi.org/10.1001/jamapsychiatry.2015.0627

30. McMahon WM, Carter AS, Fredine N, Pauls DL. Children at familial risk for Tourette's disorder: Child and parent diagnoses. *Am J Med Genet*. 2003;121B(1):105–111. https://doi.org/10.1002/ajmg.b.20065

31. Hanna PA, Janjua FN, Contant CF, Jankovic J. Bilineal transmission in Tourette syndrome. *Neurology*. 1999;53(4):813–818. https://doi.org/10.1212/wnl.53.4.813

32. Abelson JF, Kwan KY, K, O'Roak BJ, et al. Sequence variants in SLITRK1 are associated with Tourette's syndrome. *Science*.2005;310(5746):317–320.

33. Ercan-Sencicek AG, Stillman AA, Ghosh AK, et al. L-histidine decarboxylase and Tourette's syndrome. *N Engl J Med*. 2010;362(20):1901–1908. https://doi.org/10.1056/NEJMoa0907006

34. Qi Y, Zheng Y, Li Z, Liu Z, Xiong L. Genetic studies of tic disorders and Tourette syndrome. *Methods Mol Biol*. 2019;2011:547–571. https://doi.org/10.1007/978-1-4939-9554-7_32

35. Yu D, Sul JH, Tsetsos F, et al. Interrogating the genetic determinants of Tourette's syndrome and other tic disorders through genome-wide association studies. *Am J Psychiatry*. 2019;176(3):217–227. https://doi.org/10.1176/appi.ajp.2018.18070857

36. Kurlan R. Tourette's syndrome and "PANDAS": Will the relation bear out? *Neurology*. 1998;50(6):1530–1534. https://doi.org/10.1212/WNL.50.6.1530

37. Xu J, Liu R-J, Fahey S, et al. Antibodies from children with PANDAS bind specifically to striatal cholinergic interneurons and alter their activity. *Am J Psychiatry*. 2020;June 16(published online ahead of print). https://doi.org/10.1176/appi.ajp.2020.19070698

38. Walker KG, Lawrenson J, Wilmshurst JM. Neuropsychiatric movement disorders following streptococcal infection. *Dev Med Child Neurol*. 2005;47(11):771–775. https://doi.org/10.1017/S0012162205001611

39. Church AJ, Dale RC, Lees AJ, Giovannoni G, Robertson MM. Tourette's syndrome: a cross sectional study to examine the PANDAS hypothesis. *J Neurol Neurosurg Psychiatry*. 2003;74(5):602–607. https://doi.org/10.1136/jnnp.74.5.602

40. Taylor JR, Morshed SA, Parveen S, et al. An animal model of Tourette's syndrome. *Am J Psychiatry*. 2002;159(4):657–660. https://doi.org/10.1176/appi.ajp.159.4.657

41. Karp BI, Porter S, Toro C, Hallett M. Simple motor tics may be preceded by a premotor potential. *J Neurol Neurosurg Psychiatry*. 1996;61(1):103–106. https://doi.org/10.1136/jnnp.61.1.103

42. Obeso JA, Rothwell JC, Marsden CD. Simple tics in Gilles de la Tourette's syndrome are not prefaced by a normal premovement EEG potential. *J Neurol Neurosurg Psychiatry*. 1981;44(8):735–738. https://doi.org/10.1136/jnnp.44.8.735

43. Van Der Salm SMA, Tijssen MAJ, Koelman JHTM, Van Rootselaar AF. The bereitschaftspotential in jerky movement disorders. *J Neurol Neurosurg Psychiatry*. 2012;83(12):1162–1167. https://doi.org/10.1136/jnnp-2012-303081

44. Cagle JN, Okun MS, Opri E, et al. Differentiating tic electrophysiology from voluntary movement in the human thalamocortical circuit. *J Neurol Neurosurg Psychiatry*. 2020;91(5):533–539. https://doi.org/10.1136/jnnp-2019-321973

45. Ganos C, Martino D. Tics and Tourette syndrome. *Neurol Clin*. 2015;33(1):115–136. https://doi.org/10.1016/j.ncl.2014.09.008

46. Ganos C, Rothwell J, Haggard P. Voluntary inhibitory motor control over involuntary tic movements. *Mov Disord*. 2018;33(6):937–946. https://doi.org/10.1002/mds.27346

47. Greene DJ, Schlaggar BL, Black KJ. Neuroimaging in Tourette syndrome: research highlights from 2014 to 2015. *Curr Dev Disord Reports*. 2015;2(4):300–308. https://doi.org/10.1007/s40474-015-0062-6

48. Neuner I, Werner CJ, Arrubla J, et al. Imaging the where and when of tic generation and resting state networks in adult Tourette patients. *Front Hum Neurosci*. 2014;8(362):1–16. https://doi.org/10.3389/fnhum.2014.00362

49. Niccolai V, Korczok S, Finis J, et al. A peek into premonitory urges in Tourette syndrome: temporal evolution of neurophysiological oscillatory signatures. *Park Relat Disord*. 2019;65:153–158. https://doi.org/10.1016/j.parkreldis.2019.05.039

50. Tinaz S, Malone P, Hallett M, Horovitz SG. Role of the right dorsal anterior insula in the urge to tic in Tourette syndrome. *Mov Disord*. 2015;30(9);1190–1197. https://doi.org/10.1002/mds.26230

51. Jackson SR, Loayza J, Crighton M, Sigurdsson HP, Dyke K, Jackson GM. The role of the insula in the generation of motor tics and the experience of the premonitory urge-to-tic in Tourette syndrome. *Cortex*. 2020;126:119–133. https://doi.org/10.1016/j.cortex.2019.12.021

52. Kalanithi PSA, Zheng W, Kataoka Y, et al. Altered parvalbumin-positive neuron distribution in basal ganglia of individuals with Tourette syndrome. *Proc Natl Acad Sci U S A*. 2005;102(37):13307–13312. https://doi.org/10.1073/pnas.0502624102

53. Kataoka Y, Kalanithi PSA, Grantz H, et al. Decreased number of parvalbumin and cholinergic interneurons in the striatum of individuals with Tourette syndrome. *J Comp Neurol.* 2010;518(3):277–291. https://doi.org/10.1002/cne.22206

54. Xua M, Kobetsa A, Dua JC, et al. Targeted ablation of cholinergic interneurons in the dorsolateral striatum produces behavioral manifestations of Tourette syndrome. *Proc Natl Acad Sci U S A.* 2015;112(3):893–898. https://doi.org/10.1073/pnas.1419533112

55. Puts NAJ, Harris AD, Crocetti D, et al. Reduced GABAergic inhibition and abnormal sensory symptoms in children with Tourette syndrome. *J Neurophysiol.* 2015;114(2):808–817. https://doi.org/10.1152/jn.00060.2015

56. Lerner A, Bagic A, Simmons JM, et al. Widespread abnormality of the γ-aminobutyric acidergic system in Tourette syndrome. *Brain.* 2012;135(Pt6):1926–1936. https://doi.org/10.1093/brain/aws104

57. Jankovic J, Jimenez-Shahed J, Budman C, et al. Deutetrabenazine in tics associated with Tourette syndrome. *Tremor Other Hyperkinet Mov (N Y).* 2016;6. https://doi.org/10.7916/D8M32W3H

58. Fasano A, Bentivoglio AR. Tetrabenazine. *Expert Opin Pharmacother.* 2009;10(17):2883–2896. https://doi.org/10.1517/14656560903386292

59. Golden GS. The relationship between stimulant medication and tics. *Pediatr Ann.* 1988;17(6):405–406. https://doi.org/10.3928/0090-4481-19880601-08

60. Lowe TL, Cohen DJ, Detlor J, Kremenitzer MW, Shaywitz BA. Stimulant medications precipitate Tourette's syndrome. *JAMA J Am Med Assoc.* 1982;247(12):1729–1731. https://doi.org/10.1001/jama.1982.03320330064029

61. Ernst M, Zametkin AJ, Jons PH, Matochik JA, Pascualvaca D, Cohen RM. High presynaptic dopaminergic activity in children with Tourette's disorder. *J Am Acad Child Adolesc Psychiatry.* 1999;38(1):86–94. https://doi.org/10.1097/00004583-199901000-00024

62. Singer HS, Szymanski S, Giuliano J, et al. Elevated intrasynaptic dopamine release in Tourette's syndrome measured by PET. *Am J Psychiatry.* 2002;159(8):1329–1336. https://doi.org/10.1176/appi.ajp.159.8.1329

63. Müller-Vahl KR, Berding G, Brücke T, et al. Dopamine transporter binding in Gilles de la Tourette syndrome. *J Neurol.* 2000;247(7):514–520. https://doi.org/10.1007/PL00007806

64. Cheon KA, Ryu YH, Namkoong K, Kim CH, Kim JJ, Lee JD. Dopamine transporter density of the basal ganglia assessed with [123I]IPT SPECT in drug-naive children with Tourette's disorder. *Psychiatry Res - Neuroimaging.* 2004;130(1):85–95. https://doi.org/10.1016/j.pscychresns.2003.06.001

65. Albin RL, Koeppe RA, Wernette K, et al. Striatal [11C]dihydrotetrabenazine and [11C]methylphenidate binding in Tourette syndrome. *Neurology.* 2009;72(16):1390–1396. https://doi.org/10.1212/WNL.0b013e3181a187dd

66. Albin RL, Minderovic C, Koeppe RA. Normal striatal vesicular acetylcholine transporter expression in Tourette syndrome. *eNeuro.* 2017;4(4):1–6. https://doi.org/10.1523/ENEURO.0178-17.2017

67. Pourfar M, Feigin A, Tang CC, et al. Abnormal metabolic brain networks in Tourette syndrome. *Neurology.* 2011;76(11):944–952. https://doi.org/10.1212/WNL.0b013e3182104106

68. Singer HS, Hahn I -H, Moran TH. Abnormal dopamine uptake sites in postmortem striatum from patients with Tourette's syndrome. *Ann Neurol.* 1991;30(4):558–562. https://doi.org/10.1002/ana.410300408

69. Minzer K, Lee O, Hong JJ, Singer HS. Increased prefrontal D2 protein in Tourette syndrome: a postmortem analysis of frontal cortex and striatum. *J Neurol Sci*. 2004;219(1–2):55–61. https://doi.org/10.1016/j.jns.2003.12.006

70. Yoon DY, Gause CD, Leckman JF, Singer HS. Frontal dopaminergic abnormality in Tourette syndrome: a postmortem analysis. *J Neurol Sci*. 2007;255(1–2):50–56. https://doi.org/10.1016/j.jns.2007.01.069

71. Martino D, Pringsheim TM, Cavanna AE, et al. Systematic review of severity scales and screening instruments for tics: Critique and recommendations. *Mov Disord*. 2017;32(3):467–473. https://doi.org/10.1002/mds.26891

72. Baumung L, Müller-Vahl K, Dyke K, et al. Developing the Premonitory Urges for Tic Disorders Scale–Revised (PUTS-R). *J Neuropsychol*. 2020:e12216 (online ahead of print). https://doi.org/10.1111/jnp.12216

73. Jimenez-Shahed J. Medical and surgical treatments of Tourette syndrome. *Neurol Clin*. 2020;38(2):349–366. https://doi.org/10.1016/j.ncl.2020.01.006

74. Fischer JF, Mainka T, Mainka T, et al. Self-injurious behaviour in movement disorders: systematic review. *J Neurol Neurosurg Psychiatry*. 2020;91(7):712–719. https://doi.org/10.1136/jnnp-2019-322569

75. Mathews CA, Waller J, Glidden D V., et al. Self injurous behaviour in Tourette syndrome: correlates with impulsivity and impulse control. *J Neurol Neurosurg Psychiatry*. 2004;75(8):1149–1155. https://doi.org/10.1136/jnnp.2003.020693

76. Nussey C, Pistrang N, Murphy T. How does psychoeducation help? A review of the effects of providing information about Tourette syndrome and attention-deficit/hyperactivity disorder. *Child Care Health Dev*. 2013;39(5):617–627. https://doi.org/10.1111/cch.12039

77. Capriotti MR, Himle MB, Woods DW. Behavioral treatments for Tourette syndrome. *J Obsessive Compuls Relat Disord*. 2014;3(4):415–420. https://doi.org/10.1016/j.jocrd.2014.03.007

78. Wilhelm S, Peterson AL, Piacentini J, et al. Randomized trial of behavior therapy for adults with Tourette syndrome. *Arch Gen Psychiatry*. 2012;69(8):795–803. https://doi.org/10.1001/archgenpsychiatry.2011.1528

79. Rizzo R, Pellico A, Silvestri PR, Chiarotti F, Cardona F. A randomized controlled trial comparing behavioral, educational, and pharmacological treatments in youths with chronic tic disorder or Tourette syndrome. *Front Psychiatry*. 2018;9:1–9. https://doi.org/10.3389/fpsyt.2018.00100

80. Pringsheim T, Okun MS, Müller-Vahl K, et al. Practice guideline recommendations summary: treatment of tics in people with Tourette syndrome and chronic tic disorders. *Neurology*. 2019;92(19):896–906. https://doi.org/10.1212/WNL.0000000000007466

81. Jankovic J. Treatment of tics associated with Tourette syndrome. *J Neural Transm*. 2020;127(5):843–850. https://doi.org/10.1007/s00702-019-02105-w

82. Chadehumbe MA, Brown LW. Advances in the treatment of Tourette's disorder. *Curr Psychiatry Rep*. 2019;21(5):1–6. https://doi.org/10.1007/s11920-019-1018-z

83. Internet-based CBIT for children with chronic tics - full text view - ClinicalTrials.gov. https://clinicaltrials.gov/ct2/show/NCT04087616. Accessed May 24, 2020.

84. Du YS, Li HF, Vance A, et al. Randomized double-blind multicentre placebo-controlled clinical trial of the clonidine adhesive patch for the treatment of tic disorders. *Aust N Z J Psychiatry*. 2008;42(9):807–813. https://doi.org/10.1080/00048670802277222

85. Boon-yasidhi V, Kim YS, Scahill L. An open-label, prospective study of guanfacine in children with ADHD and tic disorders. *J Med Assoc Thail*. 2005;88(suppl8):156–162.

86. Scahill L, Chappell PB, Kim YS, et al. A placebo-controlled study of guanfacine in the treatment of children with tic disorders and attention deficit hyperactivity disorder. *Am J Psychiatry*. 2001;158(7):1067–1074. https://doi.org/10.1176/appi.ajp.158.7.1067

87. Murphy TK, Fernandez T V., Coffey BJ, et al. Extended-release guanfacine does not show a large effect on tic severity in children with chronic tic disorders. *J Child Adolesc Psychopharmacol*. 2017;27(9):762–770. https://doi.org/10.1089/cap.2017.0024

88. Weisman H, Qureshi IA, Leckman JF, Scahill L, Bloch MH. Systematic review: pharmacological treatment of tic disorders—efficacy of antipsychotic and alpha-2 adrenergic agonist agents. *Neurosci Biobehav Rev*. 2013;37(6):1162–1171. https://doi.org/10.1016/j.neubiorev.2012.09.008

89. Caroff SN, Hurford I, Lybrand J, Campbell EC. Movement disorders induced by antipsychotic drugs: implications of the CATIE schizophrenia trial. *Neurol Clin*. 2011;37(1):127–148. https://doi.org/10.1016/j.ncl.2010.10.002

90. Scigliano G, Ronchetti G. Antipsychotic-induced metabolic and cardiovascular side effects in schizophrenia: a novel mechanistic hypothesis. *CNS Drugs*. 2013;27(4):249–257. https://doi.org/10.1007/s40263-013-0054-1

91. Brander G, Isomura K, Chang Z, et al. Association of Tourette syndrome and chronic tic disorder with metabolic and cardiovascular disorders. *JAMA Neurol*. 2019;76(4):454–461. https://doi.org/10.1001/jamaneurol.2018.4279

92. Sallee F, Kohegyi E, Zhao J, et al. Randomized, double-blind, placebo-controlled trial demonstrates the efficacy and safety of oral aripiprazole for the treatment of Tourette's disorder in children and adolescents. *J Child Adolesc Psychopharmacol*. 2017;27(9):771–781. https://doi.org/10.1089/cap.2016.0026

93. Dion Y, Annable L, Sandor P, Chouinard G. Risperidone in the treatment of Tourette syndrome: a double-blind, placebo-controlled trial. *J Clin Psychopharmacol*. 2002;22(1):31–39. https://doi.org/10.1097/00004714-200202000-00006

94. Scahill L, Leckman JF, Schultz RT, Katsovich L, Peterson BS. A placebo-controlled trial of risperidone in Tourette syndrome. *Neurology*. 2003;60(7):1130–1135. https://doi.org/10.1212/01.WNL.0000055434.39968.67

95. Bruggeman R, Van der Linden C, Buitelaar JK, Gericke GS, Hawkridge SM, Temlett JA. Risperidone versus pimozide in Tourette's disorder: a comparative double-blind parallel-group study. *J Clin Psychiatry*. 2001;62(1):50–56. https://doi.org/10.4088/JCP.v62n0111

96. Wijemanne S, Wu LJC, Jankovic J. Long-term efficacy and safety of fluphenazine in patients with Tourette syndrome. *Mov Disord*. 2014;29(1):126–130. https://doi.org/10.1002/mds.25692

97. Goetz CG, Tanner CM, Klawans HL. Fluphenazine and multifocal tic disorders. *Arch Neurol*. 1984;41(3):271–272. https://doi.org/10.1001/archneur.1984.04050150049015

98. Eggers C, Rothenberger A, Berghaus U. Clinical and neurobiological findings in children suffering from tic disease following treatment with tiapride. *Eur Arch Psychiatry Neurol Sci*. 1988;237(4):223–229. https://doi.org/10.1007/BF00449911

99. Roessner V, Schoenefeld K, Buse J, Bender S, Ehrlich S, Münchau A. Pharmacological treatment of tic disorders and Tourette syndrome. *Neuropharmacology*. 2013;68:143–149. https://doi.org/10.1016/j.neuropharm.2012.05.043

100. Macerollo A, Martino D, Cavanna AE, et al. Refractoriness to pharmacological treatment for tics: a multicentre European audit. *J Neurol Sci*. 2016;366:136–138. https://doi.org/10.1016/j.jns.2016.05.004

101. Stahl SM. Mechanism of action of vesicular monoamine transporter 2 (VMAT2) inhibitors in tardive dyskinesia: reducing dopamine leads to less "go" and more "stop" from the motor striatum for robust therapeutic effects. *CNS Spectr.* 2018;23(1):1–6. https://doi.org/10.1017/S1092852917000621

102. Chen JJ, Ondo WG, Dashtipour K, Swope DM. Tetrabenazine for the treatment of hyperkinetic movement disorders: a review of the literature. *Clin Ther.* 2012;34(7):1487–1504. https://doi.org/10.1016/j.clinthera.2012.06.010

103. Niemann N, Jankovic J. Real-world experience with VMAT2 inhibitors. *Clin Neuropharmacol.* 2019;42(2):37–41. https://doi.org/10.1097/WNF.0000000000000326

104. Coffey B, Jankovic J, Claassen DO, et al. Efficacy and safety of deutetrabenazine treatment for Tourette syndrome in children and adolescents: results from the ARTISTS 1 and ARTISTS 2 studies. In: *Virtual Conference—Tourette Association of America.* 2020. https://tourette.org/about-tourette/virtual-conference/. Accessed July 13, 2020.

105. Jankovic J, Jimenez-Shahed J, Brown LW. A randomised, double-blind, placebo-controlled study of topiramate in the treatment of Tourette syndrome. *J Neurol Neurosurg Psychiatry.* 2010;81(1):70–73. https://doi.org/10.1136/jnnp.2009.185348

106. Yang CS, Zhang LL, Zeng LN, Huang L, Liu YT. Topiramate for Tourette's syndrome in children: a meta-analysis. *Pediatr Neurol.* 2013;49(5):344–350. https://doi.org/10.1016/j.pediatrneurol.2013.05.002

107. Awaad Y, Michon AM, Minarik S, Rizk T. Levetiracetam in Tourette syndrome: a randomized double blind, placebo controlled study. *J Pediatr Neurol.* 2009;7(3):257–263. https://doi.org/10.3233/JPN-2009-0300

108. Hedderick EF, Morris CM, Singer HS. Double-blind, crossover study of clonidine and levetiracetam in Tourette syndrome. *Pediatr Neurol.* 2009;40(6):420–425. https://doi.org/10.1016/j.pediatrneurol.2008.12.014

109. Milosev LM, Psathakis N, Szejko N, Jakubovski E, Müller-Vahl KR. Treatment of Gilles de la Tourette Syndrome with cannabis-based medicine: results from a retrospective analysis and online survey. *Cannabis Cannabinoid Res.* 2019;4(4):265–274. https://doi.org/10.1089/can.2018.0050

110. Müller-Vahl KR, Schneider U, Prevedel H, et al. Δ9-tetrahydrocannabinol (THC) is effective in the treatment of tics in Tourette syndrome: a 6-week randomized trial. *J Clin Psychiatry.* 2003;64(4):459–465. https://doi.org/10.4088/JCP.v64n0417

111. Curtis A, Clarke CE, Rickards HE. Cannabinoids for Tourette's syndrome. *Cochrane Database Syst Rev.* 2009;4:CD006565. https://doi.org/10.1002/14651858.cd006565.pub2

112. Black N, Stockings E, Campbell G, et al. Cannabinoids for the treatment of mental disorders and symptoms of mental disorders: a systematic review and meta-analysis. *Lancet Psychiatry.* 2019;6(12):995–1010. https://doi.org/10.1016/S2215-0366(19)30401-8

113. Bellows S, Jankovic J. Treatment of dystonia and tics. *Clin Park Relat Disord.* 2020;2:12–19. https://doi.org/10.1016/j.prdoa.2019.11.005

114. Pandey S, Srivanitchapoom P, Kirubakaran R, Berman BD. Botulinum toxin for motor and phonic tics in Tourette's syndrome. *Cochrane Database Syst Rev.* 2018;1:CD012285. https://doi.org/10.1002/14651858.CD012285.pub2

115. Marras C, Andrews D, Sime E, Lang AE. Botulinum toxin for simple motor tics: a randomized, double-blind, controlled clinical trial. *Neurology.* 2001;56(5):605–610. https://doi.org/10.1212/WNL.56.5.605

116. Kwak CH, Hanna PA, Jankovic J. Botulinum toxin in the treatment of tics. *Arch Neurol.* 2000;57(8):1190–1193. https://doi.org/10.1001/archneur.57.8.1190

117. Krauss JK, Jankovic J. Severe motor tics causing cervical myelopathy in Tourette's syndrome. *Mov Disord.* 1996;11(5):563–566. https://doi.org/10.1002/mds.870110512

118. Martinez-Ramirez D, Jimenez-Shahed J, Leckman JF, et al. Efficacy and safety of deep brain stimulation in Tourette syndrome: the international Tourette syndrome deep brain stimulation public database and registry. *JAMA Neurol.* 2018;75(3):353–359. https://doi.org/10.1001/jamaneurol.2017.4317

119. Kefalopoulou Z, Zrinzo L, Jahanshahi M, et al. Bilateral globus pallidus stimulation for severe Tourette's syndrome: a double-blind, randomised crossover trial. *Lancet Neurol.* 2015;14(6):595–605. https://doi.org/10.1016/S1474-4422(15)00008-3

120. Baldermann JC, Schüller T, Huys D, et al. Deep brain stimulation for Tourette-syndrome: a systematic review and meta-analysis. *Brain Stimul.* 2016;9(2):296–304. https://doi.org/10.1016/j.brs.2015.11.005

121. Mahajan U V., Purger DA, Mantovani A, et al. Deep brain stimulation results in greater symptomatic improvement in Tourette syndrome than conservative measures: a meta-analysis. *Stereotact Funct Neurosurg.* 2020:1–8. https://doi.org/10.1159/000507059

15
Huntington's Disease

Natalia Pessoa Rocha, Andy Liu, Karen Anderson, and Erin Furr Stimming

Introduction

Huntington's disease (HD) is an inherited, neurodegenerative disease that encompasses a triad of motor, cognitive, and behavioral features.[1] HD is traditionally classified as a movement disorder, as its formal diagnosis is based on the unequivocal presence of otherwise unexplained extrapyramidal motor symptoms, mainly chorea, dystonia, and parkinsonism.[1,2] Chorea is the most prominent symptom in adult- or late-onset HD. Incoordination, bradykinesia, and rigidity tend to predominate in young-onset HD and in the late stages of the more common adult-onset HD.[1] While the presence of motor symptoms is required for the clinical diagnosis of HD, cognitive impairment is also a core characteristic of the disease and can emerge years before the diagnosis.[3] Along with motor and cognitive changes, behavioral problems complete the triad of signs and symptoms that characterize HD. Psychiatric disorders can be present across all stages of HD, often preceding the development of motor symptoms. Although not universal, they are common and may be a cause of significant distress in HD. Psychiatric manifestations in HD include depression, irritability, apathy, obsessions, and occasionally psychosis.[4]

HD is an autosomal dominant disease caused by a CAG repeat expansion in the *huntingtin (HTT)* gene on chromosome 4p16.3,[5] which encodes an abnormally long polyglutamine repeat in the huntingtin protein (HTT).[6] Penetrance of HD is classified according to the number of repeats as age-dependent (36–39) or full (≥40), although intermediate alleles (27–35 repeats) are susceptible to instability and expansion, and HD phenotype and pathology have been reported in this range.[1] Therefore, a definitive CAG repeat diagnostic cut-off is not clear.

Males and females are affected equally. The incidence of HD was estimated to be of 0.38 per 100,000 per year, and the worldwide service-based prevalence of HD 2.71 per 100,000, based on a meta-analysis.[7] However, prevalence estimates vary across the world. For example, the ascertained prevalence of HD in Asia is much lower than in Western populations. The estimated prevalence of HD in North America, northwestern Europe, and Australia ranges from 5.96 to 13.7 cases per 100,000 population.[8]

The pathological hallmark of HD is the inclusion of mutant HTT aggregates in neuronal nuclei, cytoplasm, dendrites, and axon terminals. The localization of visible aggregates does not correlate well with cell death, corroborating the hypothesis that they are, at least in part, a protective cellular response to misfolded protein.[6] Striatal degeneration is the main change observed in HD brains, where neuronal loss is accompanied by prominent astrocytosis.[9] Accordingly, structural brain imaging shows a gradual constant decrease in striatal volume in HD.[10] Striatal changes occur early in the disease course, and are observed in HD gene carriers who are more than 15 years before the predicted onset of diagnosable features. In addition, the atrophy rates are significantly associated with the CAG repeat length.[11,12] Other subcortical regions (e.g., globus pallidus, thalamus, and hippocampus) and cortical gray matter also undergo atrophy in HD, although less noticeably than in the striatum.[11]

Although the mutation that causes HD was discovered almost 30 years ago, the mechanisms underlying neuronal death/dysfunction in HD are not completely understood. Similar to other neurodegenerative diseases, protein misfolding is regarded as the primary mechanism related to HD pathogenesis. However, it is not clear how the expanded HTT causes neuronal death in specific brain regions, as HTT is expressed robustly in all brain regions. Several mechanisms have been proposed to explain the selective neuronal vulnerability, including excitotoxicity, inflammation, and the quinolinic acid pathway. Yet, this topic is still a matter of debate.[6]

Natural History of HD

The course of HD can be divided into premanifest and manifest periods.[1] Manifest HD has traditionally been defined based on a motor examination that identifies the disease "motor onset," i.e., when an HD gene expansion carrier receives a score of 4 in the diagnostic confidence level (DCL) of the Huntington Disease Rating Scale (UHDRS). The UHDRS is currently the most commonly used clinical and research tool for the assessment of motor function, cognitive function, behavioral abnormalities, and functional capacity in HD. The DCL = 4 refers to the expert rater's confidence (≥99%) that the observed motor abnormalities are unequivocal signs of HD.[1,2] HD gene carriers who do not meet the DCL 4 criterion have historically been considered premanifest. It is worth mentioning that cognitive and behavioral symptoms commonly occur years before the motor onset, and the concept of "manifest HD" should not lead to the misunderstanding of actual disease onset, or a false dichotomy between sick and well, as HD onset is actually a process that occurs gradually, even over decades.[1] On the other hand, the use of motor onset to classify manifest vs. premanifest HD is justified by the fact that it is the more overt and consistently agreed disease feature among the considerable clinical phenotypic heterogeneity of the disease.[1]

More recently, a task force commissioned by the Movement Disorder Society suggested modifying the current diagnostic criteria to more broadly incorporate clinical features of HD. They proposed adding nonmotor signs, particularly cognitive signs, to current motor diagnostic criteria. Accordingly, HD gene carriers should be diagnosed as manifest HD if they present a DCL = 4 or a DCL = 3 plus minor or major neurocognitive changes.[13]

Premanifest HD can be subdivided into presymptomatic (when HD gene carriers cannot be clinically distinguished from noncarriers) and prodromal phases (characterized by subtle motor, cognitive, and behavioral changes).[1] Regarding the manifest period, there are five stages based on the total functional capacity score, which reflects independence in five domains: occupation, ability to manage finances, ability to perform domestic chores, ability to perform personal activities of daily living, and setting for the level of care.[2,14,15] However, this classification is merely a description of the continuously changing functionality, instead of reflecting biological events that can affect prognosis and treatments.[1] Therefore, experts recommend that manifest HD be divided into three phases: early, moderate, and late stages. In early-stage HD, individuals are largely functional and independent. In moderate-stage

HD, individuals lose the ability to perform complex tasks, such as work, drive, and manage finances, but will be able to perform activities of daily living, such as eat, dress, and personal hygiene. In late-stage HD, individuals require assistance in all activities of daily living.[16]

The age of motor onset in HD strongly depends on the individuals' CAG repeat length.[17] It is possible to estimate the age of motor onset by calculating the CAG-Age Product (CAP). The original study about this topic demonstrated that this index was a good predictor of striatal pathology in postmortem evaluations of brains of people with HD.[18] Later, the CAP score was improved to serve as a proxy of disease severity or disease burden, based on the cumulative exposure to mutant HTT toxicity. In this regard, the CAP score is currently used to predict time to motor symptoms onset.[19]

More recently, the CAP has been defined as:

$$CAP = AGE \times (CAG - L) / K$$

where AGE is the current age of the individual, CAG is the repeat length, and L and K are constants. L is an estimate of the lower limit of the CAG expansion at which phenotypic expression of the effects of mutant HTT could be observed, and K is a normalizing constant. In the CAP proposed by Warner and Sampaio, L = 30 and K = 6.27, and the CAP will be equal to 100 at the subject's expected age of motor symptoms onset.[20]

As previously mentioned, the decrease in volumes of the striatum (and less pronounced in other subcortical areas and in the cortex) initiates very early in the HD course, but it is faster in individuals close to predicted onset, remaining fairly constant throughout the disease course.[11,12]

Motor Symptoms in HD

Chorea is the most prominent and the most recognized symptom, but other motor abnormalities occur, such as dystonia, bradykinesia, rigidity, myoclonus, tics, and tremor.[21] Chorea predominates early in the disease course and typically progresses through the middle stages of HD, but often declines as rigidity increases in the later stages.[16]

Chorea is characterized by irregular muscle contractions in the facial muscles, trunk, and extremities. These movements can contribute to social embarrassment, sleep interruptions, falls, and physical injuries.[22] Currently, there are two approved treatments for chorea in the United States, both of which are VMAT2 inhibitors: deutetrabenazine and tetrabenazine.[23] With any VMAT2 inhibitors, there are possible increased risks of depression, suicidality, and parkinsonism.[23] Experts agree that off-label use of antipsychotics, such as haloperidol or risperidone, can be effective when chorea is accompanied by behavioral symptoms (or neuropsychiatric symptoms) or for individuals who do not tolerate VMAT2 inhibitors.[22,24] Amantadine has also been suggested as an option for chorea treatment in HD in evidence-based guidelines,[23] although the degree of benefit is still unknown. Two placebo-controlled clinical trials yielded conflicting results.[25,26] When a meta-analysis was performed as part of the Cochrane review, the pooled result did not significantly favor the use of amantadine for the control of chorea.[27] As a result there is disagreement between experts about the use of amantadine for chorea in HD.[24]

Impairments in balance and coordination eventually occur in virtually all patients with HD. Physical therapy interventions can mitigate the impact of these symptoms. Expert consensus guidelines found a high level of support for aerobic exercise, alone or in combination with resistance training and supervised gait training.[28] There is some evidence to support inspiratory and expiratory training, training of transfers, rising from the floor, and providing strategies for caregivers to facilitate patient involvement in physical activities.

Dysphagia and dysarthria are also common in HD, with onset in early or middle stages and progression as the disease advances. Both swallowing and speech therapy can be helpful for patients.[21] A speech pathologist can assist with recommendations of diet modification and safe swallow techniques to minimize the risk of aspiration. Later in the disease, discussions about percutaneous endoscopic gastrostomy (PEG) placement may be indicated, depending on patient and family preferences. Speech therapy is often implemented to address dysarthria. Word-boards to allow patients to point to what they want to say, and other communication strategies can help alleviate the frustration patients and caregivers experience when their communication is limited.

Dystonia can emerge in mid- to late-stage HD, but it is quite common in juvenile and the adult-onset rigid-dystonic variant of HD.[16] Dystonia is characterized by repetitive unwanted muscle contractions that result in a twisted appearance. Benzodiazepines, baclofen, and other muscle relaxants can be effective pharmacological treatments for dystonia and dopaminergics can treat parkinsonism, most commonly seen in juvenile HD.[22] For focal dystonia, botulinum toxin injections can be effective.[22] More recently, Saft et al. found cannabinoids effective for the treatment of dystonia in HD, which also improved mood and other physical markers such as fine motor skills and gait.[29]

Cognitive Impairment in HD

Cognitive symptoms in HD are extremely disabling for many individuals with the disease, particularly because this may begin long before the onset of motor symptoms, resulting in earlier disability. Well-characterized, large studies of people at risk for HD, but who do not have motor symptoms of the illness have shown that those with HD genetic mutation expansions have deficits in multiple cognitive domains compared to those without expansions.[30,31]

Cognitive impairment is a core feature of HD and it will occur in all HD gene carriers, yet symptoms are heterogeneous and the cognitive disorder will manifest differently in each individual. It is worth mentioning that the cognitive tests often have a motor component, and the variability of symptoms in different phases of the disease may be at least partly due to psychomotor slowing and/or other motor skill impairment.[32] The cognitive deficits in HD are characterized by cognitive slowing and difficulties in attention, planning, mental flexibility, visuospatial functions, and emotion recognition. Learning and retrieval of new information are also impaired, but language is relatively preserved in HD. The clinical picture of the cognitive impairment in HD encompasses cognitive and psychiatric realms of function, including problems with initiation, lack of awareness of deficits, and disinhibition.[1]

There is very little information, other than expert opinion, on the treatment of cognitive symptoms in HD. Unfortunately, no medications, including acetylcholinesterase inhibitors,[33,34] have been proven to improve cognitive function in HD.[22] The consensus is to decrease and stop all medication that may be sedating or add to the confusion, or to use these medications at the lowest dose possible if they must be continued. Off-label use of memantine is sometimes helpful in slowing cognitive decline.[22]

Psychiatric Syndromes in HD

Virtually all HD gene carriers will experience psychiatric and behavioral problems at some point in the disease course. These symptoms occur from early to late stages, and they are more variable than the motor and cognitive features observed in HD.[1] The neuropsychiatric and behavioral signs and symptoms of HD encompass the full spectrum of psychiatric illness, and people with HD will typically experience multiple symptoms or disorders. These can result from the underlying progressive neurodegeneration but can also be a psychological reaction to the burden posed by the possibility or knowledge of being a gene carrier. Some medications can also contribute to the development or worsening of neuropsychiatric and behavioral symptoms in HD. For example, VMAT2 inhibitors used to treat chorea may worsen apathy, depression, and other psychiatric symptoms.[35] It should also be noted that many psychiatric scales developed for general populations, when used in HD, especially those which include somatic queries, might be artificially elevated by HD-specific symptoms and signs.

Depression

Depression is a well-documented disorder among HD patients. Studies indicate that anywhere from 28.6% to 65.4% of HD patients develop depression at some point.[36,37] The risk of developing depression is not only higher than in the general population but also than other neurodegenerative disorders.[38]

There are multiple environmental and pathophysiological risk factors associated with the development of depression in HD. Environmental factors that affect patients at disease onset often include increased disability, coping with a terminal illness, and dealing with grief.[39] Marder et al.[40] showed that depression was the only psychiatric symptom in HD that was associated with the rate of decline of independence as measured on the independence scale. However, other work has not shown an association between depression in HD with cognitive impairment, motor impairment, CAG repeat length, or sex.[41,42]

Degeneration of the orbitofrontal cortices is thought to play a large role in the development of depression in HD.[38,39] In particular, specific connections associated with the default mode network and basal ganglia in premanifest HD patients seem to be involved in the development of depression.[43] Dale et al. found that depression could be predicted by the stage of disease.[42]

Depression not only affects the daily life of the patient but also has clinical significance as a potential indicator of future development of HD.[44] It is one of the first symptoms reported by family members of patients who go on to develop HD and has a significant negative impact on the prognosis of the disease.[45,46] Like many psychiatric symptoms in HD, the patient often has poor recognition and insight.

Suicidal Ideation

Suicide is the third leading cause of death in HD.[47] HD patients are more likely to commit suicide than the general population, with reported odds of the death being due to suicide in the HD individuals being as high as 8.2 times that of controls.[47–49] Not only do HD patients have a higher risk of suicide than the general population, but they also have a higher risk compared to patients of other neurological diseases such as Alzheimer's and Parkinson's.[50] Considering this well-documented risk, it is important to further understand potential risk factors for suicide ideation (SI).

Research has been varied in the role of sex on SI risk in HD patients. Hayden et al. found that among an HD population in South Africa, females were more likely to have attempted suicide while males were more likely to be successful in their suicide attempt,[51] consistent with the general population. Anderson et al. did not see a significant association between gender and suicide attempts in people at risk for HD.[52] Multiple studies have found that risk of suicide is greatest during the early stages of the disease even before diagnosis.[49,50,53]

SI is closely linked with sociodemographic factors of the patient and their quality of life.[54] Many of the psychiatric symptoms of HD have been associated with increased SI. Among patients who are at risk for HD, depression was significantly associated with SI.[52,55] Among manifest HD patients, depression continues to be strongly correlated with SI.[54,55] Other psychiatric symptoms such as anxiety, aggression, irritability, and elevated motor scores have also been associated with SI among patients at risk for HD.[52] Hubers et al. however, did not find an association between motor scores or CAG expansion length and SI among manifest HD patients.[55] Impulsivity and lack of future planning may also contribute.

Effectively querying for suicidality even in the absence of classic depressive symptoms is important. There are two critical periods for increased suicide risk in HD: just before receiving a formal diagnosis, and when independence decreases.[56]

Irritability

Irritability is a well-documented psychiatric symptom among HD patients with studies reporting anywhere from 38% to 73% of patients experiencing irritability.[57,58] Vaccarino et al. found that irritability was the most frequently recorded symptom among pre-HD and early HD patients.[59] Irritability begins before the manifestation of motor symptoms and may continue throughout the stages of HD.[60,61]

These findings suggest that irritability is more of a pathophysiological effect of HD because increasing disability due to motor difficulties does not significantly increase irritability in patients.[62] Anxiety is a symptom that is significantly linked with the development of irritability.[54] Dale and van Duijin found that suicide ideation did not have a significant influence on irritability.[63] Irritability has not been found to correlate with CAG expansion length.[57,64]

Aggression

Aggression is defined as overt behavior, physical or verbal, that threatens the individual or others.[65] Aggression is a well-documented psychiatric disorder among the HD population, with rates varying from a low of 3.6% to a high of 65.2%.[66] Studies that found lower rates only considered aggression documented as the primary reason for hospitalization and it is likely that most instances of aggression do not result in hospitalization.[66]

There are mixed reports of aggression frequency through the different stages of HD. Dewherst et al. suggested that aggression is most prominent in patients who are in the early stages of the disease.[67] In contrast, Craufurd et al. found aggression peaked toward the mid and late stages of the disease.[57] Similarly, van Duijn et al. found that aggression increased with progression of the disease.[68] Thus, the more recent consensus is that aggression increases with the stage of HD. Some studies have concluded that aggression affects both male and female patients equally.[57,69,70] However, other studies have found a higher risk of aggression in male HD patients.[66,71,72]

There are multiple studies that associate aggression in HD patients with other psychiatric symptoms that develop during the course of the disease. Anderson et al. found aggression to be positively correlated with obsessive-compulsive disorder.[73] Other studies have also found suicide ideation to be associated with aggressin.[55,74] In addition to the association with psychiatric symptoms, Grimbergen et al. found that patients who experienced more falls or dealt with more severe motor symptoms had higher rates of aggression.[75]

Apathy

Apathy is considered one of the most distressing psychiatric symptoms of HD to caregivers and a strong predictor of future genetic testing for those at risk of HD.[76] Apathy can be distinguished from depression by diminished motivation as opposed to the emotional distress and sad affect seen in depression.[77] More than 50% of patients with HD exhibit signs of apathy.[78]

Apathy seems to increase with the progression of HD. Fritz et al. found that apathy increased significantly from prodromal to manifest HD.[79] Yang et al. found a statistically significant increase in apathy with patients at later stages of HD.[80] This increase in apathy as HD progresses could potentially be explained by the influence of other HD psychiatric symptoms. CAG length may correlate positively with the risk of apathy.[79] Duff et al. found that CAG expanded premanifest patients had significantly higher levels of apathy and executive dysfunction than patients who were at risk but did not have the CAG expansion.[3] Mason et al. found that apathy was linked with depression,[81] while Bouwens et al. found that apathy had a strong correlation with irritability in patients with HD.[82] Additionally, the progression of motor impairment in HD may also be associated with the degree of apathy in the individual.[79] The positive correlation between apathy, CAG length, and motor symptoms suggests that apathy is correlated with disease progression. It is worth mentioning that apathy and lack of insight both contribute to poor care in this population. Anecdotally, it is rare for a symptomatic HD patient to seek medical attention unless compelled to by the family.

Anxiety

Anxiety is a documented psychiatric symptom of HD that is typically characterized by undue worry and unease among patients. There is a lack of expert consensus on the exact prevalence of anxiety as scales used to assess anxiety may be falsely elevated by other HD features.[35] However, some studies have roughly estimated anxiety to be present in about 50% of HD patients.[57] The prevalence of anxiety among HD patients was found to range from 34% to 61%.[58]

Anxiety often precedes the manifestation of motor symptoms of HD.[35] That said, HD patients rarely have an anxious affect and usually appear more indifferent/apathetic. Prodromal anxiety is sometimes thought to be due to anxiety about the possible development of the disease or receiving the genetic test results.[83] Orvoen et al. demonstrated that knock-in mice with the *HTT* gene show increased levels of anxiety, particularly male mice, which may hint at a potential pathophysiological link of HD to anxiety.[84] Some studies have reported that as HD progresses anxiety increases as a byproduct of communication and motor difficulties.[35] Another study reported that motor symptoms as measured by chorea and other aberrant motor behavior was not associated with anxiety.[85] Younger patients with HD tend to report higher levels of anxiety than their older counterparts.[86] Neither CAG repeat length nor sex has been correlated with the development of anxiety.[42,87]

Perseveration/Obsessive-Compulsive Symptoms

Perseveration is defined as a repetitive behavior that has outlasted the initial stimuli. Studies have found that rates of perseveration among HD patients anywhere from 24% to 75%.[57,88] These reported rates may be even lower than in practice because patients with high levels of perseveration may often choose not to participate in clinical studies. Obsessive-compulsive symptoms (OCs) are very common in the HD population. OCs are defined by the American Psychiatric Association as the persistence of thought that is distressing accompanied by repeated compulsive behaviors to help relieve the distressing thoughts. Van Djuin et al. found a prevalence of OCs varying from 10% to 52% of patients with HD.[58] Perseveration and OCs are often grouped together due to the behavioral and intervention similarities between the two.[89] The content of OCs commonly observed in HD is dissimilar from obsessive-compulsive disorder (OCD), as HD patients seldom have checking behavior or dirt/germ avoidance. In addition, unlike individuals with OCD, HD gene carriers often lack insight into the symptoms and are not troubled by them. In sum, the majority of OCs in HD are better defined as perseverative behaviors.[89]

Perseveration is often associated with frontal lobe damage. Dysfunction particularly in the orbitofrontal cortex may be responsible for the development of perseveration.[73,90] OCs, on the other hand, are believed to be caused by dysfunction of the striatum of the basal ganglia.[91] Perseveration has been linked with increased suicidal ideation and is an important consideration when treating patients with HD.[92]

Sleep Disorders

Sleep disorders are common, but can be underreported in HD. Studies using objective measures of sleep quality (e.g., polysomnography and actigraphy) have reported sleep disturbances in virtually all HD gene carriers. The sleep disturbances observed in HD include circadian rhythm disturbances,[93] increased sleep onset latency, sleep fragmentation and frequent nocturnal awakenings, reduced sleep efficiency, delayed and shortened rapid eye movement (REM) sleep, and increased periodic leg movements.[94–97] Nevertheless, self-reported sleep problems in HD might be reduced because patients with HD do not demonstrate excessive daytime sleepiness (EDS)[95,98] or do not report it, likely due to anosognosia. As a result, sleep dysfunction in HD is likely to be underdiagnosed by clinicians and underreported by patients,[98] a phenomenon that impacts directly on patients' adequate treatment. When asked directly about the quality of their sleep, almost 90% of patients with HD acknowledged having sleep problems.[99] Most of them (~60%) rated sleep difficulties as either "very important" or "moderately important" components of their overall health problems.[99] The sleep disorders are reported throughout the course of the illness, from prodromal to advanced stages, where it may be more prevalent and can adversely impact cognition.[98,100] Comorbid psychiatric symptoms can contribute to sleep impairment; the presence of chorea can interfere with sleep onset in HD. Conversely, poor sleep quality can negatively impact other disease symptoms and can further impair cognitive and functional capacities in HD.

Psychotic Symptoms

Psychosis is the presence of prominent delusions and/or hallucinations. Although the prevalence of psychosis in HD is usually considered relatively low compared to other neuropsychiatric conditions, such as Parkinson's disease, they do occur in 3%–11% of patients with HD.[58,68,78] One study, using less stringent criteria, found them to be present in nearly 18% of people with HD.[101] Psychotic symptoms may be easily missed, masked if an antipsychotic is used for another indication, or remain undiagnosed at advanced stages of disease when patients have severe impairment in communication. When psychotic symptoms occur in HD, comorbid schizophrenia spectrum or mood disorders with psychotic features may be the cause. Psychotic symptoms may also occur in HD due to delirium resulting from infections, electrolyte imbalance, and other medical conditions. It may be difficult to distinguish delusions from perseverative symptoms, particularly when perseveration is very prominent or fixated on bizarre questions or ideas.

Psychotic symptoms may be associated with worse outcomes in HD, including impaired function, cognition, and worse concomitant psychiatric symptoms, compared to patients without these symptoms.[68,101] Patients with psychotic symptoms may also have less severe chorea.[101]

Sexual Disorders

Sexual disorders may be quite common in HD, as in other neurological disorders. They were included in the original description of the condition, in 1872: "two married men with HD who are constantly making love to some ladies, not seeming to be aware that there is any impropriety in it and they never let go an opportunity to flirt with a girl."[102]

Different sexual disorders may occur in HD, and they may be caused by the progression of the disease, medication side effects, and comorbidities like depression, anxiety, or dementia. Motor symptoms, personality changes, and knowledge of possible genetic transmission of the disease to potential children may also affect sexual function.

A recent review of the literature found the following disorders were the most commonly reported by patients with HD and their caregivers: hypoactive sexual disorder (53%–83% of patients), hyperactive sexual disorder (6%–30%), erectile (48%–74%) and ejaculatory dysfunctions (30%–65%), lubrication problems (53%–83%), and orgasmic dysfunction (35%–78%).[103]

There has been little work on the impact of sexual dysfunction in HD. One small study found a significant impact of HD on women's sexual function that worsened with the disease stage and impaired quality of life.[104] Another small study by the same group found a similar worsening of sexual dysfunction with the disease stage progression in men with HD.[105]

Disinhibition and Impulsivity

Disinhibited and impulsive behaviors are reported in people with HD, even before the onset of motor symptoms. Disinhibition is more prevalent among premanifest HD gene carriers in comparison with people from HD families who do not have the expansion mutation.[3] Disinhibition is likely due to disruption of frontal-striatal circuitry, which is also related to impulsive or risky behaviors, apathy, and executive dysfunction, all of which are seen in HD.[106] Disinhibition has also been proposed as an important risk factor for suicide, although there is no data corroborating this hypothesis yet. In general, there has been little formal study of impulsivity in HD despite this anecdotally being a very prominent feature.

Treatment of Psychiatric Symptoms in HD

The management of neuropsychiatric symptoms in HD can be complex because multiple syndromes often coexist and treatment decisions should attempt to cover all symptoms while limiting polypharmacy.[35] The treatment of psychiatric symptoms in HD lacks high-quality controlled data, so most recommendations are based on case series and expert opinion. Early identification and treatment is very important for at-risk, premanifest, and manifest HD populations. There is a need to ask specifically for classically underreported symptoms (e.g., irritability and emotional dyscontrol), which are often deleterious to home and social environments.[56] Antidepressants, neuroleptics, and mood stabilizers are often used to treat the neuropsychiatric symptoms in HD. Interdisciplinary, nonpharmacological treatments are also important, these include physical, occupational, and speech therapy, psychotherapy, genetic counseling, nutrition, and social work services.[56] Behavioral adjustment, counseling, and other nonpharmacological interventions can be effective, particularly for early manifest and prodromal populations, although lack of insight in this population can be problematic. Caregiver behavioral modification and environmental adjustments can help ease symptoms such as anxiety or apathy that may have a cognitive component.[56]

The use of standard medication classes, such as selective serotonin reuptake inhibitors (SSRIs) or tricyclic antidepressants (TCAs) are applicable for depressive symptoms in the HD population. These drugs are also used for other neuropsychiatric symptoms, such as OCs (SSRIs or clomipramine) and anxiety. According to expert-based consensus guidelines, SSRIs are preferred for the treatment of anxiety as an isolated symptom or when coexisting with depression or obsessive perseverative behaviors. Alternative serotonergic drugs (nonselective serotonin reuptake inhibitors, clomipramine) are pharmacologic options if the initial SSRI is ineffective or not tolerated.[35] Sedating antidepressants such as mirtazapine or trazodone are pharmacologic options for treating sleep disorders in HD. Expert consensus is that selection of treatment for sleep disorders in HD is dependent on presence of comorbid symptoms and may vary with stage of disease. Many drugs approved for treatment of insomnia in the general population (e.g., benzodiazepines) may be associated with adverse effects in HD, including fatigue, slowing of cognitive processing, and balance impairment.[35] Indeed, the use of a benzodiazepine is discouraged in ambulatory individuals unless all other options have failed.[35] When needed, benzodiazepines should be started at a very low dose, gradually titrated, and then tapered off when no longer necessary.[56]

SSRIs are also the initial choice in the treatment of irritability. Antipsychotic drugs can also be used for mild, moderate, and severe irritability.[107] Of note, if manifestations of acute irritability are present, such as aggression and impulsivity, antipsychotics (e.g., olanzapine, risperidone, and quetiapine) may be preferred as a first-line choice. Likewise, "atypical" antipsychotic drugs that still markedly block dopamine receptors, e.g., olanzapine and risperidone, should be used when both chorea and irritability/aggression are present. However, potential side effects include weight gain, metabolic syndrome, and tardive dyskinesia.[108]

Antipsychotics are the treatment of choice for psychosis in HD. Side effect profiles usually guide medication choice—e.g., a more sedating antipsychotic for a patient with agitation and psychosis. Many practitioners choose a second-generation antipsychotic, but a first-generation antipsychotic may be preferable for patients with significant chorea.[35] Clozapine may be considered as a treatment for psychosis in HD when symptoms have not responded to adequate trials of one or two other antipsychotic drugs, as long as patients are able and willing to cooperate with agranulocytosis monitoring.

The treatment of sexual disorders in HD is similar to the approach used in the general population. This includes limiting, when possible, medications with effects on sexual function (e.g., SSRI antidepressants, which can cause hypoactive sexual disorder) and treatment of other underlying medical conditions that may contribute to sexual dysfunction. In contrast, SSRIs could be considered to treat hypersexuality.

For apathy, it is worth trying at first a nonsedating antidepressant, such as an SSRI or buproprion, even if the person does not meet the criteria for depression. Anecdotal reports have been published of the successful treatment of apathy in HD with amantadine, bromocriptine, and selegiline. Individuals with primary apathy sometimes respond to psychostimulants such as methylphenidate or dextroamphetamine. However, these medicines should be used with caution as they are highly abusable, worsen chorea, and may exacerbate irritability.[22]

Disease-Modifying Therapies and Future Treatment for Huntington's Disease

As discussed in the previous sections, a variety of symptomatic treatments are currently available for individuals with HD, and they can improve patients' functionality and quality of life. However, there is not yet an available treatment with proven efficacy to modify HD progression. Recent advances in the field promise an exciting era for clinical trials in HD. The current and future trials are focused on reducing the amount of mutant HTT (mHTT) by inhibiting the synthesis of mHTT and modulating HTT homeostasis.

Lowering mHTT levels strategies include inhibiting mRNA synthesis by blocking transcription (Zinc finger proteins, ZFP), avoiding post-transcriptional processes, and stimulating early mRNA degradation with antisense oligonucleotides (ASO) or inhibiting mRNA translation with small interfering RNA (siRNA).[109] The ASOs are clinically the farthest along in the development of disease-modifying therapies for HD. After positive results in preclinical studies, the first human clinical trial with a non-allele-specific ASO designed to lower HTT was performed by Ionis Pharmaceuticals in collaboration with Roche (NCT02519036). The results of the clinical trial suggested that the ASO was safe, well tolerated, and associated with a ~40% reduction in CSF mHTT concentration at the two highest doses (90 and 120 mg). This reduction may correspond to a 55%–85% reduction in cortical mHTT levels. In addition, there was a correlation between the reduction in the CSF levels of mHTT and improvements in the composite Unified Huntington Disease Rating Scale (cUHDRS) score.[110] These results motivated the execution of two open-label extensions (NCT03342053 and NCT03842969) and a phase 3, randomized, double-blind, placebo-controlled study that will evaluate the safety and efficacy of the same ASO (tominersen) in patients with manifest HD (NCT03761849). However, the independent data monitoring committee (iDMC) recently recommended stopping dosing in all study arms based on an overall benefit/risk assessment of data through 17 months. No new safety concerns were identified, but tominersen was found to be comparable or unfavorable to placebo in functional, motor, and cognitive assessments. Importantly, the iDMC recommended continuing the study to follow participants for safety and clinical outcomes, which will help significantly advance the understanding of HTT-lowering therapies.

Although the ASOs have demonstrated efficacy in reducing the CSF levels of HTT, the clinical relevance is still a matter of debate, especially because basal mutant protein levels are still detected and the treatment decreases both wild-type HTT and mHTT levels. Given that HTT is a highly conserved protein with several important cellular functions,[111] it is necessary to define the impact of wild-type HTT reduction in future investigations. In this regard, the use of allele-specific ASOs is an interesting alternative. There are two randomized, double-blind, placebo-controlled, phase Ia/IIb trials studying allele-specific ASOs, WVE-120101 (PRECISION-HD1) and WVE-120102 (PRECISION-HD2) (NCT03225833 and NCT03225846, respectively) sponsored by Wave Life Sciences and Takeda Pharmaceutical Company. A preliminary announcement of results from the PRECISION-HD2 trial (NCT03225846) reported that this drug was considered to be generally safe and well tolerated among patients receiving doses up to 16 mg. In comparison with placebo, the WVE-120102 treatment (all doses pooled together) resulted in a reduction of CSF mHTT by 12.4%, while CSF total HTT remained unchanged. A higher dosage cohort (32 mg) was then added to both trials.[112] However, the most recent updates from the broader PRECISION-HD program were disappointing, as the trial results did not support further development of either WVE-120102 or WVE-120101. Overall, the treatments resulted in either modest reductions or no statistically significant changes in mHTT levels in comparison with placebo. Participants still have a final follow-up visit but will receive no further doses. A final, complete set of analyses is expected soon and Wave Life Sciences has announced a new investigational oligonucleotide (WVE-003) that has been developed to target SNP3, which is associated with mHTT. This phase 1b/2a study was designed to provide proof of concept of the safety, tolerability, and pharmacodynamic effects of WVE-003 in early manifest HD, and it is expected to be launched soon.

Other strategies to silence or edit the mutant *HTT* were developed in preclinical models and are promising approaches for clinical trials in HD. These potential modalities involve the neutralization of targeted mRNA molecules by employing siRNA and artificial microRNA (miRNA), thus inhibiting gene expression or translation, a process known as RNA interference (RNAi).[113,114] A clinical trial with a gene therapy product (AMT-130) has been recently launched by UniQure Biopharma B.V. (NCT04120493). AM-130 consists of an engineered miRNA targeting human *HTT* mRNA, delivered via AAV vector serotype 5 (AAV5-miHTT). One-time intrastriatal (brain) administration of AAV5-miHTT in transgenic HD minipigs resulted in a strong, widespread, and sustained (up to 12 months) reduction of mHTT levels, supporting a proof of concept. The UniQure trial using this technology in early manifest HD patients is evaluating the safety, tolerability, of a single-time bilateral intrastriatal injection of AAV5-miHTT in adults (25 to 65 years of age), comparing with sham injection, for disease progression.

Despite the great advance in therapies lowering mHTT, many questions remain such as the long-term safety of these treatments, especially regarding the decrease in wild-type HTT levels, and the clinical significance of mHTT lowering. In this regard, the Clustered Regularly Interspaced Short Palindromic Repeats / CRISPR-associated (Cas)9 (CRISPR/Cas9) system has emerged as an option due to its potency and sequence specificity, thus mitigating the expression of the mutant allele only. Accordingly, CRISPR/Cas9 has been regarded as a promising therapy for HD and several other diseases in which DNA editing can be beneficial. The CRISPR/Cas system is used by bacterial immune systems in order to cleave foreign DNA. The CRISPR/Cas-9 technology was used in fibroblasts of an HD patient to delete the promoter regions, transcription start site, and the CAG mutation expansion of the mutant *HTT* gene, resulting in complete inactivation of the mutant allele without affecting the normal allele.[115] Recently, the method was successfully tested in an HD rodent model (HD140Q-knock-in mice). The CRISPR/Cas9-mediated inactivation efficiently depleted HTT, reversing the HD-associated neuropathology and behavioral phenotypes. The decrease of mHTT expression in striatal neuronal cells in adult HD140Q-knock-in mice did not affect cell viability but improved motor deficits.[116] Despite the positive results obtained from preclinical studies, several issues must be addressed before bringing CRISPR/Cas9 technologies into humans, such as: (1) the fact that it is an irreversible method; (2) there are ethical concerns regarding germline alteration; (3) delivery problems as with other viral-delivered approaches; and (4) immunogenicity of bacterial proteins.[117]

Conclusions

HD is a complex neurodegenerative disease that encompasses motor, cognitive, and psychiatric/behavioral syndromes. Although there is not yet an approved disease-modifying treatment for HD, there are effective available symptomatic pharmacologic and nonpharmacologic treatments. The motor and cognitive symptoms are progressive, with a less predictable trajectory for most of the psychiatric symptoms. The neurocognitive symptoms may be apparent during the prodromal period and can lead to significant personal and professional strife and therefore must be acknowledged and addressed. It is imperative that providers are aware of the frequency of anosognia in individuals with HD and therefore, make every effort to obtain information from both the patient and the caregiver when treating individuals with HD. Clinicians should address the patients' and caregivers' concerns to optimize symptom control, quality of life, and functional independence.

References

1. Ross, C. A., Aylward, E. H., Wild, E. J., et al. (2014). Huntington disease: natural history, biomarkers and prospects for therapeutics. *Nat Rev Neurol, 10*(4), 204–216.

2. Huntington Study Group. (1996). Unified Huntington's Disease Rating Scale: reliability and consistency. *Mov Disord, 11*(2), 136–142.

3. Duff, K., Paulsen, J. S., Beglinger, L. J., et al. (2010). "Frontal" behaviors before the diagnosis of Huntington's disease and their relationship to markers of disease progression: evidence of early lack of awareness. *J Neuropsychiatry Clin Neurosci, 22*(2), 196–207.

4. Epping, E. A., Kim, J. I., Craufurd, D., et al. (2016). Longitudinal psychiatric symptoms in prodromal Huntington's disease: a decade of data. *Am J Psychiatry, 173*(2), 184–192.

5. The Huntington's Disease Collaborative Research Group. (1993). A novel gene containing a trinucleotide repeat that is expanded and unstable on Huntington's disease chromosomes. *Cell, 72*(6), 971–983.

6. Ross, C. A., & Tabrizi, S. J. (2011). Huntington's disease: from molecular pathogenesis to clinical treatment. *Lancet Neurol, 10*(1), 83–98.

7. Pringsheim, T., Wiltshire, K., Day, L., Dykeman, J., Steeves, T., & Jette, N. (2012). The incidence and prevalence of Huntington's disease: a systematic review and meta-analysis. *Mov Disord, 27*(9), 1083–1091.

8. Baig, S. S., Strong, M., & Quarrell, O. W. (2016). The global prevalence of Huntington's disease: a systematic review and discussion. *Neurodegener Dis Manag, 6*(4), 331–343.

9. Vonsattel, J. P., Myers, R. H., Stevens, T. J., Ferrante, R. J., Bird, E. D., & Richardson, E. P., Jr. (1985). Neuropathological classification of Huntington's disease. *J Neuropathol Exp Neurol, 44*(6), 559–577.

10. Tabrizi, S. J., Langbehn, D. R., Leavitt, B. R., et al. (2009). Biological and clinical manifestations of Huntington's disease in the longitudinal TRACK-HD study: cross-sectional analysis of baseline data. *Lancet Neurol, 8*(9), 791–801.

11. Aylward, E. H., Nopoulos, P. C., Ross, C. A., et al. (2011). Longitudinal change in regional brain volumes in prodromal Huntington disease. *J Neurol Neurosurg Psychiatry, 82*(4), 405–410.

12. Ruocco, H. H., Bonilha, L., Li, L. M., Lopes-Cendes, I., & Cendes, F. (2008). Longitudinal analysis of regional grey matter loss in Huntington disease: effects of the length of the expanded CAG repeat. *J Neurol Neurosurg Psychiatry, 79*(2), 130–135.

13. Ross, C. A., Reilmann, R., Cardoso, F., et al. (2019). Movement Disorder Society Task Force viewpoint: Huntington's disease diagnostic categories. *Mov Disord Clin Pract, 6*(7), 541–546.

14. Shoulson, I., & Fahn, S. (1979). Huntington disease: clinical care and evaluation. *Neurology, 29*(1), 1–3.

15. Shoulson, I. (1981). Huntington disease: functional capacities in patients treated with neuroleptic and antidepressant drugs. *Neurology, 31*(10), 1333–1335.

16. Rosenblatt, A. (2011). Overview and principles of treatment. In M. Nance, J. S. Paulsen, A. Rosenblatt, & V. Wheelock (Eds.), *A Physician's Guide to the Management of Huntington's Disease* (pp. 5–13): Huntington's Disease Society of America.

17. Langbehn, D. R., Hayden, M. R., Paulsen, J. S., & and the Predict-HD Investigators of the Huntington Study Group (2010). CAG-repeat length and the age of onset in Huntington

disease (HD): a review and validation study of statistical approaches. *Am J Med Genet B Neuropsychiatr Genet, 153B*(2), 397–408.

18. Penney, J. B., Jr., Vonsattel, J. P., MacDonald, M. E., Gusella, J. F., & Myers, R. H. (1997). CAG repeat number governs the development rate of pathology in Huntington's disease. *Ann Neurol, 41*(5), 689–692.

19. Zhang, Y., Long, J. D., Mills, J. A., et al. (2011). Indexing disease progression at study entry with individuals at-risk for Huntington disease. *Am J Med Genet B Neuropsychiatr Genet, 156B*(7), 751–763.

20. Warner, J. H., & Sampaio, C. (2016). Modeling Variability in the progression of Huntington's disease a novel modeling approach applied to structural imaging markers from TRACK-HD. *CPT Pharmacometrics Syst Pharmacol, 5*(8), 437–445.

21. Wheelock, V. (2011). The motor disorder. In M. Nance, J. S. Paulsen, A. Rosenblatt, & V. Wheelock (Eds.), *A Physician's Guide to the Management of Huntington's Disease* (pp. 39–50): Huntington's Disease Society of America.

22. Nance, M., Paulsen, J. S., Rosenblatt, A., & Wheelock, V. (2011). *A Physician's Guide to the Management of Huntington's Disease* (3rd ed.): Huntington's Disease Society of America.

23. Armstrong, M. J., Miyasaki, J. M., & American Academy of Neurology. (2012). Evidence-based guideline: pharmacologic treatment of chorea in Huntington disease: report of the guideline development subcommittee of the American Academy of Neurology. *Neurology, 79*(6), 597–603.

24. Burgunder, J. M., Guttman, M., Perlman, S., Goodman, N., van Kammen, D. P., & Goodman, L. (2011). An international survey-based algorithm for the pharmacologic treatment of chorea in Huntington's disease. *PLoS Curr, 3*, RRN1260.

25. O'Suilleabhain, P., & Dewey, R. B., Jr. (2003). A randomized trial of amantadine in Huntington disease. *Arch Neurol, 60*(7), 996–998.

26. Verhagen Metman, L., Morris, M. J., Farmer, C., et al. (2002). Huntington's disease: a randomized, controlled trial using the NMDA-antagonist amantadine. *Neurology, 59*(5), 694–699.

27. Mestre, T., Ferreira, J., Coelho, M. M., Rosa, M., & Sampaio, C. (2009). Therapeutic interventions for symptomatic treatment in Huntington's disease. *Cochrane Database Syst Rev,* (3), CD006456.

28. Quinn, L., Kegelmeyer, D., Kloos, A., Rao, A. K., Busse, M., & Fritz, N. E. (2020). Clinical recommendations to guide physical therapy practice for Huntington disease. *Neurology, 94*(5), 217–228.

29. Saft, C., von Hein, S. M., Lucke, T., et al. (2018). Cannabinoids for treatment of dystonia in Huntington's disease. *J Huntingtons Dis, 7*(2), 167–173.

30. Paulsen, J. S., Langbehn, D. R., Stout, J. C., et al. (2008). Detection of Huntington's disease decades before diagnosis: the Predict-HD study. *J Neurol Neurosurg Psychiatry, 79*(8), 874–880.

31. Tabrizi, S. J., Scahill, R. I., Owen, G., et al. (2013). Predictors of phenotypic progression and disease onset in premanifest and early-stage Huntington's disease in the TRACK-HD study: analysis of 36-month observational data. *Lancet Neurol, 12*(7), 637–649.

32. Snowden, J. S., Craufurd, D., Thompson, J., & Neary, D. (2002). Psychomotor, executive, and memory function in preclinical Huntington's disease. *J Clin Exp Neuropsychol, 24*(2), 133–145.

33. Cubo, E., Shannon, K. M., Tracy, D., et al. (2006). Effect of donepezil on motor and cognitive function in Huntington disease. *Neurology, 67*(7), 1268–1271.

34. Vattakatuchery, J. J., & Kurien, R. (2013). Acetylcholinesterase inhibitors in cognitive impairment in Huntington's disease: a brief review. *World J Psychiatry, 3*(3), 62–64.

35. Anderson, K. E., van Duijn, E., Craufurd, D., et al. (2018). Clinical management of neuropsychiatric symptoms of Huntington disease: expert-based consensus guidelines on agitation, anxiety, apathy, psychosis and sleep disorders. *J Huntingtons Dis, 7*(3), 355–366.

36. Leroi, I., O'Hearn, E., Marsh, L., et al. (2002). Psychopathology in patients with degenerative cerebellar diseases: a comparison to Huntington's disease. *Am J Psychiatry, 159*(8), 1306–1314.

37. Murgod, U. A., Saleem, Q., Anand, A., Brahmachari, S. K., Jain, S., & Muthane, U. B. (2001). A clinical study of patients with genetically confirmed Huntington's disease from India. *J Neurol Sci, 190*(1–2), 73–78.

38. Kulisevsky, J., Litvan, I., Berthier, M. L., Pascual-Sedano, B., Paulsen, J. S., & Cummings, J. L. (2001). Neuropsychiatric assessment of Gilles de la Tourette patients: comparative study with other hyperkinetic and hypokinetic movement disorders. *Mov Disord, 16*(6), 1098–1104.

39. Paulsen, J. S. (2005). Depression and stages of Huntington's disease. *Journal of Neuropsychiatry, 17*(4), 496–502.

40. Marder, K., Zhao, H., Myers, R. H., et al. (2000). Rate of functional decline in Huntington's disease. Huntington Study Group. *Neurology, 54*(2), 452–458.

41. Zappacosta, B., Monza, D., Meoni, C., et al. (1996). Psychiatric symptoms do not correlate with cognitive decline, motor symptoms, or CAG repeat length in Huntington's disease. *Arch Neurol, 53*(6), 493–497.

42. Dale, M., Maltby, J., Shimozaki, S., Cramp, R., & Rickards, H. (2016). Disease stage, but not sex, predicts depression and psychological distress in Huntington's disease: a European population study. *Journal of Psychosomatic Research, 80*, 17–22.

43. McColgan, P., Razi, A., Gregory, S., et al. (2017). Structural and functional brain network correlates of depressive symptoms in premanifest Huntington's disease. *Hum Brain Mapp, 38*(6), 2819–2829.

44. Folstein, S., Abbott, M. H., Chase, G. A., Jensen, B. A., & Folstein, M. F. (1983). The association of affective disorder with Huntington's disease in a case series and in families. *Psychol Med, 13*(3), 537–542.

45. Di Maio, L., Squitieri, F., Napolitano, G., Campanella, G., Trofatter, J. A., & Conneally, P. M. (1993). Onset symptoms in 510 patients with Huntington's disease. *J Med Genet, 30*(4), 289–292.

46. Kirkwood, S. C., Su, J. L., Conneally, P., & Foroud, T. (2001). Progression of symptoms in the early and middle stages of Huntington disease. *Arch Neurol, 58*(2), 273–278.

47. Farrer, L. A. (1986). Suicide and attempted suicide in Huntington disease: implications for preclinical testing of persons at risk. *Am J Med Genet, 24*(2), 305–311.

48. Sorensen, S. A., & Fenger, K. (1992). Causes of death in patients with Huntington's disease and in unaffected first degree relatives. *J Med Genet, 29*(12), 911–914.

49. Schoenfeld, M., Myers, R. H., Cupples, L. A., Berkman, B., Sax, D. S., & Clark, E. (1984). Increased rate of suicide among patients with Huntington's disease. *J Neurol Neurosurg Psychiatry, 47*(12), 1283–1287.

50. Eliasen, A., Dalhoff, K. P., & Horwitz, H. (2018). Neurological diseases and risk of suicide attempt: a case-control study. *J Neurol, 265*(6), 1303–1309.

51. Hayden, M. R., Ehrlich, R., Parker, H., & Ferera, S. J. (1980). Social perspectives in Huntington's chorea. *S Afr Med J, 58*(5), 201–203.

52. Anderson, K. E., Eberly, S., Groves, M., et al. (2016). Risk factors for suicidal ideation in people at risk for Huntington's disease. *J Huntingtons Dis, 5*(4), 389–394.

53. Haw, C., Harwood, D., & Hawton, K. (2009). Dementia and suicidal behavior: a review of the literature. *Int Psychogeriatr, 21*(3), 440–453.

54. Honrath, P., Dogan, I., Wudarczyk, O., et al. (2018). Risk factors of suicidal ideation in Huntington's disease: literature review and data from Enroll-HD. *J Neurol, 265*(11), 2548–2561.

55. Hubers, A. A., van Duijn, E., Roos, R. A., et al. (2013). Suicidal ideation in a European Huntington's disease population. *J Affect Disord, 151*(1), 248–258.

56. Testa, C. M., & Jankovic, J. (2019). Huntington disease: a quarter century of progress since the gene discovery. *J Neurol Sci, 396*, 52–68.

57. Craufurd, D., Thompson, J. C., & Snowden, J. S. (2001). Behavioral changes in Huntington disease. *Neuropsychiatry Neuropsychol Behav Neurol, 14*(4), 219–226.

58. van Duijn, E., Kingma, E. M., & van der Mast, R. C. (2007). Psychopathology in verified Huntington's disease gene carriers. *J Neuropsychiatry Clin Neurosci, 19*(4), 441–448.

59. Vaccarino, A. L., Anonymous, Anderson, K. E., et al. (2011). Assessing behavioural manifestations prior to clinical diagnosis of Huntington disease: "anger and irritability" and "obsessions and compulsions." *PLoS Curr, 3*, RRN1241.

60. Ramos, A. R. S., & Garrett, C. (2017). Huntington's disease: premotor phase. *Neurodegener Dis, 17*(6), 313–322.

61. Diago, E. B., Martinez-Horta, S., Lasaosa, S. S., et al. (2018). Circadian rhythm, cognition, and mood disorders in Huntington's disease. *J Huntingtons Dis, 7*(2), 193–198.

62. Singh-Bains, M. K., Tippett, L. J., Hogg, V. M., et al. (2016). Globus pallidus degeneration and clinicopathological features of Huntington disease. *Ann Neurol, 80*(2), 185–201.

63. Dale, M., & van Duijn, E. (2015). Anxiety in Huntington's disease. *J Neuropsychiatry Clin Neurosci, 27*(4), 262–271.

64. Berrios, G. E., Wagle, A. C., Markova, I. S., et al. (2001). Psychiatric symptoms and CAG repeats in neurologically asymptomatic Huntington's disease gene carriers. *Psychiatry Res, 102*(3), 217–225.

65. Lane, S. D., Kjome, K. L., & Moeller, F. G. (2011). Neuropsychiatry of aggression. *Neurol Clin, 29*(1), 49–64, vii.

66. Jensen, P., Fenger, K., Bolwig, T. G., & Sorensen, S. A. (1998). Crime in Huntington's disease: a study of registered offences among patients, relatives, and controls. *J Neurol Neurosurg Psychiatry, 65*(4), 467–471.

67. Dewhurst, K., Oliver, J., Trick, K. L., & McKnight, A. L. (1969). Neuro-psychiatric aspects of Huntington's disease. *Confin Neurol, 31*(4), 258–268.

68. van Duijn, E., Craufurd, D., Hubers, A. A., et al. (2014). Neuropsychiatric symptoms in a European Huntington's disease cohort (REGISTRY). *J Neurol Neurosurg Psychiatry, 85*(12), 1411–1418.

69. Pflanz, S., Besson, J. A., Ebmeier, K. P., & Simpson, S. (1991). The clinical manifestation of mental disorder in Huntington's disease: a retrospective case record study of disease progression. *Acta Psychiatr Scand, 83*(1), 53–60.

70. Shiwach, R. S., & Patel, V. (1993). Aggressive behaviour in Huntington's disease: a cross-sectional study in a nursing home population. *Behav Neurol, 6*(1), 43–47.

71. Tamir, A., Whittier, J., & Korenyi, C. (1969). Huntington's chorea: a sex difference in psychopathological symptoms. *Dis Nerv Syst, 30*(2), 103.

72. Tyler, A., Harper, P. S., Davies, K., & Newcome, R. G. (1983). Family break-down and stress in Huntington's chorea. *J Biosoc Sci, 15*(2), 127–138.

73. Anderson, K. E., Gehl, C. R., Marder, K. S., Beglinger, L. J., Paulsen, J. S., & Huntington's Study, G. (2010). Comorbidities of obsessive and compulsive symptoms in Huntington's disease. *J Nerv Ment Dis, 198*(5), 334–338.

74. Wetzel, H. H., Gehl, C. R., Dellefave-Castillo, L., et al. (2011). Suicidal ideation in Huntington disease: the role of comorbidity. *Psychiatry Res, 188*(3), 372–376.

75. Grimbergen, Y. A. M., Knol, M. J., Bloem, B. R., Kremer, B. P. H., Roos, R. A. C., & Munneke, M. (2008). Falls and gait disturbances in Huntington's disease. *Mov Disord, 23*(7), 970–976.

76. Quaid, K. A., Eberly, S. W., Kayson-Rubin, E., et al. (2017). Factors related to genetic testing in adults at risk for Huntington disease: the prospective Huntington at-risk observational study (PHAROS). *Clin Genet, 91*(6), 824–831.

77. Levy, M. L., Cummings, J. L., Fairbanks, L. A., et al. (1998). Apathy is not depression. *J Neuropsychiatry Clin Neurosci, 10*(3), 314–319.

78. Paulsen, J. S., Ready, R. E., Hamilton, J. M., Mega, M. S., & Cummings, J. L. (2001). Neuropsychiatric aspects of Huntington's disease. *J Neurol Neurosurg Psychiatry, 71*(3), 310–314.

79. Fritz, N. E., Boileau, N. R., Stout, J. C., et al. (2018). Relationships among apathy, health-related quality of life, and function in Huntington's disease. *J Neuropsychiatry Clin Neurosci, 30*(3), 194–201.

80. Yang, J., Chen, K., Wei, Q., et al. (2016). Clinical and genetic characteristics in patients with Huntington's disease from China. *Neurol Res, 38*(10), 916–920.

81. Mason, S., & Barker, R. A. (2015). Rating apathy in Huntington's disease: patients and companions agree. *J Huntingtons Dis, 4*(1), 49–59.

82. Bouwens, J. A., van Duijn, E., van der Mast, R. C., Roos, R. A., & Giltay, E. J. (2015). Irritability in a prospective cohort of Huntington's disease mutation carriers. *J Neuropsychiatry Clin Neurosci, 27*(3), 206–212.

83. Kingma, E. M., van Duijn, E., Timman, R., van der Mast, R. C., & Roos, R. A. (2008). Behavioural problems in Huntington's disease using the Problem Behaviours Assessment. *Gen Hosp Psychiatry, 30*(2), 155–161.

84. Orvoen, S., Pla, P., Gardier, A. M., Saudou, F., & David, D. J. (2012). Huntington's disease knock-in male mice show specific anxiety-like behaviour and altered neuronal maturation. *Neurosci Lett, 507*(2), 127–132.

85. Soliveri, P., Monza, D., Piacentini, S., et al. (2002). Cognitive and psychiatric characterization of patients with Huntington's disease and their at-risk relatives. *Neurol Sci, 23 Suppl 2*, S105–106.

86. Witjes-Ane, M. N., Zwinderman, A. H., Tibben, A., van Ommen, G. J., & Roos, R. A. (2002). Behavioural complaints in participants who underwent predictive testing for Huntington's disease. *J Med Genet, 39*(11), 857–862.

87. Vassos, E., Panas, M., Kladi, A., & Vassilopoulos, D. (2008). Effect of CAG repeat length on psychiatric disorders in Huntington's disease. *J Psychiatr Res, 42*(7), 544–549.

88. Thompson, J. C., Harris, J., Sollom, A. C., et al. (2012). Longitudinal evaluation of neuropsychiatric symptoms in Huntington's disease. *J Neuropsychiatry Clin Neurosci, 24*(1), 53–60.

89. Anderson, K., Craufurd, D., Edmondson, M. C., et al. (2011). An international survey-based algorithm for the pharmacologic treatment of obsessive-compulsive behaviors in Huntington's disease. *PLoS Curr, 3*, RRN1261.

90. Nordahl, T. E., Benkelfat, C., Semple, W. E., Gross, M., King, A. C., & Cohen, R. M. (1989). Cerebral glucose metabolic rates in obsessive compulsive disorder. *Neuropsychopharmacology, 2*(1), 23–28.

91. Burguiere, E., Monteiro, P., Mallet, L., Feng, G., & Graybiel, A. M. (2015). Striatal circuits, habits, and implications for obsessive-compulsive disorder. *Curr Opin Neurobiol, 30*, 59–65.

92. Roman, O. C., Stovall, J., & Claassen, D. O. (2018). Perseveration and suicide in Huntington's disease. *J Huntingtons Dis, 7*(2), 185–187.

93. Morton, A. J. (2013). Circadian and sleep disorder in Huntington's disease. *Exp Neurol, 243*, 34–44.

94. Arnulf, I., Nielsen, J., Lohmann, E., et al. (2008). Rapid eye movement sleep disturbances in Huntington disease. *Arch Neurol, 65*(4), 482–488.

95. Aziz, N. A., Anguelova, G. V., Marinus, J., Lammers, G. J., & Roos, R. A. (2010). Sleep and circadian rhythm alterations correlate with depression and cognitive impairment in Huntington's disease. *Parkinsonism Relat Disord, 16*(5), 345–350.

96. Emser, W., Brenner, M., Stober, T., & Schimrigk, K. (1988). Changes in nocturnal sleep in Huntington's and Parkinson's disease. *J Neurol, 235*(3), 177–179.

97. Wiegand, M., Moller, A. A., Lauer, C. J., et al. (1991). Nocturnal sleep in Huntington's disease. *J Neurol, 238*(4), 203–208.

98. Goodman, A. O., Rogers, L., Pilsworth, S., et al. (2011). Asymptomatic sleep abnormalities are a common early feature in patients with Huntington's disease. *Curr Neurol Neurosci Rep, 11*(2), 211–217.

99. Taylor, N., & Bramble, D. (1997). Sleep disturbance and Huntington's disease. *Br J Psychiatry, 171*, 393.

100. Goodman, A. O., & Barker, R. A. (2010). How vital is sleep in Huntington's disease? *J Neurol, 257*(6), 882–897.

101. Connors, M. H., Teixeira-Pinto, A., & Loy, C. T. (2020). Psychosis and longitudinal outcomes in Huntington disease: the COHORT study. *J Neurol Neurosurg Psychiatry, 91*(1), 15–20.

102. Huntington, G. (2003). On chorea. George Huntington, M.D. *J Neuropsychiatry Clin Neurosci, 15*(1), 109–112.

103. Szymus, K., Bystrzynski, A., Kwasniak-Butowska, M., et al. (2020). Sexual dysfunction in Huntington's disease—a systematic review. *Neurol Neurochir Pol, 54*(4), 305–311.

104. Kolenc, M., Kobal, J., & Podnar, S. (2017). Female sexual dysfunction in presymptomatic mutation carriers and patients with Huntington's disease. *J Huntingtons Dis, 6*(2), 105–113.

105. Kolenc, M., Kobal, J., & Podnar, S. (2015). Male sexual function in presymptomatic gene carriers and patients with Huntington's disease. *J Neurol Sci, 359*(1-2), 312–317.

106. Kalkhoven, C., Sennef, C., Peeters, A., & van den Bos, R. (2014). Risk-taking and pathological gambling behavior in Huntington's disease. *Front Behav Neurosci, 8*, 103.

107. Groves, M., van Duijn, E., Anderson, K., et al. (2011). An international survey-based algorithm for the pharmacologic treatment of irritability in Huntington's disease. *PLoS Curr, 3*, RRN1259.

108. Karagas, N. E., Rocha, N. P., & Stimming, E. F. (2020). Irritability in Huntington's disease. *J Huntingtons Dis, 9*(2), 107–113.

109. Mestre, T. A. (2019). Recent advances in the therapeutic development for Huntington disease. *Parkinsonism Relat Disord, 59*, 125–130.

110. Tabrizi, S. J., Leavitt, B. R., Landwehrmeyer, G. B., et al. (2019). Targeting huntingtin expression in patients with Huntington's disease. *N Engl J Med, 380*(24), 2307–2316.

111. Saudou, F., & Humbert, S. (2016). The biology of huntingtin. *Neuron, 89*(5), 910–926.

112. Rodrigues, F. B., & Wild, E. J. (2020). Huntington's disease clinical trials corner: April 2020. *J Huntingtons Dis, 9*(2), 185–197.

113. McBride, J. L., Boudreau, R. L., Harper, S. Q., et al. (2008). Artificial miRNAs mitigate shRNA-mediated toxicity in the brain: implications for the therapeutic development of RNAi. *Proc Natl Acad Sci U S A, 105*(15), 5868–5873.

114. DiFiglia, M., Sena-Esteves, M., Chase, K., et al. (2007). Therapeutic silencing of mutant huntingtin with siRNA attenuates striatal and cortical neuropathology and behavioral deficits. *Proc Natl Acad Sci U S A, 104*(43), 17204–17209.

115. Shin, J. W., Kim, K. H., Chao, M. J., et al. (2016). Permanent inactivation of Huntington's disease mutation by personalized allele-specific CRISPR/Cas9. *Hum Mol Genet, 25*(20), 4566–4576.

116. Yang, S., Chang, R., Yang, H., et al. (2017). CRISPR/Cas9-mediated gene editing ameliorates neurotoxicity in mouse model of Huntington's disease. *J Clin Invest, 127*(7), 2719–2724.

117. Tabrizi, S. J., Ghosh, R., & Leavitt, B. R. (2019). Huntingtin lowering strategies for disease modification in Huntington's disease. *Neuron, 102*(4), 899.

16

Behavioral Abnormalities in Other Genetic and Nongenetic Causes of Chorea

Ricardo Maciel, Débora Palma Maia, and Francisco Cardoso

Introduction

Chorea, characterized by a flow of continuous and random muscle contractions, can be caused by a myriad of genetic and acquired conditions (Table 16.1). Regardless of the underlying etiology, it is related to hypoactivity of the output of the subthalamic nuclei.[1] It is not surprising, then, that the nonmotor frontal-striatal circuits of the basal ganglia are often dysfunctional in choreatic disorders. This often results in cognitive and psychiatric abnormalities. Among the former are reduced verbal fluency, dysexecutive function, and dementia. The most common behavioral changes present in choreatic disorders are obsessions, compulsions, and attention deficit and hyperactivity disorder (ADHD). Huntington's disease (HD) is arguably the most extensively studied illness associated with chorea. As described in another chapter, HD subjects invariably display a combination of motor, cognitive, and behavioral features. Importantly, the nonmotor changes are the most important source of morbidity in HD.[2] As neuropathological abnormalities in HD are widespread, it is possible that some of the clinical features result from lesions outside the basal ganglia. Many of the conditions listed in Table 16.1 also display a combination of chorea and other features. The aim of this chapter is to provide an overview of behavioral changes described in some genetic and nongenetic causes of chorea. Some of them, such as Huntington's disease-like 2 (HDL2), share with HD the presence of neuropathological changes distributed throughout the central nervous system. Others, particularly Sydenham's chorea (SC), are characterized by selective dysfunction of the basal ganglia, highlighting the important role played by these structures in nonmotor function.[3]

Huntington's Disease-Like 2

Huntington's disease-like 2 (HDL2) is an autosomal dominant disorder caused by a CAG/CTG nucleotide expansion in the *Junctophilin 3* (*JPH3*) gene, located in the long arm of chromosome 16 (16q24.3). This disease was first reported in 2001 in an African American family pedigree previously thought to have Huntington's disease (HD), but who were later found not to bear the *Huntingtin* (HTT) gene expansion typical of HD.[4] Since this original description, HDL2 has been found to be one of the most common HD phenocopies, despite its rareness. Of about 70 cases reported in the literature, all patients have an African ancestry, pointing toward a founder effect. The disease seems to be most prevalent in South Africa,

Table 16.1 Neuropsychiatric Syndromes Associated With Chorea

Central Nervous System	Peripheral Nervous System
Aseptic meningitis	Cranial neuropathy
Cerebrovascular disease	Mononeuropathy
Myelopathy	Guillain-Barré syndrome
Seizures	Myasthenia gravis
Movement disorders	Plexopathy
Demyelinating syndrome	Autonomic disorder
Cognitive dysfunction	Polyneuropathy
Psychosis	
Acute confusional state	
Severe depression	

where it accounts for 15% to 35% of cases presenting with a HD-like phenotype (HDL).[5,6] Other reported cases originate from countries with a significant population of African descent, including the United States, Haiti, Mexico, Morocco, Brazil, and Venezuela.

Clinically, HDL2 is indistinguishable from HD and classically presents with a triad of movement disorders, cognitive decline, and psychiatric manifestations. The disease is invariably progressive and culminates in death 15 to 20 years after the motor onset. In accordance with other repeat expansion disorders, age of onset is inversely correlated with the number of CAG/CTG repeats. Most patients have onset in the fourth to fifth decades of life. Chorea is the most common movement disorder, followed by parkinsonism and dystonia. Myoclonus[7] and action tremor[4] have also been reported. Other motor manifestations include abnormal saccades and ocular pursuit, dysarthria, dysphagia, apraxia, abnormal reflexes, gait abnormalities, weight loss, and postural instability.

Most information regarding the neuropsychiatric features of HDL2 come from case reports or small case series. Clinical descriptions are often incomplete, poorly detailed, and focused on the motor phenomenology of the disease to the detriment of its nonmotor features. In addition, the majority of cases have been described in developing countries with limited healthcare. This often precludes timely diagnosis and prospective evaluation of early cognitive and psychiatric symptoms, before their progression to full-blown and undifferentiated dementia. Therefore, data regarding the cognitive profile of patients with HDL2 must be interpreted with caution.

In about two-thirds of patients, neuropsychiatric symptoms predate the motor onset of the disease. The most common psychiatric manifestation is depression, followed by personality changes as well as anxiety. Psychosis with delusions and visual hallucinations can also occur. Patients are often described by family members as being emotionally labile, inflexible, and irritable. On the other hand, apathy is also often reported, especially in later stages of the disease.[8] Frontal disinhibition, obsessive-compulsive symptoms, and perseveration can also occur.[9] Interestingly, impulsivity and suicidality have not been described in HDL2, though both are common manifestations of HD. Whether this represents a true distinction between the two disorders or are only due to underreporting is currently unknown.

Cognitive complaints also occur early in the disease, akin to what is seen in HD. Dementia is a universal feature in later disease stages. In keeping with the dysfunction of basal ganglia and frontal circuits seen in both diseases, the cognitive profile of HDL2 shows marked deficits in attention, processing speed, and executive function. Detailed prospective neuropsychological data is lacking in HDL2. However, a few studies have tried to systematically evaluate cognitive deficits of HDL2 patients in comparison to HD. Ferreira-Correia and colleagues have found that psychomotor speed and visuoconstructive skills were the most severely impaired domains in HDL2 patients, followed by executive functions (including verbal fluency, judgement, concept formation, and impairment of inhibition), attention and working memory.[9] The same group also reports that, compared to HD, patients with HDL2 have worse performance in working memory, and auditory-verbal recognition tasks, however, this could be due to the small number of patients studied.[10]

C9orf72 Disease

A hexanucleotide (GGGGCC) repeat expansion in the *C9orf72* gene is the most common cause of familial amyotrophic lateral sclerosis (ALS), frontotemporal dementia (FTD), or a combination of both disorders[11] The expansion is inherited in an autosomal dominant fashion and is responsible for about 7% of sporadic ALS, 20% to 30% of cases of familial ALS, 25% of familial FTD, and the majority of ALS-FTD cases.[12] The expansion is considered pathogenic if higher than 30 repeats, but not infrequently it numbers in the thousands.[13] In contrast to what is seen in other repeat expansion diseases, there is no clear evidence of correlation between repeat length, age of onset, disease severity, or anticipation. This might be due to somatic mosaicism obscuring the "true" repeat length in affected brain areas (i.e., not corresponding to repeat length measured in blood) or other yet to be identified risk modifying polymorphisms.[14] Besides the typical clinical presentations mentioned above, the mutation has also been described in patients with atypical parkinsonism.[15] MRI can be normal, or show atrophy involving the frontotemporal regions, as typically seen in FTD, but also on the parietal cortex, thalamus and cerebellum.[16] *C9orf72* has also been identified as the most common cause of the HD-like phenotype in HTT negative cohorts,[17] which merits its inclusion in the current chapter. In 2014, Hensman Moss and colleagues reported 10 positive patients for the *C9orf72* mutation in a cohort of 514 HD phenocopy syndrome cases.[17] These are defined as patients with a clinical presentation consistent with HD according to an experienced neurologist, a negative HTT gene expansion, and the combination of a movement disorder (namely chorea, associated or not with parkinsonism, dystonia), and either cognitive decline, psychiatric symptoms, or a family history consistent with an autosomal dominant pattern. About 97% of HD phenocopies remain undiagnosed.[18] In Caucasian populations, *C9orf72* is the most common identified cause of an HDL phenotype, ranging from 1.75% to 5% of cases in European cohorts.[19-21] Compared to other HD phenocopies, patients with C9orf72 disease display more prominent psychiatric and cognitive features, as well as more frequent movement disorders and upper motor neuron signs.[17] Psychosis, depression, obsessions, apathy, and other behavioral abnormalities are the presenting features of the disease in up to 60% of patients.[17] Other behavioral symptoms include disinhibition, irritability, emotional lability, pathologic crying and laughing, and hypomania.[20,21] A history of dementia or motor neuron disease in first-degree relatives is sometimes present and can be a clue to the diagnosis.

ALS is a neurodegenerative condition in which there is progressive loss of upper and/or lower motor neurons. The disease usually starts in the limbs or bulbar regions and spreads to neighboring motor neurons, death usually occurs in 3 to 5 years after disease onset due to respiratory failure or other complications. C9orf72-related ALS motor symptoms are indistinguishable from sporadic ALS, the exception being that bulbar onset is more common,[22] which is linked to a poorer prognosis. A history of psychiatric disorder (depression, suicide, schizophrenia) in first- or second-degree relatives of patients with C9orf72-ALS is more frequent than in sporadic ALS. It is unclear, though, if this is due to incomplete penetrance in carriers or other shared risk factors.[23]

The behavioral variant is the most common presentation of C9orf72-related FTD (bvFTD). The disease is characterized by a progressive dementia with prominent executive dysfunction, personality changes, social dysfunction, and behavioral changes. Other less frequent presentations of C9orf72 include the primary progressive aphasias (a form of dementia in which language is early and prominently affected), with the nonfluent type being the second-most frequent presentation after bvFTD. As expected, motor neuron symptoms and parkinsonism are more frequent in mutation positive bvFTD cases in comparison to C9orf72-negative patients.[24] Psychotic symptoms are much more prevalent in mutation carriers (ranging from 20% to 50% of cases), and often involve somatic delusions with altered body perception (e.g., belief of infestation, foreign objects, pregnancy).[25] Visual and auditory hallucinations are also frequent.[26] Psychotic symptoms are thought to respond poorly to medications. Other reported psychiatric symptoms include hypomania, apathy, depression, anxiety, obsessive-compulsive symptoms, and catatonia.[27] Not infrequently, psychiatric manifestations precede the development of cognitive impairment by up to 5 years, which can lead to a misdiagnosis of schizophrenia.[28] There are case reports of patients with very a slow progression of cognitive symptoms and preserved insight,[29] which is unusual for FTD.

Late-onset psychosis are common presentations of all the C9orf72-related disorders described above. Also, there is a wide spectrum of reported psychiatric manifestations in C9orf72 kindreds, including depression, anxiety disorders, mania, obsessive-compulsive symptoms, and eating disorders, among others.[27,30] There is an increased risk of schizophrenia, suicide, and autism spectrum disorders in C9orf72-ALS- and FTD-positive first-degree relatives.[31,32] The risk of psychiatric disorders in kindreds of C9orf72-HDL cohorts has not been reported, possibly owing to the rarity of the condition. A number of observational studies have tried to assess if C9orf72 expansions might be a cause of primary psychiatric syndromes. Overall, however, the prevalence of C9orf72 expansions in large cohorts of patients with schizophrenia or schizoaffective disorders, obsessive-compulsive disorders (OCDs), and bipolar disorders has not been found to be higher than expected for the general population.[23,31,33–35]

ADCY5

ADCY5-related dyskinesia is an autosomal dominant disorder resulting from mutations in the *ADCY5* gene located on the short arm of chromosome 3, which encodes adenylate cyclase.[36] Previously known as familial dyskinesia with facial myokymia, ADCY5-related dyskinesia is associated with diverse phenotypes. As patients may mimic NKX2-1-related benign hereditary chorea (BHC), some authors call ADCY5 a BHC-like or one mutation of BHC's syndrome.[37]

The original description involved an early childhood to adolescent onset of paroxysmal dyskinesia and facial twitches, which progressed in frequency and severity to a constant movement disorder by the third decade before stabilizing or improving with older age.[38] Later electrophysiological studies showed that the facial dyskinesia is not myokymia.[39] Subsequent reports of ADCY5-related dyskinesia have included a syndrome of infantile to early childhood onset of chorea and dystonia, associated with pyramidal signs, with or without apparent facial twitching. Yet, facial dyskinesia is a diagnostic clue as well as exacerbation of dyskinesia during transitions between wakefulness and sleep including drowsiness and sleep arousal.[40] Other clinical features that may be present are myoclonus,[36] hypotonia, and delayed motor milestones. Regarding clinical course, there is a steady deterioration as the children grow with stabilization in adulthood. However, in some patients, the movements may be paroxysmal with bouts of hyperkinesia separated by remission lasting days to weeks. Cerebral MRI in affected individuals is normal.[41] There are reports of motor functional improvement in ADCY5 patients treated with clonazepam, clobazam, or levetiracetam.[41,42]

Cognition is often normal in carriers of the mutation, but there are occasional patients with cognitive impairment and autistic-like behavior. There are few reports of psychiatric symptoms associated with ADCY5. Psychosis and depression were mentioned in a few cases.[40] Waalkens et al. in 2018 described one of three patients with ADCY5 mutation with obsessive-compulsive and anxiety disorder with phobias. Family history revealed no psychiatric disorders.[42] Vijiaratnam and colleagues related anxiety and depressive symptoms in one 29-year-old man with onset in adolescence followed by acute psychosis in his early 20s. He evolved with mood instability and, at the age of 28, was admitted to hospital following a suicide attempt. His mother had a similar movement disorder, with anxiety and depression. She committed suicide at age 26.[39] It remains unclear if the psychiatric manifestations can be ascribed to the ADCY5 phenotype, given the prevalence of psychiatric disorders in the general population. Other reports suggest though that psychiatric symptoms may be part of the phenotype of ADCY5 mutations.[39,41]

Benign Hereditary Chorea

Benign hereditary chorea (BHC) is an autosomal dominant disorder that was first described in 1967 as a childhood onset, nonprogressive generalized chorea[43] It is caused by mutations in the *NKX2.1* gene (formerly known as TITF-1) that encodes the thyroid transcription factor-1. It is located on the long arm of chromosome 14 and regulates the activity of genes in the formation of brain, lung, and thyroid tissues.[37,44,45] This accounts for the disorder presenting with chorea and other movement disorders, congenital hypothyroidism, and respiratory problems. This triad is also named "brain-lung-thyroid syndrome."[46] The lung involvement typically manifests as neonatal respiratory failure, as well as recurrent pulmonary infections, chronic airways disease, and even lung cancer.[36] There is a slight female preponderance, with a male-to-female ratio of 0.70.[36]

Classically, the neurological features of BHC include hypotonia in infancy as well as delayed motor milestones, particularly with walking.[44] This is followed by early-childhood-onset (2.5 to 3 years) generalized chorea, although onset from infancy to late childhood and adolescence has also been described. Usually, chorea worsens with stress and improves during sleep. There is gradual improvement as the subject grows older, eventually stabilizing during adulthood. Associated movement disorders may include myoclonus, dystonia, tics, ataxia, upper limb intentional tremor, restless legs syndrome, and nonepileptic drop attacks.[36,45,47] As chorea improves with age, myoclonus often becomes the main disabling symptom in adulthood. Speech disorder has been reported in up to 40% of cases with BHC.[36,45] Structural brain imaging in BHC is typically normal. Variable success in treatment of the motor features of BHC has been reported with levodopa and tetrabenazine.[36]

There are reports of nonmotor features associated with BHC. Although normal intellectual function in adult life seems the rule, learning difficulty and lower IQ scores have been reported in carriers of BHC mutations with or without motor findings. Gras et al., for instance, reported learning difficulties in 20 of 28 patients with BHC. Formal assessment of cognitive performance performed in 14 of 20 showed that three had intellectual disability, three a borderline IQ (between 70 and 80) and eight a normal IQ.[48] It is unclear whether these deficits in cognitive function reflect an integral part of the BHC phenotype, congenital hypothyroidism, or are a consequence of social difficulties and isolation resulting in impaired formal education.[45,46] There are also descriptions of behavioral abnormalities in subjects with BHC. Depression, apathy, introverted behavior, and psychosis were described in the era prior to *TITF1* identification in two families with clinical presentations of BHC, and therefore could not be related to *TITF1* mutation.[46] In 2008, Glik et al. described a genetically confirmed case of BHC with nonprogressive chorea since birth, who developed psychosis diagnosed as schizophrenia at the age of 27 years.[49] OCD and ADHD have also been reported in patients with *NKX2.1* mutation. Gras et al., in a large, longitudinal French study, found 7 out of 28 mutation-positive cases to have a diagnosis of ADHD, six with normal IQ.[48]

Systemic Lupus Erythematosus

Systemic lupus erythematosus (SLE) is an autoimmune disease affecting various organs including the nervous system. Neuropsychiatric symptoms are important components of the disease morbidity spectrum and have been classified by the American College of Rheumatology into well-defined syndromes[50] (Table 16.1). Neuropsychiatric involvement in SLE tends to occur in the first three years of disease or even precede the development of the other systemic symptoms that are necessary for the diagnosis of SLE. The neuropsychiatric syndromes of SLE occur in a wide spectrum of morbidity, from headache, to coma, and depending on the methodology used to assess them, have a prevalence from 12% to 95%.[51] When considering only major neurologic manifestations, including seizures, stroke, myelopathy and demyelinating disease, chorea, aseptic meningitis, and acute confusional states, neuropsychiatric SLE has an estimated prevalence of 4%.[52] Their occurrence is independently associated with a more severe disease and worse prognosis.

Movement disorders are rare in SLE, with a prevalence of about 0.5%.[51] The most common movement disorder associated with lupus is chorea, which tends to occur in the third decade of life or earlier, often before the diagnosis of SLE can be made. The main differential diagnosis is with SC, especially considering that both disorders can cause arthralgia and cardiac valve abnormalities. Women are preferentially affected, as is the case with most autoimmune diseases. The presence of antiphospholipid antibodies can be detected in 60 to 90% of cases.[53,54] Other described movement disorders in SLE include parkinsonism, myoclonus, and ataxia.[55–57] Chorea in SLE patients might be accompanied by other neurological and psychiatric manifestations, including seizures, stroke, and psychosis.[58] Chorea can be unilateral or generalized. Recurrences, up to 4 years after the initial presentation, can also occur.[54] Magnetic resonance imaging might be unrevealing or show ischemic lesions, especially in patients with associated antiphospholipid syndrome. Cerebrospinal fluid and serum markers of inflammation can also be normal.

Cognitive deficits occur in up to 80% of patients with SLE, depending on methodology used for its definition, assessment, and the population studied. Subtle subclinical deficits are not specific and do not discriminate between patients with or without other neuropsychiatric manifestations. Most patients have a fluctuating course of impairment, although some patients can present with progressive deficits. Executive function, attention, memory, and learning are the most affected domains.

Psychosis occurs in about 1% of patients with SLE. In a large cohort of SLE patients, the occurrence of psychosis was associated with male sex, younger age at diagnosis, concurrent neuropsychiatric syndromes, and presence of anti-P antibodies.[59] Most patients improve with a combination of antipsychotic therapy and immunosuppression.

Depression and anxiety are also common in SLE patients, occurring in up to 75% of patients.[60] Albeit more prevalent than in the general population, they are not associated with disease activity and are most likely multifactorial in origin.[61] Obsessive-compulsive and attention deficit and hyperactivity symptoms are more common in patients with SLE than in the general population, and the severity of symptoms associates with disease activity.[62] Other studies have also found a higher prevalence of panic disorders, obsessive-compulsive symptoms and bipolar disorders in women with SLE in comparison to controls.[63–65]

Sydenham's Chorea

SC, described by Thomas Sydenham in 1686, is the neurological manifestation of acute rheumatic fever (RF), a delayed autoimmune complication of group A β-hemolytic streptococcal infection (GABHS). SC affects about 26% of patients with RF[66] and remains the most common cause of acute chorea in children worldwide.[67,68] Despite the decline of its incidence, RF remains a significant public health problem in developing areas of the world.

The usual age at onset of SC is about 9 years, with a female preponderance. Typically, patients develop this disease 4 to 8 weeks after an episode of GABHS pharyngitis. Chorea, the cardinal motor feature of the illness, rapidly spreads and becomes generalized, but 20% of patients develops hemichorea.[66,69] Hypotonia, tics, hypometric saccades, motor impersistence, and bradykinesia are other motor findings that are common in SC.[66,70–72] In severe and rare cases, the muscle tone is so decreased that the patient may become bedridden, the so-called chorea paralytica. Migraine,[73] decreased verbal fluency,[74] and prosody[75] have also been reported in SC patients.

Behavioral problems are common in SC patients and have been reported in early descriptions of the disease.[76,77] Many studies found obsessive-compulsive behavior (OCB) and

Box 16.1 Conditions Associated With Chorea

Genetic causes

- Ataxia-telangiectasia
- Ataxia associated with oculomotor apraxia
- Benign hereditary chorea
- C9orf72 expansions
- Dentatorubropallidoluysian degeneration
- Friedreich ataxia
- Glucose transporter deficiency
- Huntington disease
- Huntington disease-like illnesses
- Leigh disease and other mitochondriopathies
- Lesch-Nyhan disease
- McLeod syndrome
- Neuroacanthocytosis
- Neuroferritinopathy
- Pantothenate kinase associated degeneration
- POLG mutation
- Prion disease
- PRRT2 gene mutation
- Spinocerebellar atrophy type 2
- Spinocerebellar atrophy type 3
- Spinocerebellar atrophy type 17
- Tuberous sclerosis
- Xeroderma pigmentosum
- Wilson's disease

Immune

- Acute disseminated encephalomyelopathy
- Antiphospholipid antibody syndrome
- Behçet's disease
- Celiac disease
- Paraneoplastic syndromes
- Sarcoidosis
- Sjogren's syndrome
- Sydenham's chorea and variants (chorea gravidarum and contraceptive-induced chorea)
- Systemic lupus erythematosus

Drug-related

- Amantadine
- Amphetamine
- Anticonvulsants
- Antihistamine agents
- Carbon monoxide
- CNS stimulants (methylphenidate, pemoline, cyproheptadine)
- Cocaine
- Dopamine agonists
- Dopamine-receptor blockers
- Ethanol
- Levodopa
- Levofloxacin
- Lithium
- Sympathomimetics
- Theophylline
- Tricyclic antidepressants
- Valproic acid
- Withdrawal emergent syndrome

Infections

- AIDS related (toxoplasmosis, progressive multifocal leukoencephalopathy, HIV encephalitis)
- Bacteria
  - Diphtheria - Scarlet fever - Whooping cough
- Encephalitis
  - B19 parvovirus - Herpes-6 virus encephalitis
  - Influenza encephalitis - Japanese encephalitis - Measles - Mumps - West Nile River encephalitis - Others
- Parasites
  - Neurocysticercosis
- Protozoan
  - Malaria - Syphilis

Endocrine-metabolic dysfunction

- Adrenal insufficiency
- Hyper/hypocalcemia
- Hyper/hypoglycemia
- Hypomagnesemia
- Hypernatremia
- Liver failure
- Uremia

Vascular

- Polycitemia vera
- Postpump chorea (cardiac surgery)
- Posterior reversible encephalopathy syndrome
- Stroke
- Subdural hematoma

Miscellaneous

- Anoxic encephalopathy
- Brainstem cavernous malformation
- Brainstem glioma
- Cerebral palsy
- Cerebrospinal fluid shunt-induced
- Extrapontine myelinolysis
- Intratumoral chemotherapy catheter
- Kernicterus
- Multiple sclerosis
- Normal maturation (less than 12 months old)
- Nutritional (e.g., B12 deficiency)
- Pontine hemorrhage
- Posttraumatic (brain injury)
- Putaminal cavernous malformation

OCD in subjects with SC.[78–80] In our own study of behavioral abnormalities of 50 patients with RF without chorea, and 56 patients with SC compared with 50 normal controls, we found that OCB, OCD, and ADHD were more frequent in the SC group (19%, 23.2%, 30.4%) than in RF without chorea (14%, 6%, 8%) and controls (11%, 4%, 8%). In this study, we also showed that OCB displays little interference in the performance of the activities of daily living. Comparing patients with acute and persistent SC, OCB, OCD, and ADHD were more common among subjects with prolonged forms of SC.[81] Hounie et al., described that OCB is more frequently in patients with SC who have relatives with obsessions and compulsions. This suggests that there is an interplay between genetic and environmental factors in the development of behavioral symptoms in SC.[82] Checking (53%), cleaning (42%), and repeating (36%) are common compulsions in individuals with SC. The two most reported obsessional symptoms are aggressive obsessions (63%) and fear of contamination (34%). This is in contrast with the types of obsessions commonly seen in individuals with tic disorders,[83] which are attention to symmetry, "just right" behavior, aritmomania, and others.

The finding that behavioral problems are common in patients with RF and chorea contributed to the notion that SC is a model for childhood autoimmune neuropsychiatric disorders, the so-called Pediatric Autoimmune Neuropsychiatric Disorders Associated with Streptoccocus (PANDAS).[84] PANDAS is a controversial concept which states that infection with GABHS may induce tics, OCB, and other neuropsychiatric disorders. There is a long list of potential neurologic symptoms and signs related to streptococcus infection: dementia, dystonia, encephalitis lethargica-like syndrome, motor stereotypies, myoclonus, opsoclonus, parkinsonism, paroxysmal dyskinesia, restless-leg syndrome, and tremor. However, there is no conclusive evidence that antineuronal antibodies induced by streptococcus play a significant role in the pathogenesis of tic disorders. The only movement disorder undeniably related to streptococcus infection is SC.[68,85]

There are studies describing the occurrence of other psychiatric abnormalities in SC. For instance, the frequency of depression and anxiety is increased during and after the occurrence of motor findings in SC symptoms.[83,86] Interestingly, the frequency of psychiatric disorders does not differ between SC patients in remission and individuals with persistent chorea, except for depressive disorders which are more frequent in the later.[86] These findings suggest that SC causes an irreversible basal ganglia dysfunction in at least one subset of individuals. Finally, there are rare reports of psychosis and trichotillomania during the acute phase of SC.[87,88]

Conclusions

All genetic or acquired choreatic disorders display a combination of motor and behavioral disorders. Among the latter, the most common findings are dysexecutive function, OCB, and ADHD, although other features, such as apathy and depression, can also be present. Despite the heterogeneity of the underlying pathological abnormalities in these disorders, it is likely that these nonmotor findings are related to dysfunction of the frontostriatal circuits. Obviously, the clinician must consider these findings when providing care for these individuals.

References

1. Cardoso, F., Seppi, K., Mair, K.J., Wenning, G.K., Poewe, W. (2006). Seminar on choreas. *Lancet Neurol*, 5(7), 589–602.
2. Cardoso, F. (2017). Nonmotor symptoms in Huntington disease. *Int Rev Neurobiol*, 134, 1397–1408.
3. Cardoso, F. (2017). Autoimmune choreas. *J Neurol Neurosurg Psychiatry*, 88(5), 412–417.
4. Margolis, R.L., O'Hearn, E., Rosenblatt, A., et al. (2001). A disorder similar to Huntington's disease is associated with a novel CAG repeat expansion. *Ann Neurol*, 50(6), 373–380.
5. Krause, A., Mitchell, C., Essop, F., et al. (2015). Junctophilin 3 (JPH3) expansion mutations causing Huntington disease like 2 (HDL2) are common in South African patients with African ancestry and a Huntington disease phenotype. *Am J Med Genet*, 168(7), 573–585.
6. Anderson, D.G., Walker, R.H., Connor, M., Carr, J., Margolis, R.L., Krause, A. (2017). A systematic review of the Huntington disease-like 2 phenotype. *J Huntingtons Dis*, 6(1), 37–46.
7. Bardien, S., Abrahams, F., Soodyall, H., et al. (2007). A South African mixed ancestry family with Huntington disease-like 2: clinical and genetic features. *Mov Disord*, 22(14), 2083–2089.
8. Fischer, C.A., Licht, E.A., Mendez, M.F. (2012). The neuropsychiatric manifestations of Huntington's disease-like 2. *J Neuropsychiatry Clin Neurosci*, 24(4), 489–492.

9. Ferreira-Correia, A., Anderson, D.G., Cockcroft, K., Krause, A. (2020). The neuropsychological deficits and dissociations in Huntington disease-like 2: A series of case-control studies. *Neuropsychologia*, 136, 107238.

10. Ferreira-Correia, A., Anderson, D.G., Cockcroft, K., Krause, A. (2020). A comparison between the neurocognitive profile of Huntington disease-like 2 and Huntington disease: exploring the presence of double dissociations. *Appl Neuropsychol Adult*, 9, 1–11.

11. DeJesus-Hernandez, M., Mackenzie, I.R., Boeve, B.F., et al. (2011). Expanded GGGGCC hexanucleotide repeat in noncoding region of C9ORF72 causes chromosome 9p-linked FTD and ALS. *Neuron*, 72(2), 245–256.

12. Marogianni, C., Rikos, D., Provatas, A., et al. (2019). The role of C9orf72 in neurodegenerative disorders: a systematic review, an updated meta-analysis, and the creation of an online database. *Neurobiol Aging*, 84, 238.e25–238.e34.

13. Van Mossevelde, S., van der Zee, J., Cruts, M., Van Broeckhoven, C. (2017). Relationship between C9orf72 repeat size and clinical phenotype. *Curr Opin Genet Dev*, 44, 117–124.

14. Cooper-Knock, J., Shaw, P.J., Kirby, J. (2014). The widening spectrum of C9ORF72-related disease; genotype/phenotype correlations and potential modifiers of clinical phenotype. *Acta Neuropathol*, 127(3), 333–345.

15. Cannas, A., Solla, P., Borghero, G., et al. (2015). C9ORF72 intermediate repeat expansion in patients affected by atypical parkinsonian syndromes or Parkinson's disease complicated by psychosis or dementia in a Sardinian population. *J Neurol*, 262(11), 2498–2503.

16. Yokoyama, J.S., Rosen, H.J. (2012). Neuroimaging features of C9ORF72 expansion. *Alzheimers Res Ther*, 4(6), 45.

17. Hensman Moss, D.J., Poulter, M., Beck, J., et al. (2014). C9orf72 expansions are the most common genetic cause of Huntington disease phenocopies. *Neurology*, 82(4), 292–299.

18. Wild, E.J., Tabrizi, S.J. (2007). Huntington's disease phenocopy syndromes. *Curr Opin Neurol*, 20(6), 681–687.

19. Beck, J., Poulter, M., Hensman, D., et al. (2013). Large C9orf72 hexanucleotide repeat expansions are seen in multiple neurodegenerative syndromes and are more frequent than expected in the UK population. *Am J Hum Genet*, 92(3), 345–353.

20. Koutsis, G., Karadima, G., Kartanou, C., Kladi, A., Panas, M. (2015). C9ORF72 hexanucleotide repeat expansions are a frequent cause of Huntington disease phenocopies in the Greek population. *Neurobiol Aging*, 36(1), 547.e13–6.

21. Kostić, V.S., Dobričić, V., Stanković, I., Ralić, V., Stefanova, E. (2014). C9orf72 expansion as a possible genetic cause of Huntington disease phenocopy syndrome. *J Neurol*, 261(10), 1917–1921.

22. Stewart, H., Rutherford, N.J., Briemberg, H., et al. (2012). Clinical and pathological features of amyotrophic lateral sclerosis caused by mutation in the C9ORF72 gene on chromosome 9p. *Acta Neuropathol*, 123(3), 409–417.

23. Silverman, H.E., Goldman, J.S., Huey, E.D. (2019). Links between the C9orf72 repeat expansion and psychiatric symptoms. *Curr Neurol Neurosci Rep*, 19(12), 93.

24. Boeve, B.F., Boylan, K.B., Graff-Radford, N.R., et al. (2012). Characterization of frontotemporal dementia and/or amyotrophic lateral sclerosis associated with the GGGGCC repeat expansion in C9ORF72. *Brain*, 135(3), 765–783.

25. Snowden, J.S., Adams, J., Harris, J., et al. (2015). Distinct clinical and pathological phenotypes in frontotemporal dementia associated with MAPT, PGRN and C9orf72 mutations. *Amyotroph Lateral Scler Frontotemporal Degener*, 16(7–8), 497–505.

26. Kertesz, A., Ang, L.C., Jesso, S., et al. (2013). Psychosis and hallucinations in frontotemporal dementia with the C9ORF72 mutation: a detailed clinical cohort. *Cogn Behav Neurol Off J Soc Behav Cogn Neurol*, 26(3), 146–154.

27. Ducharme, S., Bajestan, S., Dickerson, B.C., Voon, V. (2017). Psychiatric presentations of C9orf72 mutation: what are the diagnostic implications for clinicians? *J Neuropsychiatry Clin Neurosci*, 29(3), 195–205.

28. Shinagawa, S., Naasan, G., Karydas, A.M., et al. (2015). Clinicopathological study of patients with C9ORF72-associated frontotemporal dementia presenting with delusions. *J Geriatr Psychiatry Neurol*, 28(2), 99–107.

29. Khan, B.K., Yokoyama, J.S., Takada, L.T., et al. (2012). Atypical, slowly progressive behavioural variant frontotemporal dementia associated with C9ORF72 hexanucleotide expansion. *J Neurol Neurosurg Psychiatry*, 83(4), 358–364.

30. Dobson-Stone, C., Hallupp, M., Bartley, L., et al. (2012). C9ORF72 repeat expansion in clinical and neuropathologic frontotemporal dementia cohorts. *Neurology*, 79(10), 995–1001.

31. Devenney, E.M., Ahmed, R.M., Halliday, G., Piguet, O., Kiernan, M.C., Hodges, J.R. (2018). Psychiatric disorders in C9orf72 kindreds: study of 1,414 family members. *Neurology*, 91(16), e1498–e1507.

32. Byrne, S., Heverin, M., Elamin, M., et al. (2013). Aggregation of neurologic and neuropsychiatric disease in amyotrophic lateral sclerosis kindreds: a population-based case-control cohort study of familial and sporadic amyotrophic lateral sclerosis. *Ann Neurol*, 74(5), 699–708.

33. Arthur, K.C., Rivera, A.M., Samuels, J., et al. (2017). C9orf72 hexanucleotide repeat expansions are not a common cause of obsessive-compulsive disorder. *J Neurol Sci*, 375, 71–72.

34. Meisler, M.H., Grant, A.E., Jones, J.M., et al. (2013). C9ORF72 expansion in a family with bipolar disorder. *Bipolar Disord*, 15(3), 326–332.

35. Fahey, C., Byrne, S., McLaughlin, R., et al. (2014). Analysis of the hexanucleotide repeat expansion and founder haplotype at C9ORF72 in an Irish psychosis case-control sample. *Neurobiol Aging*, 35(6), 1510.e1–5.

36. Ha, A.D., Maia, D., Fung, V.S.C., Cardoso, F. (2016). Huntington disease and other genetic causes of choreas. *DeckerMed Psychiatry*. 10.2310/NEURO.6357.

37. Mestre T.A. (2016). Chorea. *Contin (Minneap Minn)*, 22(4), 1186–1207.

38. Fernandez, M., Raskind, W., Wolff, J., et al. (2001). Familial dyskinesia and facial myokymia (FDFM): a novel movement disorder. *Ann Neurol*, 49(4), 486–492.

39. Vijiaratnam, N., Newby, R., Kempster, P.A. (2018). Depression and psychosis in ADCY5-related dyskinesia—part of the phenotypic spectrum? *J Clin Neurosci*, 57, 167–168.

40. Chang, F.C.F., Westenberger, A., Dale, R.C., et al. (2016). Phenotypic insights into ADCY5-associated disease. *Mov Disord*, 31(7), 1033–1040.

41. Raskind, W.H., Friedman, J.R., Roze, E., Méneret, A., Chen, D.H., Bird, T.D. (2017). ADCY5-related dyskinesia: comments on characteristic manifestations and variant-associated severity. *Mov Disord*, 32(2), 305–306.

42. Waalkens, A.J.E., Vansenne, F., van der Hout, A.H., et al. (2018). Expanding the ADCY5 phenotype toward spastic paraparesis. *Neurol Genet*, 4(1), e214.

43. Haerer, A.F., Currier, R.D., Jackson, J.F. (1967). Hereditary nonprogressive chorea of early onset. *N Engl J Med*, 276(22), 1220–1224.

44. Rice, J. (2014). Benign hereditary chorea: more than meets the eye. *Dev Med Child Neurol*, 56(7), 606–607.

45. Peall, K.J., Kurian, M.A. (2015). Benign hereditary chorea: an update. *Tremor Other Hyperkinet Mov*, 5, 314.

46. Inzelberg, R., Weinberger, M., Gak, E. (2011). Benign hereditary chorea: an update. *Park Relat Disord*, 17(5), 301–307.

47. Iodice, A., Carecchio, M., Zorzi, G., et al. (2018). Restless legs syndrome in NKX2-1-related chorea: an expansion of the disease spectrum. *Brain Dev*, 41(3), 250–256.

48. Gras, D., Jonard, L., Roze, E., et al. (2012). Benign hereditary chorea: phenotype, prognosis, therapeutic outcome and long term follow-up in a large series with new mutations in the TITF1/NKX2-1 gene. *J Neurol Neurosurg Psychiatry*, 83(10), 956–962.

49. Glik, A., Vuillaume, I., Devos, D., Inzelberg, R. (2008). Psychosis, short stature in benign hereditary chorea: a novel thyroid transcription factor-1 mutation. *Mov Disord*, 23(12), 1744–1747

50. Ainiala, H., Hietaharju, A., Loukkola, J., et al. (2001). Validity of the new American College of Rheumatology criteria for neuropsychiatric lupus syndromes: a population-based evaluation. *Arthritis Rheum*, 45(5), 419–423.

51. Unterman, A., Nolte, J.E.S., Boaz, M., Abady, M., Shoenfeld, Y., Zandman-Goddard, G. (2011). Neuropsychiatric syndromes in systemic lupus erythematosus: a meta-analysis. *Semin Arthritis Rheum*, 41(1), 1–11.

52. Kampylafka, E.I., Alexopoulos, H., Kosmidis, M.L., et al. (2013). Incidence and prevalence of major central nervous system involvement in systemic lupus erythematosus: a 3-year prospective study of 370 patients. *PLoS One*, 8(2), e55843–e55848.

53. Cervera, R., Asherson, R.A., Font, J., et al. (1997). Chorea in the antiphospholipid syndrome: clinical, radiologic, and immunologic characteristics of 50 patients from our clinics and the recent literature. *Medicine (Baltimore)*, 76(3), 203–212.

54. Reiner, P., Galanaud, D., Leroux, G., et al. (2011). Long-term outcome of 32 patients with chorea and systemic lupus erythematosus or antiphospholipid antibodies. *Mov Disord*, 26(13), 2422–2427.

55. García-Moreno, J.M., Chacón, J. (2002). Juvenile parkinsonism as a manifestation of systemic lupus erythematosus: case report and review of the literature. *Mov Disord*, 17(6), 1329–1335.

56. Santos, M.J., Reis, P., da Silva, J.A., de Queiroz, M.V. (1994). [Ischemic lesion of the CNS in patients with systemic lupus erythematosus]. *Acta Med Port*, 7(4), 201–206.

57. Joseph, F.G., Lammie, G.A., Scolding, N.J. (2007). CNS lupus: a study of 41 patients. *Neurology*, 69(7), 644–654.

58. Baizabal-Carvallo, J.F., Alonso-Juarez, M., Koslowski, M. (2011). Chorea in systemic lupus erythematosus. *J Clin Rheumatol Pract reports Rheum Musculoskelet Dis*, 17(2), 69–72.

59. Hanly, J.G., Li, Q., Su, L., et al. (2019). Psychosis in systemic lupus erythematosus: results from an international inception cohort study. *Arthritis Rheumatol*, 71(2), 281–289.

60. Asano, N.M.J., Coriolano, M. das G.W. de S., Asano, B.J., Lins, O.G. (2013). Psychiatric comorbidities in patients with systemic lupus erythematosus: a systematic review of the last 10 years. *Rev Bras Reumatol*, 53(5), 431–437.

61. Jarpa, E., Babul, M., Calderón, J., et al. (2011). Common mental disorders and psychological distress in systemic lupus erythematosus are not associated with disease activity. *Lupus*, 20(1), 58–66.

62. Maciel, R.O.H., Ferreira, G.A., Akemy, B., Cardoso, F. (2016). Executive dysfunction, obsessive–compulsive symptoms, and attention deficit and hyperactivity disorder in systemic lupus erythematosus: Evidence for basal ganglia dysfunction? *J Neurol Sci*, 360(C), 94–97.

63. Bachen, E.A., Chesney, M.A., Criswell, L.A. (2009). Prevalence of mood and anxiety disorders in women with systemic lupus erythematosus. *Arthritis Rheum*, 61(6), 822–829.

64. Slattery, M.J., Dubbert, B.K., Allen, A.J., Leonard, H.L., Swedo, S.E., Gourley, M.F. (2004). Prevalence of obsessive-compulsive disorder in patients with systemic lupus erythematosus. *J Clin Psychiatry*, 65(3), 301–306.

65. Garcia, R.J., Francis, L., Dawood, M., Lai, Z.-W., Faraone, S.V., Perl, A. (2013). Attention deficit and hyperactivity disorder scores are elevated and respond to N-acetylcysteine treatment in patients with systemic lupus erythematosus. *Arthritis Rheum*, 65(5), 1313–1318.

66. Cardoso, F., Silva, C.E., Mota, C.C. (1997). Chorea in fifty consecutive patients with rheumatic fever. *Mov Disord*, 12(5), 701–703.

67. Zomorrodi, A., Wald, E.R. (2006). Sydenham's chorea in western Pennsylvania. *Pediatrics*, 117(4), e675–e679.

68. Cardoso, F. (2011). Sydenham's chorea. *Handb Clin Neurol.*, 100, 221–229.

69. Nausieda, P.A., Grossman, B.J., Koller, W.C., Weiner, W.J., Klawans, H.L. (1980). Sydenham chorea: an update. *Neurology*, 30(3), 331–334.

70. Mercadante, M.T., Rosario Campos, M.C., Marques-Dias, M.J., Miguel, E.C., Leckman, J. (1997). Vocal tics in Sydenham's chorea. *J Am Acad Child Adolesc Psychiatry*, 36(3), 305–306.

71. Teixeira, A.L., Cardoso, F., Maia, D.P., Cunningham, M.C. (2003). Sydenham's chorea may be a risk factor for drug induced parkinsonism. *J Neurol Neurosurg Psychiatry*, 74(9), 1350–1351.

72. Barreto, L.B., Horta Maciel, R.O., Maia, D.P., Teixeira, A.L., Cardoso, F. (2012). Parkinsonian signs and symptoms in adults with a history of Sydenham's chorea. *Park Relat Disord*, 18(5), 595–597.

73. Teixeira, A.L., Meira, F.C., Maia, D.P., Cunningham, M.C., Cardoso, F. (2005). Migraine headache in patients with Sydenham's chorea. *Cephalalgia*, 25(7), 542–544.

74. Cunningham, M.C.Q.S., Maia, D.P., Teixeira Jr., A.L., Cardoso, F. (2006). Sydenham's chorea is associated with decreased verbal fluency. *Park Relat Disord*, 12(3), 165–167.

75. Oliveira, P.M., Cardoso, F., Maia, D.P., Cunningham, M.C.Q., Teixeira, A.L., Jr., Reis, C. (2010). Acoustic analysis of prosody in Sydenham's chorea. *Arq Neuropsiquiatr*, 68(5), 744–748.

76. Diefendorf, A.R. (1912). Mental symptoms of acute chorea. *J Nerv Ment Dis*, 39, 161–172.

77. Ebaugh, F.G. (1926). Neuropsychiatric aspects of chorea in children. *JAMA*, 87, 1083–1088.

78. Freeman, J.M., Aron, A.M., Collard, J.E., Mackay, M. C. (1965). The emotional correlates of Sydenham's chorea. *Pediatrics*, 35, 42–49.

79. Swedo, S.E., Rapoport, J.L., Cheslow, D.L., et al. (1989). High prevalence of obsessive-compulsive symptoms in patients with Sydenham's chorea. *Am J Psychiatry*, 146(2), 246–249.

80. Asbahr, F.R., Negrão, A.B., Gentil, V., et al. (1998). Obsessive-compulsive and related symptoms in children and adolescents with rheumatic fever with and without chorea: a prospective 6-month study. *Am J Psychiatry*, 155(8), 1122–1124.

81. Maia, D.P., Teixeira Jr., A.L., Cunningham, M.C.Q., Cardoso, F. (2005). Obsessive compulsive behavior, hyperactivity, and attention deficit disorder in Sydenham chorea. *Neurology*, 64(10), 1799–1801.

82. Hounie, A.G., Pauls, D.L., do Rosario-Campos, M.C., et al. (2007). Obsessive-compulsive spectrum disorders and rheumatic fever: a family study. *Biol Psychiatry*, 61(3), 266–272.

83. Punukollu, M., Mushet, N., Linney, M., Hennessy, C., Morton, M. (2016). Neuropsychiatric manifestations of Sydenham's chorea: a systematic review. *Dev Med Child Neurol*, 58(1), 16–28.

84. Swedo, S.E. (1994). Sydenham's chorea: a model for childhood autoimmune neuropsychiatric disorders. *JAMA*, 272(22), 1788–1791.

85. Bottas, A., Richter, M.A. (2002). Pediatric autoimmune neuropsychiatric disorders associated with streptococcal infections (PANDAS). *Pediatr Infect Dis J*, 21(1), 67–71.

86. Moreira, J., Kummer, A., Harsányi, E., Cardoso, F., Teixeira, A.L. (2014). Psychiatric disorders in persistent and remitted Sydenham's chorea. *Park Relat Disord*, 20(2), 233–236.

87. Kummer, A., Maia, D.P., Cardoso, F., Teixeira, A.L. (2007). Trichotillomania in acute Sydenham's chorea. *Aust N Z J Psychiatry*, 41(12), 1013–1014.

88. Teixeira, A.L., Jr., Maia, D.P., Cardoso, F. (2007). Psychosis following acute Sydenham's chorea. *Eur Child Adolesc Psychiatry*, 16(1), 67–69.

17

Parkinson's Disease and Atypical Parkinsonian Syndromes

Julia Ridgeway-Diaz and Laura Marsh

Introduction

Parkinson's disease (PD) and atypical parkinsonian syndromes (APSs), defined mostly by motor features, are frequently complicated by concurrent psychiatric disorders. PD refers specifically to the progressive neurodegenerative disease characterized by its three cardinal motor symptoms: rigidity, tremor, and bradykinesia, two of which are required for diagnosis. Parkinsonism, a less specific and nonetiologic term, is used when some of the following motor signs are present—rigidity, tremor, bradykinesia, and impaired postural reflexes.[1–3] APSs are significantly less common than PD, and include other neurodegenerative disorders that present with parkinsonism, including multiple system atrophy (MSA), progressive supranuclear palsy (PSP), corticobasal degeneration (CBD), dementia with Lewy bodies (DLB), frontotemporal dementia (FTD), and vascular parkinsonism (VP). Except for vascular parkinsonism, APSs have historically been referred to as "Parkinson's plus" syndromes in that the signs and symptoms include, but are not limited to, parkinsonism and can be difficult to distinguish from PD early in the disease course. Each of these conditions needs to be distinguished from medication-induced parkinsonism, a side effect of multiple psychiatric and non-psychiatric medications.

Given varying degrees of motor, cognitive, and psychiatric phenomena in PD or APS, collaborative and interdisciplinary care benefits both patients and clinicians. For example, when cognitive and psychiatric symptoms prompt clinical attention before motor signs are overt, psychiatrists may be on the front lines for screening and considering PD and APS in the differential diagnosis. A role for psychiatrists in longitudinal management of these conditions is underscored by the impact of mood, psychotic, behavioral, and cognitive disturbances, which can have a greater effect on quality of life than motor symptoms.[4]

This chapter provides an integrated approach to psychiatric assessment and formulation when a patient presents to psychiatric care with parkinsonism. First, we review individual diseases, then concentrate on psychiatric symptoms. We then discuss how patients may present to a psychiatrist and discuss evaluation and management.

Epidemiology of PD, APS, and Associated Psychiatric Disturbances

Parkinson's Disease

Parkinson's disease (PD) is the second-most common neurodegenerative disease after Alzheimer's disease and the most common parkinsonian syndrome. As with Alzheimer's disease, age is the most important risk factor for PD. In industrialized countries, prevalence of PD is 0.3% of the entire population and increases to 1% of the population over the age of 60, and approximately 3% of the population over the age of 70.[1] Incidence of PD is highest in patients 70–79 years of age while prevalence is highest among those ages 85–89 years.[5] Late-onset PD is often defined as motor symptom onset at age 70 or older (39% of patients), middle-onset PD begins at ages 50–69 years (51%), and young-onset PD is defined as symptom onset before age 50 (10%).[6]

Heterogeneity in PD across multiple domains adds to its complexity, and many different subtypes have been proposed. One recent proposal segregates PD into subtypes: mild motor-predominant (49% of PD patients), intermediate (35%), and diffuse malignant (16%).[7] The mild motor-predominant subtype is associated with a longer time from diagnosis to major disability milestones (frequent falls, dementia, nursing home placement, wheelchair use) (an average of 14.3 years) and better survival after diagnosis (an average of 20.2 years).[5] Patients with the intermediate subtype live on average 8.2 years until major disability and survive 13.2 years after diagnosis. Diffuse malignant PD, the most severe subtype, involves major disability an average of 3.5 years after diagnosis and an average survival time of 8.1 years after diagnosis.[5,7] The variation in PD severity and prognosis challenges traditional views of PD, which were dominated by the natural history of the diffuse malignant subtype. Long survival times of the intermediate and mild motor-predominant forms highlight the importance of maintaining each patient's quality of life, which is largely determined by their psychiatric symptom burden.

Epidemiology of Psychiatric Disorders in PD

In clinical practice, psychiatric symptoms of all types are frequently undetected by clinicians,[8] underreported by patients,[9] and, hence, undertreated in spite of their profound impact on health-related quality of life.[10] Almost all PD patients experience at least one and usually multiple psychiatric symptoms at some point in their course. Cognitive changes, depression, psychosis, anxiety, and sleep disturbances are most common though prevalence estimates vary with screening, diagnostic criteria, and population differences.

Atypical Parkinsonian Syndromes

APS, in general, are characterized by similar constellations of symptoms as PD, but with differing severities and orders of onset. In contrast to PD, motor symptoms in APS respond poorly to levodopa. Like PD, the most common psychiatric diagnoses involve depression, anxiety, psychosis, and sleep disturbances.

Multiple System Atrophy

Multiple system atrophy (MSA) is a rare, heterogeneous neurodegenerative disease characterized neuropathologically by aggregation of alpha-synuclein in oligodendrocytes, as opposed to neurons, as is seen with PD. The term MSA subsumed three other diagnoses that are no longer used: olivopontocerebellar atrophy, Shy-Drager syndrome, and striatonigral degeneration, which could not be distinguished from each other reliably. MSA is now subtyped as MSA with parkinsonian features and MSA with cerebellar features. In a European study, estimated incidence of MSA was 0.6 cases per 100,000 people per year.[11] Prevalence is thought to be 4.4 cases per 100,000, translating to approximately one living MSA case for every 40 living PD cases.[12] MSA onset, on average, is in the early 50s,[13,14] and typically progresses more rapidly than PD. Mean survival duration is 7–9 years after MSA onset.

Like PD, depressive symptoms in MSA, and anxiety to a lesser extent, are primary determinants of quality of life when compared to overall MSA severity.[15] In a multisite study, 43% of MSA patients had probable depression and 37% had probable anxiety.[15] In a single site study, nearly 40% had moderate to severe depressive symptoms.[16] Up to one-third of MSA patients show impairments in global cognition, including subclinical symptoms of dementia.[17]

Progressive Supranuclear Palsy (PSP)

PSP, recognized as a disorder distinct from PD in 1964, is a tauopathy, like Alzheimer's disease and corticobasal degeneration (CBD). Global prevalence estimates vary from 3 to 6 in every 100,000 people and mean survival time after symptom onset is about 6–8 years.[18] Onset is usually after age 60 with a typical presentation of balance complaints and frequent and early falls, followed by bulbar and oculomotor symptoms. The diagnosis may be delayed because of overlapping symptoms with PD.

Affective and behavioral presentations of PSP include emotional lability (pseudobulbar palsy), irritability, disinhibition, depressed mood or anhedonia, and "personality" changes.[19] Like PD and MSA, depression, apathy, and anxiety are the most important drivers of quality of life.[15,20] Over half of PSP patients (56%) suffer from depression and about one-third (37%) suffer from anxiety.[15] Compared to other APS, apathy is especially prominent in PSP, was the most common psychiatric disorder in several studies, and can be expected to be present or emerge in least half of patients with PSP.[19,20]

Cognitive decline can be evident early. One study showed subclinical to clinical global impairment in 57%–62% of PSP patients; though severity of cognitive impairment correlated with disease stage, 50% of early-stage PSP patients had some degree of impairment. Executive function is most often affected and memory is relatively spared.[21] When assessed specifically, executive dysfunction is seen in 70%–90% of PSP patients.[17,22]

Corticobasal Degeneration

Corticobasal degeneration (CBD), a rare neurodegenerative disease, usually presents as corticobasal syndrome (CBS), but is a frequently misdiagnosed syndrome with a heterogeneous presentation.[23,24] CBS is a markedly assymetric motor and sensory apraxia, however pathologically confirmed CBD may present with primary language dysfunction or behavioral changes, mimicking frontotemporal dementia. CBD prevalence ranges from 5 in 100,000 up to 11 in 100,000 when using more sensitive diagnostic criteria.[25,26] Depression (73%) and apathy (40%) are the most prominent psychiatric symptoms, though irritability (20%) and agitation (20%) also occur.[27] Cognitive impairment and behavioral changes occur, respectively, in 70% and 55% of patients over course of CBD.[23]

Dementia with Lewy Bodies

Dementia with Lewy bodies (DLB), a progressive neurocognitive disorder characterized by early changes in cognition with abnormal perceptions, and parkinsonism, and is the second-most common synucleinopathy after PD. Prevalence studies are wide-ranging: general population studies report 0.1% and 2.0% prevalence among those over age 65 years and 0% to 5% among people older than 70 years.[1] In a general population of people 75 years and older, DLB prevalence was approximately 5%, which is half that of Alzheimer's disease and equal to vascular dementia.[28] Naturally, DLB prevalence is higher in populations with dementia, from

2.8% to 30.5%.[1] Psychiatric symptoms of DLB include hallucinations (76%), delusions (57%), apathy (50%), depression (20-51%, up to 93% in inpatients), and anxiety (38-50%).[29-37]

Frontotemporal Dementia

Frontotemporal dementia (FTD), a notable cause of young-onset dementia (i.e., onset usually in the sixth decade of life), causes behavioral changes (primarily apathy and disinhibition) and language deficits early in its course followed by later memory and other cognitive changes. Estimated point prevalence is 15–22 cases per 100,000.[38] FTD has three subtypes: behavioral variant, semantic variant primary progressive aphasia, and nonfluent variant primary progressive aphasia. FTD is discussed in detail in another chapter.

Vascular Parkinsonism

Vascular parkinsonism (VP), a secondary form of parkinsonism, results from cerebrovascular infarcts in the thalamus and basal ganglia, diffuse white matter ischemic lesions, and, rarely, large vessel strokes.[39] Also referred to as arteriosclerotic parkinsonism, vascular pseudo-parkinsonism, and lower-body parkinsonism, VP represents an estimated 2.5% to 6% of PD cases in various population-based and clinical cohort studies.[39,40] VP can be difficult to distinguish from idiopathic PD, though, as with other APS, motor benefits from levodopa are poor. While epidemiological data on prevalence of psychiatric comorbidities in VP is scarce, depression, anxiety, apathy, and cognitive changes are reported as common.

Prodromal Features: Some Clinical Considerations

Both PD and APS may manifest with prominent psychiatric symptoms and, as discussed, some patients will present for a psychiatric evaluation before a diagnosis of PD or APS is established. This supports evidence for a discernable prodromal phase involving a variety of nonmotor symptoms, sometimes beginning up to 20 years before overt motor symptoms.[41] Prospective studies support the predictive value of olfactory loss, constipation, and rapid eye movement (REM) sleep behavior disorder (RBD), where patients act out dreams due to the loss of REM atonia, but depression, anxiety, and excessive daytime sleepiness may also be seen prior to motor onset. Accordingly, these highly predictive nonmotor prodromal phenomena, especially depression and anxiety, underscore the role for psychiatrists to screen for movement abnormalities at regular intervals in middle-aged and elderly patients with depression, anxiety, or apathy. A sleep history is particularly important. RBD screening is of particular interest, given its strong association with synucleinopathies (PD, MSA, and DLB) and portends a poor prognosis.[42] In one study, 35% to 92% of patients with RBD eventually developed a neurodegenerative disease, most commonly PD and DLB.[43] Relevant motor symptoms or findings should prompt appropriate evaluations and referrals.

Phenomenology

Motor Phenomena

Parkinson's Disease

The characteristic motor signs of PD include tremor, rigidity, and bradykinesia, of which at least two must be evident to make the clinical diagnosis. The motor signs usually begin on one side of the body and remain worse on that side, even when motor phenomena involve both sides. Its signature tremor is a slow 3–6 Hz pill-rolling tremor that occurs while those limb muscles are at rest, but absence of tremor does not exclude the diagnosis of PD. Many patients also have some postural and/or kinetic tremor.

Bradykinesia means slowness of movements and hypokinesia is smallness of movement. PD patients demonstrate decreased amplitude of movement and spontaneous movements, hypomimia (decreased facial expression), decreased blink rate, and hypophonia (soft speech). The slower speed and amplitude of finger and hand movements affect fine motor control. For example, handwriting deteriorates with smaller and more crowded letters. Akinesia refers to absence of movement, including "freezing," i.e., difficulty initiating desired movements such as taking a step forward. Rigidity is a sign seen on examination, but patients may complain of asymmetric stiffness or cramping in limbs. Having the patient perform contralateral voluntary movements can accentuate tone.

Gait phenomena include a tendency to walk in a flexed forward posture with a shorter stride and reduced arm swing that is greater on one side or evident in one limb only. With the slower gait, the patient may shuffle, festinate, i.e., take small steps with a tendency to fall forward, and turn en bloc, i.e., take multiple small steps to turn instead of pivoting on the toes. Postural instability emerges later.

Motor complications of dopaminergic therapies used to treat PD should be assessed in the psychiatric evaluation. Initially, dopaminergic therapy may completely alleviate parkinsonism. As PD progresses, "on-off" motor fluctuations result from the waning impact and duration of the dopaminergic response. With higher and more frequent dosing, patients fluctuate between "on" states, when motor function improves after taking the medication, and "off" states of reduced mobility from the medication effect "wearing off," sometimes to the point of immobility.

Abnormal involuntary hyperkinetic movements, referred to as dyskinesias, are the second long-term motor complication of dopaminergic therapy. Medication-induced dyskinesias typically emerge during "on" states, can be mild to severe in intensity, and may be aggravated by emotional tension or cognitive effort. They are similar in form to the writhing, choreo-athetoid movements of the trunk and limbs seen in tardive dyskinesia or Huntington's disease, *except* they dissipate as the dopaminergic effect wears off. Dyskinesias are more likely to appear unseemly to others, whereas patients may be unaware or grateful for the time-limited period of greater mobility.

"On–off" fluctuations can involve motor and nonmotor manifestations and occur multiple times during the day. Psychiatric features during "on" states include elevated mood, racing thoughts, hypersexuality, and hypomanic or manic phenomena. In "off" periods, nonmotor features include bradyphrenia (referred to as "clognition" by one patient), apathy, depression, dysphoria, anxiety, panic, and irritability.[44] "Off" nonmotor symptoms can be confused with panic attacks or even mimic a myocardial infarct. Other PD-specific medication-related mood and anxiety syndromes include early morning off (EMO) states with anxiety and low mood[45] and dopamine agonist withdrawal syndrome (DAWS),[46] which includes drug cravings, severe anxiety with possible panic attacks, suicidality, agitation, depression, and dysphoria in the setting of stopping dopaminergic medications.

Atypical Parkinsonian Syndromes

MSA phenomena include parkinsonism, early autonomic dysfunction, and cerebellar and pyramidal symptoms. These are manifest as rapidly progressive parkinsonism, gait ataxia with cerebellar dysarthria, limb ataxia, cerebellar oculomotor dysfunction, Babinski sign with hyperreflexia, postural instability, and dysphagia. At least one sign of autonomic dysfunction should be seen. Two subtypes, cerebellar (MSA-C, the more common form in the United States) and parkinsonian (MSA-P) also warrant distinction.

Initial parkinsonism in MSA is often difficult to distinguish from PD. Autonomic dysfunction, usually an early sign of MSA, includes fainting and lightheadedness related to orthostatic hypotension, bladder dysfunction, heart rate changes, and erectile dysfunction. Sexual dysfunction, before diagnosis of MSA, may prompt a patient to seek psychiatric care. Similarly, symptoms of RBD, evident in 69%–100% of polysomnograms of MSA patients, may be the initial complaint.[13,47] If not recognized, RBD can be interpreted as nightmares or attributed to trauma-related distress. Additional MSA characteristics that may distinguish it from PD include prominent snoring and apnea (central and obstructive), stridor, a low-pitched or quivering voice, and abnormal posture with anterocollis (Pisa syndrome). Pathological laughter and crying (pseudobulbar affect), panic attacks, and suicidal ideation also occur.

In PSP, progressive parkinsonism with prominent akinesia and axial rigidity plus early loss of postural reflexes leads to frequent falls.[48] Tremor is less common. Posture in PSP is often stiff and upright with a tendency to fall backward, in contrast to the stooped posture of PD. Progressive loss of voluntary control of eye movements, a hallmark of the disease, cause symptoms of visual blurring or tunnel vision because of reduced visual field, especially impaired upward and downward gaze. Gaze difficulties affect ability to read, i.e., scan lines on a page, make eye contact, eat, or walk downstairs. Though not diagnostic, PSP characteristically causes a fixed staring expression with reduced blink rate. Raised eyebrows (due to frontalis muscle overactivity) cause the individual to appear startled ("astonished sign") and vertical wrinkles in the glabella region ("procerus sign") make them appear worried. Speech is typically dysarthric with a soft, strained, or breathy voice that can be difficult to hear. Dysphagia develops over the disease course. PSP has a wide range of phenotypic variability, and subtypes of most interest to the psychiatrist include PSP with parkinsonism resembling idiopathic PD (PSP-P), PSP with speech/language disorders (PSP-SL), and PSP with frontal lobe cognitive or behavioral features (PSP-F).

Corticobasal syndrome involves progressive markedly asymmetric parkinsonism, motor and sensory apraxia, postural instability, unsteady gait, axial rigidity, limb dystonia, and myoclonus. Corticobasal syndrome is most commonly associated with pathologically diagnosed CBD, but CBD can also manifest as frontal-behavioral-spatial syndrome (FBS), nonfluent/agrammatic variant of primary progressive aphasia (naPPA), and progressive supranuclear palsy syndrome (PSPS). CBD typically includes progressive deficits in cortical functioning manifest as asymmetric apraxia and rigidity, alien limb syndrome, and myoclonus, and deficits related to basal ganglia degeneration, including bradykinesia, tremor, and dystonia.[49,50] Like other APS, CBD responds poorly to dopaminergic medication. In CBD, greater irritability and depression and relatively less apathy, as compared to PSP, may distinguish the two conditions. However, phenotypical features of CBD and PSP may overlap, and the underlying pathology does not always correlate with the classic phenotype.[51] Sleep disturbances are more common in CBD relative to age-matched peers, but less common than in PSP.[52]

DLB is defined by progressive disabling cognitive deficits in which the domains of attention, executive function, and visual processing are disproportionately affected relative to memory and naming. Diagnosis of probable DLB, in recent DLB consensus criteria,[53] also requires at least two core clinical features: delirium-like cognitive fluctuations, recurrent complex visual hallucinations, parkinsonism, and RBD.

Motor symptoms are less prominent in FTD and often not as impairing as in CBD and PSP. Parkinsonism is seen more in bvFTD and the nonfluent agrammatic variant. In contrast to PD, there is symmetric, axial rigidity. Tremor, while uncommon, may be postural, action, or resting.

Vascular parkinsonism presents with prominent postural instability and falls (like PSP), bradykinesia, a parkinsonian-ataxic gait (shuffling with a wider stance), pyramidal signs, and less prominent upper limb resting tremor.[40]

Cognitive Symptoms in Parkinsonian Conditions

Parkinson's Disease

Some degree of cognitive change is experienced by all patients with PD, who have a sixfold higher risk of developing dementia over the course of the disease, as compared to the general population, after controlling for age, gender, and education level.[54,55] In patients with PD, approximately 40% develop dementia (i.e., PDD); age and disease severity increase that risk dramatically.[55,56] A large Norwegian population-based study reported an 80%–90% cumulative incidence of PDD by age 90, conditional on survival.[57]

Cognitive changes in PD may be evident early in the disease course, are heterogeneous in severity and impact, and progress over time to a dementia syndrome, even if mild, in most patients. Early in PD, cognitive changes typically affect one or two domains and may impact IADLs or be evident only on formal testing or during specific tasks when cognitive abilities are challenged. Executive dysfunction, especially common, reflects disrupted basal ganglia and frontal networks. Common complaints include difficulties organizing ideas and planning and completing tasks, especially those with greater complexity that require shifting attention from one area of focus to another. In contrast to the "rapid forgetting" of Alzheimer's disease, in which information is not encoded, PD patients are typically able to learn and retain information but have difficulty retrieving or recalling stored memories. With relative preservation of recognition memory, cuing can prompt recall of that information. Visual-spatial difficulties affect depth perception and measuring distances, which can limit driving abilities. Language deficits involve difficulty retrieving words ("tip of the tongue" phenomenon) and comprehending complex sentences, such as when a question is combined with other information and details. Limiting sentence complexity can facilitate patient interviews.

Dementia (or major neurocognitive disorder) is diagnosed when deficits are present in one or more cognitive domain and are severe enough to interfere with daily living. As Alzheimer's disease is the most common cause of dementia in the United States, patients and families often raise concerns about its possible diagnosis. Generally, patients with PD who progress to dementia are assumed to have PD dementia, though Alzheimer pathology may be seen on postmortem neuropathology along with PD pathology.[58] Compared to Alzheimer's disease, delayed recall and language functions are often relatively intact, and dense aphasia, apraxia, or agnosia are less likely. In its latest stages, cognitive deficits in PDD may be difficult to distinguish from advanced Alzheimer's disease. Then, the pattern of cognitive deficits and movement abnormalities and their historical course, if available, assists in diagnosis.

Atypical Parkinsonian Syndromes

The 2008 consensus statement on diagnosis of MSA described dementia as a "red flag" suggestive of other diagnoses. However, up to 50% of MSA patients in longitudinal studies of MSA patients developed significant cognitive impairment. Executive dysfunction is more likely in MSA-P, whereas learning and visuospatial impairments are more likely in MSA-C.[59]

Cognitive presentations in PSP are that of a subcortical dementia: slow processing speed (bradyphrenia), memory impairment, and notable frontal lobe dysfunction (executive, memory retrieval, visuospatial, attentional, language, and social deficits). The key features of cortical dementias like Alzheimer's disease, i.e., aphasia, apraxia, and agnosia, are not evident. Cognitive deficits in PSP subtypes present as expected; prominent speech-language deficits in PSP-SL and dysexecutive behaviors, indicative of frontal lobe network dysfunction, in PSP-F.

CBD, like MSA, does not have a characteristic dementia syndrome, but cognitive impairment is prevalent. Nearly half of CBD patients have general cognitive impairment at diagnosis and 70% become impaired over the disease course.[23] One study showed deficits in learning, word fluency, verbal comprehension, cognitive flexibility, and perceptual organization, while another showed executive, language, and visuospatial deficits.[60,61] However, a small study of pathologically confirmed CBD reported dementia as the most common presentation.[62] Since CBD pathology is very asymmetric, neuropsychiatric dysfunction can vary, depending on the more impacted side, e.g. primary aphasia when it impacts the left cortex initially.

DLB, defined by the fundamental presence of major neurocognitive disorder (dementia), involves a decline in more than one cognitive domain that interferes with ability to perform usual functions. Cognitive impairment first affects the domains of attention, executive function, and visuoperceptual ability.[53] Cross-sectionally, cognitive phenomena of DLB and PDD may overlap. DLB is diagnosed when the dementia and other psychiatric symptoms have their onset a year or more before the emergence of motor symptoms. Memory deficits usually emerge later, though they can occur earlier. Pronounced fluctuations in attention and alertness in DLB mimic delirium, yet a delirium work-up will be negative. Still, DLB, like all dementias, carries increased risk for developing a delirium superimposed on baseline dementia. Mental status changes that deviate from a patient's usual DLB-type cognitive fluctuations can be indicative of delirium. Teaching families and care givers to monitor for relatively subtle changes can facilitate early interventions, e.g., treatment of a urinary tract infection.

Behavioral variant FTD presents with a pronounced dysexecutive profile and relative sparing of episodic memory and visuospatial skills.[63] Anosognosia and indifference toward their cognitive and social deficits are often the most striking cognitive change in FTD.

Damage to subcortical structures in vascular parkinsonism results in an early subcortical dementia characterized by bradyphrenia, frontal lobe dysfunction, and, to a lesser extent, memory impairment. There is a high risk of concurrent vascular dementia in vascular parkinsonism.

Psychiatric Phenomena

When psychiatric symptoms are evident in a neurological disease, a first step is to characterize what clinical phenomena are present and determine if there is evidence for a psychiatric syndrome versus isolated symptoms or signs. Psychiatric syndromes, defined as a combination of distinct clinical signs and symptoms that correlate with one another, tend to be associated with discrete disorders, e.g., major depressive disorder, and delimited from others, e.g., panic disorder. The psychiatric disorder provides a basis for anticipating prognosis and planning treatment.[64] In PD and APS, the phenomena of psychiatric syndromes often resemble their counterpart idiopathic psychiatric syndromes, e.g., mood disorders and anxiety disturbances. However, some conditions, e.g., "off-related" anxiety in PD, impulse control disorders, visual hallucinations are specifically related to the neurological disease or its treatment.

A common misconception among medical professionals and the lay public is that depression and anxiety in the context of a diagnosis of PD or APS are unavoidable psychological reactions to such news, and thus do not require or even respond to psychiatric treatment. To the contrary, multiple lines of evidence suggest that depression, anxiety, and apathy are etiologically related to the consequences of neurodegeneration caused by the underlying disease.[65,66] However, intermittent low mood, frustration, demoralization, and even embarrassment or shame can be part of the normal psychological reactions to these illnesses. In this setting, a period of "watchful waiting," combined with support, education, and rehabilitative therapies as indicated, rather than immediate pharmacotherapy.

Parkinson's Disease

Depressive Disorders

Clinically significant depressive symptoms occur in 40%–50% of PD patients. Population-based studies show that depression determines 54% of the variance in quality-of-life scores[67,68] and approximately 25% of affected patients experience major depressive disorder.[69-71] While a longitudinal study of PD showed that remission of depressive episodes restored functional abilities to the level of never-depressed PD patients,[72] several studies showed that as few as 20% of diagnosed patients receive treatment for depression, representing an enormous lost opportunity to improve quality of life for patients and caregivers.[71,73,74] Additionally, untreated depression in PD is associated with earlier initiation of dopaminergic therapy, faster progression of physical and cognitive deterioration, greater disability, increased mortality, and greater caregiver burden.[72,75] Similar impacts on physical aspects of movement disorders are seen with anxiety, psychosis, and sleep disturbances.[76,77]

Major depression, minor depression, and dysthymia in PD resemble idiopathic mood disorders phenomenologically, i.e., they do not have distinct clinical profiles. In both, core features are a persistent and pervasive low mood or sadness, a reduced ability to enjoy activities that would otherwise be pleasurable, or a decline in interests from a usual baseline. Anhedonia frequently occurs in absence of sadness, leading some patients to conclude they are "not depressed." Whereas a nondepressed PD patient will find new activities to enjoy when motor symptoms limit function, one with a depressive disorder will fail to find alternate activities to enjoy, even when their physical abilities are not limiting. Earlier studies suggested that self-blame, negative self-attitude, and beliefs of decreased self-worth were less likely in PD with major depression, but that is not substantiated.[78,79] Other emotional and ideational features of depression include excessive and inappropriate feelings of guilt, feelings of failure, pessimism, helplessness, hopelessness, and suicidal or death ideation.

A diagnosis of a depressive disorder should be considered when self-reported disability exceeds what is expected from the examination. Coping and adaptation are extremely difficult in the face of an unremitted mood disorder. This is evident in patients with mild PD and depression, which can be profoundly disabling and more problematic than motor symptoms. Following treatment for depression, such individuals are able to face their challenges associated with PD, a sign the mood disorder is improved; many patients say, "I can cope with PD, but not when depressed."

In addition to mood changes, depressive syndromes involve persistent nonaffective changes, such as disturbances in sleep, appetite, energy or fatigue, psychomotor activity, or cognition. Because such symptoms can occur in PD, mood disorders can be overlooked when they are attributed to PD only and ideational features of depression are not elicited. Diagnosis of depressive disorders in PD may also be confounded by concerns as to whether phenomena such as psychomotor and cognitive changes should be attributed, or explained, by PD or by the mood disorder. Since such attributions are not always possible, an inclusive approach to the diagnosis of depressive disorders is recommended.[75] For example, during a depressive episode, the bradykinesia and hypomimia of PD and psychomotor retardation and flat affect of the mood disorder can be indistinguishable.

Suicidal ideation is probably elevated in PD compared to age matched controls. However, it is not clear that suicide is more common in PD, as various studies show, less, similar, and greater suicide rates.[80] Risk factors for suicide within the PD population include depression and male sex, but not PD severity. Both dopaminergic medications and deep brain stimulation have been reported to increase suicidality, possibly via increased impulsivity, but larger studies have not supported those observations.[80]

Pseudobulbar affect (PBA), also known as pathological laughter and crying, involves exaggerated, involuntary, emotional outbursts that are inappropriate and fleeting with excessive crying or laughter in the absence of feelings of sadness or mirth. The increased emotionality often occurs in the absence of a prevailing mood disorder, but it can still cause distress, embarrassment, and social difficulties. Patients or families may think the person has a depressive disorder because of frequent crying in response to sad or poignant stimuli. When prominent in early PD, an APS, particularly PSP, should be considered in the differential diagnosis, as PBA is probably more common in APS.

Apathy, both a symptom and a syndrome, is manifest by diminished motivation and reduced self-initiated and goal-directed emotional, cognitive, and behavioral activity. Up to 30% of patients demonstrate apathy in the early course of PD. Over 5–10 years, prevalence increases to 40% among nondemented patients and 60% of those with PDD.[20,71,81] It can be a feature of a depressive disorder or an isolated symptom. Apathy may also develop after reduction in dopaminergic medications following subthalamic nucleus deep brain stimulation. Patients with syndromic apathy may appear depressed with little interest in their surroundings or themselves, or engagement in activities, including spontaneous conversation. However, when apathy is not a symptom of a depressive disorder, low mood and distress are typically absent. For example, an apathetic patient may participate in an activity once facilitated or prompted to engage, whereas the depressed or anhedonic patient does not. While apathetic patients rarely complain, their behavior distresses families, who may misattribute the patient's inaction as deliberate. Apathy worsens clinical outcomes because of reduced self-care, treatment adherence, and exercise.

Mania and *hypomania* are not well characterized in PD. Bipolar disorder, a chronic affective disorder that includes depressive and hypomanic or manic episodes, develops long before PD onset in some patients. However, use of dopamine-blocking medications, lithium, and valproic acid for mood stabilization can cause drug-induced parkinsonism. More often in PD, manic phenomena are associated with dopamine replacement therapy or neurosurgical treatments.[82] Hypomanic features can occur in the "on state" with increased irritability and goal-directed activities. Aside from the associations with fluctuating mood and motor states, mania and hypomania present similarly to non-PD patients. Features include elevated mood and sense of self, irritability, hyperactivity, increased goal-directed activity, including risky behaviors, and mood-congruent psychotic phenomena.

Anxiety disorders, in PD and in the general population, are heterogeneous in nature and involve somatic, emotional, and cognitive phenomena. Somatic and vegetative symptoms, e.g., tremors, diaphoresis, gastrointestinal upset, racing heart, and autonomic symptoms, overlap with PD and complicate diagnosis. As with depressive disorders, a focus on emotional phenomena improves recognition of anxiety disorders. Pathological anxiety should be distinguished from "understandable" anxiety, such as reactive anxiety resulting from akinesia while crossing a street. Anxiety disorder symptoms are usually stereotyped and regarded as excessive. Common symptoms include excessive worry, fatigue, concentration problems, sleep disturbances, restlessness, panic, fear of specific objects or situations and avoidance, including phobic avoidance.

Anxiety may occur in up to 55% of PD patients, and up to 40% meet diagnostic criteria for a specific anxiety disorder.[74,83] In a phenomenon unique to PD and APS (when the latter is treated with dopaminergic medications), anxiety can fluctuate with the "on-off" motor states associated with levodopa dosing and may occur multiple times daily, typically when the medicines wear off. Many anxiety disturbances in PD do not fall into classic DSM categories, though they are often comorbid with depressive disorders. Panic disorders involve episodic attacks, but the panic attacks may be associated with motor deficits or on-off fluctuations. Whereas panic attacks are unprovoked, claustrophobia, social phobia, and other phobias involve extreme apprehension precipitated by specific circumstances. Panic features can develop when anxiety is more severe. Severe situational anxiety can aggravate motor deficits. Generalized anxiety disorder involves excessive anxiety and worry over many aspects of life. Avoidance may be more subtle and not readily discerned without query. For example, fears of falling, despite no history of such, can lead to avoidance of walking independently. Drug-induced and fluctuating mood states related to antiparkinsonian medications often involve significant anxiety.

Psychosis in the form of hallucinations, delusions, or both, is often associated with dopaminergic medications but is also a feature of PD itself.[84,85] Up to 60% of PD patients experience psychosis over their disease course; the risk is fourfold in PDD.[86,87] Psychosis remains arguably the greatest predictor of nursing home placement, caregiver burden and stress, and death.[88-91]

Sleep fragmentation, daytime sleepiness, vivid dreams, and nightmares can be early signs of impending PD psychosis.[92] Psychotic disorders that occur with either depression or mania in PD would be associated with mood congruent hallucinations or delusions, such as Cotard's syndrome (i.e., belief that the person is dead or has lost his/her blood or internal organs). More often, hallucinations and delusions present as independent nonaffective phenomena. Delusions and hallucinations may also be present concurrently, but the content of each may be unrelated.

Hallucinations in PD can involve any sensory modality (i.e., visual, auditory, olfactory, gustatory, tactile, or kinesthetic), but visual hallucinations are most common.[93] They may be fleeting simple images, such as a shadow, or complex scenes with well-formed people who often present in a stereotyped manner when they occur, e.g., a little girl sitting at the edge of the bed. Minor hallucinations include a sensation of presence (e.g., a person), brief images of something (usually a person or an animal) passing in the peripheral visual field, and sensory distortions or illusions, which are misperceptions of actual stimuli (versus true hallucinations). In early-stage PD, patients usually have insight into the non-real nature of hallucinations. When insight is absent, there may be suspiciousness, agitation, fear over intruders, or, conversely, a desire to feed unexpected "houseguests." Up to 50% of patients with visual hallucinations experience other types of hallucinations, with auditory hallucinations next most common.

Delusions in PD are typically distressing and can lead to hostile, aggressive, or violent behavior. Most often, there are paranoid, persecutory, or infidelity themes that focus on a single subject or theme, such as spousal infidelity, fears of being poisoned, robbed, injured, or abandoned, or elaborate conspiracies.[94] Grandiose, somatic, erotomanic, and delusions of reference are much less common. Delusional misidentification syndromes (Capgras, i.e., belief that a familiar person is replaced by an impostor, and Fregoli, i.e., belief that a single person, usually a persecutor, repeatedly changes their appearance) and first rank symptoms can also rarely occur.[95]

Impulse control disorders (ICDs) involve an inability to resist the drive to behave in ways that create immediate gratification, but are ultimately harmful to oneself or others. In PD, the most common ICDs involve eating, gambling, shopping, and sexual behaviors. Prevalence estimates range from 3.5% to 42.8%.[96]

ICDs in PD are strongly associated with antiparkinsonian treatment, especially dopamine agonists (pramipexole, ropinirole, and rotigotine) or, less commonly, neurosurgery.[97] Common forms include hypersexuality, paraphilias, pathologic gambling, excessive shopping, and compulsive eating; many patients have more than one ICD. Psychosis or mood disorders may be present, but ICDs are not necessarily associated with mania or hypomania. Poor or absent insight regarding the scope of the ICDs can result in devastating legal, financial, and social consequences. Accordingly, patients should be monitored for development of ICDs.

Additional pathological and repetitive behaviors seen in PD are punding and hobbyism.[98] *Punding*, a syndrome first associated with amphetamine addiction, involves complex, seemingly purposeless, and sustained stereotyped behaviors such as repetitive handling or sorting of objects, dissembling and reassembling items at home, such as flashlights or appliances, cataloging items such as jewelry, or moving things about in a desk drawer. In contrast to ICDs, which are driven by the prospect of an award, punding is often calming. The behaviors are more upsetting to others, particularly when a patient is asked to stop, but resists and may even neglect their need to sleep or eat. *Hobbyism* includes excessive engagement in more complex behaviors, such as a new interest that soon dominates and consumes the life of the patient with PD.

Some Psychiatric Manifestations in Atypical Parkinsonian Syndromes

The only neuropsychiatric symptom included in diagnostic guidelines for MSA is pathological laughing and crying (i.e., pseudobulbar affect, PBA), which is considered a supporting feature.[99] However, depression, anxiety, panic attacks, and suicidal ideation are also seen, and should be assessed and treated appropriately.

PSP is associated with higher rates of depression, anxiety, and apathy. Studies show that PSP patients have increased rates of disinhibition, psychosis, and PBA.[88] Research on distinct depressive profiles in neurodegenerative diseases describe PSP patients as reporting depressive symptoms of hopelessness, dysphoria, and withdrawal at significantly higher rates than healthy age-matched controls.[100]

CBD can lead to depression, apathy, irritability, and agitation. CBD patients are particularly prone to experiencing hopelessness and dysphoria in their clinical presentation of depression.[100]

DLB is particularly associated with REM sleep behavior disorder, now considered a core clinical feature of DLB. Recurrent visual hallucinations are also a core clinical feature of DLB, especially if present in the absence of dopaminergic medications.[53] They are typically well formed, detailed, and not always distressing to the patient. Paranoia is a supportive clinical feature. As in PD, paranoia may involve beliefs that one has been the victim of theft or infidelity or more systematized delusions. Other supportive clinical features include depression, apathy, anxiety, and hallucinations in other domains. All APS have greater sensitivity to antipsychotic-induced parkinsonism; this sensitivity is severe in DLB and poses a management challenge.

The psychiatric profile of the patient with VP varies and is dependent on the location and severity of the patient's cerebrovascular infarcts. Depression and apathy, including abulia at times, are most common.[101]

Presentation to a Psychiatrist, Evaluation, and Management

Approach to Clinical Assessment

Psychiatric comorbidities in PD and APS are often challenging to discern or diagnose; their clinical features are subject to misinterpretation and more than one psychiatric disorder may be present. When motor and psychiatric features overlap, definitive attribution to either the movement disorder or the psychiatric disorder can be impossible. As such, one or the other diagnosis may not be recognized. Phenotypically, for example, psychomotor retardation, poor concentration, and restricted affect in a patient with melancholic depression and known PD can look the same as bradykinesia, bradyphrenia, and hypomimia. If the movement disorder is not already diagnosed, the parkinsonian signs might be overlooked and attributed to a mood disorder only. Motor signs can also be misattributed to a psychiatric basis. A notable example is seen in PSP, where the characteristic facial expression, manifest by a reduced blink rate, furrowed eyebrows, and a wrinkled forehead, causes a patient to appear startled or worried and interpreted as having significant anxiety.

A comprehensive and accurate history, as always, is key to the clinical diagnosis and helps distinguish among differential diagnoses. The gold standard for assessment remains the patient interview, mental status and neurological exam, and review of other medical records to obtain a detailed clinical history of motor, cognitive, and psychiatry phenomena, their intersection over time, and treatment. Whenever possible, an informant should be interviewed because cognitive deficits, lack of insight regarding psychiatric symptoms, or unawareness of motor signs affect a patient's report of their history.[102] When evaluating psychiatric complaints, it can be helpful to restructure the interview by first systematically screening for and obtaining details and timelines of cognitive and motor phenomena (along with other elements of the history) before eliciting the details of the psychiatric disorder. This facilitates an appreciation of when and how the present psychiatric problem relates to the underlying movement and/or cognitive disorder and other aspects of the medical, family, and psychosocial history.[103] Accurate medication reconciliation is critical because polypharmacy is common and medications that treat the movement disorder can cause confusion or psychosis and medicines used to treat psychiatric conditions can cause or exacerbate parkinsonism.

A second goal of the motor exam, in the context of psychiatric assessment, is to evaluate the extent that motor deficits relate to reported impairment. In a major depressive episode, somatic complaints, including motor symptoms and dysfunction, are often increased or disproportionate to the objective evidence. This disparity resolves when the mood disorder remits. By contrast, anosognosia, or lack of awareness of deficits, as in frontotemporal dementia, contributes to denial of illness. Such patients may deny movement abnormalities, report better function than their exam suggests, or demonstrate impulsive behaviors that increase the risk of falls. Additionally, psychiatric symptoms can directly impact motor features. For example, dyskinesias in a PD patient may begin or intensify while discussing a distressing topic. Finally, the psychiatrist should always conduct baseline and serial, focused motor exams to monitor for side effects of prescribed psychiatric medications. History of drug-induced parkinsonism may reflect, in some cases, a preclinical sign of PD, with the offending medications simply unmasking pre-existing deficits in the dopaminergic system.[104]

Some psychiatrists raise concerns that evaluating movement abnormalities and their history is outside their purview, except when prescribing psychiatric medications that can cause movement disorders. Others may resist the practice, citing a lack of time. Fortunately, many motor abnormalities are evident upon casual observation of the patient and do not require additional time.

An important caveat for the psychiatrist, at least on initial assessment, is to resist any propensity to attribute abnormal movements to emotional etiologies. Rather, reported or observed movement phenomena should be recorded and an effort made to identify associated features, how and when they manifest, and patterns of accompanying signs and symptoms. For example, a patient eventually diagnosed with PD described initial symptoms of new onset fine motor difficulties, such as when buttoning, donning a pierced earring, or hanging a framed picture. As the patient was in the midst of relationship difficulties, her general practitioner (perhaps influenced by unconscious biases) attributed her motor difficulties to "nerves" or stress, though clinical exam suggested early stage PD with right hemiparkinsonism including slowed gait, dragging of her right leg, and decreased arm swing.

Prevailing subcortical neuropathology in PD and APS renders cognitive deficits relatively subtle, especially in early stages. This contrasts with Alzheimer's disease, in which clinical manifestations of widespread cortical and hippocampal involvement are generally more overt, e.g., "rapid forgetting," expressive and receptive aphasia, and agnosia, and limited ability to convey history. Still, even subtle deficits in PD and APS may be disabling, progress to overt dementia, and are aggravated by comorbid psychiatric symptoms. Executive dysfunction, especially common, may be evident only with specific inquiry. Patients can be asked about changes or trouble in ability to make decisions, focus, maintain a conversation, or carry out higher-level tasks as part of instrumental activities of daily living (IADLs) that require them to process new information and anticipate, plan, initiate, maintain, or change behaviors. With computerization of many IADL tasks, e.g., automated bill-pay and navigation, deficits may not be apparent until a problem occurs that requires *new* information processing and adaptation. Visuospatial skills, information processing speed, and verbal abilities are also affected, whereas memory and language are relatively preserved in parkinsonism compared to AD. Open-ended questions and allowing a patient time to respond freely and fully without assistance can reveal memory, language, and attention deficits, abnormal thought content or perceptions such as delusions or hallucinations, or irritability or anxiety that arise when the patient is cognitively challenged. Bradyphrenia is manifest by slowed thought processes and speech latency. Its severity may be disproportionately greater than other cognitive deficits and frustrate communications and discourse. Patience is encouraged as the degree of impairment caused by bradyphrenia may belie a patient's social awareness.

Clinical scales or symptom checklists, such as *DSM* criteria, are not diagnostic tools or substitutes for history-taking and clinical evaluation. Clinical scales, often used as objective cross-sectional measures in research, are also used to screen for new or emergent psychiatric, cognitive, and motor symptoms and signs, measure disease and symptom severity, and track treatment response and longitudinal change of motor, cognitive, or psychiatric phenomena. In clinical practice, longitudinal measurement of clinical severity and symptom profiles may reveal treatment nonresponse or signs of psychiatric relapse before subjective concerns are evident. Several self-report scales are suitable to screen for depressive disorders in PD,[105] and other neuropsychiatric disorders including depression, sleep disturbances, and psychosis.[106,107] PD screening scales have variable sensitivity and specificity depending on demographic and clinical characteristic of the study population.[3] Like psychiatric scales, they are not diagnostic tools.

Additional Evaluations

Laboratory
There is no definitive biological marker for PD or APS; they are clinical diagnoses. Typical laboratory tests for a new patient with new or worsening psychiatric phenomena include a complete blood count, comprehensive metabolic panel, thyroid function tests, urinalysis, urine toxicology screen, vitamin D, vitamin B12 and folate levels, and any indicated infectious disease tests. Additionally, depending on patient demographics and presentation, one can consider laboratory tests to exclude Wilson disease, Niemann-Pick disease type C, hypoparathyroidism, neuroacanthocytosis, and neurosyphillis. A rapidly progressive course warrants consideration of laboratory tests to investigate prion disease, paraneoplastic encephalitis, and Whipple disease.

Imaging
Brain MRI imaging is recommended to evaluate new motor or cognitive symptoms. Brain MRI is expected to be normal in PD. Functional imaging with dopamine transporter single photon emission computerized tomography (DaT SPECT) can be useful in diagnosis of PD versus essential tremor or PD versus parkinsonism from dopamine antagonist drugs, though guidelines indicate its use only after emergence of motor signs. DaT SPECT scans,

and probably other dopamine imaging, cannot reliably distinguish PD from CBD, PSP, or MSA, or monitor disease progression.

Imaging findings are not a core diagnostic feature in MSA,[99] though certain findings can support a diagnosis of MSA including atrophy of the putamen, middle cerebellar peduncle, or pons. Brain MRI should be obtained to rule out other etiologies. Hypometabolism in cerebellum, putamen, or brainstem on 18-F fluorodeoxyglucose-positron emission tomography (FDG-PET) is a supportive feature for possible MSA with predominant parkinsonism.

As in MSA, brain imaging does not play a definitive role in diagnosis of PSP, but midbrain atrophy ("Mickey Mouse sign" or "hummingbird sign") can be seen. Findings of midbrain atrophy or hypometabolism or postsynaptic dopaminergic degeneration in the striatum are considered supportive features for the diagnosis of PSP.[48]

Imaging of CBD can show marked cortical asymmetry. Parietal lesions of any type sometimes mimic CBD.

In DLB, indicative biomarkers for diagnosis include reduced DaT uptake in basal ganglia on PET or SPECT and low uptake of [123]iodine-MIBG myocardial scintigraphy. Reduced perfusion on SPECT and reduced metabolism on PET, with especially low occipital lobe activity, is a potentially useful marker of DLB.[53] Brain MRI, in which prominent hippocampal atrophy is suggestive of AD, can be used to raise or lower suspicion for AD as an alternate diagnosis to DLB.

A diagnosis of VP over PD can be supported by the presence of diffuse white matter ischemic lesions and/or specific subcortical gray matter infarcts on MRI (substantia nigra, striatum, or ventromedial or ventrolateral nuclei of the thalamus).[39]

Treatment of Neuropsychiatric Disorders in PD and APS

General Principles

Absent cures for PD or APS, the cornerstones of effective psychiatric management are judicious pharmacotherapy, detection and optimal management of other medical conditions, illness education, skills training to maintain activity levels and manage stressors, and emotional support. Ideally, the treatments are feasible, have no or a beneficial impact on other psychiatric symptoms, cognition, or motor function, and integrate stepped-care measurement-informed care models to assist with evaluating progress or relapse.[108] Interdisciplinary and patient-centered approaches include a range of medical specialists; rehabilitative services such as occupational therapy, physical therapy, and speech language pathology; psychotherapists; social workers; and home health services.[109] Local, national, and international movement disorder and dementia organizations offer educational programs and support groups, including on-line emotional support, information on resources and coping with PD and APS, and recreational, exercise, and educational programs for patients, families, and caregivers. Examples include the Parkinson Foundation, Alzheimer's Association (addresses all dementias), Lewy Body Dementia Association, Lewy Body Society, Multiple System Atrophy Coalition, PSP Association, CurePSP, Association for Frontotemporal Degeneration, and Family Caregiver Alliance.

Guiding principles for pharmacotherapy are the same as those for the elderly: simplify and minimize medication regimens across all medical conditions, eliminate polypharmacy if possible, and maximize behavioral and supportive strategies. New medications should be started one at a time at low doses and titrated slowly given susceptibility to adverse effects and decreased medication clearance with age. Importantly, constipation, common in PD, also affects drug absorption, general well-being, and comportment, and should be treated routinely or prevented as a mainstay of care. Anticholinergic, opiate, and benzodiazepine medications should be avoided or used cautiously given adverse cognitive effects and risk of overdose. Antipsychotics are associated with increased risk of death in patients with dementia. When other approaches fail for psychosis, agitation, or aggression, selected antipsychotics are used following a discussion of potential risks and benefits. Similarly, treatment with dopamine repletion therapy or dopamine agonists, should start with a discussion of their potential side effects.

Motor Symptoms

The role of movement, exercise, and physical therapy cannot be understated at any stage of disease. Physiotherapy is efficacious for treating general motor symptoms in PD, and exercise-based movement strategy training, formalized patterned exercises, speech therapy, and occupational therapy should all be strongly considered.[110]

Treatment of PD and APS motor phenomena is symptomatic and aimed at restoring function, reducing disability, and improving quality of life. With no disease modifying, regenerative, or neuroprotective agents identified to date, levodopa, combined with carbidopa to prevent metabolism of levodopa before it reaches the brain, remains the gold standard of pharmacotherapy. Levodopa is often tried in APS, but typically only has any benefit in early MSA. There are no established treatments for PSP, CBD, FTD, or VP, although immune modulation antibody therapies have been studied for PSP and FTD.

Levodopa dramatically improves PD motor symptoms, but more frequent dosing is needed as PD progresses and response duration shortens. There are several longer acting L-dopa versions, but these still have a relatively short duration of effect. Catecho-o-methyltransferase inhibitors (e.g., tolcapone, opicapone, and entacapone) inhibit L-dopa metabolism and are paired with levodopa to extend duration of the motor response and reduce motor fluctuations.[110] The MAO-I agents rasagiline, safinamide, and selegiline inhibit dopamine metabolism and are used with and without L-dopa.[110] Whether they provide long-term benefits or neuroprotection is debated.

The non-ergot dopamine agonists pramipexole, rotigotine, and ropinirole are used to treat motor symptoms that cause disability[110] and are sometimes used initially to delay use of L-dopa. Older ergot dopamine agonists like cabergoline, DHEC, pergolide, and bromocriptine carry a risk of cardiac fibrosis and are rarely used. Anticholinergic medications, including trihexyphenidyl or benztropine, are used in a minority of PD patients for tremor and rigidity. Amantadine increases dopamine release, blocks dopamine reuptake, and antagonizes NMDA-type glutamate receptors and is the only medication that can improve PD features and dyskinesia. Istradefylline antagonizes adenosine alpha$_2$-a receptors, which seems to potentiate dopamine-2 receptor function.

Psychiatric side effects are one of the greatest limitations of antiparkinsonian therapy. Anticholinergics worsen cognition. Dopamine agonists cause hallucinations, daytime somnolence, and ICDs. Amantadine is a major contributor to hallucinations. L-dopa may contribute to punding, manic-like behaviors, and a variety of wearing off symptoms (apathy, fatigue, anxiety, etc.).

Neurosurgical therapies for PD include high-frequency deep brain stimulation (DBS), usually of the subthalamic nucleus (STN) and globus pallidus pars interna (GPi). Ablation of GPi, thalamus (pallidotomy and thalamotomy), and sometimes STN, is also available through several techniques. Such procedures usually improve quality of life and benefit most motor features of PD and on-off fluctuations. However, acute DBS stimulation can have psychiatric consequences, including severe depression or mania, including in patients with no history of such symptoms, mirthless laughter, and possibly suicidality. STN DBS may also modestly worsen cognition. While psychiatric symptoms associated with on-off fluctuations may improve, depression, anxiety, interpersonal deficits, and most other psychiatric symptoms do not.

Treatment of Cognitives Symptoms

Patient self-efficacy and ability to cope with motor and nonmotor aspects of PD or APS is achieved when patients and care givers know how and when to play to a patient's relative cognitive strengths and compensate for deficits. Education about cognitive changes should include a focus on executive functioning as those deficits are disabling but subtle. Planning for individualized support as deficits progress should be encouraged. Review of cognitive screens or formal neuropsychological evaluations with family, care givers, and patients provides a basis for understanding the unique impact on that patient. That data along with functional assessments, informs cognitive rehabilitation approaches that target everyday functions.[111] Speech-language therapists address voice, speech, and swallowing impairments, and develop strategies and skills to enhance cognition and communication, thus enhancing socialization and quality of life.[112]

Pharmacologic approaches to mild cognitive impairment and major neurocognitive impairment in PD, also referred to as mild cognitive impairment in PD (MCI-PD) and Parkinson's disease dementia (PDD) focus largely on cholinergic deficits.[113] There is no evidence-based treatment for MCI-PD at present. Randomized trials of donepezil and rivastigmine in PDD and DLB show modestly improved cognition and psychiatric symptoms (including psychosis) to similar degrees as seen in AD.[107,114] Trials of galantamine showed mixed results with high drop-out rates due to gastrointestinal side effects and self-reported exacerbation of PD symptoms.[115] The side effect profile of cholinesterase inhibitors includes nausea, vomiting, dizziness, sedation, anorexia, insomnia, and vivid dreams. Slow titration and administration with food can mitigate some of these effects.

Memantine appears to have a modest effect on tests of global cognitive function, but efficacy in studies in PDD and DLB were inconsistent.[116] An early randomized placebo-controlled trial of memantine in PDD showed improved clinical global impression of change, but no improvement on secondary cognitive measures.[117] Consistent with those findings, systematic review showed improved clinical global impression of change with both cholinesterase inhibitors and memantine, but only cholinesterase inhibitors improved cognitive test performance.[118]

Other studies report benefits on quality of life and RBD.[116] Memantine has a favorable safety and tolerability profile, however it can precipitate confusion and hallucinations.[119]

Treatment of Psychiatric Symptoms

Depression

Depressive disorders in PD range from mild to severe, and treatment can be customized accordingly. When treated deliberately and assiduously, depressive disorders in PD respond effectively to medications, other somatic treatments, psychotherapies and rehabilitative therapies, or combinations of these.[120] An algorithm for treating depression in PD has been suggested.[121] "Watchful waiting" and problem-solving strategies are appropriate first steps for demoralization, nonmajor forms of depression, or when life stressors prevail and it is unclear if the patient has a mood disorder. Follow-up no later than 2–3 weeks should evaluate for a persistent mood disorder. Early use of rehabilitative therapies assists with problem-solving, enhances positive disease self-management, increases patient and caregiver knowledge about how PD affects them specifically, and provides support. Together, these interventions can reduce the impact of stressors that may become overwhelming and contribute to depressed or anxious moods. Exercise, adequate sleep hygiene, healthy emotional activities, and engagement in peer support programs, e.g., through local and national PD organizations, should be encouraged.

Cognitive-behavioral therapy (CBT), a skills-based approach for individual or groups, addresses thoughts and behaviors that contribute to an individual's distress and problems. Flexibility of the CBT approach is ideal for treating patients with health-related concerns across a variety of medical conditions. Thus, it is especially useful in PD, in which symptoms of depression and anxiety overlap with those of PD itself. In addition, CBT protocols can be individualized to patient preferences, incorporate behavioral activation, anxiety management techniques, sleep hygiene, cognitive restructuring, and caregiver support in the context of cognitive impairment.[71] A randomized controlled trial of CBT for PD depression demonstrated efficacy of individual CBT as monotherapy or in combination with antidepressant medication, including for reducing residual symptoms in patients already treated with antidepressants.[122] In-person and remote telephone- or video-based modalities for delivering CBT are also efficacious.[123]

When depressive symptoms persist, are prolonged, and are at least moderately disruptive, antidepressant or other pharmacotherapies should be considered. There are relatively few controlled trials of antidepressant medications in PD. Selective serotonin reuptake inhibitors (SSRIs) are first line medications to treat idiopathic depression due to their efficacy, safety, and tolerability, and are also commonly used for depressive disorders in PD. The serotonin-norepinephrine reuptake inhibitor (SNRI) venlafaxine extended release was also shown to be efficacious.[124] A metanalysis of 13 trials testing antidepressant medications in PD revealed that treatment with standard antidepressants had a significant effect on depression; further stratification implicated SSRIs as most efficacious.[125] Randomized, placebo-controlled studies of antidepressant medications also demonstrate efficacy for nortriptyline and desipramine.[126]

Dosing strategies resemble practices in geriatric psychiatry, starting with low doses to assess tolerance (e.g., sertraline 25 mg daily, escitalopram 5 mg daily, venlafaxine 37.5 mg daily, bupropion 50 mg daily, nortriptyline 10 mg daily). When symptoms persist, it is important to advance to typical target doses or switch antidepressants if there is an inadequate response after 12 weeks at a maximum dose. Notably, most antidepressant treatment trials are 8 to 12 weeks in duration and there is a strong early placebo response. In clinical practice, patients are expected to remain on a medication for at least that long before seeing a full response, with the expectation that they would see further response afterward. There are no data on duration of antidepressant treatment in PD. Chronic maintenance therapy is often warranted because depressive symptoms return when the antidepressant is reduced or discontinued. As in treatment of depressive disorders in general, antidepressant medications plus psychotherapy may be required to achieve and sustain remission, though this has not been studied in PD.[71]

Antidepressant selection is similar to practices for the general population, with consideration of the specific needs of that patient and medication side effect profiles. For example, paroxetine is more anticholinergic than other SSRIs and can lead to undesirable side effects. Additionally, paroxetine, fluoxetine, and fluvoxamine can precipitate drug–drug interactions via their influence on the CYP 450 system, a potential problem in patients who are often on multiple medications.[125] Bupropion, a noradrenergic and dopaminergic atypical antidepressant, has not been studied in controlled blinded trials, though case reports show positive effects on mood symptoms.[127,128] Mirtazapine is often used for depression with insomnia, anxiety, or weight loss, but has not been studied in PD-depression. Alternative medications for depression, including atomoxetine, trazadone, and memantine have not proven efficacious for depression, though they can be used for other symptoms.[125,129] Reports on efficacy of dopamine agonists for improving depressive symptoms in PD are difficult to interpret as subjects did not necessarily have clinical diagnoses of depression, but are anecdotally effective for anhedonia.[130]

Repetitive transcranial magnetic stimulation is being investigated as a new modality for treatment of PD depression. A recent multicenter, double-blind, sham-controlled study did not find it superior to placebo for depression, though, interestingly, it improved motor function,[131] consistent with findings of a systematic review.[132] Electroconvulsive therapy (ECT) is well-known to be useful for PD depression. A recent systematic review confirmed its efficacy for both depression (improved in 93% of patients) and motor symptoms (improved in 83% of patients), leading the authors to conclude that ECT is underused in PD and should be offered earlier in the treatment algorithm.[133] Of note, ECT can improve motor symptoms of PD even in the absence of mood symptoms.[132] ECT is also the gold-standard treatment for catatonia.

Apathy

Several lines of evidence suggest that cholinergic medications may impact cognitive features of apathy and dopaminergic medications may improve behavioral and emotional features of apathy.[134] In PD patients without dementia or comorbid depression, apathy improved in double-blind placebo-controlled trials of medications that either enhance acetylcholine (rivastigmine),[135] or stimulate dopamine D2 or D3 receptors (piribedil).[136] SSRIs were shown to increase apathy in PD,[134] though bupropion, which is not serotonergic, can be used for both depression and apathy.[137] Methylphenidate, a dopaminergic stimulant, may benefit apathy in PD.[138,139] Dopamine agonists ropinirole, pramipexole, and rotigotine resulted in significant improvements in apathy after subthalamic nucleus DBS,[134] and anecdotally can be effective in many PD patients. In the nondepressed patient, other dopaminergic agents including levodopa, dopamine receptor agonists, selegiline, amphetamines, and amantadine have some evidence for use.[140]

Anxiety

Despite high rates of anxiety in PD, the evidence-base to guide treatment decisions is sparse. There are no randomized clinical treatment trials[74] though a treatment algorithm was recently proposed.[121] CBT, the gold standard of psychotherapies for anxiety, was supported in a systematic literature review as a useful treatment for both depression and anxiety in PD.[141] Clinical trials of CBT for anxiety in PD have been small and showed improved depression and anxiety symptoms as compared to controls, while others showed a benefit on depression but not anxiety.[142] Results of DBS are inconsistent, showing improved anxiety in some patients and worsened anxiety in others after DBS.[143] Anecdotally, off-anxiety may improve when DBS is targeted for motor fluctuations. Pharmacotherapy for anxiety in PD resembles depression treatment. SSRI and SNRI medications are considered first line and benzodiazepines should be avoided given their adverse side effect profile, especially in older adults. A clinical trial of buspirone for anxiety in PD is underway. An innovative Spanish study on the effect of resistance exercise training as an adjunctive therapy for anxiety in PD showed significant improvement in anxiety and quality of life.[144] This is consistent with the large body of literature supporting use of exercise in the treatment of depression and anxiety in various patient populations.

Psychosis

Treating psychosis in PD requires achieving a reduction in psychotic symptoms without aggravating motor symptoms from reduced dopaminergic tone in the central nervous system. A judicious first step is to reduce or simplify the antiparkinsonian medication regimen, starting with discontinuation or reduction of anticholinergics, amantadine, and MAO-B inhibitors. Levodopa therapy is preferred over dopamine agonists. If antipsychotic treatment is not urgent, a reasonable second step is to treat cognition. Donepezil was shown to reduce the development of psychotic symptoms in PD patients with and without dementia, and rivastigmine may reduce psychosis in PDD.[145,146]

Antipsychotic medications are necessary when patients cannot tolerate further reductions in antiparkinsonian medications and insight is lost and behavior is disruptive, aggressive, or combative, such as paranoia toward the family or medications. Clozapine, which does not antagonize D2 receptors, is the gold standard treatment for psychosis in PD and is effective at small doses (12.5–75 mg per day, usually given at night). Despite its superior efficacy, required hematologic monitoring discourages its use. Clozapine-induced agranulocytosis in PD appears rare, but weekly CBCs are required for six months, then every other week for the next six months, and monthly tests indefinitely. Quetiapine is often used as an alternative, despite it not showing efficacy in multiple controlled trials and potential side effects of orthostasis and sedation.[147] Low starting doses are recommended, e.g., quetiapine 12.5 mg nightly. Second-generation antipsychotics with more potent D2 antagonism (olanzapine, risperidone, aripiprazole, ziprasidone) can greatly aggravate parkinsonism, thus precluding their use. Worsening motor features can be gradual, with gait, posture, and balance being most problematic. Pimavanserin, a potent inverse agonist at 5-HT2A receptors with a highly selective affinity for 5-HT$_{2C}$ receptors, is the first FDA-approved atypical antipsychotic for PD psychosis. Studies show equal improvement in both hallucinations and delusions, and the drug may also improve cognition and sleep.[148] The standard dose of 34 mg daily does not worsen motor function in PD, but there is a delay in psychiatric benefit as the long half-life of pimavanserin requires 1–2 weeks of administration before achieving a steady state. ECT is an effective treatment for parkinsonism, major depression with psychosis, and nonpsychotic depression.

Impulse Control Disorders

The primary treatment for medication induced ICDs is reduction or withdrawal of the offending drug. This can be complicated by the dopamine agonist withdrawal syndrome, which cannot be alleviated with levodopa and can lead to worse motor symptoms. In such cases, alternative agents, extended release formulations, doses, and scheduling are tried. Families and care givers play a critical role in creating an environment that limits the ability of the patient to engage in these behaviors, such as removing access to money, credit cards, transportation, or the Internet. The management of problematic sexual behavior is especially challenging. The Movement Disorder Society review of medication treatments for medication-induced ICD concluded there was only sufficient evidence to recommend amantadine as a treatment of pathological gambling,[149] but that single study reporting benefit has not been replicated. DBS has mixed results regarding ICDs in PD, as it has been known to precipitate new symptoms.[150]

Harmless punding often does not require treatment. Other treatment is challenging, given that the behavior is related to dopaminergic replacement therapy and often occurs in patients with advanced PD. A proposed treatment algorithm, based on postulated involvement of medications acting on dopamine D1 and D2 receptors, suggests careful reductions of these medications, starting with bedtime doses, and adding a COMT inhibitor to extend the duration of the levodopa effect.[151] Dopamine agonists can be substituted for motor control but carry the risk of triggering or worsening ICDs. Quetiapine can be used when there is psychosis or reduced sleep time. Amantadine is recommended if there are also dyskinesias, but it may cause psychosis. Clozapine is indicated when there are both dyskinesias and psychosis. Subthalamic DBS can reduce the daily dose of dopaminergic medications and may improve punding, but this has not been studied.

Atypical Parkinsonian Syndromes

There is little high-quality published data demonstrating symptomatic benefit in motor or nonmotor symptoms in APS, and many commonly attempted therapeutics are extrapolated from PD data and experience.

MSA

Motor symptoms of MSA can be treated with levodopa, amantadine, physiotherapy, occupational therapy, and speech therapy. Dystonia can be alleviated with botulinum toxin injections. There are no recommended treatments for cognitive changes though acetylcholinesterase inhibitors can be tried. Mood symptoms may respond to levodopa early in the course, though the effect is incomplete and transient (as with motor symptoms). SSRIs are recommended over tricyclic antidepressants due to risks of orthostasis and urinary retention with tricyclics. ECT can be safely used. Treatments for autonomic orthostatic hypotension include fluids, salt, fludrocortisone, droxidopa, midodrine, pyridostigmine, and physical measures.

PSP

Levodopa responsiveness was once an exclusionary criterion for diagnosis of PSP; this changed given some evidence for mild to moderate benefit from levodopa in some PSP patients.[152] Transdermal rotigotine also improved parkinsonism in PSP without increasing behavioral disturbances.[153] Amantadine trials showed limited benefit.[50] Focal dystonia can be treated with baclofen or botulinum toxin injections.[154] Zolpidem transiently improved speech and some aspects of motor function in a PSP case study, but its short action and association with adverse benzodiazepine effects discourages its use.[155] There are no approved treatments for cognitive changes in PSP. Cholinesterase inhibitors and memantine may improve cognition but are associated with worse motor symptoms and other adverse effects. Similarly, there are no PSP-specific guidelines for treatment of depression, anxiety, or other psychiatric symptoms, though tricyclic and SSRIs are used. In an older retrospective study, amitriptyline and imipramine improved depression in about one-third of subjects.[156] Pedunculopontine nucleus DBS was of interest until a randomized controlled trial showed no improvement in gait, postural instability, or falls.[157] ECT is used for both motor and mood symptoms though there is limited evidence for its efficacy and treatment-related confusion can limit use.

CBD

Levodopa provides little benefit for parkinsonism in CBD. In a case study, levetiracetam, which can be associated with an increased risk of depression, reduced severe myoclonus in CBD.[158] Use of amantadine in CBD has little support.[159] Transdermal rotigotine was effective and safe in a study of 51 patients with APS, including CBD.[153] There are no recommended treatments for cognitive or psychiatric symptoms. Results from studies of acetylcholinesterase inhibitors and memantine are variable.[160] Tricyclic antidepressants and SSRIs are medications of choice for depression and anxiety, though use is off-label. Literature on ECT in CBD is scarce.

DLB

Parkinsonism in DLB can be difficult to treat given the propensity for psychotic symptoms, but trials of low doses of levodopa, which is preferred over dopamine agonists, with appropriate monitoring can improve function and ease care burdens.[161] Zonisamide has been used adjunctively with levodopa, and a recent controlled, multisite trail of zonisamide monotherapy was efficacious for parkinsonism in DLB.[162,163] With the prominent cholinergic deficit in DLB, acetylcholinesterase inhibitors are useful for cognition and psychosis.[161,162] Studies of memantine yielded mixed results. Low doses of clonazepam, used for RBD, carry the usual risks of benzodiazepines. Pimavanserin, quetiapine, and clozapine have all been used for psychotic symptoms. In a case study, clozapine successfully treated visual hallucinations and agitation in a patient who had failed multiple treatment options. There is little published research on use of clozapine in DLB,[164] but psychosis seems to respond to the same agents as used for PD with psychosis. Off-label use of SSRIs and SNRIs for depression and anxiety yield unclear benefits. Rivastigmine may improve depression along with cognition, representing an opportunity to reduce polypharmacy.[165] ECT and TMS may be efficacious and underused somatic, nonpharmacologic treatments.[34]

FTD

FTD is challenging to manage and has no definitive treatments. Once diagnosis is established, education, problem-solving assistance, and support to the family are critical components of care to help them weather the course of the disease. Families need to hear, often repeatedly, that the patient's profound apathy, impulsivity, and reduced capacity for empathy are features of a degenerative brain disease, rather than their true sentiments.

When parkinsonism in FTD is severe enough to warrant treatment, levodopa may be used judiciously for akinesis and rigidity; amantadine can be used for dystonia and fatigue, with careful monitoring.[166] For nonmotor symptoms, trazodone is often used in FTD and has demonstrated efficacy for reducing problematic behaviors and other neuropsychiatric symptoms.[167] It is not thought to improve cognition. Rivastigmine may improve behavior and caregiver burden, though an open label study failed to impact cognitive deterioration.[153] Donepezil is not recommended in FTD as it is associated with worse behavior without improved cognition. Galantamine failed to benefits behavior or language symptoms in bvFTD and primary progressive aphasia.[168] SSRIs may improve behavioral symptoms, though evidence is limited. A randomized controlled trial of paroxetine in 35 patients with FTD significantly reduced anxiety and ritualistic behaviors, though other studies of paroxetine failed to benefit behavioral symptoms and worsened cognition.[169] A small open label study of citalopram reduced neuropsychiatric symptoms and improved behavior.[170] In a case series of three patients, clomipramine improved compulsive behaviors.[171]

An uncontrolled unblinded study of rTMS for cognition in FTD showed improved performance on the Montreal Cognitive Assessment test, letter and digit cancellation test, and Stroop test and improved caregiver impression of daily functioning.[172] There was no change in mood. ECT has been used in FTD to treat comorbid depression or bipolar disorder but not the symptoms of FTD itself.[173,174]

Vascular Parkinsonism

The basis of treatment for vascular parkinsonism is secondary prevention of further cerebrovascular events. Imaging can inform treatment decisions, i.e., levodopa may be useful when lesions primarily affect nigrostriatal pathways, though most patients have damage elsewhere.[175] Parkinsonism due to white matter lesions does not typically respond to levodopa or subthalamic DBS.[175] Given pathophysiological and symptom similarities between VP and normal pressure hydrocephalus, therapeutic cerebrospinal fluid drainage has been used in VP with positive results.[175–177] A prospective pilot study of rTMS for gait dysfunction in VP showed promising results, though further research is needed.[178] There is no literature on use of ECT in VP, though ECT is useful for mood symptoms and catatonia in patients with vascular dementia.

Conclusions

PD and APS are complex neuropsychiatric conditions in which the motor phenotype is the basis for diagnosis, but may have prominent or even dominant psychiatric and cognitive phenomena. They may present as initial signs of PD or APS before motor abnormalities are evident, overlap with nonmotor somatic aspects of the movement disorder (e.g., autonomic dysfunction and anxiety), and impact function and quality of life to an extent that is more adverse than motor dysfunction. In this context, it is remarkable that psychiatric disorders in PD and APS are frequently unrecognized or, even when detected, may be undertreated.

Integration of psychiatric specialists into the multidisciplinary care team can benefit patients by providing experts with a specific focus on psychiatric aspects of movement disorders. To facilitate that, psychiatrists must also recognize the clinical phenomena of PD and APS syndromes and be familiar with differences, associated features, and treatments of associated motor, cognitive, and psychiatric phenomena.

References

1. Savica R, Boeve BF, Logroscino G. Epidemiology of alpha-synucleinopathies: from Parkinson disease to dementia with Lewy bodies. Handb Clin Neurol 2016;138:153–158.

2. Bower JH, Maraganore DM, McDonnell SK, Rocca WA. Incidence and distribution of parkinsonism in Olmsted County, Minnesota, 1976–1990. Neurology 1999;52(6):1214–1220.

3. Dahodwala N, Karlawish J, Siderowf A, Duda JE, Mandell DS. Delayed Parkinson's disease diagnosis among African-Americans: the role of reporting of disability. Neuroepidemiology 2011;36(3):150–154.

4. Hely MA, Morris JGL, Reid WGJ, Trafficante R. Sydney multicenter study of Parkinson's disease: non-L-dopa-responsive problems dominate at 15 years. Mov Disord 2005;20(2):190–199.

5. Armstrong MJ, Okun MS. Time for a new image of Parkinson disease. JAMA Neurol 2020;77(11):1345–1346.

6. Mehanna R, Moore S, Hou JG, Sarwar AI, Lai EC. Comparing clinical features of young onset, middle onset and late onset Parkinson's disease. Parkinsonism Relat Disord 2014;20(5):530–534.

7. De Pablo-Fernández E, Lees AJ, Holton JL, Warner TT. Prognosis and neuropathologic correlation of clinical subtypes of Parkinson disease. JAMA Neurol 2019;76(4):470–479.

8. Shulman LM, Taback RL, Rabinstein AA, Weiner WJ. Non-recognition of depression and other non-motor symptoms in Parkinson's disease. Parkinsonism Relat Disord 2002;8(3):193–197.

9. Chaudhuri KR, Prieto-Jurcynska C, Naidu Y, et al. The nondeclaration of nonmotor symptoms of Parkinson's disease to health care professionals: an international study using the nonmotor symptoms questionnaire. Mov Disord 2010;25(6):704–709.

10. Gallagher DA, Lees AJ, Schrag A. What are the most important nonmotor symptoms in patients with Parkinson's disease and are we missing them? Mov Disord 2010;25(15):2493–2500.

11. Vanacore N, Bonifati V, Fabbrini G, et al. Epidemiology of multiple system atrophy. ESGAP Consortium. European Study Group on Atypical Parkinsonisms. Neurol Sci Off J Ital Neurol Soc Ital Soc Clin Neurophysiol 2001;22(1):97–99.

12. NORD. Multiple system atrophy. Multiple System Atrophy. https://rarediseases.org/rare-diseases/multiple-system-atrophy/. Published 2021. Accessed June 6, 2021.

13. Flabeau O, Meissner WG, Tison F. Multiple system atrophy: current and future approaches to management. Ther Adv Neurol Disord 2010;3(4):249–263.

14. Schrag A, Wenning GK, Quinn N, Ben-Shlomo Y. Survival in multiple system atrophy. Mov Disord 2008;23(2):294–296.

15. Schrag A, Sheikh S, Quinn NP, et al. A comparison of depression, anxiety, and health status in patients with progressive supranuclear palsy and multiple system atrophy. Mov Disord 2010;25(8):1077–1081.

16. Benrud-Larson LM, Sandroni P, Schrag A, Low PA. Depressive symptoms and life satisfaction in patients with multiple system atrophy. Mov Disord 2005;20(8):951–957.

17. Brown RG, Lacomblez L, Landwehrmeyer BG, et al. Cognitive impairment in patients with multiple system atrophy and progressive supranuclear palsy. Brain 2010;133(Pt 8):2382–2393.

18. National Institute for Neurological Disorders and Stroke. Progressive supranuclear palsy fact sheet 2020. https://www.ninds.nih.gov/Disorders/Patient-Caregiver-Education/Fact-Sheets/Progressive-Supranuclear-Palsy-Fact-Sheet.

19. Belvisi D, Berardelli I, Suppa A, et al. Neuropsychiatric disturbances in atypical parkinsonian disorders. Neuropsychiatr Dis Treat 2018;14:2643–2656.

20. Stanton BR, Leigh PN, Howard RJ, Barker GJ, Brown RG. Behavioural and emotional symptoms of apathy are associated with distinct patterns of brain atrophy in neurodegenerative disorders. J Neurol 2013;260(10):2481–2490.

21. Gerstenecker A, Mast B, Duff K, Ferman TJ, Litvan I. Executive dysfunction is the primary cognitive impairment in progressive supranuclear palsy. Arch Clin Neuropsychol Off J Natl Acad Neuropsychol 2013;28(2):104–113.

22. Cotelli M, Borroni B, Manenti R, et al. Action and object naming in frontotemporal dementia, progressive supranuclear palsy, and corticobasal degeneration. Neuropsychology 2006;20(5):558–565.

23. Armstrong MJ, Litvan I, Lang AE, et al. Criteria for the diagnosis of corticobasal degeneration. Neurology 2013;80(5):496–503.

24. Bruns MB, Josephs KA. Neuropsychiatry of corticobasal degeneration and progressive supranuclear palsy. Int Rev Psychiatry 2013;25(2):197–209.

25. NORD. Corticobasal degeneration. https://rarediseases.org/rare-diseases/corticobasal-degeneration/. Published 2012.

26. Coyle-Gilchrist ITS, Dick KM, Patterson K, et al. Prevalence, characteristics, and survival of frontotemporal lobar degeneration syndromes. Neurology. 2016;86(18):1736–1743.

27. Cummings JL, Litvan I. Neuropsychiatric aspects of corticobasal degeneration. Adv Neurol 2000;82:147–152.

28. Rahkonen T, Eloniemi-Sulkava U, Rissanen S, Vatanen A, Viramo P, Sulkava R. Dementia with Lewy bodies according to the consensus criteria in a general population aged 75 years or older. J Neurol Neurosurg & Psychiatry 2003;74(6):720 LP–724.

29. Chiu P-Y, Wang C-W, Tsai C-T, Li S-H, Lin C-L, Lai T-J. Depression in dementia with Lewy bodies: A comparison with Alzheimer's disease. PLoS One 2017;12(6):e0179399.

30. Aarsland D, Ballard C, Larsen JP, McKeith I. A comparative study of psychiatric symptoms in dementia with Lewy bodies and Parkinson's disease with and without dementia. Int J Geriatr Psychiatry 2001;16(5):528–536.

31. Andreasen P, Lönnroos E, von Euler-Chelpin MC. Prevalence of depression among older adults with dementia living in low- and middle-income countries: a cross-sectional study. Eur J Public Health 2014;24(1):40–44.

32. Ballard C, Bannister C, Solis M, Oyebode F, Wilcock G. The prevalence, associations and symptoms of depression amongst dementia sufferers. J Affect Disord 1996;36(3-4):135–144.

33. Ferran J, Wilson K, Duran M, et al. The early onset dementias: a study of clinical characteristics and service use. Int J Geriatr Psychiatry 1996;11:863–869.
34. Takahashi S, Mizukami K, Yasuno F, Asada T. Depression associated with dementia with Lewy bodies (DLB) and the effect of somatotherapy. Psychogeriatrics 2009;9(2):56–61.
35. Ballard C, Holmes C, McKeith I, et al. Psychiatric morbidity in dementia with Lewy bodies: a prospective clinical and neuropathological comparative study with Alzheimer's disease. Am J Psychiatry 1999;156(7):1039–1045.
36. Kuring JK, Mathias JL, Ward L. Prevalence of depression, anxiety and PTSD in people with dementia: a systematic review and meta-analysis. Neuropsychol Rev 2018;28(4):393–416.
37. Breitve MH, Brønnick K, Chwiszczuk LJ, Hynninen MJ, Aarsland D, Rongve A. Apathy is associated with faster global cognitive decline and early nursing home admission in dementia with Lewy bodies. Alzheimers Res Ther. 2018;10(1):83.
38. Onyike CU, Diehl-Schmid J. The epidemiology of frontotemporal dementia. Int Rev Psychiatry 2013;25(2):130–137.
39. Vale TC, Barbosa MT, Caramelli P, Cardoso F. Vascular Parkinsonism and cognitive impairment: literature review, Brazilian studies and case vignettes. Dement Neuropsychol 2012;6(3):137–144.
40. Gupta D, Kuruvilla A. Vascular parkinsonism: what makes it different? Postgrad Med J 2011;87(1034):829–836.
41. Postuma RB, Berg D. Prodromal Parkinson's disease: the decade past, the decade to come. Mov Disord 2019;34(5):665–675.
42. Kim Y, Kim YE, Park EO, Shin CW, Kim H-J, Jeon B. REM sleep behavior disorder portends poor prognosis in Parkinson's disease: a systematic review. J Clin Neurosci Off J Neurosurg Soc Australas 2018;47:6–13.
43. Iranzo A, Fernández-Arcos A, Tolosa E, et al. Neurodegenerative disorder risk in idiopathic REM sleep behavior disorder: study in 174 patients. PLoS One 2014;9(2):e89741.
44. Racette BA, Hartlein JM, Hershey T, Mink JW, Perlmutter JS, Black KJ. Clinical features and comorbidity of mood fluctuations in Parkinson's disease. J Neuropsychiatry Clin Neurosci 2002;14(4):438–442.
45. Rizos A, Martinez-Martin P, Odin P, et al. Characterizing motor and non-motor aspects of early-morning off periods in Parkinson's disease: an international multicenter study. Parkinsonism Relat Disord 2014;20(11):1231–1235.
46. Rabinak CA, Nirenberg MJ. Dopamine agonist withdrawal syndrome in Parkinson disease. Arch Neurol 2010;67(1):58–63.
47. Plazzi G, Corsini R, Provini F, et al. REM sleep behavior disorders in multiple system atrophy. Neurology 1997;48(4):1094–1097.
48. Höglinger GU, Respondek G, Stamelou M, et al. Clinical diagnosis of progressive supranuclear palsy: the movement disorder society criteria. Mov Disord 2017;32(6):853–864.
49. Boeve BF. The multiple phenotypes of corticobasal syndrome and corticobasal degeneration: implications for further study. J Mol Neurosci 2011;45(3):350–353.
50. Lamb R, Rohrer JD, Lees AJ, Morris HR. Progressive supranuclear palsy and corticobasal degeneration: pathophysiology and treatment options. Curr Treat Options Neurol 2016;18(9):42.
51. Litvan I, Cummings JL, Mega M. Neuropsychiatric features of corticobasal degeneration. J Neurol Neurosurg Psychiatry 1998;65(5):717–721.

52. Abbott SM, Videnovic A. Sleep disorders in atypical parkinsonism. Mov Disord Clin Pract 2014;1(2):89–96.

53. McKeith IG, Boeve BF, Dickson DW, et al. Diagnosis and management of dementia with Lewy bodies: fourth consensus report of the DLB consortium. Neurology 2017;89(1):88–100.

54. Aarsland D, Andersen K, Larsen JP, Lolk A, Nielsen H, Kragh-Sørensen P. Risk of dementia in Parkinson's disease: a community-based, prospective study. Neurology 2001;56(6):730–736.

55. Emre M. Dementia associated with Parkinson's disease. Lancet Neurol 2003;2(4):229–237.

56. Levy G, Schupf N, Tang M-X, et al. Combined effect of age and severity on the risk of dementia in Parkinson's disease. Ann Neurol 2002;51(6):722–729.

57. Buter TC, van den Hout A, Matthews FE, Larsen JP, Brayne C, Aarsland D. Dementia and survival in Parkinson disease: a 12-year population study. Neurology 2008;70(13):1017–1022.

58. Miyasaki JM, Shannon K, Voon V, et al. Practice parameter: evaluation and treatment of depression, psychosis, and dementia in Parkinson disease (an evidence-based review): report of the Quality Standards Subcommittee of the American Academy of Neurology. Neurology 2006;66(7):996–1002.

59. Stankovic I, Krismer F, Jesic A, et al. Cognitive impairment in multiple system atrophy: a position statement by the Neuropsychology Task Force of the MDS Multiple System Atrophy (MODIMSA) study group. Mov Disord 2014;29(7):857–867.

60. Vanvoorst WA, Greenaway MC, Boeve BF, et al. Neuropsychological findings in clinically atypical autopsy confirmed corticobasal degeneration and progressive supranuclear palsy. Parkinsonism Relat Disord 2008;14(4):376–378.

61. Murray R, Neumann M, Forman MS, et al. Cognitive and motor assessment in autopsy-proven corticobasal degeneration. Neurology 2007;68(16):1274–1283.

62. Grimes DA, Lang AE, Bergeron CB. Dementia as the most common presentation of cortical-basal ganglionic degeneration. Neurology 1999;53(9):1969–1974.

63. Rascovsky K, Hodges JR, Knopman D, et al. Sensitivity of revised diagnostic criteria for the behavioural variant of frontotemporal dementia. Brain 2011;134(Pt 9):2456–2477.

64. Robins E, Guze SB. Establishment of diagnostic validity in psychiatric illness: its application to schizophrenia. Am J Psychiatry 1970;126(7):983–987.

65. Dickson DW, Fujishiro H, Orr C, et al. Neuropathology of non-motor features of Parkinson disease. Parkinsonism Relat Disord 2009;15 Suppl 3:S1–5.

66. Wen M-C, Chan LL, Tan LCS, Tan EK. Depression, anxiety, and apathy in Parkinson's disease: insights from neuroimaging studies. Eur J Neurol 2016;23(6):1001–1019.

67. Schrag A, Jahanshahi M, Quinn N. What contributes to quality of life in patients with Parkinson's disease? J Neurol Neurosurg Psychiatry 2000;69(3):308–312.

68. Sławek J, Derejko M, Lass P. Factors affecting the quality of life of patients with idiopathic Parkinson's disease—a cross-sectional study in an outpatient clinic attendees. Parkinsonism Relat Disord 2005;11(7):465–468.

69. Reijnders JSAM, Ehrt U, Weber WEJ, Aarsland D, Leentjens AFG. A systematic review of prevalence studies of depression in Parkinson's disease. Mov Disord 2008;23(2):183–189; quiz 313.

70. Goodarzi Z, Mrklas KJ, Roberts DJ, Jette N, Pringsheim T, Holroyd-Leduc J. Detecting depression in Parkinson disease: a systematic review and meta-analysis. Neurology 2016;87(4):426–437.

71. Marsh L. Depression and Parkinson's disease: current knowledge. Curr Neurol Neurosci Rep 2013;13(12):409.

72. Pontone GM, Bakker CC, Chen S, et al. The longitudinal impact of depression on disability in Parkinson disease. Int J Geriatr Psychiatry 2016;31(5):458–465.

73. Frisina PG, Borod JC, Foldi NS, Tenenbaum HR. Depression in Parkinson's disease: health risks, etiology, and treatment options. Neuropsychiatr Dis Treat 2008;4(1):81–91.

74. Goodarzi Z, Mele B, Guo S, et al. Guidelines for dementia or Parkinson's disease with depression or anxiety: a systematic review. BMC Neurol 2016;16(1):244.

75. Marsh L, Dobkin R. Depression and anxiety in Parkinson's disease. In: A. I. Tröster (Ed.), Clinical neuropsychology and cognitive neurology of Parkinson's disease and other movement disorders (pp. 265–290). Oxford University Press..

76. Mack J, Rabins P, Anderson K, et al. Prevalence of psychotic symptoms in a community-based Parkinson disease sample. Am J Geriatr psychiatry Off J Am Assoc Geriatr Psychiatry 2012;20(2):123–132.

77. Chen JJ, Marsh L. Anxiety in Parkinson's disease: identification and management. Ther Adv Neurol Disord 2014;7(1):52–59.

78. Gotham AM, Brown RG, Marsden CD. Depression in Parkinson's disease: a quantitative and qualitative analysis. J Neurol Neurosurg Psychiatry 1986;49(4):381–389.

79. Merschdorf U, Berg D, Csoti I, et al. Psychopathological symptoms of depression in Parkinson's disease compared to major depression. Psychopathology 2003;36(5):221–225.

80. Shepard MD, Perepezko K, Broen MPG, et al. Suicide in Parkinson's disease. J Neurol Neurosurg & Psychiatry 2019;90(7):822 LP–829.

81. Pagonabarraga J, Kulisevsky J. Apathy in Parkinson's disease. Int Rev Neurobiol 2017;133:657–678.

82. Maier F, Merkl J, Ellereit AL, et al. Hypomania and mania related to dopamine replacement therapy in Parkinson's disease. Parkinsonism Relat Disord 2014;20(4):421–427.

83. Broen MPG, Narayen NE, Kuijf ML, Dissanayaka NNW, Leentjens AFG. Prevalence of anxiety in Parkinson's disease: a systematic review and meta-analysis. Mov Disord 2016;31(8):1125–1133.

84. Ravina B, Marder K, Fernandez HH, et al. Diagnostic criteria for psychosis in Parkinson's disease: report of an NINDS, NIMH work group. Mov Disord 2007;22(8):1061–1068.

85. Pagonabarraga J, Martinez-Horta S, Fernández de Bobadilla R, et al. Minor hallucinations occur in drug-naive Parkinson's disease patients, even from the premotor phase. Mov Disord 2016;31(1):45–52.

86. Fénelon G, Soulas T, Zenasni F, Cleret de Langavant L. The changing face of Parkinson's disease-associated psychosis: a cross-sectional study based on the new NINDS-NIMH criteria. Mov Disord 2010;25(6):763–766.

87. Weintraub D. Progress regarding Parkinson's disease psychosis: it's no illusion. Mov Disord Clin Pract 2016;3(5):431–434.

88. Aarsland D, Litvan I, Larsen JP. Neuropsychiatric symptoms of patients with progressive supranuclear palsy and Parkinson's disease. J Neuropsychiatry Clin Neurosci 2001;13(1):42–49.

89. Aarsland D, Larsen JP, Tandberg E, Laake K. Predictors of nursing home placement in Parkinson's disease: a population-based, prospective study. J Am Geriatr Soc 2000;48(8):938–942.

90. Goetz CG, Stebbins GT. Mortality and hallucinations in nursing home patients with advanced Parkinson's disease. Neurology 1995;45(4):669–671.

91. Schrag A, Hovris A, Morley D, Quinn N, Jahanshahi M. Caregiver-burden in parkinson's disease is closely associated with psychiatric symptoms, falls, and disability. Parkinsonism Relat Disord 2006;12(1):35–41.

92. Chahine LM, Amara AW, Videnovic A. A systematic review of the literature on disorders of sleep and wakefulness in Parkinson's disease from 2005 to 2015. Sleep Med Rev 2017;35:33–50.

93. Lee AH, Weintraub D. Psychosis in Parkinson's disease without dementia: common and comorbid with other non-motor symptoms. Mov Disord 2012;27(7):858–863.

94. Factor SA, Molho ES, Podskalny GD, Brown D. Parkinson's disease: drug-induced psychiatric states. Adv Neurol 1995;65:115–138.

95. Marsh L. Psychosis in Parkinson's disease. Curr Treat Options Neurol 2004;6(3):181–189.

96. Antonini A, Barone P, Bonuccelli U, Annoni K, Asgharnejad M, Stanzione P. ICARUS study: prevalence and clinical features of impulse control disorders in Parkinson's disease. J Neurol Neurosurg Psychiatry 2017;88(4):317–324.

97. Evans AH, Strafella AP, Weintraub D, Stacy M. Impulsive and compulsive behaviors in Parkinson's disease. Mov Disord 2009;24(11):1561–1570.

98. Weintraub D, Papay K, Siderowf A. Screening for impulse control symptoms in patients with de novo Parkinson disease: a case-control study. Neurology 2013;80(2):176–180.

99. Gilman S, Wenning GK, Low PA, et al. Second consensus statement on the diagnosis of multiple system atrophy. Neurology 2008;71(9):670–676.

100. Shdo SM, Ranasinghe KG, Sturm VE, et al. Depressive symptom profiles predict specific neurodegenerative disease syndromes in early stages. Front Neurol 2020;11:446.

101. Rektor I, Bohnen NI, Korczyn AD, et al. An updated diagnostic approach to subtype definition of vascular parkinsonism—recommendations from an expert working group. Parkinsonism Relat Disord 2018;49:9–16.

102. Hirsch ES, Adler G, Amspoker AB, Williams JR, Marsh L. Improving detection of psychiatric disturbances in Parkinson's disease: the role of informants. J Parkinsons Dis 2013;3(1):55–60.

103. Peters ME, Taylor J, Lyketsos CG, Chisolm MS. Beyond the DSM: the perspectives of psychiatry approach to patients. Prim care companion CNS Disord 2012;14(1): PCC.11m01233..

104. Shin H-W, Chung SJ. Drug-induced parkinsonism. J Clin Neurol 2012;8(1):15–21.

105. Williams JR, Hirsch ES, Anderson K, et al. A comparison of nine scales to detect depression in Parkinson disease: which scale to use? Neurology 2012;78(13):998–1006.

106. Martinez-Martin P, Leentjens AFG, de Pedro-Cuesta J, Chaudhuri KR, Schrag AE, Weintraub D. Accuracy of screening instruments for detection of neuropsychiatric syndromes in Parkinson's disease. Mov Disord 2016;31(3):270–279.

107. Dubois B, Burn D, Goetz C, et al. Diagnostic procedures for Parkinson's disease dementia: recommendations from the movement disorder society task force. Mov Disord 2007;22(16):2314–2324.

108. Breland JY, Mignogna J, Kiefer L, Marsh L. Models for treating depression in specialty medical settings: a narrative review. Gen Hosp Psychiatry 2015;37(4):315–322.

109. Taylor J, Anderson WS, Brandt J, Mari Z, Pontone GM. Neuropsychiatric complications of Parkinson disease treatments: importance of multidisciplinary care. Am J Geriatr psychiatry Off J Am Assoc Geriatr Psychiatry 2016;24(12):1171–1180.

110. Fox SH, Katzenschlager R, Lim S-Y, et al. International Parkinson and movement disorder society evidence-based medicine review: update on treatments for the motor symptoms of Parkinson's disease. Mov Disord 2018;33(8):1248–1266.

111. Alzahrani H, Venneri A. Cognitive rehabilitation in Parkinson's disease: a systematic review. J Parkinsons Dis 2018;8(2):233–245.

112. Armstrong MJ, Okun MS. Diagnosis and treatment of Parkinson disease: a review. JAMA 2020;323(6):548–560.

113. Zhang Q, Aldridge GM, Narayanan NS, Anderson SW, Uc EY. Approach to cognitive impairment in Parkinson's disease. Neurother J Am Soc Exp Neurother 2020;17(4):1495–1510.

114. Emre M, Aarsland D, Albanese A, et al. Rivastigmine for dementia associated with Parkinson's disease. N Engl J Med 2004;351(24):2509–2518.

115. Grace J, Amick MM, Friedman JH. A double-blind comparison of galantamine hydrobromide ER and placebo in Parkinson disease. J Neurol Neurosurg Psychiatry 2009;80(1):18–23.

116. Brennan L, Pantelyat A, Duda JE, et al. Memantine and cognition in parkinson's disease dementia/dementia with Lewy bodies: a meta-analysis. Mov Disord Clin Pract 2016;3(2):161–167.

117. Aarsland D, Ballard C, Walker Z, et al. Memantine in patients with Parkinson's disease dementia or dementia with Lewy bodies: a double-blind, placebo-controlled, multicentre trial. Lancet Neurol 2009;8(7):613–618.

118. Wang B-S, Wang H, Wei Z-H, Song Y-Y, Zhang L, Chen H-Z. Efficacy and safety of natural acetylcholinesterase inhibitor huperzine A in the treatment of Alzheimer's disease: an updated meta-analysis. J Neural Transm 2009;116(4):457–465.

119. Ridha BH, Josephs KA, Rossor MN. Delusions and hallucinations in dementia with Lewy bodies: worsening with memantine. Neurology 2005;65(3):481–482.

120. Price A, Rayner L, Okon-Rocha E, et al. Antidepressants for the treatment of depression in neurological disorders: a systematic review and meta-analysis of randomised controlled trials. J Neurol Neurosurg Psychiatry 2011;82(8):914–923.

121. Pontone GM, Mills K. Optimal treatment of depression and anxiety in Parkinson's disease. Am J Geriatr Psychiatry 2021;29(6):530–540.

122. Dobkin RD, Menza M, Allen LA, et al. Cognitive-behavioral therapy for depression in Parkinson's disease: a randomized, controlled trial. Am J Psychiatry 2011;168(10):1066–1074.

123. Dobkin RD, Mann SL, Gara MA, Interian A, Rodriguez KM, Menza M. Telephone-based cognitive behavioral therapy for depression in Parkinson disease: a randomized controlled trial. Neurology 2020;94(16):e1764–e1773.

124. Richard IH, McDermott MP, Kurlan R, et al. A randomized, double-blind, placebo-controlled trial of antidepressants in Parkinson disease. Neurology 2012;78(16):1229–1236.

125. Ryan M, Eatmon C V, Slevin JT. Drug treatment strategies for depression in Parkinson disease. Expert Opin Pharmacother 2019;20(11):1351–1363.

126. Troeung L, Egan SJ, Gasson N. A meta-analysis of randomised placebo-controlled treatment trials for depression and anxiety in Parkinson's disease. PLoS One 2013;8(11):e79510.

127. Leentjens AF, Verhey FR, Vreeling FW. [Successful treatment of depression in a Parkinson disease patient with bupropion]. Ned Tijdschr Geneeskd 2000;144(45):2157–2159.

128. Załuska M, Dyduch A. Bupropion in the treatment of depression in Parkinson's disease. Int Psychogeriatrics 2011;23(2):325–327.

129. Weintraub D, Mavandadi S, Mamikonyan E, et al. Atomoxetine for depression and other neuropsychiatric symptoms in Parkinson disease. Neurology 2010;75(5):448–455.

130. Assogna F, Pellicano C, Savini C, et al. Drug choices and advancements for managing depression in Parkinson's disease. Curr Neuropharmacol 2020;18(4):277–287.

131. Brys M, Fox MD, Agarwal S, et al. Multifocal repetitive TMS for motor and mood symptoms of Parkinson disease: a randomized trial. Neurology 2016;87(18):1907–1915.

132. Fregni F, Simon DK, Wu A, Pascual-Leone A. Non-invasive brain stimulation for Parkinson's disease: a systematic review and meta-analysis of the literature. J Neurol Neurosurg Psychiatry 2005;76(12):1614–1623.

133. Borisovskaya A, Bryson WC, Buchholz J, Samii A, Borson S. Electroconvulsive therapy for depression in Parkinson's disease: systematic review of evidence and recommendations. Neurodegener Dis Manag 2016;6(2):161–176.

134. Pagonabarraga J, Kulisevsky J, Strafella AP, Krack P. Apathy in Parkinson's disease: clinical features, neural substrates, diagnosis, and treatment. Lancet Neurol 2015;14(5):518–531.

135. Devos D, Moreau C, Maltête D, et al. Rivastigmine in apathetic but dementia and depression-free patients with Parkinson's disease: a double-blind, placebo-controlled, randomised clinical trial. J Neurol Neurosurg Psychiatry 2014;85(6):668--674.

136. Thobois S, Lhommée E, Klinger H, et al. Parkinsonian apathy responds to dopaminergic stimulation of D2/D3 receptors with piribedil. Brain 2013;136(Pt 5):1568–1577.

137. Corcoran C, Wong ML, O'Keane V. Bupropion in the management of apathy. J Psychopharmacol 2004;18(1):133–135.

138. Moreau C, Delval A, Defebvre L, et al. Methylphenidate for gait hypokinesia and freezing in patients with Parkinson's disease undergoing subthalamic stimulation: a multicentre, parallel, randomised, placebo-controlled trial. Lancet Neurol 2012;11(7):589–596.

139. Herrmann N, Rothenburg LS, Black SE, et al. Methylphenidate for the treatment of apathy in Alzheimer disease: prediction of response using dextroamphetamine challenge. *J Clin Psychopharmacol* 2008;28(3):296–301.

140. Krishnamoorthy A, Craufurd D. Treatment of apathy in Huntington's disease and other movement disorders. Curr Treat Options Neurol 2011;13(5):508–519.

141. Armento MEA, Stanley MA, Marsh L, et al. Cognitive behavioral therapy for depression and anxiety in Parkinson's disease: a clinical review. J Parkinsons Dis 2012;2(2):135–151.

142. Pontone GM, Dissanayka N, Apostolova L, et al. Report from a multidisciplinary meeting on anxiety as a non-motor manifestation of Parkinson's disease. NPJ Park Dis 2019;5:30.

143. Couto MI, Monteiro A, Oliveira A, Lunet N, Massano J. Depression and anxiety following deep brain stimulation in Parkinson's disease: systematic review and meta-analysis. Acta Med Port 2014;27(3):372–382.

144. Ferreira RM, Alves WMG da C, de Lima TA, et al. The effect of resistance training on the anxiety symptoms and quality of life in elderly people with Parkinson's disease: a randomized controlled trial. Arq Neuropsiquiatr 2018;76(8):499–506.

145. Sawada H, Oeda T, Kohsaka M, et al. Early use of donepezil against psychosis and cognitive decline in Parkinson's disease: a randomised controlled trial for 2 years. J Neurol Neurosurg Psychiatry 2018;89(12):1332–1340.

146. Hasnain M. Psychosis in Parkinson's disease: therapeutic options. *Drugs Today (Barc)* 2011;47(5):353–367.

147. Chen JJ, Hua H, Massihi L, et al. Systematic literature review of quetiapine for the treatment of psychosis in patients with parkinsonism. J Neuropsychiatry Clin Neurosci 2019;31(3):188–195.

148. Cummings J, Isaacson S, Mills R, et al. Pimavanserin for patients with Parkinson's disease psychosis: a randomised, placebo-controlled phase 3 trial. Lancet (London, England) 2014;383(9916):533–540.

149. Seppi K, Ray Chaudhuri K, Coelho M, et al. Update on treatments for nonmotor symptoms of Parkinson's disease-an evidence-based medicine review. Mov Disord 2019;34(2):180–198.

150. Bhattacharjee S. Impulse control disorders in Parkinson's disease: Review of pathophysiology, epidemiology, clinical features, management, and future challenges. Neurol India 2018;66(4):967–975.

151. Fasano A, Petrovic I. Insights into pathophysiology of punding reveal possible treatment strategies. Mol Psychiatry 2010;15(6):560–573.

152. Armstrong MJ. Progressive supranuclear palsy: an update. Curr Neurol Neurosci Rep 2018;18(3):12.

153. Moretti DV, Binetti G, Zanetti O, Frisoni GB. Behavioral and neurophysiological effects of transdermal rotigotine in atypical parkinsonism. Front Neurol 2014;5:85.

154. Stamelou M, Höglinger G. A review of treatment options for progressive supranuclear palsy. CNS Drugs 2016;30(7):629–636.

155. Chang AY, Weirich E. Trial of zolpidem, eszopiclone, and other GABA agonists in a patient with progressive supranuclear palsy. Case Rep Med 2014;2014:107064.

156. Nieforth KA, Golbe LI. Retrospective study of drug response in 87 patients with progressive supranuclear palsy. Clin Neuropharmacol 1993;16(4):338–346.

157. Scelzo E, Lozano AM, Hamani C, et al. Peduncolopontine nucleus stimulation in progressive supranuclear palsy: a randomised trial. J Neurol Neurosurg Psychiatry 2017;88(7):613–616.

158. Cho JW, Lee JH. Suppression of myoclonus in corticobasal degeneration by levetiracetam. J Mov Disord 2014;7(1):28–30.

159. Mahapatra RK, Edwards MJ, Schott JM, Bhatia KP. Corticobasal degeneration. Lancet Neurol 2004;3(12):736–743.

160. Armstrong MJ. Diagnosis and treatment of corticobasal degeneration. Curr Treat Options Neurol 2014;16(3):282.

161. Fernandez HH, Wu C-K, Ott BR. Pharmacotherapy of dementia with Lewy bodies. Expert Opin Pharmacother 2003;4(11):2027–2037.

162. Hershey LA, Coleman-Jackson R. Pharmacological management of dementia with Lewy bodies. Drugs Aging 2019;36(4):309–319.

163. Murata M, Odawara T, Hasegawa K, et al. Effect of zonisamide on parkinsonism in patients with dementia with Lewy bodies: a phase 3 randomized clinical trial. Parkinsonism Relat Disord 2020;76:91–97.

164. Bhamra M, Rajkumar AP, Ffytche DH, Kalafatis C. Successful management of persistent distressing neuropsychiatric symptoms by clozapine in a patient suffering from dementia with Lewy bodies. BMJ Case Rep 2018; 2018:bcr2018224710.

165. McKeith I, Del Ser T, Spano P, et al. Efficacy of rivastigmine in dementia with Lewy bodies: a randomised, double-blind, placebo-controlled international study. Lancet (London, England) 2000;356(9247):2031–2036.

166. Rowe JB. Parkinsonism in frontotemporal dementias. Int Rev Neurobiol 2019;149:249–275.

167. Lebert F, Stekke W, Hasenbroekx C, Pasquier F. Frontotemporal dementia: a randomised, controlled trial with trazodone. Dement Geriatr Cogn Disord 2004;17(4):355–359.

168. Kertesz A, Morlog D, Light M, et al. Galantamine in frontotemporal dementia and primary progressive aphasia. Dement Geriatr Cogn Disord 2008;25(2):178–185.

169. Moretti R, Torre P, Antonello RM, Cazzato G, Bava A. Frontotemporal dementia: paroxetine as a possible treatment of behavior symptoms. a randomized, controlled, open 14-month study. Eur Neurol 2003;49(1):13–19.

170. Herrmann N, Black SE, Chow T, Cappell J, Tang-Wai DF, Lanctôt KL. Serotonergic function and treatment of behavioral and psychological symptoms of frontotemporal dementia. Am J Geriatr Psychiatry 2012;20(9):789–797.

171. Furlan JC, Henri-Bhargava A, Freedman M. Clomipramine in the treatment of compulsive behavior in frontotemporal dementia: a case series. Alzheimer Dis Assoc Disord 2014;28(1):95–98.

172. Antczak J, Kowalska K, Klimkowicz-Mrowiec A, et al. Repetitive transcranial magnetic stimulation for the treatment of cognitive impairment in frontotemporal dementia: an open-label pilot study. Neuropsychiatr Dis Treat 2018;14:749–755.

173. Paul S, Goetz J, Bennett J, Korah T. Efficacy of electroconvulsive therapy for comorbid frontotemporal dementia with bipolar disorder. Case Rep Psychiatry 2013;2013:124719.

174. Borisovskaya A, Augsburger J, Pascualy M. Electroconvulsive therapy for frontotemporal dementia with comorbid major depressive disorder. J ECT 2014;30(4):e45–e46.

175. Korczyn AD. Vascular parkinsonism—characteristics, pathogenesis and treatment. Nat Rev Neurol 2015;11(6):319–326.

176. Tisell M, Tullberg M, Hellström P, Edsbagge M, Högfeldt M, Wikkelsö C. Shunt surgery in patients with hydrocephalus and white matter changes. J Neurosurg 2011;114(5):1432–1438.

177. Ondo WG, Chan LL, Levy JK. Vascular parkinsonism: clinical correlates predicting motor improvement after lumbar puncture. Mov Disord 2002;17(1):91–97.

178. Yip CW, Cheong PWT, Green A, et al. A prospective pilot study of repetitive transcranial magnetic stimulation for gait dysfunction in vascular parkinsonism. Clin Neurol Neurosurg 2013;115(7):887–891.

18

Frontotemporal Dementia

Symptoms, Distinguishing Features, Genetics, Pathology, and Associated Movement Disorders

Albert Y. Amran, Avram S. Bukhbinder, and Paul E. Schulz

Definition of FTD

Frontotemporal dementia (FTD) is a term given to a heterogeneous group of clinical syndromes whose unifying feature is that they predominantly involve the frontal and/or temporal lobes. Because of the wide-ranging functions of these lobes, the clinical picture in FTD is very diverse, often including cognitive, mood, and behavioral changes. Nonetheless, a careful clinical history, corroborated by relevant neuroimaging and neuropsychological testing, leads to a correct diagnosis of FTD. FTD has traditionally been suggested to present in one of three forms: behavioral-variant FTD (bvFTD), nonfluent variant primary progressive aphasia (nfvPPA), and semantic-variant PPA (svPPA). However, FTD has more recently been recognized as a spectrum of disorders. To the above three, then, other disorders are often added, including corticobasal degeneration (CBD), progressive supranuclear palsy (PSP), and FTD with motor neuron disease. The pathology underlying these diseases is now known to include at least several different proteinopathies, including tau deposition, tar DNA binding protein 43 (TDP-43), and several less common ones. Perhaps because the classification of these diseases was initially done clinically, followed later by identifying their underlying neuropathology and then many underlying genetic mutations, the nomenclature for FTD can be confusing.

Neurologic and Psychiatric Symptoms

The hypernym "FTD," as noted, is classically divided into three clinical syndromes: bvFTD and two types of primary progressive aphasia (PPA): nfvPPA and svPPA. The third subtype of PPA, logopenic PPA, is pathologically related to Alzheimer's disease (AD) and is therefore not conventionally considered to be an FTD syndrome, but it is a cause of the PPA phenotype. Among patients with any of the three main FTD syndromes, approximately 15%–20% have a concomitant motor neuron disease (MND).[1,2] Relevant to this book, movement disorders, especially parkinsomism and stereotype, are also common in FTD.[2] The mean age of onset for FTD is approximately 58 years, with the onset for most cases occurring between 25 and 83 years of age.[3]

Behavioral Variant FTD (bvFTD)

Behavioral variant FTD accounts for approximately 55% of clinically diagnosed FTD cases.[4,5] The average age at presentation is 58 years.[4] The neuropsychiatric symptoms commonly seen in the early-to-mid stages of bvFTD (i.e., within approximately three years of onset) include apathy; loss of sympathy, empathy, and prosociality; poor insight; disinhibition; alterations in musical and/or dietary preferences, often with hyperorality and a predilection for candies and other sweets; rigid or inflexible thinking; development of compulsive, perseverative, or stereotyped behaviors (although hygiene-related compulsions, like those commonly seen in obsessive-compulsive disorder, are uncommon in bvFTD); development of new hobbies or interests, especially those related to religion or spirituality, which are "pursued obsessively"; distractibility or impersistence; and psychotic features.[6]

Although patients with bvFTD often develop simple stereotypies and/or compulsive rituals early in the disease course, the frequency of these behaviors typically diminishes in the later stages of the disease as patients' apathy progresses toward abulia and, ultimately, toward akinetic mutism. Relatedly, in the later stages of the disease, patients with bvFTD often develop a progressive logopenia; the extent to which this language impairment is caused by behavioral mutism versus a true primary aphasia is unclear.[7,8]

Patients with bvFTD typically have a normal motor, sensory, and cranial nerve examination at presentation, though they can have increased deep tendon reflexes and frontal release signs, such as snout or grasp reflexes, but these signs are neither sensitive nor specific to FTD.[6] Pyramidal syndromes, ataxia, and/or oculomotor control issues are possible, albeit infrequent, abnormalities that can occur in late-stage bvFTD.[9]

Cases associated with certain genetic mutations (e.g., *C9ORF72*) have a higher probability of presenting with concomitant parkinsonism more resembling progressive supranuclear palsy (PSP) (see "Genetics" section below).[8] As the disease progresses, the majority of patients with bvFTD will develop an atypical parkinsonism, most commonly in the form of bradykinesia, symmetrical muscle rigidity, parkinsonian gait, and/or generalized hypokinesia.[4] In addition, antipsychotic use is a common cause for extrapyramidal signs. Medication review should be conducted at every visit with FTD patients to assess for such unfavorable adverse medication effects.

Nonfluent Variant PPA (nfvPPA)

Nonfluent variant PPA accounts for approximately 25% of clinically diagnosed FTD cases.[4,5] The average age at presentation for nfvPPA is 63 years.[4]

The characteristic neuropsychiatric symptoms of nfvPPA are agrammatism and apraxia of speech, manifesting as effortful, halting speech with inconsistent phonetic errors and distortions. Types of grammatical errors observed in the speech of a patient with nfvPPA include omission of small, closed-class words (e.g., a, in, the, and) and the presence of subject-verb disagreement. While comprehension of syntactically complex sentences may be impaired early in the course of nfvPPA, single word comprehension and object knowledge are typically unaffected until much later in the disease course.[6,8] This timeline may assist in differentiating nfvPPA from svPPA, which classically has impaired object naming earlier in the disease.[10]

Unlike bvFTD, patients with nfvPPA typically possess insight into their condition. This may relate to the increased rates of depression seen in patients with nfvPPA, which is not seen in patients with bvFTD. Most patients with nfvPPA will begin to develop behavioral changes associated with bvFTD (e.g., apathy, hyperorality, disinhibition) within three years of nfvPPA onset.[7]

Parkinsonism rarely occurs in patients with nfvPPA, even in later stages of the disease.[2] Motor abnormalities that might occur in nfvPPA are typically subtle and include right-sided fine-motor bradykinesia and pronator drift.[8]

Semantic Variant PPA (svPPA)

Semantic variant PPA accounts for approximately 20% of clinically diagnosed FTD cases.[4,5] The average age at presentation for svPPA is 59 years.[4]

Characteristic neuropsychiatric symptoms of svPPA include impairments in object naming (i.e., anomia) and single-word comprehension. Impaired object knowledge as well as impairment of written word recognition or the production of written words (dysgraphia) may be present early in the disease and are increasingly likely to be seen as the disease progresses. svPPA typically spares grammar, fluency, and repetition until much later in the disease course. Although the speech in svPPA is usually fluent, it is often tangential or circumlocutory, with very little specific content and frequent use of imprecise terms (i.e., "filler words") such as "stuff" and "thing."[6,8] This habit may reflect the impairment in object knowledge.

Similar to nfvPPA, patients with svPPA typically possess insight in the early stages of the disease, and probably because of this, mood disorders, such as depression, are common. As with nfvPPA, most patients with svPPA will also begin to develop behavioral changes (e.g., apathy, hyperorality, and disinhibition) within three years of svPPA onset.[7] In addition to this gradual onset of behavioral changes, patients with svPPA frequently also develop prosopagnosia, visual agnosia, and/or impairments in gustation and olfaction.[6]

Parkinsonism or other motor abnormalities rarely occur in patients with isolated svPPA, even in the later stages of the disease.[2,6,8]

FTD With Motor Neuron Disease (FTD-MND)

Approximately 15%–20% of patients with FTD also develop motor neuron disease (MND).[1] Most patients with both FTD and MND (FTD-MND) display behavioral changes consistent with bvFTD; however, some display symptoms more closely resembling PPA, with aphasia, mild executive dysfunction, and absent or relatively minor behavioral changes.[8,11]

Regardless of whether frontotemporal dysfunction is more consistent with bvFTD or PPA, the motor abnormalities seen in patients with FTD-MND usually closely resembles those observed in patients with classical, isolated ALS. One exception, however, is the increased rate of bulbar onset (versus limb onset) in patients with PPA-MND compared to patients with ALS without FTD.[12] Bulbar onset refers to the impairment of the 9th–12th cranial nerves and includes swallowing and speech difficulties. It is unclear whether there is an increased rate of bulbar onset in patients with bvFTD-MND versus those with isolated ALS.

Comparing isolated bvFTD without MND to bvFTD-MND, patients with bvFTD-MND more frequently experience psychotic symptoms such as hallucinations or delusions.

Hallucinations may be somatic, visual, or auditory, while delusions are typically somatic, bizarre, and/or paranoid. Psychotic symptoms are significantly more common in patients with bvFTD-MND due to a *C9ORF72* repeat expansion.[8]

Not surprisingly, FTD-MND is associated with a significant reduction in average life expectancy. The average life expectancy for FTD without MND is 7–10 years after symptom onset (3–4 years after clinical diagnosis),[5] while for patients with FTD and MND, the average life expectancy after symptom onset is only 2–3 years, which is similar to that of ALS without FTD.[8]

Recognition of the link between MND and FTD led to an expansive investigation into the pathophysiological relatedness between both diseases. Genetic evidence indicates that these diseases are closely related such that the same mutation (*C9orf72*) may lead to the development of MND in one family member and FTD in another. Furthermore, some MND patients evaluated at presentation meet FTD criteria prompting an evaluation of motor symptoms in FTD.[13] An analysis of a random sample of 36 sporadic FTD patients demonstrated that several met criteria for the diagnosis of MND confirmed by electromyography testing.[14] Conversely, another study in which a random sample of 279 sporadic MND patients were assessed for cognitive impairment resulted in 51% being found to have cognitive impairment.[15] Of the total MND patients, examination resulted in a diagnosis of FTD in 15% of them. There is clearly a need, then, to screen both patients with MND and FTD for symptoms of the other.[16] Characterization of these MND symptoms in FTD patients included muscular weakness, fasciculations, and dysphagia.

Neuropathologically, FTD-ALS is most frequently associated with TDP-43 deposition, which was demonstrated microscopically by Trojanowski and Lee in 2007 following papers documenting the co-occurrence of ALS in FTD patients.[15,17] But, FTD-ALS can occur with other pathologies, including tauopathies.

Movement Disorder Symptoms in FTD

The spectrum of movement disorders in FTD varies widely based on the genetic mutations involved. Heterogeneous phenotypes are common as well, even among patients with similar mutations. Genetically linked FTD is associated with mixed presentations, including features of parkinsonism, atypical parkinsonism, PSP, CBD, and multiple system atrophy (MSA). Estimation of the course of the patient's disease, including expected later features following diagnosis, may require genetic testing or an accurate family history. However, it is likely that the manifestation of these symptoms occurs as the disease involves areas of the brain that produce the clinical phenotype.

Certain genetic mutations are also linked to parkinsonism in FTD. These have been characterized and described in 2014 by Siuda et al., who identified the most common movement features among bvFTD patients as parkinsonism.[3] In fact, akinesia, rigidity, and tremor were supportive symptoms for the diagnosis of FTD in the 1998 diagnostic criteria for FTD, before being removed in 2011 as the diagnosis focused more on neuropsychological symptoms such as behavior and cognition.[18,19] More recent characterization of parkinsonism in FTD has identified bradykinesia and rigidity as the most common presentations, with resting tremor being rare.[20] Gait and balance impairment is also seen.

Atypical parkinsonism seen in FTD includes features of PSP and CBS. PSP is associated with vertical gaze palsy as well as the difficulty initiating saccades.[3] The most common CBS manifestation in FTD is apraxia, the inability to perform movements on command despite normal strength, though both cortical sensory loss and the alien limb phenomenon have been documented as well.[21] Other movement disorders observed in FTD included myoclonus and dystonia.

Mutations in the chromosome 17 microtubule-associated protein tau (*MAPT*) gene account for over 50% of heritable FTD cases, and are highly varied in presentation. *MAPT* mutations have nearly 100% penetrance and follow an autosomal dominant inheritance pattern. Movement disorders associated with mutations in this gene (see Table 18.2) can manifest at any time during the disease course, though typically occur late in the disorder. The appearance of movement disorder symptoms in *MAPT* patients is unrelated to disease progression. The course of cognitive degeneration and lifespan remain independent of the onset of movement disorder in these patients.[3] Parkinsonism in these patients is typically symmetrical, if it appears, and may respond to symptomatic management early in the disease. The initial response to treatment can lead to an incorrect diagnosis of Parkinson's disease. This differentiates it from parkinsonism related to other genetic FTD variants, which usually do not respond to dopaminergic treatment, including the second-most common gene where mutations have been identified leading to FTD, progranulin (*PGRN*; Table 18.2). It should be noted that parkinsonism arising in *MAPT*-derived cases may present on average about 10 years before *PGRN*-derived cases. An initial diagnosis of a movement disorder may be made, but the appearance of dementia-like symptoms or a negative response to symptomatic management may prompt screening for FTD or FTLD-related pathologies.

Lastly, cases of *C9orf72*, *PGRN*, and *TARDBP* FTD patients may exhibit a Huntington's disease (HD) phenotype, including stereotype, chorea, cognitive decline, and behavioral changes. Their genetic FTD variants were found after failed genetic tests for HD.[22,23] These patients tend to display more movement symptoms than solely chorea. Concomitant symptoms include dystonia, myoclonus, tremor, and rigidity. Of these HD phenocopies, the most common FTD genetic variant has been reported to be *C9orf72*.[24]

Epidemiology

FTD incidence varies with age, ranging from the lowest 2.2/100,000 for ages 40–49 to peaking around 8.9/100,000 in adults 60–69.[25,26] Men have a greater prevalence of bvFTD or svPPA, while women are more likely to develop nfvPPA. Genetics contributes significantly to FTD cases, with 40% having a known family history.[27]

Movement disorders are the initial manifestation in only 27% of genetic FTD cases, according to a 2016 systematic review of the phenomenology of motor issues in FTD.[2] Prevalence of movement disorders in genetic FTD syndromes varies, depending on the mutation; however, statistical testing proved to be of limited utility in this respect. Generally, it appears that parkinsonism is the most common motor manifestation.

Etiology/Genetics

Approximately 40% of FTD cases are associated with an autosomal dominant pattern of inheritance. Although the remaining 60% of FTD cases are considered to be sporadic, studies have found that a genetic mutation may be found in about 6% of patients with no family history of FTD.[8]

bvFTD and the nonfluent, agrammatic variant of PPA are the most common phenotypes in genetic FTD, although CBS presentations can also occur. Semantic variant PPA is almost always sporadic.[8]

Diagnostic Tests

Diagnosis of FTD and its variant subtypes, like that of other dementias, is made through a combination of history, neuropsychological evaluation, genetic testing, and imaging. The neuropsychological evaluation of FTD will reveal symptoms described above in the presentation section and imaging findings are found in the next section.

Imaging

Imaging findings, like that of the presentation of this disease, also can vary significantly, Nevertheless, patterns of imaging findings can assist clinicians in making diagnoses of FTD and its various subtypes. Additionally, there are imaging findings that reveal clinically helpful information about the diagnosis and projected disease course.

Structural magnetic resonance imaging (MRI) and (18F)–fluorodeoxyglucose positron emission tomography (FDG-PET) are two techniques used in the evaluation of FTD. However, newer molecular PET ligands capable of binding to tau proteins within the brain have resulted in further characterization of the pathology of this disease.

Despite the heterogeneity in both cognitive, behavioral, and motor symptoms seen in FTD, neuroimaging findings tend to pattern based on the genetic defect involved, as well as the clinical syndromes (Table 18.1).

Table 18.1 Patterns of Atrophy on MRI or Hypometabolism on FDG PET in Different Regions of the Brain in FTD

	Prefrontal Cortex	Premotor Cortex	Medial Temp. L	Lateral Temp L.	Parietal L.	Occipital L.	Striatum	Cerebellum
Clinical Syndromes								
bvFTD	+++	+	++	++	+	–	+	+
nfPPA	–	++	–	–	–	–	+	–
svPPA	+	–	+++	+++	–	–	+	–
Genetic Mutations								
MAPT	++	–	+++	+++	+	–	+	–
PGRN	++	–	+	++	++	–	–	++
C9orf72	+++	++	+	++	++	+	+	++

(–) indicates little involvement, (+) minor involvement, (++) moderate involvement, and (+++) major involvement. L = lobe. Modified from references 3 and 28.

Table 18.2 Genetics of FTD with Associated Clinicopathologic Phenotypes

	MAPT	PGRN	C9ORF72	CHMP2B	TARDBP	VCP	FUS
Penetrance	Almost 100%	90% by 70 years	Probably high	UKN	UKN	Incomplete	UKN
Anticipation	0	+	++	UKN	UKN	UKN	UKN
Estimated mutation frequency in FTD	0%–50%	3%–26%	14%–48%	<1%	<1%	<1%	UKN
Mean AAO (range)	49 years (25–76)	59 years (48–83)	55 years (33–75)	58 years (46–65)	54 years (40–69)	55 years (46–79)	43 years (30–60)
Mean DD (range)	7 years (2–30)	7 years (1–14)	4.5 years (3–10)	10 years (5–21)	3 years (1–5)	6 years (5–8)	43 years (30–60)
Most frequent initial Dx.	bvFTD ±P	bvFTD ±P	FTD/ALS	ALS, FTD	ALS, bvFTD	IBMPFD	FTD, ALS
Possible Motor Features	Parkinsonism, PSP, CBD	CBD, Huntington's-like phenotype	ALS; parkinsonism, Huntington's-like phenotype		ALS; Huntington's-like phenotype; rarely parkinsonism	Weak association with parkinsonism & ALS	Rigid-akinetic parkinsonism late in the disease; postural tremor
Clinical Dx. During disease course — Most frequent Dx.	FTD Parkinsonism	FTD CBS	FTD MND*	FTD Dementia	MND*	FTD MND*	FTD MND*
Common Dx.	Pyramidal signs, PSP	Parkinsonism, Pyramidal signs	Parkinsonism	Parkinsonism	FTD, Parkinsonism	Dementia	Dementia
Rare Dx.	CBS, MND	MND, Hallucinations	CBS	MND*, Epilepsy	Dementia	Language impairment, Parkinsonism	Parkinsonism
Prominent neuropathology	Tau	TDP-43	TDP-43, Ubiq	Ubiq	TDP-43	TDP-43	FUS
Levodopa responsiveness	Possibly temporarily effective	Usually not effective	Possibly temporarily effective	UKN	Effective	Possibly effective	UKN

Modified from reference 3.

*-including upper and lower motor neuron signs.

AAO = age at onset; ALS = amyotrophic lateral sclerosis; bvFTD = behavioral variant frontotemporal dementia; CBS = corticobasal syndrome; DD = disease duration; Dx. = Diagnosis; FTD = frontotemporal dementia; FUS = fused in sarcoma; IBMPFD = inclusion body myopathy with Paget disease of bone and frontotemporal dementia; MND = motor neuron disease; P = parkinsonism; TDP-43 = TAR DNA-binding protein 43; Ubiq = ubiquitin; UKN = unknown; 0 = not present; "+" = present in some cases; "++" = frequently occurs.

Evaluation of FTD based on MRI should only be done in concert with clinical examination and neuropsychological interview, as patients with clinical FTD syndromes may appear grossly normal on structural imaging.[29,30] bvFTD patients can be diagnosed based on MRI compared to controls with about 85% accuracy, but this often requires special expertise on part of the interpreter.[31,32]

The FDG PET, which measures glucose uptake, has proven to be invaluable for the diagnosis of FTD. FDG-PET is more sensitive and specific than MRI, more able to discriminate from Alzheimer's disease, and has been demonstrated to be helpful in differentiating between types of FTD.[33,34]

Tau PET imaging has emerged as a new avenue of diagnostic exploration, though biological isoforms of mutant tau in the large spectrum of FTLD pathologies underpinning the clinical disease, make finding a valuable universal ligand difficult. To be more specific, a point or frame-shift mutation in an exon of *MAPT* could result in differently gene products, and thus different isoforms of tau.

Functional MRI has been proposed as a potentially useful measure of clinical functioning, though standardization across studies remains a challenge.[35] Famously, neuroscientist Craig Bennett and his colleagues used fMRI to scan a dead salmon's "emotional" response to different pictures of humans in social settings and found that the standard scanning analytics at the time (2009) were invariably returning false positives.[36] Since then, studies of fMRI have only demonstrated value in combination with conventional testing such as structural MRI.[37] At present, fMRI is not helpful for the diagnosis of FTD.

Diffusion tensor imaging (DTI), which studies the structural connectivity of the brain may also be useful for the study of FTD. While DTI appears more sensitive in the detection of FTD, it may not be as useful as FDG-PET on an individual patient-level for diagnosis.[38-40]

In summary, in bvFTD, imaging generally reveals right greater than left frontal lobe changes, in right-handers, with sparing the posterior lobes. svFTD stereotypically affects the anterior temporal region, left-greater-than right. Finally, nfFTD involves the left posterior frontal lobe, including Broca's area.[41] Commonly, widening of the left perisylvian fissure is observed.[28] Imaging changes correlate anatomically with the areas of the brain responsible for the disease phenotypes, but it is important to note that structural MRI may show no changes, despite clinical impairment. FDG-PET is generally more sensitive in these cases.

Treatments

No curative treatment exists for FTD at the current time, but strides in disease-modifying therapies have been made due to advances in the understanding of the pathology and genetics of this disease spectrum. Most current treatment for FTD centers around symptomatic management, but new areas of investigation will be discussed here as well.

The wide spectrum of cognitive and motor symptoms that can arise over the course of the disease makes a strict treatment regimen difficult but generally management can be divided into pharmacological treatment and lifestyle management.

Neuropsychological presentations of FTD across the spectrum require close communication with caregivers and patients to track progression of the disease as new symptoms may arise. Furthermore, caregiver burnout can reduce quality of life for dementia patients.[42]

Pharmacological Management

Cholinesterase inhibitors, traditionally used in for Alzheimer's disease and more recently shown to have some effect in LBD and Parkinson's dementia, have been associated with temporary worsening of cognitive and behavioral symptoms in patients with FTD.[43,44] Overall, the evidence considering these drugs in the treatment of FTD is poor and they are not recommended.

The N-methyl-D-aspartic acid receptor (NMDA) antagonist memantine is another medication indicated in the treatment of Alzheimer's disease. In FTD, there has been poor evidence for the effectiveness of memantine in controlling symptoms. The first study in this area was done as an open-label, uncontrolled trial of 6 months that included 16 patients. There was no evidence of change with regard to the Neuropsychiatric Inventory (NPI) score or Frontal Behavioral Inventory (FBI), and cognitive performance was worse at the end of the observation period.[45] Evidence supporting the use of memantine was isolated to a case series of three patients demonstrating improvements in the NPI, though one 8.5-month open-label study in 2009 found transient cognitive improvement in patients with FTD.[46,47] Two later, more powered and randomized studies found no benefit of memantine use, at least with respect to neuropsychiatric score endpoints. More frequent cognitive adverse advents were observed in the memantine groups vs. placebo. These results were consistent between both studies.[47,48]

Selective serotonin reuptake inhibitors (and similar medications) may improve behavioral and psychological symptoms of FTD, including disinhibition and irritability, which are common in bvFTD. However, most studies to date have been open-label or case series. Trazodone in particular can improve irritability, agitation, and symptoms of depression 12 weeks after treatment in one double-blind, randomized, placebo-controlled study. Citalopram, sertraline, fluoxetine, and paroxetine improve symptoms in open-label trials and case series, though paroxetine failed to demonstrate improvement when studied in a double-blind, placebo-controlled, cross over trial.[49-51]

Antipsychotics mitigate behavioral disturbances and improve caregiver stress, though particular attention should be paid to possible extrapyramidal side effects of these drugs. Aripiprazole, risperidone, and olanzapine have been documented as potentially beneficial in FTD.[52-54] Case reports and case series are the strongest evidence available in this area with few open-label studies.[55] More rigorously-designed trials fail to demonstrate effectiveness. Moreover, atypical antipsychotics have been associated with higher mortality rates compared to placebo.[56] Hence, one needs to carefully weigh the potential risk of mortality, due to heart or infectious etiologies, against the potential behavioral benefits of this drug class. Quetiapine is commonly used as a first-line therapy to treat behavioral disturbances in FTD and has the most favorable side effect profile, though formal evidence as to its benefits in FTD does not currently exist.[57]

The evidence supporting antiepileptic agents is also too poor to recommend their use. Given the wide array of unfavorable side effects with these medications, careful considerations must be given before prescribing them. Mood stabilization is traditionally the goal of treatment with these medications in the context of FTD. Abatement of FTD-related disinhibited behaviors has been observed in at least one case report of carbamazepine use.[58] Valproic acid, another common mood stabilizer, was associated with increased brain atrophy in Alzheimer's dementia at the one-year mark in a two-year randomized trial of 89 partici-pants.[59] At the two-year mark, however, no cognitive, functional, or behavioral changes were observed vs. the placebo.

Dopaminergic therapy for the neuropsychiatric symptoms of FTD has been suggested in light of the demonstrated dopamine deficits in FTD-affected patients.[60] Interestingly, dopa-minergic therapies have shown to improve behavior in two small, double-blind, randomized studies.[56,61] However, adverse effects that may include behavioral disturbances and hallucinations on a background of a disease associated with altered cognition may not be favorable. Furthermore, the later need for anti-psychotic therapies, which utilize dopamine-blockade as the mechanism of action, may warrant the discontinuation of the medications as well.

Motor symptom management must be tailored to symptoms. As reviewed earlier in the motor symptoms section and Table 18.2, FTD-associated parkinsonism may or may not re-spond to dopaminergic therapies. Some patients do respond or may respond only initially. Movement disorders specialists can be helpful for their motor management. MND associated with *C9orf72* FTD can be treated with riluzole. The "Parkinson's-plus" syndromes associated with FTD, such as CBD or PSP, are particularly poorly responsive to dopamine therapies.[62]

Physical, speech, and occupational therapy are indicated for FTD patients based on symp-tomology. Gait and balance training can be conducted by a physical therapist. A home safety evaluation and ADL-assistance will need to be done by an occupational therapist. Speech therapy has been demonstrated to help in PPA variants of FTD and cases where patients later develop hypophonia, apraxia, and dysarthria.[63]

Emerging therapies have been derived to affect aberrant tau, manipulate genetic expres-sion, or modify neurotransmitter signaling in the brain. Anti-tau antibodies, antisense oli-gonucleotides to limit genetic expression, and pharmacotherapies such as methylene blue derivatives are all under investigation. Antibodies against compounds that metabolize ac-tive PRGN, in order to increase circulating PRGN levels, are undergoing trials. Adenoviral vectors have also been developed to replace mutant genes *in vivo* and are also undergoing clinical trials.

References

1. Burrell JR, Kiernan MC, Vucic S, Hodges JR. Motor neuron dysfunction in frontotemporal de-mentia. *Brain*. 2011;134(9):2582–2594. https://doi.org/10.1093/brain/awr195.

2. Baizabal-Carvallo JF, Jankovic J. Parkinsonism, movement disorders and genetics in fron-totemporal dementia. *Nat Rev Neurol*. 2016;12(3):175–185. https://doi.org/10.1038/nrneu rol.2016.14.

3. Siuda J, Fujioka S, Wszolek ZK. Parkinsonian syndrome in familial frontotemporal de-mentia. *Parkinsonism Relat Disord*. 2014;20(9):957–964. https://doi.org/10.1016/j.parkrel dis.2014.06.004.

4. Johnson JK, Diehl J, Mendez MF, et al. Frontotemporal lobar degeneration: Demographic characteristics of 353 patients. *Arch Neurol*. 2005;62(6):925–930. https://doi.org/10.1001/ archneur.62.6.925.

5. Ghosh S, Lippa CF. Clinical subtypes of frontotemporal dementia. *Am J Alzheimers Dis Other Demen*. 2015;30(7):653–661. https://doi.org/10.1177/1533317513494442

6. Warren JD, Rohrer JD, Rossor MN. Frontotemporal dementia. *BMJ*. 2013;347:f4827. https://doi.org/10.1136/bmj.f4827.

7. Banks SJ, Weintraub S. Neuropsychiatric symptoms in behavioral variant frontotemporal dementia and primary progressive aphasia. *J Geriatr Psychiatry Neurol*. 2008;21(2):133–141. https://doi.org/10.1177/0891988708316856

8. Finger E. C. Frontotemporal dementias. *Continuum*. 2016; *22*(2), 464–489. https://doi.org/10.1212/CON.0000000000000300

9. Seeley WW. Behavioral variant frontotemporal dementia. *Continuum*. 2019;25(1):76. https://doi.org/10.1212/CON.0000000000000698.

10. Hillis AE, Oh S, Ken L. Deterioration of naming nouns versus verbs in primary progressive aphasia. *Ann Neurol*. 2004;55(2):268–275. https://doi.org/https://doi.org/10.1002/ana.10812.

11. Strong MJ, Grace GM, Freedman M, et al. Consensus criteria for the diagnosis of frontotemporal cognitive and behavioural syndromes in amyotrophic lateral sclerosis. *Amyotrophic Lateral Sclerosis*. 2009;10(3):131–146. https://doi.org/10.1080/17482960802654364. https://doi.org/10.1080/17482960802654364.

12. Coon EA, Sorenson EJ, Whitwell JL, Knopman DS, Josephs KA. Predicting survival in frontotemporal dementia with motor neuron disease. *Neurology*. 2011;76(22):1886–1892. https://doi.org/10.1212/WNL.0b013e31821d767b.

13. Lomen-Hoerth C, Murphy J, Langmore S, Kramer JH, Olney RK, Miller B. Are amyotrophic lateral sclerosis patients cognitively normal? *Neurology*. 2003;60(7):1094–1097. https://doi.org/10.1212/01.wnl.0000055861.95202.8d.

14. Lomen-Hoerth C, Anderson T, Miller B. The overlap of amyotrophic lateral sclerosis and frontotemporal dementia. *Neurology*. 2002;59(7):1077–1079. https://doi.org/10.1212/wnl.59.7.1077.

15. Ringholz GM, Appel SH, Bradshaw M, Cooke NA, Mosnik DM, Schulz PE. Prevalence and patterns of cognitive impairment in sporadic ALS. *Neurology*. 2005;65(4):586–590.

16. Lillo P, Caramelli P, Musa G, et al. Inside minds, beneath diseases: social cognition in amyotrophic lateral sclerosis-frontotemporal spectrum disorder. *J Neurol Neurosurg Psychiatry*. 2020;91(12):1279–1282. doi: 10.1136/jnnp-2020-324302.

17. Cairns NJ, Neumann M, Bigio EH, et al. TDP-43 in familial and sporadic frontotemporal lobar degeneration with ubiquitin inclusions. *Am J Pathol*. 2007;171(1):227–240. https://doi.org/S0002-9440(10)61957-8 [pii].

18. Neary D, Snowden JS, Gustafson L, et al. Frontotemporal lobar degeneration: A consensus on clinical diagnostic criteria. *Neurology*. 1998;51(6):1546–1554. https://doi.org/10.1212/wnl.51.6.1546.

19. Rascovsky K, Hodges JR, Knopman D, et al. Sensitivity of revised diagnostic criteria for the behavioural variant of frontotemporal dementia. *Brain*. 2011;134(9):2456–2477. https://doi.org/10.1093/brain/awr179.

20. Padovani A, Agosti C, Premi E, Bellelli G, Borroni B. Extrapyramidal symptoms in frontotemporal dementia: prevalence and clinical correlations. *Neurosci Lett*. 2007;422(1):39–42. https://doi.org/10.1016/j.neulet.2007.05.049.

21. Pan X, Chen X. Clinic, neuropathology and molecular genetics of frontotemporal dementia: a mini-review. *Transl Neurodegener*. 2013;2:8. https://doi.org/10.1186/2047-9158-2-8.

22. Kovacs GG, Murrell JR, Horvath S, et al. TARDBP variation associated with frontotemporal dementia, supranuclear gaze palsy, and chorea. *Mov Disord*. 2009;24(12):1843–1847. https://doi.org/10.1002/mds.22697.

23. Wider C, Uitti RJ, Wszolek ZK, et al. Progranulin gene mutation with an unusual clinical and neuropathologic presentation. *Mov Disord*. 2008;23(8):1168–1173. https://doi.org/10.1002/mds.22065.

24. Hensman Moss DJ, Poulter M, Beck J, et al. C9orf72 expansions are the most common genetic cause of Huntington disease phenocopies. *Neurology*. 2014;82(4):292–299. https://doi.org/10.1212/WNL.0000000000000061.

25. Bott NT, Radke A, Stephens ML, Kramer JH. Frontotemporal dementia: diagnosis, deficits and management. *Neurodegener Dis Manag*. 2014;4(6):439–454. https://doi.org/10.2217/nmt.14.34.

26. Onyike CU, Diehl-Schmid J. The epidemiology of frontotemporal dementia. *Int Rev Psychiatry*. 2013;25(2):130–137. https://doi.org/10.3109/09540261.2013.776523.

27. Shpilyukova YA, Fedotova EY, Illarioshkin SN. [Genetic diversity in frontotemporal dementia]. *Mol Biol (Mosk)*. 2020;54(1):17–28. https://doi.org/10.31857/S0026898420010139.

28. Whitwell JL. Neuroimaging across the FTD spectrum. *Prog Mol Biol Transl Sci*. 2019;165:187–223. https://doi.org/10.1016/bs.pmbts.2019.05.009.

29. Davies RR, Kipps CM, Mitchell J, Kril JJ, Halliday GM, Hodges JR. Progression in frontotemporal dementia: identifying a benign behavioral variant by magnetic resonance imaging. *Arch Neurol*. 2006;63(11):1627–1631. https://doi.org/10.1001/archneur.63.11.1627.

30. Kipps CM, Davies RR, Mitchell J, Kril JJ, Halliday GM, Hodges JR. Clinical significance of lobar atrophy in frontotemporal dementia: application of an MRI visual rating scale. *Dement Geriatr Cogn Disord*. 2007;23(5):334–342. https://doi.org/10.1159/000100973.

31. Meyer S, Mueller K, Stuke K, et al. Predicting behavioral variant frontotemporal dementia with pattern classification in multi-center structural MRI data. *Neuroimage Clin*. 2017;14:656–662. https://doi.org/10.1016/j.nicl.2017.02.001.

32. Möller C, Pijnenburg YAL, van der Flier, Wiesje M., et al. Alzheimer disease and behavioral variant frontotemporal dementia: automatic classification based on cortical atrophy for single-subject diagnosis. *Radiology*. 2016;279(3):838–848. https://doi.org/10.1148/radiol.2015150220.

33. Nazem A, Tang CC, Spetsieris P, et al. A multivariate metabolic imaging marker for behavioral variant frontotemporal dementia. *Alzheimers Dement (Amst)*. 2018;10:583–594. https://doi.org/10.1016/j.dadm.2018.07.009.

34. Foster NL, Heidebrink JL, Clark CM, et al. FDG-PET improves accuracy in distinguishing frontotemporal dementia and Alzheimer's disease. *Brain*. 2007;130(Pt 10):2616–2635. https://doi.org/10.1093/brain/awm177.

35. Beisteiner R, Pernet C, Stippich C. Can we standardize clinical functional neuroimaging procedures? *Front Neurol*. 2019; 9: 1153. https://doi.org/10.3389/fneur.2018.01153.

36. Bennett CM, Miller MB, Wolford GL. Neural correlates of interspecies perspective taking in the post-mortem Atlantic salmon: an argument for multiple comparisons correction. *NeuroImage*. 2009;47:S125. https://doi.org/10.1016/S1053-8119(09)71202-9.

37. Bouts, Mark J. R. J., Möller C, Hafkemeijer A, et al. Single subject classification of Alzheimer's disease and behavioral variant frontotemporal dementia using anatomical, diffusion tensor, and resting-state functional magnetic resonance imaging. *J Alzheimers Dis*. 2018;62(4):1827–1839. https://doi.org/10.3233/JAD-170893.

38. Elahi FM, Marx G, Cobigo Y, et al. Longitudinal white matter change in frontotemporal dementia subtypes and sporadic late onset Alzheimer's disease. *Neuroimage Clin*. 2017;16:595–603. https://doi.org/10.1016/j.nicl.2017.09.007.

39. Yu J, Lee TMC. The longitudinal decline of white matter microstructural integrity in behavioral variant frontotemporal dementia and its association with executive function. *Neurobiol Aging.* 2019;76:62–70. https://doi.org/10.1016/j.neurobiolaging.2018.12.005.

40. Krämer, J., Lueg, G., Schiffler, P., Vrachimis, A., Weckesser, M., Wenning, C., Pawlowski, M., Johnen, A., Teuber, A., Wersching, H., Meuth, S. G., & Duning, T. (2018). Diagnostic value of diffusion tensor imaging and positron emission tomography in early stages of frontotemporal dementia. *J Alzheimers Dis.* 63(1), 239–253. https://doi.org/10.3233/JAD-170224

41. Josephs KA, Duffy JR, Strand EA, et al. Clinicopathological and imaging correlates of progressive aphasia and apraxia of speech. *Brain.* 2006;129(Pt 6):1385–1398. https://doi.org/10.1093/brain/awl078.

42. Takai M, Takahashi M, Iwamitsu Y, et al. The experience of burnout among home caregivers of patients with dementia: relations to depression and quality of life. *Arch Gerontol Geriatr.* 2009;49(1):e1–e5. https://doi.org/10.1016/j.archger.2008.07.002.

43. Mendez, M. F., Shapira, J. S., McMurtray, A., & Licht, E. (2007). Preliminary findings: behavioral worsening on donepezil in patients with frontotemporal dementia. *Am J Geriatr Psychiatry.* 15(1), 84–87. https://doi.org/10.1097/01.JGP.0000231744.69631.33

44. Arciniegas, D. B., & Anderson, C. A. (2013). Donepezil-induced confusional state in a patient with autopsy-proven behavioral-variant frontotemporal dementia. *J Neuropsychiatr Clin Neurosci,* 25(3), E25–E26.

45. Diehl-Schmid J, Förstl H, Perneczky R, Pohl C, Kurz A. A 6-month, open-label study of memantine in patients with frontotemporal dementia. *Int J Geriatr Psychiatry.* 2008;23(7):754–759. https://doi.org/10.1002/gps.1973.

46. Swanberg MM. Memantine for behavioral disturbances in frontotemporal dementia: a case series. *Alzheimer Dis Assoc Disord.* 2007;21(2):164–166. https://doi.org/10.1097/WAD.0b013e318047df5d.

47. Boxer AL, Knopman DS, Kaufer DI, et al. Memantine in frontotemporal lobar degeneration: a multicenter, randomised, double-blind, placebo-controlled trial. *Lancet Neurol.* 2013;12(2):149–156. https://doi.org/10.1016/S1474-4422(12)70320-4.

48. Vercelletto M, Boutoleau-Bretonnière C, Volteau C, et al. Memantine in behavioral variant frontotemporal dementia: negative results. *J Alzheimers Dis.* 2011;23(4):749–759. https://doi.org/10.3233/JAD-2010-101632.

49. Herrmann N, Black SE, Chow T, Cappell J, Tang-Wai DF, Lanctôt KL. Serotonergic function and treatment of behavioral and psychological symptoms of frontotemporal dementia. *Am J Geriatr Psychiatry.* 2012;20(9):789–797. https://doi.org/10.1097/JGP.0b013e31823033f3.

50. Swartz JR, Miller BL, Lesser IM, Darby AL. Frontotemporal dementia: treatment response to serotonin selective reuptake inhibitors. *J Clin Psychiatry.* 1997;58(5):212–216.

51. Chow TW, Mendez MF. Goals in symptomatic pharmacologic management of frontotemporal lobar degeneration. *Am J Alzheimers Dis Other Demen.* 2002;17(5):267–272. https://doi.org/10.1177/153331750201700504

52. Curtis RC, Resch DS. Case of pick's central lobar atrophy with apparent stabilization of cognitive decline after treatment with risperidone. *J Clin Psychopharmacol.* 2000;20(3):384–385. https://doi.org/10.1097/00004714-200006000-00018.

53. Reeves RR, Perry CL. Aripiprazole for sexually inappropriate vocalizations in frontotemporal dementia. *J Clin Psychopharmacol.* 2013;33(1):145–146. https://doi.org/10.1097/01.jcp.0000426190.64916.3b.

54. Moretti R, Torre P, Antonello RM, Cazzato G, Griggio S, Bava A. Olanzapine as a treatment of neuropsychiatric disorders of Alzheimer's disease and other dementias: a 24-month follow-up of 68 patients. *Am J Alzheimers Dis Other Demen*. 2003;18(4):205–214. https://doi.org/10.1177/153331750301800410.

55. Tsai RM, Boxer AL. Treatment of frontotemporal dementia. *Curr Treat Options Neurol*. 2014;16(11):319. https://doi.org/10.1007/s11940-014-0319-0.

56. Huey ED, Garcia C, Wassermann EM, Tierney MC, Grafman J. Stimulant treatment of frontotemporal dementia in 8 patients. *J Clin Psychiatry*. 2008;69(12):1981–1982. https://doi.org/10.4088/jcp.v69n1219a.

57. Asmal L, Flegar SJ, Wang J, Rummel-Kluge C, Komossa K, Leucht S. Quetiapine versus other atypical antipsychotics for schizophrenia. *Cochrane Database Syst Rev*. 2013(11):CD006625. https://doi.org/10.1002/14651858.CD006625.pub3.

58. Poetter CE, Stewart JT. Treatment of indiscriminate, inappropriate sexual behavior in frontotemporal dementia with carbamazepine. *J Clin Psychopharmacol*. 2012;32(1):137–138. https://doi.org/10.1097/JCP.0b013e31823f91b9.

59. Fleisher AS, Truran D, Mai JT, et al. Chronic divalproex sodium use and brain atrophy in Alzheimer disease. *Neurology*. 2011;77(13):1263–1271. https://doi.org/10.1212/WNL.0b013e318230a16c.

60. Huey ED, Putnam KT, Grafman J. A systematic review of neurotransmitter deficits and treatments in frontotemporal dementia. *Neurology*. 2006;66(1):17–22. https://doi.org/10.1212/01.wnl.0000191304.55196.4d.

61. Rahman S, Robbins TW, Hodges JR, et al. Methylphenidate ("Ritalin") can ameliorate abnormal risk-taking behavior in the frontal variant of frontotemporal dementia. *Neuropsychopharmacology*. 2006;31(3):651–658. https://doi.org/10.1038/sj.npp.1300886.

62. Birdi S, Rajput AH, Fenton M, et al. Progressive supranuclear palsy diagnosis and confounding features: Report on 16 autopsied cases. *Mov Disord*. 2002;17(6):1255–1264. https://doi.org/10.1002/mds.10211.

63. Kortte KB, Rogalski EJ. Behavioral interventions for enhancing life participation in behavioral variant frontotemporal dementia and primary progressive aphasia. *Int Rev Psychiatry*. 2013;25(2):237–245. https://doi.org/10.3109/09540261.2012.751017.

19

Restless Legs Syndrome and Psychiatric Issues

Emmanuel H. During and John W. Winkelman

Restless Legs Syndrome

Restless legs syndrome (RLS) is a sensorimotor syndrome characterized by unpleasant sensations associated with an urge to move the legs, with onset at rest, worse (or only occurring) in the evening or at night, and transiently relieved by counterstimulation such as standing and walking.[1] RLS affects 5%–10% of the general population and can severely impact sleep, quality of life, and well-being. This condition is also associated with a number of psychiatric conditions, use of psychotropic drugs, and clinical scenarios in mental health practice that we will attempt to cover in this chapter.

RLS is a clinical diagnosis. It is not equivalent to periodic limb movements (PLM), which are stereotyped dorsiflexion of the toes and ankles and/or flexion of knee and hip in either or both legs, rarely arms, occurring every 15–40 seconds, predominantly during the first cycle of non–rapid eye movement (NREM) sleep. Although 80%–90% of patients with RLS have PLM during sleep and even during wake when symptoms are severe, PLM in sleep are common in older males and may be associated with neurologic and cardiovascular disease. Common mimics of RLS include neuropathy (which is not associated with an urge to move), akathisia (which has no circadian pattern and tends to affect the entire body), and leg cramps (involuntary painful muscle contractures) which can be distinguished with a careful history.

A family history is common in RLS, especially in those with early-onset RLS (i.e., before age 45), with a number of well identified genetic polymorphisms (*BTBD9*, *MEIS1*, and *MAP2K5/SKOR1*).[2] Neurotransmitter pathways contributing to RLS include the dopaminergic, adenosinergic, glutamatergic, and opioid systems. RLS is characterized by a dopaminergic dysregulation, which explains why dopaminergic drugs are very effective. In addition, the adenosine 1 receptor (A1R) is downregulated in RLS, which contributes to both a presynaptic hyperdopaminergic and hyperglutamatergic state. The opioid system (mu receptor) is also implicated in RLS and the efficacy of opioids could be due to enhanced dopaminergic transmission. Possibly central in the pathogenesis, a state of low central nervous system iron (brain iron deficiency) is well described in patients with RLS and associated with the dysregulation of all key neurotransmitter pathways cited above.[3] Low CNS iron in RLS is not a mere reflection of peripheral iron status since peripheral iron levels are not different than in the general population. However, low peripheral iron stores (fasting ferritin <75 mcg/L and/or transferrin saturation index <20%) within the RLS population are associated with more severe symptoms and periodic testing of peripheral iron status is standard-of-care practice in RLS.

RLS is seen in several other conditions including kidney disease, especially those requiring dialysis; pregnancy; and possibly neuropathy, and is referred to as secondary RLS in these settings. Low systemic iron can also induce RLS.

Nonpharmacologic management of RLS includes preventive evening leg stretching, use of warm water on the legs, regular moderate exercise, and limitation of alcohol in addition to the avoidance of exacerbating medications such as antihistamine and antidopaminergic and serotonergic drugs. Daily oral iron supplementation (325 mg ferrous sulfate with 200 mg vitamin C without food) should be considered in most cases with low-normal iron status, while high-dose iron infusions (1 g low molecular weight iron dextrose, ferrous carboxymaltose, or ferumoxytol) should be considered for those who do not tolerate (gastric side effects are common), or do not respond to, oral therapy (e.g., due to malabsorption).[4] The pharmacological management of RLS includes gabapentinoids (gabapentin, pregabalin, and gabapentin enacarbil), dopaminergic agonists (pramipexole, ropinirole, and transdermal rotigotine) and, when other treatments fail, low-dose opioids. Augmentation of RLS symptoms is a common complication in patients using chronic dopaminergic drugs and is defined as paradoxical worsening of symptom, especially earlier onset, necessitating escalating doses after an initial response to therapy. This complication is common after months or years of daily use, and thus current guidelines recommend that, after nonpharmacological interventions, gabapentinoids be used first-line.[5]

Restless Legs Syndrome and Psychiatric Issues

Restless Legs Syndrome and Anxiety

The co-occurrence of RLS symptoms and anxiety and depression has been documented since the 19th century by Wittmaack, who in fact described RLS as "anxietas tibiarum."[6] A first large study conducted in Germany comparing 130 patients with RLS and over 2,000 non-RLS community participants with at least one medical illness, using clinical interviews for psychiatric diagnoses, showed a strong association with panic disorder and general anxiety disorder (GAD) with odds ratios (ORs) of 4.7 and 3.5, respectively.[7] This study also showed that in most of these patients, RLS appeared first, i.e., preceded the psychiatric disorder. Recent studies also found significantly higher rates of anxiety in RLS. Among 74 patients with RLS recruited in Spain and in the United Kingdom (mean age 64, mean IRLSSG rating scare 24.8), almost half of them reported feeling anxious or frightened.[8] This is consistent with findings from another large study in elderly French participants showing association of RLS symptoms and general anxiety disorder (GAD) in isolation or associated with depression, with odds ratio [OR] of 2.17 (95% confidence interval [CI] 1.01–4.68) and OR 3.26, 95% CI 1.14–9.29, respectively.[9] Higher rates of anxiety symptoms were also found in the hemodialysis population with RLS.[10]

Restless Legs Syndrome and Depression

Several studies in community- and clinic-dwelling patients have reported a strong association between RLS and depression. In their seminal 2005 study, Winkelmann et al. found an OR of 2.6 for major depressive disorder (MDD) within 12 months of the interview in RLS patients vs. controls without RLS.[7] The association between depression and RLS was also found in the population of patients with chronic kidney disease, even after accounting for insomnia.[11] According to a recent study in a clinic population with RLS, as many as 59% reported feeling sad, and nearly 50% reported symptoms of forgetfulness, difficulty concentrating, and unexplained pain.[8] The presence of depressive symptoms was not a function of disease duration. A large general population study conducted in 11,831 adolescents in China found a 2.2% prevalence of RLS symptoms at least 3 days per week. In those patients, RLS was associated with a 28% prevalence of hopelessness, compared to 13% in individuals without RLS and 17% in those with RLS up to two days per week, suggesting a dose-response association between RLS and depressive thoughts.[12] A similar association between moderate-to-severe RLS and the number of depressive symptoms (OR 2.85, 95% CI 1.23–6.64) was found in a large community-dwelling study (the Osteoporotic Fractures in Men [MrOS] study) following 982 men over a mean duration of 6.5 years.[13] Finally, a recent study in 192 RLS and 158 control participants recruited from the community and RLS Foundation advertisements reported the lifetime depression history was three times higher in RLS patients (65.6% vs. 22.8%).[14]

The temporal sequence between depression and RLS is variable. Patients themselves can attribute a large part of their psychiatric burden to RLS symptoms when they are both present.[7] A large prospective study in over 56,000 women free of depression at baseline, found that those with RLS at baseline were significantly more likely to develop depression over time, with a relative risk (RR) of 1.5.[15] Similarly, the results of another large prospective study analyzing data from two independent cohorts totaling nearly 4,500 individuals followed over 5 years supported the RLS to depression longitudinal direction (OR = 1.82) and in addition described the reverse directionality, with ORs of about 2 for developing new-onset RLS when depression was present at baseline.[16] Illustrating the variable temporal and possible causal relation between RLS and depression, a recent Indian sleep clinic population study in 112 consecutive RLS patients among which 37 were found to have concomitant MDD, 51% of them reported that RLS symptoms came first while 38% reported the reverse time sequence.[17]

Restless Legs Syndrome and Suicide

There is increased suicidal risk in patients with RLS. Para et al. found significantly higher lifetime suicidal ideation or behavior in patients with RLS (27.1%) vs. controls (7.0%).[14] Although the association was stronger in those with lifetime depression (OR = 7.37), after controlling for depression and other confounders, the OR was still 2.80, suggesting that the association is not solely explained by depressive symptoms. In their recent large prospective study conducted in over 24,000 patients with RLS vs. 145,000 controls over 6 years, Zhuang et al. found an OR of 2.66 for suicide and self-harm with RLS.[18] Again, excluding those with depression and insomnia, the association persisted, with adjusted hazard ratio of 4.14.[14]

Pathophysiologic Link Between Restless Legs Syndrome and Psychiatric Illness

As reported above, there is evidence of a bidirectional relationship between RLS and psychiatric symptoms. Insomnia is reported by nearly 90% of patients with RLS,[19] and this complication when left untreated is associated with an increased risk of developing a mood disorder.[20] Similarly, insomnia itself is associated with a twofold risk of developing anxiety disorders later in life.[21] A questionnaire-based study examining the determinants of reduced daytime alertness and emotional distress (moodiness, irritability) using structural equation modeling in patients with RLS found that those daytime consequences appear to be mostly secondary to the sleep disturbance associated with RLS.[22]

Daytime RLS symptoms may also contribute to psychiatric complications. The anxious anticipation of RLS symptoms when they occur day after day can be accompanied by a feeling of doom and misery. Although some patients report that RLS symptoms preceded and contributed to their psychiatric symptoms,[7] which is supported by prospective data,[15] the reverse sequence can also occur.[16] This is particularly relevant when we consider that many psychotropic drugs can trigger or aggravate RLS.

Serotonergic and antihistamine treatments used to treat depression, chronic anxiety, and insomnia, have the potential to unmask or worsen RLS. These include tricyclic agents (with the possible exception of desipramine), selective serotonergic reuptake inhibitors (SSRIs), and serotonergic and noradrenergic reuptake inhibitors (SNRIs), in addition to antidepressants that have antihistamine properties (H_1 antagonists) such as mirtazapine and low dose doxepin, often used to treat insomnia at low dose. Among the antidepressant drugs, mirtazapine may present the highest risk of treatment-induced RLS, since it occurs in up to 28% of patients receiving treatment.[23] Pre-existing or new symptoms of RLS should ideally be screened in patients who are prescribed these drugs, especially if a complaint of insomnia paradoxically worsens during treatment. Similarly, hydroxyzine or diphenhydramine are occasionally used off label to treat anxiety and pose the risk of unmasking or aggravating RLS symptoms.

Additionally, the majority of antidopaminergic antipsychotic drugs have the potential of triggering or worsening RLS. Aripiprazole, brexpiprazole, and cariprazine may have a more neutral effect on RLS possibly due to their partial dopamine agonism. Similarly, the two antidepressant drugs trazodone (minimal serotonergic effect) and bupropion (dopamine and norepinephrine reuptake inhibitor) are notable exceptions in the antidepressant class since they are not thought to be associated with RLS exacerbation.

As akathisia is another common complication in patients receiving neuroleptic treatments, it is important to distinguish it from RLS. Akathisia does not have a circadian pattern and tends to affect the entire body, while RLS mostly or only occurs in the later part of the day or only at night, and in the majority of cases affects the legs more than arms or other body parts.

When used daily for RLS, dopaminergic treatments have the potential to cause impulse control disorders (ICD), resulting in impulsive gambling, shopping, irrepressible impulses toward food and sex. This complication affects about 10% of patients with a predominance in women[24,25] and a mean delayed onset of nine months after treatment initiation.[26] Patients with augmentation of RLS symptoms on DA have an increased risk of developing ICD symptoms (OR 5.64, 95% CI 1.59–20.02),[27] potentially related to higher DA doses in such patients. The treatment of ICD is dose reduction or discontinuation of the DA drug.

Dopamine Agonists Withdrawal Syndrome

Although discontinuation of DA drugs is the optimal intervention when augmentation occurs, it occasionally results in a cluster of psychiatric and somatic symptoms known as "dopamine agonists withdrawal syndrome" (DAWS), which has mostly been reported in Parkinson's disease.[28] The wide range of possible manifestations in DAWS include anxiety, low mood ranging from dysphoria to frankly depressed mood, suicidal ideation, irritability, insomnia, agitation, generalized pain, diaphoresis and drug craving, asthenia, orthostatic hypotension, nausea, and vomiting.[29] The course of symptom is generally limited to days or weeks, but in some cases can persist months to years. The risk of DAWS is significantly increased in individuals who have developed an ICD during dopaminergic treatment, as well as those at higher doses.[30] While patient education and psychological support is the mainstay in acute DAWS, there is no specific treatment or consensus for managing the rare chronic form of DAWS. Nonetheless, the main manifestation after withdrawing DA in patients with augmentation of RLS symptoms is a marked exacerbation of RLS, which often lasts up to a week before improving.

Management of Restless Legs Syndrome in Psychiatric Patients

As outlined above, RLS is a common occurrence in psychiatric patients due to at least three factors: RLS symptoms (most prominently sleep disturbance) themselves contribute to psychiatric illness, RLS treatments can result in psychiatric symptoms, and certain psychotropic drugs can cause iatrogenic RLS. In psychiatric practice, when a patient complains or displays symptoms of RLS, it is important to first evaluate whether this could be due to a serotonergic, antidopaminergic, or antihistamine drug (see Figure 19.1). Additionally, when symptoms are frequent (occur at least 2 days per week), a fasting iron panel including ferritin and

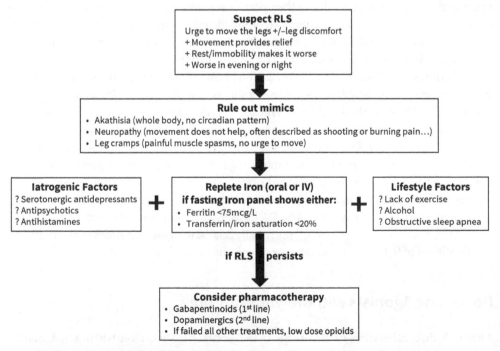

Figure 19.1 Management algorithm of restless legs syndrome.

transferrin saturation should be obtained, and iron should be supplemented at least orally in cases of low-normal levels. However, normal or elevated ferritin, even if elevated secondary to inflammation inhibits iron salt absorption, such that iron pills are probably not helpful if the ferritin is >75, even if iron-binding percentage is low. Lifestyle interventions should be explained and emphasized to patients as their systematic implementation can significantly relieve symptom burden. In the event that RLS persists despite iron optimization and lifestyle changes, dose reduction of the offending drug(s) can be considered and could start with those having the most antihistamine and antidopaminergic effects.

Once this is achieved and if symptoms persist, RLS-targeting pharmacotherapy can be considered (see Figure 19.1). Due to the common occurrence of augmentation and ICD with chronic DA use, gabapentinoids should be considered first. Their main side effects include sedation, which is usually mild and self-limited, balance problems, and weight gain with chronic use. In some individuals, gabapentinoids can contribute to depressed mood and thus the benefits of RLS treatment must be weighed against the occasional side effect of mood disturbance. There have been historical concerns regarding suicide risk with gabapentin.[31] However, this was later contradicted by a large retrospective study in 130,000 patients, suggesting that gabapentin is not associated with an increased risk of suicide attempts, or may even be associated with a lower risk in psychiatric populations.[32]

In cases of treatment-resistant severe RLS failing gabapentinoids or DA treatment, low-dose opioids can be considered as they have shown strong efficacy and good long-term safety data in the RLS population.[33-35] Opioids efficacy, as a pharmacological class, is not strictly related to an analgesic effect but could be mediated by a regulation of dopamine transmission. Methadone (5–20 mg) and oxycodone (10–30 mg) are the most commonly used opioids for RLS in the United States. Patients considered for opioid therapy should have their risk of misuse or abuse evaluated with the opioid risk assessment tool.[36] In addition, an opioid contract needs to be established with the patient.[37] These steps are common practice when prescribing opioids but are even more important in the psychiatric population who need even closer monitoring. Patients already treated with benzodiazepines present a higher risk of developing CNS depression on opioids. Although usually well tolerated at the doses used for RLS, opioids can also have psychiatric side effects on mood and anxiety. Among them, methadone presents a higher risk of causing depression. Despite the overall excellent efficacy and safety profile of opioids in the RLS population, all the above considerations need to be weighed against potential harm or complications in a patient with psychiatric comorbidity.

Conclusion

RLS is a common disorder in the general population and even more so in psychiatric populations. RLS being a potentially severe and lifelong condition, it also contributes to psychiatric comorbidity, especially anxiety, depression and risk of suicide or self-harm. RLS treatments can have iatrogenic psychiatric effects, especially with chronic dopaminergic use and withdrawal. Conversely, many psychotropic drugs can aggravate or unmask RLS symptoms. Understanding these various scenarios and frequently overlapping conditions is paramount for appropriate management of patients with RLS and psychiatric issues. Although a number of such patients can be managed by a non–sleep specialist, comanagement by a psychiatrist and a sleep physician is appropriate in more complex situations involving polypharmacy and/or refractory RLS.

References

1. American Academy of Sleep Medicine. (2014). *International Classification of Sleep Disorders, 3rd ed. (ICSD-3): Diagnostic and Coding Manual* (3rd ed). Westchester, IL: American Academy of Sleep Medicine.

2. Jiménez-Jiménez, F. J., Alonso-Navarro, H., García-Martín, E., & Agúndez, J. A. G. (2018). Genetics of restless legs syndrome: An update. *Sleep Medicine Reviews.* 39:108–121. https://doi.org/10.1016/j.smrv.2017.08.002

3. Earley, C. J., Connor, J. R., Beard, J. L., Malecki, E. A., Epstein, D. K., & Allen, R. P. (2000). Abnormalities in CSF concentrations of ferritin and transferrin in restless legs syndrome. *Neurology.* 54(8):1698–700. https://doi.org/10.1212/WNL.54.8.1698

4. Allen, R. P., Picchietti, D. L., Auerbach, M., Cho, Y. W., Connor, J. R., Earley, C. J., . . . Winkelman, J. W. (2018). Evidence-based and consensus clinical practice guidelines for the iron treatment of restless legs syndrome/Willis-Ekbom disease in adults and children: an IRLSSG task force report. *Sleep Medicine.* 41:27–44. https://doi.org/10.1016/j.sleep.2017.11.1126

5. Garcia-Borreguero, D., Silber, M. H., Winkelman, J. W., Högl, B., Bainbridge, J., Buchfuhrer, M., Allen, R. P. (2016). Guidelines for the first-line treatment of restless legs syndrome/Willis-Ekbom disease, prevention and treatment of dopaminergic augmentation: A combined task force of the IRLSSG, EURLSSG, and the RLS-foundation. *Sleep Medicine, 21,* 1–11. https://doi.org/10.1016/j.sleep.2016.01.017

6. Wittmaack, T. (1861). *Pathologie und Therapie der Sensibilitäts-Neurosen* (E. Schäfer, Ed.). Leipzig.

7. Winkelmann, J., Prager, M., Lieb, R., Pfister, H., Spiegel, B., Wittchen, H. U., . . . Ströhle, A. (2005). "Anxietas tibiarum": Depression and anxiety disorders in patients with restless legs syndrome. *Journal of Neurology,* 252(1):67–71 https://doi.org/10.1007/s00415-005-0604-7

8. Sauerbier, A., Sivakumar, C., Klingelhoefer, L., Martinez-Martin, P., Perkins, L., Inniss, R., . . . Chaudhuri, K. R. (2019). Restless legs syndrome—the under-recognised non-motor burden: a questionnaire-based cohort study. *Postgraduate Medicine.* 131(7):473–478. https://doi.org/10.1080/00325481.2019.1658506

9. Tully, P. J., Kurth, T., Elbaz, A., & Tzourio, C. (2020). Convergence of psychiatric symptoms and restless legs syndrome: A cross-sectional study in an elderly French population. *Journal of Psychosomatic Research.* 128:109884 https://doi.org/10.1016/j.jpsychores.2019.109884

10. Dikici, S., Bahadir, A., Baltaci, D., Ankarali, H., Eroglu, M., Ercan, N., & Sav, T. (2014). Association of anxiety, sleepiness, and sexual dysfunction with restless legs syndrome in hemodialysis patients. *Hemodialysis International.* 18(4):809–18. https://doi.org/10.1111/hdi.12175

11. Szentkiralyi, A., Molnar, M. Z., Czira, M. E., Deak, G., Lindner, A. V., Szeifert, L., . . . Novak, M. (2009). Association between restless legs syndrome and depression in patients with chronic kidney disease. *Journal of Psychosomatic Research.* 67(2), 173–180 https://doi.org/10.1016/j.jpsychores.2009.05.004

12. Liu, X., Chen, H., Liu, Z. Z., & Jia, C. X. (2018). Insomnia and psychopathological features associated with restless legs syndrome in Chinese adolescents. *Journal of Clinical Psychiatry.* 79(1):16m11358. https://doi.org/10.4088/JCP.16m11358

13. Koo, B. B., Blackwell, T., Lee, H. B., Stone, K. L., Louis, E. D., & Redline, S. (2016). Restless legs syndrome and depression: Effect mediation by disturbed sleep and periodic limb movements. *American Journal of Geriatric Psychiatry.* 24(11): 1105–1116. https://doi.org/10.1016/j.jagp.2016.04.003

14. Para, K. S., Chow, C. A., Nalamada, K., Kakade, V. M., Chilakamarri, P., Louis, E. D., & Koo, B. B. (2019). Suicidal thought and behavior in individuals with restless legs syndrome. *Sleep Medicine.* 54:1–7. https://doi.org/10.1016/j.sleep.2018.09.019

15. Li, Y., Mirzaei, F., O'Reilly, E. J., Winkelman, J., Malhotra, A., Okereke, O. I., . . . Gao, X. (2012). Prospective study of restless legs syndrome and risk of depression in women. *American Journal of Epidemiology.* 176(4):279–88. https://doi.org/10.1093/aje/kws016

16. Szentkiralyi, A., Völzke, H., Hoffmann, W., Baune, B. T., & Berger, K. (2013). The relationship between depressive symptoms and restless legs syndrome in two prospective cohort studies. *Psychosomatic Medicine.* 75(4):359–65. https://doi.org/10.1097/PSY.0b013e31828bbbf1

17. Gupta, R., Lahan, V., & Goel, D. (2013). A study examining depression in restless legs syndrome. *Asian Journal of Psychiatry.* 6(4):308–12. https://doi.org/10.1016/j.ajp.2013.01.011

18. Zhuang, S., Na, M., Winkelman, J. W., Ba, D., Liu, C. F., Liu, G., & Gao, X. (2019). Association of restless legs syndrome with risk of suicide and self-harm. *JAMA Network Open.* 2(8): e199966. https://doi.org/10.1001/jamanetworkopen.2019.9966

19. Hening, W., Walters, A. S., Allen, R. P., Montplaisir, J., Myers, A., & Ferini-Strambi, L. (2004). Impact, diagnosis and treatment of restless legs syndrome (RLS) in a primary care population: The REST (RLS epidemiology, symptoms, and treatment) primary care study. *Sleep Medicine.* 5(3):237–46. https://doi.org/10.1016/j.sleep.2004.03.006

20. Baglioni, C., Battagliese, G., Feige, B., Spiegelhalder, K., Nissen, C., Voderholzer, U., . . . Riemann, D. (2011). Insomnia as a predictor of depression: A meta-analytic evaluation of longitudinal epidemiological studies. *Journal of Affective Disorders.* 135(1–3):10–9. https://doi.org/10.1016/j.jad.2011.01.011

21. Breslau, N., Roth, T., Rosenthal, L., & Andreski, P. (1996). Sleep disturbance and psychiatric disorders: A longitudinal epidemiological study of young adults. *Biological Psychiatry.* 39(6), 411–418. https://doi.org/10.1016/0006-3223(95)00188-3

22. Kushida, C. A., Allen, R. P., & Atkinson, M. J. (2004). Modeling the causal relationships between symptoms associated with restless legs syndrome and the patient-reported impact of RLS. *Sleep Medicine.* 5(5):485–488 https://doi.org/10.1016/j.sleep.2004.04.004

23. Rottach, K. G., Schaner, B. M., Kirch, M. H., Zivotofsky, A. Z., Teufel, L. M., Gallwitz, T., & Messer, T. (2008). Restless legs syndrome as side effect of second generation antidepressants. *Journal of Psychiatric Research.* 43(1):70–5. https://doi.org/10.1016/j.jpsychires.2008.02.006

24. Driver-Dunckley, E. D., Noble, B. N., Hentz, J. G., Evidente, V. G. H., Caviness, J. N., Parish, J., . . . Adler, C. H. (2007). Gambling and increased sexual desire with dopaminergic medications in restless legs syndrome. *Clinical Neuropharmacology.* 30(5), 249–255. https://doi.org/10.1097/wnf.0b013e31804c780e

25. Voon, V., Schoerling, A., Wenzel, S., Ekanayake, V., Reiff, J., Trenkwalder, C., & Sixel-Döring, F. (2011). Frequency of impulse control behaviours associated with dopaminergic therapy in restless legs syndrome. *BMC Neurology.* 11: 117. https://doi.org/10.1186/1471-2377-11-117

26. Cornelius, J. R., Tippmann-Peikert, M., Slocumb, N. L., Frerichs, C. F., & Silber, M. H. (2010). Impulse control disorders with the use of dopaminergic agents in restless legs syndrome: A case-control study. *Sleep,* 33(1), 81–87. https://doi.org/10.1016/j.yneu.2010.12.010

27. Heim, B., Djamshidian, A., Heidbreder, A., Stefani, A., Zamarian, L., Pertl, M. T., . . . Högl, B. (2016). Augmentation and impulsive behaviors in restless legs syndrome. *Neurology.* 87(1):36–40. https://doi.org/10.1212/WNL.0000000000002803

28. Rabinak, C. A., & Nirenberg, M. J. (2010). Dopamine agonist withdrawal syndrome in Parkinson disease. *Archives of Neurology.* 67(1):58–63. https://doi.org/10.1001/archneu rol.2009.294

29. Nirenberg, M. J. (2013). Dopamine agonist withdrawal syndrome: Implications for patient care. *Drugs and Aging.* 30(8):587–92. https://doi.org/10.1007/s40266-013-0090-z

30. Yu, X. X., & Fernandez, H. H. (2017). Dopamine agonist withdrawal syndrome: A comprehensive review. *Journal of the Neurological Sciences.* 374:53–55. https://doi.org/10.1016/j.jns.2016.12.070

31. Patorno, E., Bohn, R. L., Wahl, P. M., Avorn, J., Patrick, A. R., Liu, J., & Schneeweiss, S. (2010). Anticonvulsant medications and the risk of suicide, attempted suicide, or violent death. *JAMA—Journal of the American Medical Association.* 303(14):1401–1409 https://doi.org/10.1001/jama.2010.410

32. Gibbons, R. D., Hur, K., Brown, C. H., & Mann, J. J. (2010). Gabapentin and suicide attempts. *Pharmacoepidemiology and Drug Safety,* 19(12), 1241–1247. https://doi.org/10.1002/pds.2036

33. Silver, N., Allen, R. P., Senerth, J., & Earley, C. J. (2011). A 10-year, longitudinal assessment of dopamine agonists and methadone in the treatment of restless legs syndrome. *Sleep Medicine,* 12(5), 440–444. https://doi.org/10.1016/j.sleep.2010.11.002

34. Trenkwalder, C., Beneš, H., Grote, L., García-Borreguero, D., Högl, B., Hopp, M., . . . Kohnen, R. (2013). Prolonged release oxycodone-naloxone for treatment of severe restless legs syndrome after failure of previous treatment: A double-blind, randomised, placebo-controlled trial with an open-label extension. *Lancet Neurology,* 12(12), 1141–1150. https://doi.org/10.1016/S1474-4422(13)70239-4

35. Mackie, S. E., & Winkelman, J. W. (2017). Therapeutic utility of opioids for restless legs syndrome. *Drugs.* 77(12):1337–1344. https://doi.org/10.1007/s40265-017-0773-6

36. Webster, L. R., & Webster, R. M. (2005). Predicting aberrant behaviors in opioid-treated patients: Preliminary validation of the opioid risk tool. *Pain Medicine.* 6(6):432–42. https://doi.org/10.1111/j.1526-4637.2005.00072.x

37. Silber, M. H., Becker, P. M., Buchfuhrer, M. J., Earley, C. J., Ondo, W. G., Walters, A. S., & Winkelman, J. W. (2018). The appropriate use of opioids in the treatment of refractory restless legs syndrome. *Mayo Clinic Proceedings.* 93(1):59–67. https://doi.org/10.1016/j.mayocp.2017.11.007

20

Neurometabolic Diseases

Nivedita Thakur, Moira Black, Sam Nicholas Russo, and Mary Kay Koenig

Introduction

Neurometabolic diseases are a group of disorders that lead to a disruption in the normal metabolism within the body and nervous system. Abnormalities of metabolic processes at any level can lead to a wide spectrum of clinical features and pathologies. The nervous system is particularly susceptible to metabolic derangements, either inborn or acquired. Early diagnosis can prevent or delay damage to the nervous system through appropriate treatment when possible. Many neurometabolic disorders have poor prognoses, and patients often present and succumb within months to the early years of life; however, some disorders can present later in life with varying levels of severity. In many later onset cases, the diagnosis is preceded by nonspecific symptoms including psychiatric manifestations. In addition to psychiatric manifestations, various neurological features often occur at some point in the course of the disease. Of these features, movement disorders are particularly common. In fact, many neurometabolic diseases will present with subtle movement disorders that are often missed or overlooked. Many congenital metabolic diseases are rapidly neurodegenerative and, due to the nature of such diseases, result in early demise or severe cognitive decline. While by no means exhaustive, this chapter aims to outline and discuss some of the neurometabolic diseases that present with both psychiatric and movement disorders as prominent features (Table 20.1)

Amino Acid Disorders

Hartnup Disease

Hartnup disease is an autosomal recessive[1,2] condition characterized by intestinal malabsorption and decreased renal reabsorption of tryptophan and other neutral amino acids.[3] It is caused by a mutation in the *SLC6A19* gene located on chromosome 5q15.33,[4] which encodes a sodium-dependent neutral amino acid transporter that is predominantly expressed in the intestines and kidneys.[1,2] In the kidneys this leads to decreased reabsorption of neutral amino acids and therefore elevated levels in the urine. In the intestines there is limited absorption of tryptophan, a precursor of niacin.[5] It is the lack of niacin in the body that is believed to cause the majority of symptoms.[6]

The initial presentation varies, and is usually preceded by a period of nutritional deficiency. To a neurologist, patients present with an unsteady, ataxic, wide-based gait. To a psychiatrist, patients present with intermittent psychotic episodes, which improve with niacin

Table 20.1 Overview of Metabolic Disorders and Related Movement and Psychiatric Features

	Disorder	Movement Features	Psychiatric Features
Aminoacidurias			
	Hartnup Disease	Ataxia, wide-based gait[9]	intermittent psychosis[8]
	Maple Syrup Urine Disease (infant, children)	opisthotonos, "fencing," "bicycling"[137]	irritability, fussiness, ADHD[138]
	Maple Syrup Urine Disease (adult)	tremor, dystonia, parkinsonism[139]	anxiety, depression, panic disorder[138]
	Phenylketonuria (PKU)	parkinsonism[140]	anxiety, depression, panic disorder[141]
Creatine Metabolism Disorders			
	Guanidinoacetate Methyltransferase Deficiency (GAMT)	choreoathetosis, ataxia, dystonia[11–13]	autism, self-injury, aggression[11–13]
Lysosomal Storage Diseases			
	Gaucher	opisthotonus, trismus, spasticity[142]	depression, somatization[143]
	Krabbe Disease	spasticity, hypotonia[144]	ADHD, mood d/o, irritability[145]
	Metachromic Leukodystrophy	gait disturbance, spasticity[45]	emotional lability, psychosis[45]
	Neimann-Pick	ataxia, dystonia[17,24]	dementia, bipolar, schizophrenia[26,27]
	Neuronal Ceroid Lipofucionosis (AKA Batten Disease)	ataxia, myoclonus, parkinsonism[53]	depression, psychosis[49,50]
	Tay-Sach Disease, Sadhoff Disease (Adult Onset)	ataxia[146]	psychosis[146]
Mineral Metabolism Disorders			
	Neurodegeneration With Brain Iron Accumulation (NBIA)	gait abnormalities, progressive dystonia, dysarthria, tremor, rigidity, spasticity, chorea, motor tic disorders[85,87]	obsessive-compulsive disorder, speech anomalies, behavioral problems, vocal tic disorders[85,87]
	Wilson's Disease	chorea, dysarthria, parkinsonism, ataxia, cervical and oromandibular dystonia, tremor[70–77,82]	bipolar disorder, schizophrenia, psychosis, personality changes, frontal syndromes, early subcortical dementia[70,72–77,79–83]
Mitochondrial Diseases			
	Coenzyme Q10 Deficiency	ataxia, myoclonus[90,91]	intellectual delay, bipolar disorder, schizophrenia, psychosis[92,93]
	Leber Hereditary Optic Neuropathy (LHON)	parkinsonism, myoclonus, dystonia, spasticity, tremor[90,91]	mood disorder, circadian rhythm disorder[92,93]

Table 20.1 Continued

	Disorder	Movement Features	Psychiatric Features
	Leigh Syndrome	dystonia, spasticity, ataxia, myoclonus[90,91]	intellectual delay, cognitive regression[92,93]
	Kearns-Sayre Syndrome	cerebellar ataxia[90,91]	cognitive decline[92]
	Mitochondrial Encephalomyopathy, Lactic Acidosis, and Stroke-like Episodes (MELAS)	parkinsonism, myoclonus[90,91]	cognitive regression, bipolar disorder[92,93]
	Myoclonus Epilepsy with Ragged Red Fibers (MERRF)	cerebellar ataxia, myoclonus, parkinsonism[90,91]	cognitive decline[92]
Neurotransmitter Metabolism Disorders			
	Aromatic L-Amino Acid Decarboxylase Deficiency	athetosis, oculogyric crisis, dystonia[147,148]	irritability, agitation[147]
	GABA-Transaminase Deficiency	choreoathetosis, hypotonia[135,136]	autistic features, intellectual disability, mood and behavior fluctuations[135,136]
	Tyrosine Hydroxylase Deficiency	parkinsonism, dystonia[100]	ADHD, OCD, anxiety, depression[101]
Organic Acidemias			
	Glutaric Aciduria	dyskinesia, dystonia, choreoathetosis, opisthotonus and nystagmus[113,114]	episodes of irritability, dementia[113]
	Methylmalonic Acidemia	hypotonia, tremor, dystonia[149]	intellectual disability[150]
Purine Metabolism Disorders			
	Lesch-Nyhan Disease	dystonia (often oromandibular), ballismus, choreoathetosis, spasticity, opisthotonus[123–128]	mood disorder, self-mutilation, cognitive impairment[123,124,132]
	Adenosine Deaminase Deficiency	hypotonia (axial and appendicular), nystagmus[133]	intellectual delay, hyperactivity, attention deficits, aggressive behavior, social behavioral problems[134]

replacement. Patients can also exhibit episodes of emotional instability such as rapid mood changes, depression, confusion, anxiety, delusions, and/or hallucinations,[7,8] which improve with niacin replacement.[6] The initial presentation may also include a pellagra-like skin rash. This rash is scaly, red, worsens with exposure to sunlight and usually is found on the hands, arms, and face. This rash is also seen in dietary niacin deficiency, however the neutral amino acids will not be elevated in the urine if diet is the culprit.

The diagnosis relies on the clinical presentation and confirmation of aminoaciduria.[9] The cornerstone of management is prevention of symptomatic episodes by ensuring a high-protein diet and niacin replacement.[6] Acute flares of both psychiatric and movement symptoms can also be treated with nicotinamide.[6] The overall prognosis is favorable with proper treatment.

Creatine Metabolism Disorders

Guanidinoacetate Methyltransferase (GAMT) Deficiency

GAMT deficiency is an autosomal recessive cerebral creatine deficiency that primarily affects the nervous system and muscles. It occurs due to deficient activity of guanidinoacetate methyltransferase, an enzyme involved in the synthesis of creatine. The onset varies but is typically between early infancy (around 3 months) to age three. Onset after age 12 years is unusual but has been reported as late as 17 years.[10]

Symptom onset includes movement and behavioral issues along with mild to severe intellectual disability, developmental delay, and epilepsy.[11-13] Observed in about 30% of individuals, movement disorders can include chorea, athetosis, dystonia, or ataxia.[11-13] Behavioral disorders, present in about 77% of individuals, include hyperactivity, autism spectrum disorder, aggressive behavior, or self-injurious behavior.[11,12]

Diagnosis can be made based on elevated GAA (guanidinoacetate) in the urine and confirmatory genetic testing.[11] MRI with spectroscopy is useful for measuring creatine levels in the brain.[14] Treatment consists of dietary adjustments with oral creatine and ornithine and dietary restriction of arginine or protein.[13,15] The treatment can be effective if started early in life, improving developmental delay, seizures, and movement disorders in patients that are symptomatic.[11,13]

Lysosomal Storage Disorders

Neimann Pick Disease Type C

Neimann Pick disease type C (NPD-C) is an autosomal recessive lipid storage disorder characterized by impaired cellular processing of low density lipoprotein (LDL) and other macromolecules. It is caused by genetic mutations in either the *NPC1* or *NPC2* genes.[16] *NPC1* is located on chromosome 18q11-q12[17] and encodes a large membrane glycoprotein localized mostly to late endosomes and facilitates the trafficking, levels, and distribution of LDL-cholesterol.[18] *NPC2*, located on chromosome 14q24.3, encodes a small lysosomal protein (previously referred to as cholesterol-binding protein).[19] When either of these proteins do not function properly, unesterified cholesterol and glycolipids accumulate in the lysosomal and late endosomal systems leading to neuronal degeneration.[20]

The initial presentation of NPD-C varies based on age of onset. Fetal onset is usually associated with ultrasound findings of organomegaly, ascites, or fetal hydrops.[21] Neonatal onset typically presents with severe hepatic disease, prolonged jaundice, and respiratory failure secondary to alveolar proteinosis or similar disease.[22,23] Infants typically present with hypotonia and developmental delay with or without liver and lung involvement. The childhood and adult onset form of NPD-C typically presents with ataxia, dystonia, supranuclear vertical gaze palsy, cognitive impairment, and seizures as well as the symptoms mentioned above.[17,24] Up to 20% of children can have gelastic cataplexy.[25] Some adults may present with cognitive dysfunction or psychiatric conditions alone. The most common psychiatric presentations are dementia, depression, bipolar disease, or schizophrenia.[26,27] Often, adults will have had subtle signs in childhood including organomegaly, learning difficulties, deafness, or impaired vertical gaze.[16]

The first step in diagnosing NPD-C is considering the diagnosis. Wijburg et al. created a suspicion index tool which can be referenced for diagnostic assistance. They found that the clinical features most strongly associated with NPD-C were vertical supranuclear gaze palsy, gelastic cataplexy, isolated unexplained splenomegaly, prolonged neonatal jaundice or cholestasis, and premature cognitive decline or dementia. Gelastic cataplexy is highly specific but not sensitive for NPD-C, and is rare among adults. Premature cognitive decline or dementia is common in NPD-C but not highly specific.[28] Once clinical suspicion is established, the practitioner should screen with levels of oxysterols,[29] the preferred being cholestane triol,[30] and confirm with genetic testing.[29] If diagnosis remains uncertain, skin biopsy with fibroblast cell culture and filipin taining[31] or electron microscopy[24] can be obtained. Brain MRI shows reduced gray matter volume involving the thalamus, hippocampus, striatum, cerebellum, and insular cortex, as well as reduced white matter involving the corpus callosum and other areas.[16] No treatment exists for NPD-C that has been proven to modify the onset or neurologic progression of the disease, nor prolong life. Supportive care should be initiated and managed by various specialists. For the neurologist management of seizures, cataplexy, and dystonia is key. Patients should be referred to physical therapy to improve or maintain mobility, and swallowing should be evaluated periodically to prevent aspiration and ensure adequate nutrition. Miglustat, an investigational drug, inhibits the biosynthesis of glycosphingolipids and was found to decrease lipid storage, improve endosomal uptake, and normalize lipid trafficking in B lymphocytes.[32] However, it is unclear if miglustat reduces disease progression in NPD-C, and data are limited and conflicting.[33-41] Other experimental therapies including stem cell transplantation are ongoing in humans and mice.

Metachromatic Leukodystrophy

Metachromatic leukodystrophy (MLD), also referred to as arylsulfatase A deficiency, is an autosomal recessive neurometabolic disease. It is characterized by accumulation of sulfatides that lead to damage of the nervous system (brain and spinal cord) and myelin breakdown.[42] MLD is most commonly caused by mutations in the *ARSA* gene, located on chromosome 22q13.33, which encodes the enzyme that breaks down these sulfatides, Arylsulfatase A.

There are three clinical subtypes: late-infantile MLD, juvenile MLD, and adult MLD. Late-infantile MLD occurs before age 30 months and can present with weakness, hypotonia, clumsiness, frequent falls, toe walking, and dysarthria. The disease progresses with motor, speech, and developmental regression and symptoms include pain, spasticity, seizures, and vision and hearing impairments. In the final stages, individuals have general unawareness of their surroundings and have tonic spasms along with decerebrate posturing.[43] Juvenile MLD presents between age 30 months and 16 years with decline in school performance, behavioral problems, and gait disturbances,[43] and progression is similar to but slower than the late-infantile form.[44] Adult MLD occurs after age 16 years and sometimes not until the fourth or fifth decade. Individuals present with problems in school or job performance, personality changes, emotional lability, or psychosis. Neurologic symptoms including weakness and loss of coordination progressing to spasticity and seizures initially predominate in some late presentations.[45] Disease course is variable with periods of stability interspersed with periods of decline and may extend over two to three decades.[43] MRI shows evidence of a leukodystrophy with diffuse symmetric abnormalities of periventricular myelin. Initial parieto-occipital preponderance is observed in most individuals with late-infantile MLD, with subcortical U-fibers and cerebellar white matter spared.[43] The abnormal white matter is often described as having a tigroid pattern or radial stripes. As the disease progresses, MRI abnormalities become more pronounced in a rostral-to-caudal progression and cerebral atrophy develops.[46] Anterior lesions may be more common initially in individuals with later onset and not all individuals with MLD show white matter lesions initially.[43]

Diagnosis based on clinical presentation, imaging, increased urinary excretion of sulfatides and genetic testing. Hematopoietic stem cell transplantation (HSCT) is the only therapy for primary central nervous system manifestations and best results are achieved by early intervention prior to symptom onset.[43,47] Physical therapy and other supportive interventions with a multidisciplinary team helps to prevent decline and maximize mobility and quality of life.

Neuronal Ceroid Lipofuscinosis

Neuronal ceroid lipofuscinosis (NCL) is a heterogeneous group of progressive disorders presenting with movement disorders, dementia, vision loss, and epilepsy and due to storage of ceroid lipofuscin in neurons. However each disease has a distinct genotypic cause and phenotypic variation.[48] Only two of the NCL disorders (CLN1 and CLN3) have prominent psychiatric complaints outside of the dementia and developmental delay, which are common to all of them.[48–50] It is important to find a balance with the movement symptoms when treating the mood disturbances associated with these diseases. There are 14 derivatives of CLN, with type 9 questionably miscategorized and actually belonging with CLN5.[51] For the purposes of this chapter, we will focus on CLN1 and CLN3.

CLN1 disease is due to a mutation of the *CLN1* gene which encodes palmitoyl-protein thioesterase 1 (PPT1).[52] CLN1 is generally associated with infantile onset consisting of rapid developmental regression around six months to two years of age. The children also have the typical NCL disease components of seizures, ataxia, and visual loss in addition to myoclonus. Prognosis is poor with complete vision loss by age two and progression to severe spasticity and decreased level of consciousness prior to early demise.[53] There are later onset variations of the disease which both progress to shortened life span with the classic ataxia, visual loss, and epilepsy but with a more protracted course. These include the late infantile form which presents at age two to four years and the juvenile form which presents between age five and ten years.[54–56] A very rare adult onset form of CLN1 exists that presents with cognitive decline and depression with the movement symptoms including ataxia and parkinsonism along with visual loss presenting later.[49,50] Although all of these phenotypes are caused by mutation of the same gene, evidence supports that the amount of gene lost and the degree to which

PPT1 is diminished predict severity and onset of disease.[55,57] MRI demonstrates cerebellar atrophy and sometimes thalamic T2 hypointensity.[58-61]

CLN3 disease is caused by mutations of the *CLN3* gene, which encodes a lysosomal transmembrane protein of unknown function and is associated with juvenile-onset NCL. There is only one phenotype associated with this disease,[62,63] which typically presents at age 4–7 years. The presenting symptoms include the typical vision loss which progresses rapidly and children are typically functionally blind within the year. This is followed by the defining features of NCL including parkinsonism, dementia, and epilepsy. The psychiatrist should note that adolescents can develop behavioral problems,[64-66] psychosis, and hallucinations. Females tend to have more rapid decline.[64,67] Cerebellar atrophy may not be seen on MRI until much later in the disease course, but can also show T2 hypodensities similar to CLN1.[5-61] MRI can be normal into adolescence.[68] Genetic testing is the mainstay of diagnosis. Management is largely symptomatic. The movement disorders seen in NCL are often complex and medically refractory. It is important that the psychiatrist and neurologist work together as treating the psychiatric components can worsen the parkinsonism. Therapies can also be tried for developmental regression to slow loss of skills and muscle development. One must remember that the disease is progressive and prognosis is poor when counseling families.[69]

Mineral Metabolism

Wilson's Disease

Wilson's disease, also known as hepatolenticular degeneration, is an autosomal recessive condition that results from a mutation in the *ATP7B* gene. This gene encodes a liver protein that functions to transport copper across organelle membranes and bile canaliculi. In Wilson's disease, this process is defective and results in elevation of serum copper, which subsequently accumulates in many different organs. The most commonly affected organs include the liver, brain, and cornea. There is a wide spectrum of clinical heterogeneity depending on the level of copper accumulation in affected organ systems.

Though the presenting symptoms of Wilson's disease vary, the liver is always affected to some degree, as it is the first site of accumulation. In fact, cirrhosis is present at diagnosis in 35%–45% of patients. Children tend to present with hepatic manifestations such as jaundice, abdominal pain, or abnormal labs. Teens and adults are more likely to present with neurologic symptoms, with chorea as the presenting feature in 20% of young teens.[70,71] Common neurologic symptoms include dysarthria and parkinsonism. Less commonly, cerebellar/gait ataxia, cervical and oromandibular dystonia, choreoathetosis, autonomic dysfunction, seizures, and cognitive impairment are also seen. Patients can develop intention tremors, atypical essential tremors, and a postural tremor that is often described as "wing-beating."[71-74] As this is a systemic disorder, many other pathologies can occur such as Fanconi syndrome, nephrolithiasis, arthropathy, cardiomyopathy, pancreatitis, and an array of skin conditions.[70,74-77] Ocular copper deposition can give the appearance of a brown ring around the peripheral cornea. These Kayser-Fleischer rings are present in almost all patients with Wilson's disease that have neurologic symptoms and in about half of patients with only hepatic disease. MRI of the brain often demonstrates T2 hyperintensities of the basal ganglia, tectum, thalamus, and brainstem.[78] Patients often have psychological and behavioral disturbances including irritability, personality changes (sometimes even personality disorders), major depression, bipolar disorder, and sometimes psychosis. Cognitive decline can occur and patients can develop frontal syndromes with symptoms of impulsivity, sexual promiscuity, poor executive dysfunction, and judgment impairment. Over time, patients can develop signs of subcortical dementia such as memory loss or slowed thought processing. Importantly, diagnosis is often delayed in teenage patients with psychiatric manifestations of Wilson disease as their symptoms get attributed to puberty and psychosocial factors.[77, 79–83]

Diagnosis can be made by various methods, often in combination, such as measuring serum ceruloplasmin concentration, serum and urine copper concentration, obtaining a liver biopsy to determine hepatic copper concentration, or by targeted genetic testing.[70,72,74,75] Treatment aims to either reduce copper absorption with interfering agents such as zinc or to bind and eliminate copper with chelating agents such as penicillamine or trientene. In cases of acute liver failure, severe progressive liver disease, or failed drug therapy, patients often need liver transplant. Without any treatment, Wilson disease is invariably fatal as the patients develop worsening cirrhosis and neurologic deterioration. Otherwise, with treatment adherence patients have an excellent prognosis.[70,84]

Neurodegeneration with Brain Iron Accumulation

Neurodegeneration with brain iron accumulation (NBIA) is a spectrum of disorders characterized by accumulation of iron in the central nervous system due to varying dysfunctional mechanisms of metabolic regulation. There are many subtypes of NBIA, the most common of which is pantothenate kinase-associated neurodegeneration (PKAN), which accounts for 50% of cases[85] and will be discussed here.

NBIA can present at any age although most present in childhood. Classically, PKAN presents within the first 10 years of life with severe symptoms and rapid progression to disability. Atypically, symptoms present in young adults in which case the course is often less severe.[86] Clinically, patients with PKAN present with gait abnormalities, psychomotor delay, and difficulty with fine motor skills. Many neurologic symptoms can develop such as progressive dystonia, dysarthria, tremor, rigidity, spasticity, and chorea. Classically, patients with PKAN can also develop disorders with psychiatric overlap such as behavioral problems, tics (both motor and vocal), obsessive-compulsive disorder, and speech anomalies such as palilalia, which is characterized by involuntary repetition of words and phrases. In NBIA in general, cognition remains relatively intact but patients with certain subtypes can cognitively decline over time.[1] The spectrum of brain iron accumulation can be seen within the globus pallidus and substantia nigra of the basal ganglia. Radiographically, this is demonstrated by T2 hypointensity of the bilateral globus pallidi on MRIs of the brain.[87] An interesting radiologic difference seen on brain MRI in PKAN is the addition of bilateral T2 hyperintensities within the aforementioned hypointense region of the globus pallidi, demonstrating the so-called "eye-of-the-tiger sign."[88]

Diagnosis depends on the subtype of NBIA but typically involves a combination of clinical and radiologic findings as well as genetic testing. In most cases of NBIA, treatment is driven by the specific or most distressing symptoms. Anticholinergics, baclofen, dopaminergics, and tetrabenazine have been used with some benefit as have surgical interventions such as deep brain stimulation of the globus pallidus internus, specific lesioning, and even pallidotomy. None of these pharmacologic or surgical treatments has changed the course of the disease,[89] and the progressive nature of the disease should be considered when counseling families.

Mitochondrial Diseases

The mitochondrial respiratory chain functions to support many physiologic metabolic processes at the most basic level—adenosine triphosphate (ATP), or energy, production; thus, dysfunction at any point in this complex process can lead to disease. The vast spectrum of mitochondrial diseases contains many subtypes. Examples include, but are certainly not limited to, mitochondrial encephalomyopathy, lactic acidosis, and stroke-like episodes (MELAS), Leber's hereditary optic neuropathy (LHON), coenzyme Q10 deficiency, and Leigh syndrome. Symptoms can present at any age and there is often striking phenotypic heterogeneity, even in patients with the same genetic mutation.

Mitochondrial diseases are often multisystemic with varying levels of severity. Generally, organ systems that require high amounts of energy, such as the brain and muscle, are more severely affected. The brain uses a disproportionate amount of oxygen and glucose to properly function. When in states of stress, more resources are needed to keep up with higher demand. In mitochondrial diseases, capacity to meet these higher demands is limited and can result in end-organ damage, especially in high energy-consuming organs. The basal ganglia, cerebellum, and brainstem commonly suffer repeated damage, and this typically manifests with movement disorders. Myoclonus and ataxia are the most frequent movement abnormalities in patients with mitochondrial diseases; however, chorea, dystonia, restless legs, parkinsonism, tremor, tics, and spasticity are also well-documented occurrences.[90,91] Neuropsychiatric disorders in mitochondrial disease include schizophrenia, major depression, and bipolar disorder. [92,93]

The diagnosis of mitochondrial diseases is a complex topic and is beyond the scope of this text. Generally, treatment for mitochondrial diseases is supportive and preventative. This includes supplying glucose and nutrients during times of crisis, such as a febrile illness, in order to help the body meet the higher demand for resources. Treatments for both movement and psychiatric disorders are symptomatic and, with the exception of avoidance of valproic acid in depletion syndromes, follow the same treatment algorithms as used for other conditions.[94]

Neurotransmitter Disorders

Tyrosine Hydroxylase Deficiency

Tyrosine hydroxylase (TH) deficiency, also known as autosomal recessive dopa-responsive dystonia and tyrosine hydroxylase-deficiency dopa-responsive dystonia, is a rare autosomal recessively inherited condition due to diminished activity of the enzyme tyrosine hydroxylase.[95] The gene coding for TH is located on chromosome 11p15.5[96] and converts TH to dopamine, a neurotransmitter critical to neurologic function.[95]

There are two recognized subtypes of TH deficiency. The first presents in infancy as an infantile Parkinsonism (type A),[97-99] and the second presents as a more severe complex encephalopathy in neonates (type B).[95] To the neurologist, patients will often present with abnormal gait ranging from children who walk on their toes to frank ataxia, dystonia that typically affects the legs, and autonomic dysfunction. Other neurologic complaints include postural tremor, spasticity, and abnormal eye movements. These abnormal eye movements can consist of brief episodes of up gaze to full oculogyric crises in which the eyes are locked in upward gaze for hours. Infantile parkinsonism is similar to parkinsonism seen in adults consisting of tremors, bradykinesia, and postural instability.[100,101] Of note, lack of sleep and prolonged exercise can worsen motor symptoms, while rest and sleep improve them.[102,103] To the psychiatrist, a child may present with attention deficit hyperactivity disorder, impulsivity, anxiety, depression, and obsessive-compulsive disorder.[103] More severely affected individuals will have developmental disabilities and learning delays.[101]

The diagnosis of TH deficiency is supported by low levels of CSF dopamine metabolite levels, especially homovanillic acid,[104] and confirmed with genetic testing.[105,106] Treatment strategies are aimed at normalizing dopamine levels in the brain. L-dopa crosses the blood-brain barrier to the central nervous system, where it is metabolized to the active form, dopamine. However it can also be metabolized to dopamine systemically, which cannot cross the blood-brain barrier, and thus can't act on the CNS. Carbidopa can be added to decrease systemic metabolism of L-dopa. The response to L-dopa varies from rapid complete reversal of symptoms to a slower effect with overall improvement but incomplete resolution of motor symptoms. Overall, most patients have a favorable motor outcome and prognosis when treated with L-dopa.[100,107,108] Investigation into other therapies also continues. Selegiline, an MAO-B inhibitor that slows the breakdown of dopamine, has shown some promise.[95,102,109–111] Anticholinergic drugs including amantadine have also been used to increase L-dopa and carbidopa effectiveness.[112] Additionally supportive care with physical and speech therapy should be pursued as needed.

Organic Acidurias

Glutaric Aciduria Type 1

Glutaric aciduria type 1 is an autosomal recessive disorder of the *GCDH* gene, which encodes for glutaryl-CoA dehydrogenase, a mitochondrial enzyme that metabolizes lysine. GCDH deficiency leads to increased concentrations of potentially neurotoxic metabolites, glutaric acid (GA), 3-hydroxy glutaric acid (3-OH-GA), and glutaconic acid within body tissues.

Most newborns are asymptomatic and present following their first encephalopathic crisis, which leads to irreversible damage in the brain. The phenotypic spectrum ranges from the infantile-onset disease to the later-onset disease (after age 6 years). In the infantile-onset disease, patients present with irritability, lack of energy/sleepy, poor appetite/difficulty feeding, jitteriness, vomiting, diarrhea, hypotonia, and macrocephaly.[113] Without treatment, most affected children develop an acute encephalopathic crisis following febrile illness episodes or other catabolic conditions resulting in bilateral striatal injury and subsequent movement disorders including dyskinesia, dystonia, choreoathetosis, opisthotonus and nystagmus.[113,114] For the psychiatrist, it is important to note the acute episodes of irritability are caused by the encephalopathic crisis. Some individuals can also have cognitive impairment and developmental regression, but these are usually mild. Untreated late-onset forms may manifest as nonspecific neurologic abnormalities including headaches, vertigo, ataxia, and dementia.[113] Brain MRI findings based on a study of 18 Dutch individuals ages 11 months to 33 years with GA-1 (most of whom were diagnosed prior to universal GA-1 NBS) included the following:[115] Open opercula, widening of CSF spaces/ventriculomegaly, attenuated signal from basal ganglia, white matter abnormalities, subdural hemorrhage, probably due to stretching of bridging veins in the enlarged extra-axial fluid spaces, subdural hemorrhage is typically associated with frontotemporal hypoplasia.[113,115]

Newborn screening (NBS) which measures glutarylcarnitine (C5DC) in dried blood spots and has shown to have 96% sensitivity helps diagnose individuals early on prior to a crisis.[116-119] Individuals can also have significantly elevated concentrations of glutaric acid, 3-hydroxyglutaric acid, glutarylcarnitine (C5DC), and glutaconic acid.[117,118,120,121] In addition, genetic testing is available.[119] The goal of treatment is to reduce lysine oxidation and enhance physiologic detoxification of glutaryl-CoA.[122] Combined therapy includes low-lysine diet with carnitine supplementation. Emergency treatment during episodes relies on averting catabolism and minimizing CNS exposure to lysine and its toxic metabolic byproducts.[113] Avoidance of encephalopathic crisis improves prognosis.

Purine Metabolism Disorders

Lesch-Nyhan Disease

Lesch-Nyhan disease (LND) is an X-linked recessive condition that results from a mutation in the *HPRT1* gene. This gene codes for the enzyme hypoxanthine-guanine phosphoribosyltransferase (HPRT), which functions within the purine metabolism cycle. Purines, along with pyrimidines, serve as building blocks for DNA and RNA. Normally, nucleic acids are broken down and their components are recycled to be used again. When HPRT is absent or scarce, this recycling process cannot occur and results in elevated serum uric acid levels which precipitate in the joints, kidneys, and brain. This leads to gout, kidney stones, and neuropsychiatric abnormalities, respectively.[123-125]

Most patients present around 3–6 months of age with motor delay due to hypotonia. Involuntary movements are typically noticed within the first year of life as well. The motor disease tends to progress over the first several years of life but often stagnates after age 5–6 years. To the neurologist, the most predominant symptom is dystonia and the oromandibular dystonia that occurs in these cases has been likened to that of tardive syndromes due to chronic dopamine antagonist use.[126-128] Additionally, patients with LND can develop ballismus, choreoathetosis, spasticity, opisthotonus, and cognitive impairment. To the psychiatrist, these patients are most likely to present for self-mutilation behavior such as head banging and biting. Neuroimaging typically shows cerebral atrophy without specific structural abnormalities. However, PET scans and biochemical studies have demonstrated loss of dopaminergic fibers and reduced levels of dopamine in the basal ganglia. The mechanism by which HPRT dysfunction disrupts brain activity is not currently clear.[126,129]

Diagnosis rests on genetic testing, however (HPRT) enzyme activity less than 1.5% of normal in cells from any tissue (e.g., blood, cultured fibroblasts, lymphoblasts) is also diagnostic.[125,127,130,131] Treatment for LND is largely symptomatic. Allopurinol is used to control uric acid levels. Muscle relaxants such as baclofen and dantrolene are used to reduce tone, as are benzodiazepines which can also help with mood lability. Dopamine antagonists such as risperidone or olanzapine can be used to help control self-injurious behavior. Paroxetine, carbamazepine, clomipramine, sertraline, and gabapentin have been used for mood stabilization or treatment for depression in these cases as well. Unfortunately, treatment does not change the course of disease and patients often succumb to renal failure within the first decade or two of life.[125,127,132]

Conclusion

Neurometabolic disorders can present at nearly any point in life with variable signs and symptoms that can often go unnoticed at first. Those with inborn or congenital etiologies often present earlier in life as detailed in the preceding account. Notably, some conditions with the same etiology can have different clinical features depending on the age of presentation as is the case in Wilson's disease, where children tend to present with hepatic features such as jaundice or abdominal pain while teenagers and adults often present with neurologic features such as chorea or parkinsonism. In many cases of neurometabolic disease, the initial signs and symptoms can be subtle or may be primarily cognitive in nature and attributed to an underlying psychiatric disorder. This can lead to delays in diagnosis and treatment, where available, and further progression of the neurodegenerative disease.

References

1. Kleta, R., Romeo, E., Ristic, Z., Ohura, T., Stuart, C., Arcos-Burgos, M., . . . Koizumi, A. (2004). Mutations in SLC6A19, encoding B0AT1, cause Hartnup disorder. *Nat Gen*, *36*(9), 999–1002. https://doi.org/10.1038/ng1405

2. Bröer, S. (2009). The role of the neutral amino acid transporter B0AT1 (SLC6A19) in Hartnup disorder and protein nutrition. *IUBMB life*, *61*(6), 591–599. https://doi.org/10.1002/iub.210

3. Scriver, C. R. (1965). Hartnup disease: a genetic modification of intestinal and renal transport of certain neutral alpha-amino acids. *N Engl J Med*, *273*, 530–532. https://doi.org/10.1056/NEJM196509022731005

4. Nozaki, J., Dakeishi, M., Ohura, T., Inoue, K., Manabe, M., Wada, Y., & Koizumi, A. (2001). Homozygosity mapping to chromosome 5p15 of a gene responsible for Hartnup disorder. Biochem Biophys Res Commun., *284*(2), 255–260. https://doi.org/10.1006/bbrc.2001.4961

5. Shih, V. E., Bixby, E. M., Alpers, D. H., Bartoscas, C. S., & Thier, S. O. (1971). Studies of intestinal transport defect in Hartnup disease. *Gastroenterol*, *61*(4), 445–453.

6. Milne, M. D., Crawford, M. A., Girao, C. B., & Loughridge, L. W. (1960). The metabolic disorder in Hartnup disease. *Q J Med*, *29*, 407–421.

7. Navab, F., & Asatoor, A. M. (1970). Studies on intestinal absorption of amino acids and a dipeptide in a case of Hartnup disease. *Gut*, *11*(5), 373–379. https://doi.org/10.1136/gut.11.5.373

8. Hersov, L. A., & Rodnight, R. (1960). Hartnup disease in psychiatric practice: clinical and biochemical features of three cases. *J Neurol Neurosurgery Psychiatry*, *23*(1), 40–45. https://doi.org/10.1136/jnnp.23.1.40

9. Baron, D. N., Dent, C. E., Harris, H., Hart, E. W., & Jepson, J. B. (1956). Hereditary pellagra-like skin rash with temporary cerebellar ataxia, constant renal amino-aciduria, and other bizarre biochemical features. *Lancet, 271*(6940), 421–428. https://doi.org/10.1016/s0140-6736(56)91914-6

10. O'Rourke, D. J., Ryan, S., Salomons, G., Jakobs, C., Monavari, A., & King, M. D. (2009). Guanidinoacetate methyltransferase (GAMT) deficiency: late onset of movement disorder and preserved expressive language. *Dev Med Child Neurol, 51*, 404–407.

11. Mercimek-Mahmutoglu, S., Stoeckler-Ipsiroglu, S., Adami, A., Appleton, R., Araujo, H. C., Duran, M., & Jakobs, C. (2006). GAMT deficiency: features, treatment, and outcome in an inborn error of creatine synthesis. *Neurology, 67*, 480–484.

12. Mercimek-Mahmutoglu, S., Ndika, J., Kanhai, W., de Villemeur, T. B., Cheillan, D., Christensen, E., . . . Salomons, G. S. (2014). Thirteen new patients with guanidinoacetate methyltransferase deficiency and functional characterization of nineteen novel missense variants in the GAMT gene. *Hum Mutat, 35*, 462–469.

13. Stockler-Ipsiroglu, S., van Karnebeek, C., Longo, N., Korenke, G. C., Mercimek-Mahmutoglu, S., Marquart, I., . . . Schulze, A. (2014). Guanidinoacetate methyltransferase (GAMT) deficiency: outcomes in 48 individuals and recommendations for diagnosis, treatment and monitoring. *Mol Genet Metab, 111*, 16–25.

14. Stöckler, S., Isbrandt, D., Hanefeld, F., Schmidt, B., & von Figura, K. (1996). Guanidinoacetate methyltransferase deficiency: the first inborn error of creatine metabolism in man. *Am J Hum Genet, 58*, 914–922.

15. Schulze, A., Ebinger, F., Rating, D., & Mayatepek, E. (2001). Improving treatment of guanidinoacetate methyltransferase deficiency: reduction of guanidinoacetic acid in body fluids by arginine restriction and ornithine supplementation. *Mol Genet Metab, 74*, 413–419.

16. Vanier, M. T. (2010). Niemann-Pick disease type C. *Orphanet J Rare Dis, 5*, 16. https://doi.org/10.1186/1750-1172-5-16

17. Vanier, M. T., Duthel, S., Rodriguez-Lafrasse, C., Pentchev, P., & Carstea, E. D. (1996). Genetic heterogeneity in Niemann-Pick C disease: a study using somatic cell hybridization and linkage analysis. *Am J Human Genet, 58*(1), 118–125.

18. Morris, J. A., Zhang, D., Coleman, K. G., Nagle, J., Pentchev, P. G., & Carstea, E. D. (1999). The genomic organization and polymorphism analysis of the human Niemann-Pick C1 gene. *Biochem Biophys Res Commun , 261*(2), 493–498. https://doi.org/10.1006/bbrc.1999.1070

19. Naureckiene, S., Sleat, D. E., Lackland, H., Fensom, A., Vanier, M. T., Wattiaux, R., Jadot, M., & Lobel, P. (2000). Identification of HE1 as the second gene of Niemann-Pick C disease. *Science, 290*(5500), 2298–2301. https://doi.org/10.1126/science.290.5500.2298

20. Cruz, J. C., Sugii, S., Yu, C., & Chang, T. Y. (2000). Role of Niemann-Pick type C1 protein in intracellular trafficking of low density lipoprotein-derived cholesterol. *J Biol Chem, 275*(6), 4013–4021. https://doi.org/10.1074/jbc.275.6.4013

21. Kelly, D. A., Portmann, B., Mowat, A. P., Sherlock, S., & Lake, B. D. (1993). Niemann-Pick disease type C: diagnosis and outcome in children, with particular reference to liver disease. *J Pediatr, 123*(2), 242–247. https://doi.org/10.1016/s0022-3476(05)81695-6

22. Bjurulf, B., Spetalen, S., Erichsen, A., Vanier, M. T., Strøm, E. H., & Strømme, P. (2008). Niemann-Pick disease type C2 presenting as fatal pulmonary alveolar lipoproteinosis: morphological findings in lung and nervous tissue. *Med Sci Monit, 14*(8), CS71–CS75.

23. Griese, M., Brasch, F., Aldana, V. R., Cabrera, M. M., Goelnitz, U., Ikonen, E., . . . Lezana, F. J. (2010). Respiratory disease in Niemann-Pick type C2 is caused by pulmonary alveolar proteinosis. *Clin Genet*, 77(2), 119–130. https://doi.org/10.1111/j.1399-0004.2009.01325.x

24. Vanier, M. T., Wenger, D. A., Comly, M. E., Rousson, R., Brady, R. O., & Pentchev, P. G. (1988). Niemann-Pick disease group C: clinical variability and diagnosis based on defective cholesterol esterification; a collaborative study on 70 patients. *Clin Genet*, 33(5), 331–348. https://doi.org/10.1111/j.1399-0004.1988.tb03460.x

25. Kandt, R. S., Emerson, R. G., Singer, H. S., Valle, D. L., & Moser, H. W. (1982). Cataplexy in variant forms of Niemann-Pick disease. *Ann Neurol*, 12(3), 284–288. https://doi.org/10.1002/ana.410120313

26. Sullivan, D., Walterfang, M., & Velakoulis, D. (2005). Bipolar disorder and Niemann-Pick disease type C. *Am J Psychiatry*, 162(5), 1021–1022. https://doi.org/10.1176/appi.ajp.162.5.1021-a

27. Josephs, K. A., Van Gerpen, M. W., & Van Gerpen, J. A. (2003). Adult onset Niemann-Pick disease type C presenting with psychosis. *J Neurol Neurosurgery Psychiatry*, 74(4), 528–529. https://doi.org/10.1136/jnnp.74.4.528

28. Wijburg, F. A., Sedel, F., Pineda, M., Hendriksz, C. J., Fahey, M. C., Walterfang, M., Patterson, M.C., Wraith, J.E., & Kolb, S. (2012). Development of a suspicion index to aid diagnosis of Niemann-Pick disease type C. *Neurology*, 78, 1560–1567.

29. Patterson, M. C., Hendriksz, C. J., Walterfang, M., Sedel, F., Vanier, M. T., Wijburg, F., & NP-C Guidelines Working Group (2012). Recommendations for the diagnosis and management of Niemann-Pick disease type C: an update. *Mol Genet Metab*, 106(3), 330–344. https://doi.org/10.1016/j.ymgme.2012.03.012

30. Giese, A. K., Mascher, H., Grittner, U., Eichler, S., Kramp, G., Lukas, J., . . . Rolfs, A. (2015). A novel, highly sensitive and specific biomarker for Niemann-Pick type C1 disease. *Orphanet J Rare Dis*, 10, 78. https://doi.org/10.1186/s13023-015-0274-1

31. Pentchev, P. G., Comly, M. E., Kruth, H. S., Vanier, M. T., Wenger, D. A., Patel, S., & Brady, R. O. (1985). A defect in cholesterol esterification in Niemann-Pick disease (type C) patients. *Proc Natl Acad Sci USA*, 82(23), 8247–8251. https://doi.org/10.1073/pnas.82.23.8247

32. Lachmann, R. H., te Vruchte, D., Lloyd-Evans, E., Reinkensmeier, G., Sillence, D. J., Fernandez-Guillen, L., . . . Platt, F. M. (2004). Treatment with miglustat reverses the lipid-trafficking defect in Niemann-Pick disease type C. *Neurobiol Dis*, 16(3), 654–658. https://doi.org/10.1016/j.nbd.2004.05.002

33. Pineda, M., Wraith, J. E., Mengel, E., Sedel, F., Hwu, W. L., Rohrbach, M., . . . Patterson, M. C. (2009). Miglustat in patients with Niemann-Pick disease Type C (NP-C): a multicenter observational retrospective cohort study. *Mol Genet Metab*, 98(3), 243–249. https://doi.org/10.1016/j.ymgme.2009.07.003

34. Wraith, J. E., & Imrie, J. (2009). New therapies in the management of Niemann-Pick type C disease: clinical utility of miglustat. *Ther Clin Risk Manag*, 5, 877–887. https://doi.org/10.2147/tcrm.s5777

35. Patterson, M. C., Vecchio, D., Jacklin, E., Abel, L., Chadha-Boreham, H., Luzy, C., Giorgino, R., & Wraith, J. E. (2010). Long-term miglustat therapy in children with Niemann-Pick disease type C. *J Child Neurol*, 25(3), 300–305. https://doi.org/10.1177/0883073809344222

36. Pineda, M., Perez-Poyato, M. S., O'Callaghan, M., Vilaseca, M. A., Pocovi, M., Domingo, R., . . . Coll, M. J. (2010). Clinical experience with miglustat therapy in pediatric patients with

Niemann-Pick disease type C: a case series. *Mol Genet Metab*, *99*(4), 358–366. https://doi.org/
10.1016/j.ymgme.2009.11.007

37. Wraith, J. E., Vecchio, D., Jacklin, E., Abel, L., Chadha-Boreham, H., Luzy, C., Giorgino, R., &
Patterson, M. C. (2010). Miglustat in adult and juvenile patients with Niemann-Pick disease
type C: long-term data from a clinical trial. *Mol Genet Metab*, *99*(4), 351–357. https://doi.org/
10.1016/j.ymgme.2009.12.006

38. Fecarotta, S., Amitrano, M., Romano, A., Della Casa, R., Bruschini, D., Astarita, L., . . . Andria,
G. (2011). The videofluoroscopic swallowing study shows a sustained improvement of dys-
phagia in children with Niemann-Pick disease type C after therapy with miglustat. *Am J Med
Genet A*, *155A*(3), 540–547. https://doi.org/10.1002/ajmg.a.33847

39. Usui, M., Miyauchi, A., Nakano, Y., Nakamura, S., Jimbo, E., Itamura, S., . . . Osaka, H. (2017).
Miglustat therapy in a case of early-infantile Niemann-Pick type C. *Brain Dev*, *39*(10), 886–
890. https://doi.org/10.1016/j.braindev.2017.05.006

40. Héron, B., Valayannopoulos, V., Baruteau, J., Chabrol, B., Ogier, H., Latour, P., . . . Vanier, M.
T. (2012). Miglustat therapy in the French cohort of paediatric patients with Niemann-Pick
disease type C. *Orphanet J Rare Dis*, *7*, 36. https://doi.org/10.1186/1750-1172-7-36

41. Chien, Y. H., Peng, S. F., Yang, C. C., Lee, N. C., Tsai, L. K., Huang, A. C., . . . Hwu, W. L. (2013).
Long-term efficacy of miglustat in paediatric patients with Niemann-Pick disease type C. *J
Inherit Metab Dis*, *36*(1), 129–137. https://doi.org/10.1007/s10545-012-9479-9

42. Von Figura, K., Gieselmann, V., & Jacken, J. (2001). Metachromatic leukodystrophy.
In: Scriver, C. R., Beaudet, A. L., Sly, W. S., & Valle, D., eds. *The Metabolic and Molecular Bases
of Inherited Disease* (pp. 3695–724). New York, NY: McGraw-Hill.

43. Gomez-Ospina N. (2006 May 30). Arylsulfatase A deficiency. [Updated 2020 Apr 30]. In: Adam,
M. P., Ardinger, H. H., Pagon, R. A., et al., eds. *GeneReviews® [Internet]*. Seattle: University of
Washington; 1993–2020. https://www.ncbi.nlm.nih.gov/books/NBK1130/

44. Kehrer, C., Blumenstock, G., Gieselmann, V., Krägeloh-Mann, I., et al. (2011a). The natural
course of gross motor deterioration in metachromatic leukodystrophy. *Dev med child neurol*,
53, 850–855.

45. Mahmood, A., Berry, J., Wenger, D. A., Escolar, M., Sobeih, M., Raymond, G., & Eichler, F. S.
(2010). Metachromatic leukodystrophy: a case of triplets with the late infantile variant and a
systematic review of the literature. *J child neurol*, *25*, 572–580.

46. Groeschel, S., Kehrer, C., Engel, C. I., Dali, C., Bley, A., Steinfeld, R., . . . Krägeloh-Mann, I.
(2011). Metachromatic leukodystrophy: natural course of cerebral MRI changes in relation to
clinical course. *J inherit metab dis*, *34*, 1095–102.

47. Boelens, J. J., & van Hasselt, P. M. (2016). Neurodevelopmental outcome after hematopoietic
cell transplantation in inborn errors of metabolism: current considerations and future perspectives. *Neuropediatrics*, *47*, 285–292.

48. Mole, S., Williams, R., & Goebel, H. (2011). Chapter 2 NCL Nomenclature and classification.
In: Sara Mole, Ruth Williams, Hans Goebel, eds. *The Neuronal Ceroid Lipofuscinoses (Batten
Disease)* (2nd ed., p. 20). Oxford: Oxford University Press.

49. Ramadan, H., Al-Din, A. S., Ismail, A., Balen, F., Varma, A., Twomey, A., . . . Mole, S.
E. (2007). Adult neuronal ceroid lipofuscinosis caused by deficiency in palmitoyl protein thioesterase 1. *Neurology*, *68*(5), 387–388. https://doi.org/10.1212/01.wnl.0000252
825.85947.2f

50. van Diggelen, O. P., Thobois, S., Tilikete, C., Zabot, M. T., Keulemans, J. L., van Bunderen,
P. A., . . . Voznyi, Y. V. (2001). Adult neuronal ceroid lipofuscinosis with palmitoyl-protein

thioesterase deficiency: first adult-onset patients of a childhood disease. *Ann Neuro*, *50*(2), 269–272. https://doi.org/10.1002/ana.1103

51. Haddad, S. E., Khoury, M., Daoud, M., Kantar, R., Harati, H., Mousallem, T., . . . Boustany, R. M. (2012). CLN5 and CLN8 protein association with ceramide synthase: biochemical and proteomic approaches. *Electrophoresis*, *33*(24), 3798–3809. https://doi.org/10.1002/elps.201200472

52. Vesa, J., Hellsten, E., Verkruyse, L. A., Camp, L. A., Rapola, J., Santavuori, P., . . . Peltonen, L. (1995). Mutations in the palmitoyl protein thioesterase gene causing infantile neuronal ceroid lipofuscinosis. *Nature*, *376*(6541), 584–587. https://doi.org/10.1038/376584a0

53. Santavuori, P., Haltia, M., & Rapola, J. (1974). Infantile type of so-called neuronal ceroid-lipofuscinosis. *Dev Med Child Neurol*, *16*(5), 644–653. https://doi.org/10.1111/j.1469-8749.1974.tb04183.x

54. Becker, K., Goebel, H. H., Svennerholm, L., Wendel, U., & Bremer, H. J. (1979). Clinical, morphological, and biochemical investigations on a patient with an unusual form of neuronal ceroid-lipofuscinosis. *Eur J Pediatr*, *132*(3), 197–206. https://doi.org/10.1007/BF00442436

55. Das, A. K., Becerra, C. H., Yi, W., Lu, J. Y., Siakotos, A. N., Wisniewski, K. E., & Hofmann, S. L. (1998). Molecular genetics of palmitoyl-protein thioesterase deficiency in the U.S. *J Clin Invest*, *102*(2), 361–370. https://doi.org/10.1172/JCI3112

56. Wisniewski, K. E., Connell, F., Kaczmarski, W., Kaczmarski, A., Siakotos, A., Becerra, C. R., & Hofmann, S. L. (1998). Palmitoyl-protein thioesterase deficiency in a novel granular variant of LINCL. *Pediatr Neurol*, *18*(2), 119–123. https://doi.org/10.1016/s0887-8994(97)00173-2

57. Das, A. K., Lu, J. Y., & Hofmann, S. L. (2001). Biochemical analysis of mutations in palmitoyl-protein thioesterase causing infantile and late-onset forms of neuronal ceroid lipofuscinosis. *Hum Mol Genet*, *10*(13), 1431–1439. https://doi.org/10.1093/hmg/10.13.1431

58. Jadav, R. H., Sinha, S., Yasha, T. C., Aravinda, H., Gayathri, N., Rao, S., . . . Satishchandra, P. (2014). Clinical, electrophysiological, imaging, and ultrastructural description in 68 patients with neuronal ceroid lipofuscinoses and its subtypes. *Pediatr Neurol*, *50*(1), 85–95. https://doi.org/10.1016/j.pediatrneurol.2013.08.008

59. Vanhanen, S. L., Puranen, J., Autti, T., Raininko, R., Liewendahl, K., Nikkinen, P., . . . Häkkinen, A. M. (2004). Neuroradiological findings (MRS, MRI, SPECT) in infantile neuronal ceroid-lipofuscinosis (infantile CLN1) at different stages of the disease. *Neuropediatrics*, *35*(1), 27–35. https://doi.org/10.1055/s-2004-815788

60. Baker, E. H., Levin, S. W., Zhang, Z., & Mukherjee, A. B. (2017). MRI brain volume measurements in infantile neuronal ceroid lipofuscinosis. *Am J Neuroradiol*, *38*(2), 376–382. https://doi.org/10.3174/ajnr.A4978

61. Autti, T., Joensuu, R., & Aberg, L. (2007). Decreased T2 signal in the thalami may be a sign of lysosomal storage disease. *Neuroradiol*, *49*(7), 571–578. https://doi.org/10.1007/s00234-007-0220-6

62. Adams, H. R., Beck, C. A., Levy, E., Jordan, R., Kwon, J. M., Marshall, F. J., . . . Mink, J. W. (2010). Genotype does not predict severity of behavioural phenotype in juvenile neuronal ceroid lipofuscinosis (Batten disease). *Dev Med Child Neurol*, *52*(7), 637–643. https://doi.org/10.1111/j.1469-8749.2010.03628.x

63. Kwon, J. M., Adams, H., Rothberg, P. G., Augustine, E. F., Marshall, F. J., Deblieck, E. A., . . . Mink, J. W. (2011). Quantifying physical decline in juvenile neuronal ceroid lipofuscinosis (Batten disease). *Neurology*, *77*(20), 1801–1807. https://doi.org/10.1212/WNL.0b013e318237f649

64. Cialone, J., Adams, H., Augustine, E. F., Marshall, F. J., Kwon, J. M., Newhouse, N., . . . Mink, J. W. (2012). Females experience a more severe disease course in Batten disease. *J Inherit Metab Dis*, *35*(3), 549–555. https://doi.org/10.1007/s10545-011-9421-6

65. Marshall, F. J., de Blieck, E. A., Mink, J. W., Dure, L., Adams, H., Messing, S., . . . Pearce, D. A. (2005). A clinical rating scale for Batten disease: reliable and relevant for clinical trials. *Neurology*, *65*(2), 275–279. https://doi.org/10.1212/01.wnl.0000169019.41332.8a

66. Kuper, W., van Alfen, C., Rigterink, R. H., Fuchs, S. A., van Genderen, M. M., & van Hasselt, P. M. (2018). Timing of cognitive decline in CLN3 disease. *J Inherit Metab Dis*, *41*(2), 257–261. https://doi.org/10.1007/s10545-018-0143-x

67. Nielsen, A. K., & Østergaard, J. R. (2013). Do females with juvenile ceroid lipofuscinosis (Batten disease) have a more severe disease course? The Danish experience. *Eur J Paediatr Neurol*, *17*(3), 265–268. https://doi.org/10.1016/j.ejpn.2012.10.011

68. Autti, T., Raininko, R., Vanhanen, S. L., & Santavuori, P. (1996). MRI of neuronal ceroid lipofuscinosis. I. Cranial MRI of 30 patients with juvenile neuronal ceroid lipofuscinosis. *Neuroradiol*, *38*(5), 476–482. https://doi.org/10.1007/BF00607283

69. Mink, J. W., Augustine, E. F., Adams, H. R., Marshall, F. J., & Kwon, J. M. (2013). Classification and natural history of the neuronal ceroid lipofuscinoses. *J Child Neurol*, *28*(9), 1101–1105. https://doi.org/10.1177/0883073813494426

70. European Association for the Study of the Liver. (2012). EASL clinical practice guidelines: Wilson's disease. *J Hepatol*, *56*(3), 671–685.

71. Manolaki, N., Nikolopoulou, G., Daikos, G. L., Panagiotakaki, E., Tzetis, M., Roma, E., . . . Syriopoulou, V. P. (2009). Wilson disease in children: analysis of 57 cases. *J Pediatr Gastroenterol Nutr*, *48*(1), 72–77.

72. Lorincz, M. T. (2010). Neurologic Wilson's disease. *Ann N Y Acad Sci*, *1184*(1), 173–187.

73. Machado, A., Fen Chien, H., Mitiko Deguti, M., Cançado, E., Soares Azevedo, R., Scaff, M., & Reis Barbosa, E. (2006). Neurological manifestations in Wilson's disease: report of 119 cases. *Mov Dis*, *21*(12), 2192–2196.

74. Taly, A. B., Meenakshi-Sundaram, S., Sinha, S., Swamy, H. S., & Arunodaya, G. R. (2007). Wilson disease: description of 282 patients evaluated over 3 decades. *Medicine*, *86*(2), 112–121.

75. Ferenci, P. (2004). Pathophysiology and clinical features of Wilson disease. *Metab Brain Dise*, *19*(3-4), 229–239.

76. Lin, L. J., Wang, D. X., Ding, N. N., Lin, Y., Jin, Y., & Zheng, C. Q. (2014). Comprehensive analysis on clinical features of Wilson's disease: an experience over 28 years with 133 cases. *Neurol Res*, *36*(2), 157–163.

77. Merle, U., Schaefer, M., Ferenci, P., & Stremmel, W. (2007). Clinical presentation, diagnosis and long-term outcome of Wilson's disease: a cohort study. *Gut*, *56*(1), 115–120.

78. Van Wassenaer-van Hall, H. N., Van den Heuvel, A. G., Algra, A., Hoogenraad, T. U., & Mali, W. P. (1996). Wilson disease: findings at MR imaging and CT of the brain with clinical correlation. *Radiology*, *198*(2), 531–536.

79. Akil, M., & Brewer, G. J. (1995). Psychiatric and behavioral abnormalities in Wilson's disease. *Adv Neurol*, *65*, 171.

80. Dening, T. R., & Berrios, G. E. (1990). Wilson's disease: a longitudinal study of psychiatric symptoms. *Biol Psychiatry*, *28*(3), 255–265.

81. Dening, T. R., & Berrios, G. E. (1989). Wilson's disease: psychiatric symptoms in 195 cases. *Arch Gen Psychiatry*, *46*(12), 1126–1134.

82. Oder, W., Grimm, G., Kollegger, H., Ferenci, P., Schneider, B., & Deecke, L. (1991). Neurological and neuropsychiatric spectrum of Wilson's disease: a prospective study of 45 cases. *J Neurol*, *238*(5), 281–287.

83. Shanmugiah, A., Sinha, S., Taly, A. B., Prashanth, L. K., Tomar, M. B. B. S. M., Arunodaya, G. R., . . . Khanna, S. (2008). Psychiatric manifestations in Wilson's disease: a cross-sectional analysis. *J Neuropsychiatry Clin Neurosci*, *20*(1), 81–85.

84. Wiggelinkhuizen, M., Tilanus, M. E. C., Bollen, C. W., & Houwen, R. H. J. (2009). Systematic review: clinical efficacy of chelator agents and zinc in the initial treatment of Wilson disease. *Aliment Pharmacol Ther*, *29*(9), 947–958

85. Christensen, C. K., & Walsh, L. (2018). Movement disorders and neurometabolic diseases. *Semin Pediatr Neurology*,25, 82–91.

86. Pellecchia, M. T., Valente, E. M., Cif, L., Salvi, S., Albanese, A., Scarano, V., . . . Di Giorgio, A. (2005). The diverse phenotype and genotype of pantothenate kinase-associated neurodegeneration. *Neurology*, *64*(10), 1810–1812.

87. Tonekaboni, S. H., & Mollamohammadi, M. (2014). Neurodegeneration with brain iron accumulation: an overview. *Iran J Child Neurol*, *8*(4), 1.

88. Hayflick, S. J., Westaway, S. K., Levinson, B., Zhou, B., Johnson, M. A., Ching, K. H., & Gitschier, J. (2003). Genetic, clinical, and radiographic delineation of Hallervorden–Spatz syndrome. *N Engl J Med*, *348*(1), 33–40.

89. Schneider, S. A., Zorzi, G., & Nardocci, N. (2013). Pathophysiology and treatment of neurodegeneration with brain iron accumulation in the pediatric population. *Curr Treat Options Neurol*, *15*(5), 652–667.

90. Ghaoui, R., & Sue, C. M. (2018). Movement disorders in mitochondrial disease. *J Neurol*, *265*(5), 1230–1240.

91. Martikainen, M. H., Ng, Y. S., Gorman, G. S., Alston, C. L., Blakely, E. L., Schaefer, A. M., . . . Turnbull, D. M. (2016). Clinical, genetic, and radiological features of extrapyramidal movement disorders in mitochondrial disease. *JAMA Neurol*, *73*(6), 668–674.

92. Rezin, G. T., Amboni, G., Zugno, A. I., Quevedo, J., & Streck, E. L. (2009). Mitochondrial dysfunction and psychiatric disorders. *Neurochem Res*, *34*(6), 1021.

93. Garcia, G. A., Khoshnevis, M., Gale, J., Frousiakis, S. E., Hwang, T. J., Poincenot, L., . . . Sadun, A. A. (2017). Profound vision loss impairs psychological well-being in young and middle-aged individuals. *Clin Ophthalmol*, *11*, 417.

94. De Vries, M. C., Brown, D. A., Allen, M. E., Bindoff, L., Gorman, G. S., Karaa, A., . . . O'Callaghan, M. (2020). Safety of drug use in patients with a primary mitochondrial disease: An international Delphi-based consensus. *J Inherit Metab Dis*. 43(4): 800–818.

95. Hoffmann, G. F., Assmann, B., Bräutigam, C., Dionisi-Vici, C., Häussler, M., de Klerk, J. B., . . . Wevers, R. A. (2003). Tyrosine hydroxylase deficiency causes progressive encephalopathy and dopa-nonresponsive dystonia. *Ann Neurol*, *54*(Suppl 6), S56–S65. https://doi.org/10.1002/ana.10632

96. Knappskog, P. M., Flatmark, T., Mallet, J., Lüdecke, B., & Bartholomé, K. (1995). Recessively inherited L-DOPA-responsive dystonia caused by a point mutation (Q381K) in the tyrosine hydroxylase gene. *Hum Mol Genet*, *4*(7), 1209–1212. https://doi.org/10.1093/hmg/4.7.1209

97. Castaigne, P., Rondot, P., Ribadeau-Dumas, J. L., & Saïd, G. (1971). Affection extrapyramidale évoluant chez deux jeunes frères; effects remarquables du traitement par la L-Dopa [Progressive extra-pyramidal disorder in 2 young brothers. Remarkable effects of treatment with L-dopa]. *Rev Neurol*, *124*(2), 162–166.

98. Rondot, P., & Ziegler, M. (1983). Dystonia--L-dopa responsive or juvenile parkinsonism? *J Neural Transm, 19 (suppl)*, 273–281.

99. Rondot, P., Aicardi, J., Goutières, F., & Ziegler, M. (1992). Dystonies dopa-sensibles [Dopa-sensitive dystonias]. *Rev Neurol, 148*(11), 680–686.

100. de Rijk-Van Andel, J. F., Gabreëls, F. J., Geurtz, B., Steenbergen-Spanjers, G. C., van Den Heuvel, L. P., Smeitink, J. A., & Wevers, R. A. (2000). L-dopa-responsive infantile hypokinetic rigid parkinsonism due to tyrosine hydroxylase deficiency. *Neurology, 55*(12), 1926–1928. https://doi.org/10.1212/wnl.55.12.1926

101. Willemsen, M. A., Verbeek, M. M., Kamsteeg, E. J., de Rijk-van Andel, J. F., Aeby, A., Blau, N., . . . Wevers, R. A. (2010). Tyrosine hydroxylase deficiency: a treatable disorder of brain catecholamine biosynthesis. *Brain, 133*(Pt 6), 1810–1822. https://doi.org/10.1093/brain/awq087

102. Yeung, W. L., Wong, V. C., Chan, K. Y., Hui, J., Fung, C. W., Yau, E., . . . Low, L. (2011). Expanding phenotype and clinical analysis of tyrosine hydroxylase deficiency. *J Child Neurol, 26*(2), 179–187. https://doi.org/10.1177/0883073810377014

103. Van Hove, J. L., Steyaert, J., Matthijs, G., Legius, E., Theys, P., Wevers, R., . . . Casaer, P. (2006). Expanded motor and psychiatric phenotype in autosomal dominant Segawa syndrome due to GTP cyclohydrolase deficiency. *J Neurol Neurosurg Psychiatry, 77*(1), 18–23. https://doi.org/10.1136/jnnp.2004.051664

104. Bräutigam, C., Steenbergen-Spanjers, G. C., Hoffmann, G. F., Dionisi-Vici, C., van den Heuvel, L. P., Smeitink, J. A., & Wevers, R. A. (1999). Biochemical and molecular genetic characteristics of the severe form of tyrosine hydroxylase deficiency. *Clin Chem, 45*(12), 2073–2078.

105. Addison, G. M. (1997). Physician's guide to the laboratory diagnosis of metabolic diseases. *J Clin Pathol, 50*(9), 797–798.

106. Scriver C. R. (2000). Mutation analysis in metabolic (and other genetic) disease: how soon, how useful. *Eur J Pediatr, 159*(Suppl 3), S243–S245. https://doi.org/10.1007/pl00014412

107. Lüdecke, B., Knappskog, P. M., Clayton, P. T., Surtees, R. A., Clelland, J. D., Heales, S. J., . . . Flatmark, T. (1996). Recessively inherited L-DOPA-responsive parkinsonism in infancy caused by a point mutation (L205P) in the tyrosine hydroxylase gene. *Hum Mol Genet, 5*(7), 1023–1028. https://doi.org/10.1093/hmg/5.7.1023

108. Surtees, R., & Clayton, P. (1998). Infantile parkinsonism-dystonia: tyrosine hydroxylase deficiency. *Mov Disord, 13*(2), 350. https://doi.org/10.1002/mds.870130226

109. Dionisi-Vici, C., Hoffmann, G. F., Leuzzi, V., Hoffken, H., Bräutigam, C., Rizzo, C., . . . Wevers, R. A. (2000). Tyrosine hydroxylase deficiency with severe clinical course: clinical and biochemical investigations and optimization of therapy. *J Pediatr, 136*(4), 560–562. https://doi.org/10.1016/s0022-3476(00)90027-1

110. Häussler, M., Hoffmann, G. F., & Wevers, R. A. (2001). L-dopa and selegiline for tyrosine hydroxylase deficiency. *J Pediatr, 138*(3), 451–452. https://doi.org/10.1067/mpd.2001.110776

111. Leuzzi, V., Mastrangelo, M., Giannini, M. T., Carbonetti, R., & Hoffmann, G. F. (2017). Neuromotor and cognitive outcomes of early treatment in tyrosine hydroxylase deficiency type B. *Neurology, 88*(5), 501–502. https://doi.org/10.1212/WNL.0000000000003539

112. Furukawa, Y., Kish, S. J., & Fahn, S. (2004). Dopa-responsive dystonia due to mild tyrosine hydroxylase deficiency. *Ann Neurol, 55*(1), 147–148. https://doi.org/10.1002/ana.10820

113. Larson, A., & Goodman, S. (2019 Sep 19). Glutaric acidemia type 1. In: Adam, M. P., Ardinger, H. H., Pagon, R. A., et al., eds. *GeneReviews® [Internet]*. Seattle: University of Washington; 1993–2020.

114. Kölker, S., Garbade, S., Greenberg, C. R., Leonard, J. V., Saudubray, J. M., Ribes, A., . . . Hoffmann, G. F. (2006). Natural history, outcome, and treatment efficacy in children and adults with glutaryl-CoA dehydrogenase deficiency. *Pediatr res*, *59*, 840–847.

115. Vester, M. E., Visser, G., Wijburg, F., van Spronsen, F. J., Williams, M., & van Rijn, R. R. (2016). Occurrence of subdural hematomas in Dutch glutaric aciduria type 1 patients. *Eur j pediatr*, *175*, 1001–1006.

116. Boy, N., Mühlhausen, C., Maier, E. M., Heringer, J., Assmann, B., Burgard, P., et al. (2017). Proposed recommendations for diagnosing and managing individuals with glutaric aciduria type I: second revision. *J inherit metab dis*, *40*, 75–101.

117. Baric, I., Wagner, L., Feyh, P., Liesert, M., Buckel, W., & Hoffmann, G. F. (1999). Sensitivity and specificity of free and total glutaric acid and 3-hydroxyglutaric acid measurements by stable-isotope dilution assays for the diagnosis of glutaric aciduria type I. *J inherit metab dis*, *22*, 867–881.

118. Chace, D. H., Kalas, T. A., & Naylor, E. W. (2003). Use of tandem mass spectrometry for multianalyte screening of dried blood specimens from newborns. *Clin chem*, *49*, 1797–1817.

119. Boy, N., Mengler, K., Thimm, E., Schiergens, K. A., Marquardt, T., Weinhold, N., . . . Kölker, S. (2018). Newborn screening: a disease-changing intervention for glutaric aciduria type 1. *Ann neurol*, *83*, 970–979.

120. Baric, I., Wagner, L., Feyh, P., Liesert, M., Buckel, W., & Hoffmann, G. F. (1999). Sensitivity and specificity of free and total glutaric acid and 3-hydroxyglutaric acid measurements by stable-isotope dilution assays for the diagnosis of glutaric aciduria type I. *J inherit metab dis*, *22*, 867–881.

121. Chace, D. H., Kalas, T. A., &Naylor, E. W. (2003). Use of tandem mass spectrometry for multianalyte screening of dried blood specimens from newborns. *Clin chem*, *49*, 1797–1817.

122. Boy, N., Haege, G., Heringer, J., Assmann, B., Mühlhausen, C., Ensenauer, R., . . . Kölker, S. (2013). Low lysine diet in glutaric aciduria type I—effect on anthropometric and biochemical follow-up parameters. *J inherit metab dis*, *36*, 525–33.

123. Lesch, M., & Nyhan, W. L. (1964). A familial disorder of uric acid metabolism and central nervous system function. *Am j med*, *36*(4), 561–570.

124. Nyhan, W. L., Oliver, W. J., & Lesch, M. (1965). A familial disorder of uric acid metabolism and central nervous system function. II. *J pediatr*, *67*(2), 257–263.

125. Seegmiller, J. E., Rosenbloom, F. M., & Kelley, W. N. (1967). Enzyme defect associated with a sex-linked human neurological disorder and excessive purine synthesis. *Science*, *155*(3770), 1682–1684.

126. Jankovic, J., Caskey, T. C., Stout, J. T., & Butler, I. J. (1988). Lesch-Nyhan syndrome: a study of motor behavior and cerebrospinal fluid neurotransmitters. *Ann Neurol*, *23*(5), 466–469.

127. Jinnah, H. A., Visser, J. E., Harris, J. C., Verdu, A., Larovere, L., Ceballos-Picot, I., . . . Desguerre, I. (2006). Delineation of the motor disorder of Lesch–Nyhan disease. *Brain*, *129*(5), 1201–1217.

128. Tan, E. K., & Jankovic, J. (2000). Tardive and idiopathic oromandibular dystonia: a clinical comparison. *J Neurol Neurosurg Psychiatry*, *68*(2), 186–190.

129. Saito, Y., & Takashima, S. (2000). Neurotransmitter changes in the pathophysiology of Lesch–Nyhan syndrome. *Brain Dev*, *22*, 122–131.

130. Fu, R., Chen, C. J., & Jinnah, H. A. (2014). Genotypic and phenotypic spectrum in attenuated variants of Lesch–Nyhan disease. *Mol Genet Metab, 112*(4), 280–285.

131. Fu, R., Sutcliffe, D., Zhao, H., Huang, X., Schretlen, D. J., Benkovic, S., & Jinnah, H. A. (2015). Clinical severity in Lesch–Nyhan disease: the role of residual enzyme and compensatory pathways. *Mol Genet Metab, 114*(1), 55–61.

132. Allen, S. M., & Rice, S. N. (1996). Risperidone antagonism of self-mutilation in a Lesch-Nyhan patient. *Prog Neuropsychopharmacol Biol Psychiatry, 5*(20), 793–800.

133. Nofech-Mozes, Y., Blaser, S. I., Kobayashi, J., Grunebaum, E., & Roifman, C. M. (2007). Neurologic abnormalities in patients with adenosine deaminase deficiency. *Pediatr Neurol, 37*(3), 218–221.

134. Rogers, M. H., Lwin, R., Fairbanks, L., Gerritsen, B., & Gaspar, H. B. (2001). Cognitive and behavioral abnormalities in adenosine deaminase deficient severe combined immunodeficiency. *J Pediatr, 139*(1), 44–50.

135. Hegde, A. U., Karnavat, P. K., Vyas, R., DiBacco, M. L., Grant, P. E., & Pearl, P. L. (2019). GABA transaminase deficiency with survival into adulthood. *J child neurol,* 34(4), 216––220.

136. Koenig, M. K., Hodgeman, R., Riviello, J. J., et al. (2017). Phenotype of GABA-transaminase deficiency. *Neurology,* 88(20), 1919–1924.

137. Strauss K.A., Puffenberger E.G., Carson V.J. (2006 Jan 30 [Updated 2020 Apr 23]). Maple Syrup Urine Disease. In: Adam M.P., Mirzaa G.M., Pagon R.A., et al., eds. GeneReviews® [Internet]. Seattle (WA): University of Washington, Seattle; 1993–2022. Available from: https://www.ncbi.nlm.nih.gov/books/NBK1319/

138. Muelly, E. R., Moore, G. J., Bunce, S. C., Mack, J., Bigler, D. C., Morton, D. H., & Strauss, K. A. (2013). Biochemical correlates of neuropsychiatric illness in maple syrup urine disease. *J Clin Invest* 123(4), 1809–1820. https://doi.org/10.1172/JCI67217

139. Carecchio, M., Schneider, S. A., Chan, H., Lachmann, R., Lee, P. J., Murphy, E., & Bhatia, K. P. (2011). Movement disorders in adult surviving patients with maple syrup urine disease. *Mov Disord, 26*(7), 1324–1328. https://doi.org/10.1002/mds.23629

140. Regier D.S., Greene C.L. (2000 Jan 10 [Updated 2017 Jan 5]). Phenylalanine Hydroxylase Deficiency. In: Adam MP, Mirzaa GM, Pagon RA, et al., editors. GeneReviews® [Internet]. Seattle (WA): University of Washington, Seattle; 1993–2022. Available from: https://www.ncbi.nlm.nih.gov/books/NBK1504/

141. Koch, R., Burton, B., Hoganson, G., Peterson, R., Rhead, W., Rouse, B., . . . Azen, C. (2002). Phenylketonuria in adulthood: a collaborative study. *J Inherit Metabol Dis, 25*(5), 333–346. https://doi.org/10.1023/a:1020158631102

142. Pastores G.M., Hughes D.A. (2000 Jul 27 [Updated 2018 Jun 21]). Gaucher Disease. In: Adam MP, Mirzaa GM, Pagon RA, et al., editors. GeneReviews® [Internet]. Seattle (WA): University of Washington, Seattle; 1993–2022. Available from: https://www.ncbi.nlm.nih.gov/books/NBK1269/

143. Packman, W., Wilson Crosbie, T., Riesner, A., Fairley, C., & Packman, S. (2006). Psychological complications of patients with Gaucher disease. *J Inherit Metabol Dis, 29*(1), 99–105. https://doi.org/10.1007/s10545-006-0154-x

144. Orsini J.J., Escolar M.L., Wasserstein M.P., et al. (2000 Jun 19 [Updated 2018 Oct 11]). Krabbe Disease. In: Adam MP, Mirzaa GM, Pagon RA, et al., editors. GeneReviews® [Internet]. Seattle (WA): University of Washington, Seattle; 1993–2022. Available from: https://www.ncbi.nlm.nih.gov/books/NBK1238/

145. Fiumara, A., Barone, R., Arena, A., Filocamo, M., Lissens, W., Pavone, L., & Sorge, G. (2011). Krabbe leukodystrophy in a selected population with high rate of late onset forms: longer survival linked to c.121G>A (p.Gly41Ser) mutation. *Clin Genet*, *80*(5), 452–458. https://doi.org/10.1111/j.1399-0004.2010.01572.x

146. Toro C., Shirvan L., Tifft C. (1999 Mar 11 [Updated 2020 Oct 1]). HEXA Disorders. In: Adam MP, Mirzaa GM, Pagon RA, et al., editors. GeneReviews® [Internet]. Seattle (WA): University of Washington, Seattle; 1993–2022. Available from: https://www.ncbi.nlm.nih.gov/books/NBK1218/

147. Brun, L., Ngu, L. H., Keng, W. T., Ch'ng, G. S., Choy, Y. S., Hwu, W. L., . . . Blau, N. (2010). Clinical and biochemical features of aromatic L-amino acid decarboxylase deficiency. *Neurology*, *75*(1), 64–71. https://doi.org/10.1212/WNL.0b013e3181e620ae

148. Maller, A., Hyland, K., Milstien, S., Biaggioni, I., & Butler, I. J. (1997). Aromatic L-amino acid decarboxylase deficiency: clinical features, diagnosis, and treatment of a second family. *J Child Neurol*, *12*(6), 349–354. https://doi.org/10.1177/088307389701200602

149. Korf, B., Wallman, J. K., & Levy, H. L. (1986). Bilateral lucency of the globus pallidus complicating methylmalonic acidemia. *Ann Neurol*, *20*(3), 364–366. https://doi.org/10.1002/ana.410200317

150. Baumgarter, E. R., & Viardot, C. (1995). Long-term follow-up of 77 patients with isolated methylmalonic acidaemia. *J Inherit Metabol Dis*, *18*(2), 138–142. https://doi.org/10.1007/BF00711749

21

Autoimmune and Paraneoplastic Encephalopathies

James F. Rini, Bradley T. Peet, and Michael D. Geschwind

Introduction

The discovery of novel autoimmune-mediated neuropsychiatric syndromes and their associated autoantibodies has made neuroimmunology one of the most rapidly evolving areas in neurology and psychiatry over the past decade.[1,2] Movement disorders are a prominent and common feature in many autoantibody-mediated neuropsychiatric disorders and are caused by an expanding spectrum of antibodies. Depending on the presenting and early symptoms, patients with these disorders are often referred to psychiatrists or general, movement disorder and/or behavioral neurologists. It is imperative not to miss diagnosing these disorders as many are potentially treatable, if not curable. Furthermore, in some cases, the autoantibody can alert the clinician to specific types of occult neoplasia underlying some of these disorders.[3–5]

This chapter will focus on the most common autoimmune, especially antibody-mediated, syndromes associated with psychiatric and movement disorders. Many of the autoimmune-mediated movement disorders discussed in this chapter are often associated with other features, including psychiatric/behavioral disorders, limbic encephalitis, and other symptoms. Autoimmune limbic encephalitis (ALE) is a syndrome in which parts of the limbic system are involved and classically presents with features including short-term memory loss, irritability, depression, hallucinations, sleep disturbances, and/or seizures.

For a helpful, detailed review specifically on antibody-mediated syndromes associated with movement disorders, please see Balint et al. 2018.[5,6]

Background

Since the 1980s, detailed clinical and immunological studies have revealed several autoantibodies against intracellular targets, such as cytoplasmic and nuclear antigens (e.g., Hu, Yo, Ri, Ma, etc.), that are associated with specific paraneoplastic neurological syndromes.[7] Many of these antibodies initially were named based on the first two letters of the last name of an index patient or the discoverer of the antibody and its target antigen. In some cases, when the specific antigenic target of the antibody was later identified, another, more scientifically appropriate name was given to the same antibody (e.g., CV2 vs. CRMP5).[8,9] Later, the discovery of another class of central nervous system (CNS) disorders associated with autoantibodies, but against nonintracellular, or extracellular, targets, such as cell surface or synaptic proteins

Antibodies against neuronal surface antigens	**Antibodies against intracellular synaptic antigens**	**Antibodies against intracellular cytoplasmic/ nuclear antigens**
Considered pathogenic as they target proteins that are accessible *in vivo* and, typically, play an important role in synaptic transmission, plasticity or excitability	Controversial role in pathogenesis (see text); their antigen could be transiently accessible during synaptic vesicle fusion and uptake	Considered markers of paraneoplastic syndromes with poor prognosis and treatment response, in which autoimmunity is mainly effected by cytotoxic T cells; the antigens are deemed to be inaccessible *in vivo*
Examples: Caspr2, DPPX, D2R, GABA$_A$R, GABA$_B$R, GlyR, LGI1, NMDAR	Examples: GAD, Amphiphysin	Examples: Hu, Yo, Ri CRMP5/CV2, Zic4, Ma2

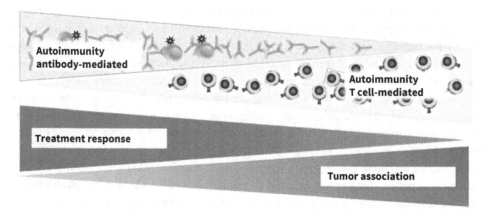

Figure 21.1 Comparison of the three groups of neuronal antibodies and their pathogenic roles, examples, treatment responses, and tumor associations.

Legend: The three groups of neuronal antibodies and their pathogenic roles, examples, treatment responses and tumor associations. AMPAR = a-amino-3-hydroxy-5-methyl-4-isoxazolepropionic acid receptor; CASPR2 = contactin associated protein like 2; D2R = dopamine 2 receptor; DPPX = dipeptidyl peptidase like protein 6; GABAAR and GABABR = gamma aminobutyric acid type A and type B receptors; GlyR = glycine receptor; LGI1 = leucine rich glioma inactivated protein 1; NMDAR = N-methyl-D-aspartate receptor.

Source: Balint B, Vincent A, Meinck H-M, Irani SR, Bhatia KP. Movement disorders with neuronal antibodies: syndromic approach, genetic parallels and pathophysiology. *Brain*. 2018;*141*(1):13–36. https://doi.org/10.1093/brain/awx189

(e.g., LGI1, CASPR2, NMDA receptor, AMPA receptor, etc.) has dramatically expanded the types of syndromes caused by autoantibodies and radically changed concepts about CNS autoimmunity.[10–13] This group with extracellular targets is the greatest expanding category for autoimmune/antibody-mediated causes of neuropsychiatric movement disorders, with new antibodies and targets continually being identified. There is yet another group in which the target antigens are not purely intra- or extracellular but rather the intracellular cytoplasmic surface of synaptic proteins (e.g., GAD and amphiphysin). Figure 21.1 shows a schematic comparing these three types of antibody-mediated disorders. The main clinical features and treatments for these disorders are summarized in Table 21.1, whereas Table 21.2 summarizes the autoantibody target, syndrome frequency, and oncological association(s) with each

Table 21.1 Autoantibody Clinical Syndrome and Treatment Considerations

Antibody target	Movement Disorder Features	Neuropsychiatric Features	Other Clinical Features	Specific Treatment Considerations
Neuronal surface antibodies				
NMDAR	Orofacial and limb dyskinesia, chorea, dystonia, myoclonus, ataxia, parkinsonism, paroxysmal dyskinesias, catatonia, stereotypies, OMS	Auditory/visual hallucinations, delusions, negative symptoms, depression, mania, disinhibition, agitation, aggression, catatonia, mutism, antipsychotic intolerance	Prodromal infectious-like symptoms, neuropsychiatric disturbance, encephalopathy with epilepsy, cognitive deficits, reduced consciousness, dysautonomia, central hypoventilation	1st-line therapies followed by 2nd-line therapies, as needed. 3rd-line therapies include proteasome inhibitors and IL-6 receptor antagonists, though evidence supporting their use is limited.
LGI1 (formerly VGKC complex)	Faciobrachial dystonic seizures, chorea, parkinsonism, ataxia, myoclonus,	Cognitive impairment, disorientation, confusion, auditory/visual hallucinations, delusions, agitation, anxiety, and depression	Limbic/brainstem encephalitis; hyponatremia, bradycardia, REM sleep, temporal lobe seizures.	1st-line therapies followed by 2nd-line therapies, as needed although IVMP as 1st line and rituximab as 2nd line seem to be most effective overall. Maintenance therapy with intermittent IVMP, IVIG, or other 2nd-line therapies.
CASPR2 (formerly VGKC complex)	Cerebellar ataxia, chorea, neuromyotonia, myokymia	Cognitive impairment, disorientation, confusion, auditory/visual hallucinations, delusions, agitation, anxiety, and depression	Morvan syndrome, limbic encephalitis, neuropathy (rarely Guillain-Barré-like syndrome), neuropathic pain.	Similar to LGI1 but given higher paraneoplastic association, greater need for cancer work-up and surveillance
AMPAR	Ataxia, involuntary movements, and upper motor neuron signs	Memory impairment, psychosis, confusion, agitation, insomnia, bradyphrenia	Seizures	1st-line therapies followed by 2nd-line therapies, as needed.
DPPX	SPSD, myoclonus, startle, ataxia, tremor, parkinsonism, opsoclonus myoclonus, myoclonus, parasomnias, PERM	Cognitive and mental dysfunction, CNS hyperexcitability (e.g. agitation)	Prominent gastrointestinal symptoms (diarrhea, constipation), urinary or erectile dysfunction, cardiac arrhythmia, Raynaud's phenomenon, allodynia, paresthesia	1st-line therapies followed by 2nd-line therapies, as needed. Majority show substantial response to first-line therapy, but often require 2nd-line therapies. Consider workup for Whipple's disease given clinical overlap.

(continued)

Table 21.1 Continued

Antibody target	Movement Disorder Features	Neuropsychiatric Features	Other Clinical Features	Specific Treatment Considerations
D2R	Basal ganglia encephalitis in children with dystonia, chorea or parkinsonism; Sydenham's chorea	Agitation, psychosis, emotional lability, anxiety, compulsions, aggression, somnolence, insomnia	Psychiatric and sleep disturbance	Abrupt onset of neuropsychiatric symptoms with evidence of a recent GAS infection should be treated promptly with antistreptococcal antibiotics; azithromycin or azithromycin plus clindamycin is the treatment of choice. 1st-line therapies have been found to be effective in those with severe or relapsing/ remitting symptoms; IVIG may be a good choice if immunocompromised.
GABA$_A$R	Chorea, dystonia or ataxia (as part of a more widespread encephalopathy), opsoclonus myoclonus syndrome; possible association with SPSD	Behavioral changes, visual hallucinations, delusions, depression, catatonia	Encephalopathy with epilepsy, reduced consciousness	1st-line therapies followed by 2nd-line therapies, as needed. Outcome seems to be improved following both 1st- and 2nd-line treatments.
GABA$_B$R	OMAS, cerebellar ataxia	Memory impairment, confusion, agitation, auditory/visual hallucinations, catatonia, personality change	Limbic encephalitis with prominent seizures	Similar to GABA$_A$R.
Glycine receptor	SPSD, myoclonus, hyperekplexia, ataxia, PERM, SPS, and variants	Visual hallucinations, synesthesia, personality change	Brainstem encephalitis, optic neuritis; limbic/epileptic encephalopathy, epilepsy, steroid-responsive deafness	1st-line therapies followed by 2nd-line therapies, as needed.
IgLON5	Gait instability, cerebellar ataxia, chorea in patients with tau brain pathology; parkinsonism, parasomnias	Depression, memory impairment, hallucinations, anxiety, confusion	REM and non-REM sleep behavior disorder; sleep apnea, stridor, dysphagia, oculomotor disturbance, cognitive decline, dysautonomia	Most cases show a lack of response to immunotherapy.
mGluR1	Cerebellar ataxia	Emotional lability, anxiety, depression, psychosis, memory/ cognitive dysfunction, visual hallucinations, prosopagnosia, sleep disturbances	Memory or attention deficits, dysgeusia, psychiatric problems (auditory hallucinations, paranoia)	1st-line therapies followed by 2nd-line therapies, as needed.

Antibody	Neurological syndrome	Psychiatric presentation	Other features	Treatment
SEZ6L2	Gait and limb ataxia, parkinsonism, oculomotor disturbances, dysarthria	Bradyphrenia	Multidomain cognitive impairment (memory, executive, language), apraxia, echolalia	Most cases show a lack of response to immunotherapy.
VGCC P/Q type	Cerebellar ataxia, myoclonus		Lambert-Eaton myasthenic syndrome, encephalopathy, neuropathy	3,4 diaminopyridine for symptoms; 1st-line immunotherapy, although best evidence for combination of steroids and azathioprine and intermittent IVIG for exacerbations.
Antibodies targeting intracellular, synaptic proteins				
Amphiphysin	SPSD, SPS	Generally, does not have significant psychiatric presentation	Sensory ganglionopathy, myelopathy	1st-line therapies followed by 2nd-line therapies, as needed. Anecdotal evidence suggests poor response to IVIG. Case reports propose PLEX with steroids, and tumor excision with chemotherapy may produce profound benefits.
GAD	SPSD, cerebellar ataxia, SPS, stiff-man phenomena, ataxia, chorea, ophthalmoplegia, parkinsonism	Depression, irritability, agitation	Limbic encephalitis, focal epilepsy, concomitant diabetes type 1, thyroid disease, vitiligo, pernicious anemia	1st-line therapies followed by 2nd-line therapies, as needed. Anti-GAD SPS responds modestly to IVIG, whereas anti-GAD cerebellar ataxia variably responds to other 1st- or 2nd-line therapies.
Antibodies targeting cytoplasmic and nuclear antigens				
ANNA-1 (Hu)	Chorea, cerebellar ataxia, opsoclonus, myoclonus, ataxia syndrome	Depression, memory impairment, confusion, agitation	Encephalomyelitis, limbic encephalitis, brainstem encephalitis, sensory neuropathy, gastrointestinal pseudo-obstruction	1st-line therapies followed by 2nd-line therapies, as needed. Prognosis is generally considered poor with the most effective treatment often targeting the associated tumor itself.
ANNA-2 (Ri)	Dystonia (jaw closing dystonia, laryngospasms), opsoclonus myoclonus ataxia syndrome, cerebellar ataxia, SPSD, pyramidal signs, rigidity	Exaggerated startle response, anxiety	Brainstem encephalitis with cranial nerve palsies, nystagmus, dysarthria, trismus,	Similar to ANNA-1

(continued)

Table 21.1 Continued

Antibody target	Movement Disorder Features	Neuropsychiatric Features	Other Clinical Features	Specific Treatment Considerations
ANNA-3	Cerebellar ataxia	similar to ANNA-1	Sensory/sensorimotor neuropathy, myelopathy, brainstem or limbic encephalitis	Similar to ANNA-1
CRMP5/CV2	Chorea, ataxia	Memory impairment, behavioral changes, deficits in social functioning	Optic neuritis, myelitis, cognitive decline, neuropathy	Role of immunotherapy unclear as symptoms often only improve following anticancer therapy
GFAP	Cerebellar ataxia, tremor, undefined movement disorders	Depression, anxiety, psychosis, insomnia, vivid dreams	Encephalomyelitis, headache, cognitive decline, optic papillitis, sensory disturbance, gastrointestinal and urogenital dysautonomia, neuropathy	1st-line therapies followed by 2nd-line therapies, as needed. Anecdotal evidence of rapid improvements upon treatment with corticosteroids. High rate of relapses often requires prolonged immunosuppression therapy
KLHL11	Cerebellar ataxia, opsoclonus-myoclonus, diplopia	Chronic psychosis	Encephalitis (limbic and extralimbic), Subacute encephalopathy, hearing loss, seizures, vertigo	1st-line therapies followed by 2nd-line therapies, as needed. Limited or moderate response to treatment
Ma1	Parkinsonism	Memory impairment, anxiety, obsessive-compulsive features	Limbic, diencephalic, or brainstem encephalitis	1st-line therapies followed by 2nd-line therapies, as needed. Treatment often includes orchiectomy in males, immunotherapy, and chemotherapy
Ma2/Ta	Parkinsonism, opsoclonus, supranuclear gaze palsy	Memory impairment, anxiety, obsessive-compulsive features	Limbic, diencephalic, or brainstem encephalitis, myelopathy, radiculoplexopathy, endocrine dysfunction, prominent sleep disorders, dysphagia, muscular atrophy, fasciculations	Similar to MA1. Remarkably high response rate to treatment
PCA1 (Yo)	Cerebellar ataxia	Mild memory and cognitive deficits with inappropriate/disinhibited behavior	Limbic encephalitis, rhombencephalitis, peripheral neuropathy	1st-line therapies followed by 2nd-line therapies, as needed. Early diagnosis, immunotherapy, and cancer treatment are crucial for stabilization of symptoms. PCD symptoms are often irreversible.

PCA2	Cerebellar ataxia	similar to PCA1	Similar to PCA-1
PCA-Tr	Cerebellar ataxia	similar to PCA1	Encephalitis, neuropathy	Similar to PCA-1. Much better prognosis than other forms of PCA.

Table modified with permission.[6]

*1st-line therapies usually include high-dose corticosteroids (e.g., 1 g/day × 3–5 days of intravenous methylprednisolone [IVMP]), intravenous gamma globulin (IVIG), and plasma exchange (PLEX), in addition to tumor resection if paraneoplastic. 2nd-line therapies usually include rituximab and cyclophosphamide.

AMPAR = α-amino-3-hydroxy-5-methyl-4-isoxazolepropionic acid (e.g., kainate) receptor; ANNA-1(Hu) = Hu proteins (HuD, HuC)/antineuronal nuclear autoantibody 1; ANNA-2 (Ri) = antineuronal nuclear autoantibody 2 (Ri); ANNA-3 = antineuronal nuclear autoantibody 3; BSRPA = brain-specific receptor-like protein A; CASPR2 = contactin associated protein 2; CBA = cell-based assay; CDR = cerebellar degeneration-related protein; CRMP5/CV2 = collapsin response mediator protein 5 (anti-CV2); D1R = dopamine 1 receptor; D2R = dopamine 2 receptor; DNER = Delta/notch-like EGF-related receptor; DNER = Delta/notch-like epidermal growth factor-related receptor; DPPX = dipeptidyl peptidase-like protein 6; FBDS = faciobrachial dystonic seizures; $GABA_AR$ = γ-aminobutyric acid A receptor; $GABA_BR$ = γ-aminobutyric acid B receptor; GAD = glutamic acid decarboxylase; GFAP = glial fibrillary acidic protein; GluA1 = Glutamate receptor 1; GluR-δ2 = glutamate receptor delta 2; GlyRα1 = glycine receptor alpha 1; GlyT2 = glycine transporter 2; IgLON5 = IgLON family member 5; IL-6 = Interleukin 6; IVIG = intravenous immunoglobulin; IVMP = IV methylprednisolone; KLHL11 = Kelch-like protein 11; KV4 = potassium channel, voltage dependent; LA/IB = line assay/immunoblot; LGI1 = leucine-rich glioma-inactivated 1; mGluR1 = metabotropic glutamate receptor type 1; NMDAR = N-methyl-D-aspartate receptor; OMS = opsoclonus myoclonus syndrome; OMAS = opsoclonus myoclonus ataxia syndrome; PCA1 (Yo) = Purkinje cell antibody 1; PCA2 = Purkinje cell antibody 2; PCA-Tr (Tr represents Dr. Trotter, who discovered the antibody); PLEX = plasma exchange; RIA = radioimmunoassay; SEZ6L2 = seizure-related 6 homolog like 2; SPSD = stiff person spectrum disorders; TBA = tissue-based assay; VGCC P/Q = voltage gated calcium channel P/Q-type; VGKC complex = voltage gated potassium channel complex; Zic4 = Zinc finger protein 4.

Table 21.2 Autoantibody Target, Syndrome Frequency, and Oncological Association

Antibody	Target	Relative frequency in clinical practice	Tumor association	Most widely used test method
Neuronal surface antibodies				
AMPAR	GluA1 or 2 receptors	+	Thymic tumors, lung carcinomas, breast carcinoma	Unfixed TBA; live/fixed CBA
LGI1	LGI1	+++	Liver carcinoid, neuroendocrine pancreas tumor, mesothelioma, rectal carcinoma	Unfixed TBA; live/fixed CBA
CASPR2	CASPR2	++	Thymoma ≫ lung, prostate, sigmoid or thyroid cancer, myeloma	Unfixed TBA; live/fixed CBA
DPPXR	DPPX subunit of Kv4 channel	++	B-cell lymphomas/leukemia	Unfixed TBA; live/fixed CBA
D2R	D2R	+	None reported	Unfixed TBA; live CBA
GABA$_A$R	GABA$_A$R α1 and γ2 subunits	++	Thymoma, lung carcinoma, rectal cancer, myeloma	Unfixed TBA; live CBA
GABA$_B$R	GABA$_B$R R-1 subunit	++	Small cell lung cancer ≫ breast cancer multiple myeloma, rectal carcinoma, esophageal carcinoma, other neuroendocrine neoplasia	Unfixed TBA; live/fixed CBA
GlyRα1	a$_1$ subunit GlyR	+++	Thymoma > small cell lung cancer, breast cancer, Hodgkin lymphoma,8chronic lymphocytic leukemia	Unfixed TBA; live CBA
IgLON5	IgLON5	+	None reported	Unfixed TBA; live/fixed CBA
mGluR	mGluR1	+	Hodgkin lymphoma ≫ prostate adenocarcinoma	Unfixed TBA; live/fixed CBA
NMDAR	NMDAR	++++	Ovarian teratoma ≫ extra ovarian teratoma, ovarian carcinomas; lung, breast, testicular and pancreatic tumors	Unfixed TBA; live/fixed CBA
SEZ6L2	SEZ6L2/BSRPA	+	Of four cases reported, one was diagnosed with stage four ovarian cancer 4 years after symptom onset	Unfixed TBA; live/fixed CBA

VGCC	P/Q and N-type CCA receptor	++	Tumor association varies in different studies between 20% and 90%, mostly small cell lung cancer, breast or gynecologic adenocarcinoma	RIA
Antibodies targeting intracellular, synaptic proteins				
Amphiphysin	Amphiphysin	++	Breast cancer, small cell lung cancer	Fixed/unfixed TBA, LA/IB
GAD	GAD65/GAD67	++++	Very rare, but thymoma; renal cell, breast, or colon adenocarcinoma reported.	Fixed TBA, LA/IB, fixed CBA, RIA, ELISA
Antibodies targeting cytoplasmic and nuclear antigens				
ANNA-1 (Hu)	ELAVL (Hu)	+++	Small cell lung cancer ≫ neuroblastoma or intestinal, prostate, breast, bladder, and ovary carcinoma	Fixed TBA, LA/IB
ANNA-2 (Ri)	NOVA 1, 2 (Ri)	++	Gynecological tumors, mainly breast cancer, and lung cancer	Fixed TBA, LA/IB
CRMP5/CV2	CRMP-5	++	Small cell lung cancer, thymoma	Fixed TBA, LA/IB, fixed CBA
GFAP	GFAP	+	Prostate and gastroesophageal adenocarcinomas, myeloma, melanoma, colonic carcinoid, parotid pleomorphic adenoma, teratoma	Fixed TBA, LA/IB
KLHL11	Kelch-like protein 11	+	Seminoma, teratoma (ovary or testicular), small-cell lung cancer	Fixed/unfixed TBA, LA/IB, fixed CBA
Ma1	PNMA1,	+	Breast, colon, testicular	Fixed TBA, LA/IB
Ma2/Ta	PNMA2 (Ma2)	++	Testis ≫ lung cancer; rarely no neoplasia	Fixed TBA, LA/IB
PCA-1 (Yo)	CDR2, L/FLEDVE, CDR3, CDR2L (CDR2-like)	+++	Gynecological tumors, Mullerian adenocarcinoma, breast	Fixed TBA, LA/IB

(continued)

Table 21.2 Continued

Antibody	Target	Relative frequency in clinical practice	Tumor association	Most widely used test method
PCA-Tr	DNER	+++	Hodgkin lymphoma ≫ lung carcinoma	Fixed/unfixed TBA, LA/IB, fixed CBA
Zic4	ZIC4	+++	Small cell lung cancer ≫ ovarian adenocarcinoma	Fixed TBA, LA/IB

Table modified with permission.[6]

+ = rare; ++ = occasional; +++ = frequent; ++++ = very frequent; AMPAR = α-amino-3-hydroxy-5-methyl-4-isoxazolepropionic acid (e.g., kainate) receptor; ANNA-1(Hu) = Hu proteins (HuD, HuC)/antineuronal nuclear autoantibody 1; ANNA-2 (Ri) = antineuronal nuclear autoantibody 2 (Ri); ANNA-3 = antineuronal nuclear autoantibody 3; BSRPA = brain-specific receptor-like protein A; CASPR2 = contactin associated protein 2; CBA = cell-based assay; CDR = cerebellar degeneration-related protein; CRMP5/CV2 = collapsin response mediator protein 5 (anti-CV2); D1R = dopamine 1 receptor; D2R = dopamine 2 receptor; DNER = Delta/notch-like EGF-related receptor; DNER = Delta/notch-like epidermal growth factor-related receptor; DPPX = dipeptidyl peptidase-like protein 6; FBDS = faciobrachial dystonic seizures; GABA$_A$R = γ-aminobutyric acid A receptor; GABA$_B$R = γ-aminobutyric acid B receptor; GAD = glutamic acid decarboxylase; GFAP = glial fibrillary acidic protein; GluA1 = Glutamate receptor 1; GluR-δ2 = glutamate receptor delta 2; GlyRα1 = glycine receptor alpha 1; GlyT2 = glycine transporter 2; IgLON5 = IgLON family member 5; IL-6 = Interleukin 6; IVIG = intravenous immunoglobulin; IVMP = IV methylprednisolone; KLHL11 = Kelch-like protein 11; KV4 = potassium channel, voltage dependent; LA/IB = line assay/immunoblot; LGI1 = leucine-rich glioma-inactivated 1; mGluR1 = metabotropic glutamate receptor type 1; NMDAR = N-methyl-D-aspartate receptor; OMS = opsoclonus myoclonus syndrome; OMAS = opsoclonus myoclonus ataxia syndrome; PCA1 (Yo) = Purkinje cell antibody 1; PCA2 = Purkinje cell antibody 2; PCA-Tr (Tr represents Dr. Trotter who discovered the antibody); PLEX = plasma exchange; RIA = radioimmunoassay; SEZ6L2 = seizure-related 6 homolog like 2; SPSD = stiff person spectrum disorders; TBA = tissue-based assay; VGCC P/Q = voltage gated calcium channel P/Q-type; VGKC complex = voltage gated potassium channel complex; Zic4 = Zinc finger protein 4.

disorder. In the text of this chapter, we will discuss in detail the more common syndromes listed in Tables 21.1 and 21.2. The fourth and final groups discussed in this chapter include syndromes associated with a known systemic autoimmune condition that do not have an identified autoantibody. We also will review the diagnostic challenge when an antibody-mediated condition or an autoimmune encephalitis is suspected, but commercially available autoantibodies in the serum and cerebrospinal fluid (CSF) are negative, as well as the treatment of these disorders at the end of this chapter. Due to space limitations, treatments for each antibody-mediated syndrome are presented briefly in Table 21.1, but comprehensive reviews on management can be found elsewhere.[14,15]

Neuronal Surface Antibody-Mediated Autoimmune Encephalitis

The proper functioning of neurons and supporting cells depend on the interactions of ion channels and synaptic receptors, such as excitatory glutamate NMDA and AMPA, and inhibitory $GABA_A$ and $GABA_B$ receptors.[16,17] Antibodies that bind to cell-surface or synaptic receptors may act initially in a stimulatory manner—causing overexcitation of the receptor or channel—or conversely may block its function, by causing internalization of the receptor or blocking the channel. Antineuronal cell-surface encephalitis typically presents with prominent psychiatric, behavioral, and memory problems, often accompanied by seizures, likely due to overstimulation. In most cases, the antibodies implicated in these disorders over time cause a decrease in the amounts of the target receptor in neurons in vitro, suggesting the antibodies are pathogenic.[3] These syndromes are important to recognize as they usually respond very well to treatment, particularly when diagnosed and treated early.[18] Some of these antibodies more commonly occur as a paraneoplastic syndrome (e.g., NMDA receptor in younger women), whereas other antibodies are less commonly paraneoplastic (e.g., LGI1).[3,4]

Voltage-Gated Potassium Channel Complex (VGKC-Complex) Associated Disorders: LGI1 and CASPR2

Voltage-gated potassium channels (VGKCs) are a diverse group of transmembrane ion channels with a wide array of molecular permutations, neuronal locations, and distinct functions.[19] VGKCs play a crucial role in action potential initiation and propagation, control of neuronal excitability, and regulation of neuronal firing pattern.[20,21]

Antibodies associated with a wide variety of neurological manifestations, including but not limited to limbic encephalitis, facial brachial dystonic spells (FBDS; see below), neuromyotonia,[22-24] and Morvan's syndrome (neuromyotonia accompanied by autonomic disturbance, sleep disturbance, and limbic encephalitis) were initially thought be binding to the VGKC, as this channel complex was pulled down in radioimmunoassays.[10,12,13,22-26] In 2010, two laboratories independently reported that the antibodies in these syndromes were not directed against VGKC itself, but against VGKC-associated proteins, namely, leucine-rich glioma inactivated 1 protein (LGI1) and contactin-associated protein-like 2 (CASPR2).[27,28] Thus, the terms LGI1 and CASPR2 should be used to refer to these specific disorders, rather than VGKC.

Leucine-Rich Glioma Inactivated 1 (LGI1) Protein

The LGI1 protein plays a role in the transsynaptic stabilization of the presynaptic VGKC and postsynaptic AMPAR. In anti-LGI1 encephalitis, the antibodies cause disruption of the transsynaptic complex,[27–29] resulting in a reduction of presynaptic VGKCs and postsynaptic AMPARs in inhibitory interneurons. This ultimately leads to excessive neuronal excitation, potentially resulting in seizures and neuronal damage.[29–32]

Perhaps, the most common clinical syndrome with anti-LGI1 antibodies is ALE, although involvement of the peripheral nervous system may be seen in a minority of cases, often presenting as Morvan's syndrome.[27,28,33,34] Seizures and cognitive impairment are the two most common initial symptoms in anti-LGI1 encephalitis.[35] Faciobrachial dystonic seizures (FBDS) are sudden, spastic, jerking movements of the face, arm, leg, or body, can be uni- or bilateral and are virtually pathognomonic for anti-LGI1 encephalitis, but are present in only about 25%–50% of cases.[27,35] Importantly, when FBDS occur in anti-LGI1 encephalitis, this is often the first symptom and if treated early with immunosuppression, the full spectrum syndrome of ALE often will not develop.[18] Other seizures, particularly simple partial and complex, are common in anti-LGI1 encephalitis.[4,27,33,35] Most patients with anti-LGI1 ALE develop memory deficits and behavioral disturbances, such as apathy and disinhibition.[27,33,35] Other common symptoms include sleep disturbance, spatial disorientation, and autonomic dysfunction.[27,33,35] Psychiatric manifestations, including visual and auditory hallucinations, paranoia, anxiety, and depression, can also be prominent features.[4,36] The incidence of anti-LGI1 syndromes is estimated to be 0.63–0.83 per million and typically presents in the early to mid-60s with a male to female ratio of 2:1.[14,35,37]

Diagnostic evaluations commonly used to assess encephalitis, such as serum electrolytes, MRI, EEG, and CSF, often show abnormalities. Hyponatremia is a common serological finding, occurring in approximately 45%–65% of anti-LGI1 cases in the acute phase[4,18,35] and seems to be more common in patients with cognitive impairment.[18] The hyponatremia in anti-LGI1 is thought to be due to a syndrome of inappropriate antidiuretic hormone secretion (SIADH) from an effect of anti-LGI1 antibodies on ADH-secreting hypothalamic neurons.[38]

Brain MRI in the acute phase of the encephalitis demonstrates unilateral or bilateral T2-weighted signal hyperintensity in the medial temporal lobes (MTL) in more than 70% of cases (Figure 21.2), although a minority have a normal brain MRI at presentation.[18,35,39–42] Chronically, hippocampal atrophy and sclerosis are common features.[35,39,41,43]

CSF analysis is generally unremarkable in the majority of cases. A 2010 study with 46 patients with anti-LGI1 encephalitis found at least one CSF abnormality in 41%, including pleocytosis in 17% and elevated protein in 28% of cases. A later study by another group had similar results with 32 patients reported pleocytosis in 16% and elevated protein in 16% of cases.[35] Unfortunately, neither study reported the range of pleocytosis, protein elevation or on any IgG index abnormalities.

Contactin-Associated Protein-Like 2 (CASPR2)

CASPR2 is a transmembrane cell adhesion molecule expressed in the cerebral cortex, basal ganglia, limbic structures, and peripheral nervous system (PNS).[44–46] It is found predominately in the juxtaparanodal region of myelinated axons, where it interacts with Contactin-2 to form a transmembrane complex. This facilitates the clustering and organization of VGKCs

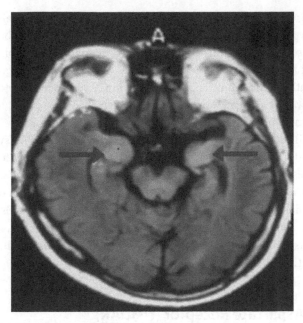

Figure 21.2 Anti-LG1I limbic encephalitis brain MRI.

Legend: 69-year-old male who presented with faciobrachial dystonia that progressed over a number of weeks to amnesia, seizure, and coma. MRI brain FLAIR demonstrates abnormal signal in bilateral hippocampus.

Source: Wang D, Hao Q, He L, Wang Q. LGI1 antibody encephalitis and psychosis. *Australas Psychiatry Bull R Aust N Z Coll Psychiatr*. 2018;26(6):612–614. doi:10.1177/1039856218771513.

and is necessary for the maintenance of the internodal resting potential and the efficient propagation of action potentials.[47–49]

Antibodies against CASPR2 disrupt the interaction between CASPR2 and Contactin-2, which interferes with the clustering of VGKC and leads to neuronal hyperexcitability.[50] As such, anti-CASPR2 antibodies are associated with a wide array of central and peripheral manifestations, although peripheral findings are much more common in anti-CASPR2 than in anti-LGI1 antibody-mediated disorders.[4,27,51] In a comprehensive meta-analysis of anti-CASPR2 cases in the literature, Boyko et al.[51] summarized the features among 667 cases from 106 publications. As we discuss this data below, an important caveat regarding frequencies reported for various features below is that this meta-analysis only included in denominators for a feature those cases/papers which mentioned that particular feature; they did not assume that the feature was not present in publications that did not mention the feature. This methodology might result in an overestimation of each feature's prevalence, so these values should be interpreted with this caution. With this caveat in mind, Boyko et al. noted the most common clinical syndromes were autoimmune encephalitis (AE) (52%) or autoimmune limbic encephalitis (ALE) (39%), isolated peripheral nerve hyperexcitability/neuromyotonia (38%), Morvan's syndrome (23%), and a cerebellar syndrome (15%). Morvan's syndrome is typically characterized by peripheral nerve hyperexcitability, autonomic instability, and encephalopathy, which historically was called Morvan's fibrillary chorea because of the appearance of the muscle movements or neuromyotonia. Movement disorders are present in at least ¼ of patients and can include gait disturbances, cerebellar dysfunction/ataxia, myoclonus, tremor, chorea, and parkinsonism, but not FBDS, which appears only in anti-LGI1 disorders.[51] The most common presenting symptoms for anti-CASPR2 encephalitis include seizures or epilepsy (38%–48%), neuropathic pain (35%), cognitive impairment (33%), peripheral nerve hyperexcitability/neuromyotonia (27%), and ataxia/cerebellar signs (19%). During the disease course, cognitive and psychiatric symptoms are prominent. Cognitive disturbances are present in about 33%–66% of cases. Behavioral disorders are common and include hallucinations, delusions, anxiety, depression, and other symptoms. Patients are often misdiagnosed as having new onset primary psychiatric disorders, such as bipolar disorder, schizophrenia, and other delusional disorders.[51]

Unlike anti-LGI1 syndromes, malignancy is more with anti-CASPR2 syndromes, occurring in about one-third of cases. Thymoma is the most common, present in about 20%, with other malignancies, including prostate cancer, lung adenocarcinoma, and melanoma, occurring in about 10% of cases.[51] Similar to anti-LGI1, there is a significant male predominance, with a male to female ratio of 4:1 and a median age of onset in the late-60s.[4,34,52] Diagnostic evaluation includes analysis of serum and CSF for anti-CASPR2 antibodies, although serum antibody testing is about twice as sensitive as CSF for detecting antibodies (100% vs. 50% sensitivity, respectively).[51,53,54]

N-Methyl-D-Aspartate Receptor (NMDAR)

For many years, patients whom we now know had anti-NMDA receptor (NMDAR) encephalitis were mistakenly thought to have viral encephalitis without an identifiable virus. In 2007, Dalmau and colleagues[11] however, discovered that this syndrome was an autoimmune-mediated disorder due to antibodies against the GluN1 subunit of the NMDA receptor. These autoantibodies lead to the downregulation of NMDAR, resulting in a complex neuropsychiatric syndrome followed by a very unusual movement disorder and other features.[3]

The typical disease course is characterized by progression through several stages over weeks to months.[3] The initial phase, typically occurring over the first week of illness, consists of a nonspecific viral prodrome, including headache and fever.[55,56] The second phase involves neuropsychiatric symptoms—such as auditory or visual hallucinations, delusions, depression, mania, agitation, and catatonia—often appearing within the first or second week.[55,57] Neurological features follow and can progress over weeks to months. Movement disorders are common and characteristic, manifesting as orofacial dyskinesias, limb and trunk choreoathetosis, oculogyric crisis, dystonia, and/or rigidity. Other features commonly appearing during the course of the illness include seizures, memory impairment, reduced speech output, autonomic instability, and a decreased level of consciousness.[3,14,55] Recovery can be protracted, taking months to years despite aggressive treatment. In some cases, behavioral changes, sleep disturbance, and deficits in executive functioning may persist indefinitely.[3]

Since the antibodies were determined to be the cause of this syndrome in 2007, anti-NMDAR encephalitis has been found to be one of the most common causes of encephalitis, with an incidence of 1.5 per million per year.[14] The relative high frequency of anti-NMDAR encephalitis was demonstrated by Gable et al.[58] showing in a retrospective analysis of banked samples from the California Encephalitis Project (CEP) that 41% of referred patients had anti-NMDAR antibodies as the cause of their encephalitis and not an infection. Caveats to this study are that 1) the CEP project accepts samples from and tracks cases of mostly undiagnosed (at the time samples are sent) encephalitis in California, so they are underrepresented by encephalitides that are routinely tested for and identified in the hospital, such as

HSV-1, VZV, and WNV, and 2) some viral encephalitides, such as HSV, might result in the development of NMDAR antibodies.[59] Nevertheless, this data highlights the high degree of clinical phenotypic overlap of this syndrome with viral encephalitis and supports its relatively high occurrence.

Approximately 65% of cases of anti-NMDAR encephalitis occur in persons age 18 or younger,[3] whereas presentations occurring after age 45 account for less than 5% of cases.[60] Under 30 years of age, the majority of cases occur in females (F:M, 4:1), however, in those over 30, this ratio is less pronounced (F:M, 1.2:1).[60]

Anti-NMDAR encephalitis is associated with teratoma in more than 50% of cases of females younger than age 45. In women older than age 45, the incidence of teratoma decreases to about 25%.[60] In adult men, only about 5%–8% have germ cell tumors, often testicular teratoma or less commonly perineal schwannoma.[55,60,61] Other cancers are associated with anti-NMDAR, including breast cancer, neuroendocrine tumors, pancreatic carcinoma, sex cord-stromal tumors, testicular germ-cell tumors, and small-cell lung carcinoma (SCLC).[55]

Diagnostic evaluations commonly used to assess encephalitides, such as CSF, EEG, and MRI, often show abnormalities. About 1/3 to just over ½ of cases have abnormalities on brain MRI, often with T2/FLAIR hyperintensity in the temporal lobes, cerebral cortex, cerebellum, and brainstem.[3,62] Deep structures, including the basal ganglia and thalamus, are less frequently involved[3] and brain MRI is unremarkable in about ½ to 2/3 of cases during the acute period.[3,62,63]

Electroencephalogram (EEG) is abnormal in more than 80% of cases, most commonly demonstrating diffuse background slowing consistent with encephalopathy.[64] Focal abnormalities are present in about 18% of cases and are most commonly localized to the temporal frontotemporal, or frontal regions.[64] Epileptiform discharges are present in 15% and seizures in about 9% of cases, with status epilepticus occurring in less than 3% of cases.[64] Almost 1/3 of cases have the unique finding of an "extreme delta brush" characterized by rhythmic delta activity at 1–3 Hz with superimposed bursts of beta activity at rhythmic 20–30 Hz.[65]

CSF is abnormal in about 80%–95% of cases, and includes moderate lymphocytic pleocytosis in about 70%–90% (Dalmau et al. 2019), oligoclonal bands in about 2/3 of cases,[66] and protein elevation in about ¼ to 1/3 of cases.[67] CSF findings may initially be unremarkable, but abnormalities typically arise as the disease progresses.[55] Anti-NMDAR antibodies are readily found in the CSF with a sensitivity of 100% on cell-binding assay versus a serum sensitivity of about 85%, indicating that testing CSF is necessary if the syndrome is suspected and serum testing is negative.[63,68]

Gamma-Aminobutyric Acid A Receptor (GABA$_A$R) and Gamma-Aminobutyric Acid B Receptor (GABA$_B$R)

In this section, we discuss both anti-GABA$_A$R and anti-GABA$_B$R, due to their many clinical similarities. The first case of anti-GABA$_B$R autoimmune encephalitis was identified in 2010 in association with limbic encephalitis, seizures, status-epilepticus, amnesia, disorientation, and psychiatric disturbances.[69] Four years later, a syndrome of encephalitis, seizures, and refractory status epilepticus was associated with high titers of serum and/or CSF anti-GABA$_A$R antibodies.[70] Since their initial description, GABAR antibody-associated syndromes have grown to include cerebellar ataxia, rapidly progressive dementia, catatonia, hallucinations, and opsoclonus myoclonus.[71-75]

In a recent review by Guo et al., of all 50 cases of anti-$GABA_AR$ encephalitis identified in the literature, the median age at presentation was 47 years (range, 2.5 months–88 years), 64% were adults, 36% were children, and there was no clear gender predilection.[76] Eighty-two percent of patients ($n = 41/50$) presented with seizures, 72% ($n = 36/50$) with encephalopathy, and 58% ($n = 29/50$) with both. Of those presenting with seizures, 42% developed status epilepticus during their disease course.[70,76-78] Almost 1/3 of all cases, 28% (14/50), had an associated malignancy detected by the time of diagnosis, 64% (9/14) of which was thymoma,[76] although previous reviews have also demonstrated a strong association with small cell lung cancer (SCLC).[79]

Compared to anti-$GABA_AR$, anti-$GABA_BR$ encephalitis also commonly presents with seizures but less commonly has status epilepticus and has a broader clinical presentation. In a recent meta-analysis of 94 cases of antibody-confirmed anti-$GABA_BR$ encephalitis by McKay et al.,[80] the median age of onset was slightly older than for anti-$GABA_AR$ encephalitis, at 60 years (range, 16 to 84 years, although this review excluded pediatric patients given their rarity in the literature) with a somewhat higher proportion of males to females (1.7:1). Similar to anti-$GABA_AR$, most patients present with a nonspecific seizure in 84% ($n = 79/94$) but with status epilepticus in only 10% ($n = 9/94$). Unlike anti-$GABA_AR$, anti-$GABA_BR$ has an expanded clinical spectrum that can include limbic symptoms (characterized by confusion, disorientation, or behavioral change) in 67% ($n = 51/76$) and gait ataxia/instability in 12% ($n = 11/94$). A neoplasm was detected in 50% ($n = 46/93$) of cases, slightly more common than anti-$GABA_AR$, but with 91% ($n = 42/46$) of the neoplastic cases being SCLC.[75,80]

Ancillary testing with MRI, CSF analysis, and EEG in both anti-$GABA_AR$ and anti-$GABA_BR$ often show some abnormalities. The vast majority of anti-$GABA_AR$ cases show MRI abnormalities (96%; $n = 48/50$), with most (83%; $n = 40/48$) being abnormal on the initial MRI and the majority (89%; 34/40) showing characteristic multifocal/diffuse cortical and subcortical nonenhancing T2/FLAIR hyperintense lesions (Figure 21.3) with variable involvement of the cerebellum, brainstem, and/or basal ganglia.[76] Unlike in anti-$GABA_AR$, MRI abnormalities in anti-$GABA_BR$ encephalitis are less common and less specific. MRI in anti-$GABA_BR$ encephalitis may show temporal lobe T2/FLAIR hyperintense lesions (55%; $n = 51/94$), which often are bilateral (60%; $n = 25/42$).[80] The CSF findings are much more commonly abnormal in anti-$GABA_BR$ encephalitis. A recent meta-analysis by Blinder and Lewerenz,[67] which compared anti-$GABA_AR$ and anti-$GABA_BR$ CSF abnormalities demonstrated lymphocytic pleocytosis in 33% (8/24) and 61% (68/112), elevated protein in 18% (4/22) and 43% (31/72), and the presence of oligoclonal bands in 25% (6/24) and 74% (14/19) of cases for anti-$GABA_AR$ and anti-$GABA_BR$, respectively.[67] We are not aware of data regarding the IgG index in either disorder.[76,80] The vast majority of anti-$GABA_AR$ encephalitis cases (94%) show abnormal EEG findings, with 77% having epileptiform discharges, 47% having focal or diffuse slowing, and 27% with both.[76] EEG abnormalities are much less frequent in anti-$GABA_BR$ encephalitis, with 58% (38/66) having temporal lobe seizures, interictal epileptiform abnormalities, or focal temporal slowing.[80]

Outcomes in both disorders appear similar. Based on 44 cases with reported outcomes for anti-$GABA_AR$ encephalitis, 80% have partial to full recovery, and the remaining 20% have a poor outcome, with 11% of all cases resulting in death. Outcomes seemed to be improved following both first- and second-line treatments.[76] Based on 73 cases of anti-$GABA_BR$

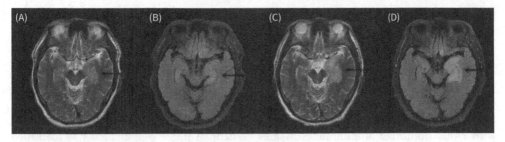

Figure 21.3 Anti-GABA_B receptor encephalitis brain MRI.

Legend: Patient presented with memory deterioration. A-B Magnetic resonance imaging (FLAIR) shows abnormal signals in the left hippocampus, as indicated by the red arrow. C-D One month later, the clinical symptoms of the patient were aggravated, and repeated magnetic resonance imaging shows an enlargement of the lesion.

Source: Zhang X, Lang Y, Sun L, Zhang W, Lin W, Cui L. Clinical characteristics and prognostic analysis of anti-gamma-aminobutyric acid-B (GABA-B) receptor encephalitis in Northeast China. *BMC Neurol*. 2020;20(1):1. doi:10.1186/s12883-019-1585-y.

encephalitis, there was a strong response to immunotherapy, with 86% resulting in partial or full recovery; 34% of these patients have a complete response.[80] Early treatment (Table 21.1) is vital to avoid severe complications and neurological sequelae.[78,81]

Glycine Receptor α1 (GlyRα1)

Anti-GlyRα1 AE was first described in 2008 in a patient with a syndrome of progressive encephalomyelitis, rigidity, and myoclonus (PERM).[82] PERM falls within a clinical spectrum that includes conditions such as "stiff-person syndrome" (SPS); both PERM and SPS historically have been associated with anti-glutamic-acid decarboxylase (GAD) 65 or 67 antibodies and are discussed in detail in the section "Glutamic Acid Decarboxylase". [83] This case was the first to show antibodies bound to GlyRα1 subunits (GlyRα1), and negative serology for anti-GAD antibodies, causing PERM.[82] Since then there have been several reports and a few series of anti-GlyR antibody-mediated encephalitis, but unfortunately, many papers do not indicate to which of the five subunits of this receptor (α1-4 and β) the antibodies were directed against. Therefore, we will use the term "glycine receptor" (GlyR) henceforth, except when papers specified the subunit.

The anti-GlyR clinical spectrum has expanded and now includes spinal/brainstem disorders and stiff person syndrome plus (SPS-plus) phenotypes. Anti-GlyR PERM/SPS-plus symptomatology includes partial or complete PERM, upper or lower motor neuron symptoms, sensory and/or autonomic dysfunction, seizures, visual hallucinations/illusions, parkinsonism, and cognitive dysfunction.[84-93] Anti-GlyR PERM/SPS syndromes are usually associated with elevated CSF anti-GlyR antibodies.[93] Although some neurologic disorders– including oculomotor disturbance, encephalopathy, and epilepsy have been reported with only serum, but negative CSF, anti-GlyR antibodies, the significance of these serum antibodies remains uncertain.[93]

In a retrospective review of 187 anti-GlyR encephalitis cases by Swayne et al. 2018, the most common presenting syndromic presentations were: PERM/SPS (painful spasms/stiffness/rigidity) (48%), epilepsy (22%), and other (30%), which included demyelination/

inflammatory lesions (12%), cerebellar ataxia/ocular motor disorders (12%), encephalitis (4%) and miscellaneous other features (2%).[94] The review implied these subgroupings were mutually exclusive, but it was not clear if some patients had mixed presentations. A comparison of the PERM/SPS with all "other" subgroups showed similar ages of onset (means 43 and 41, ranges 1–75 and 8–70, years respectively), however, the epilepsy subgroup was on average about 15 years younger (mean 27, range 1–58 years). Males and females seemed to be approximately equally represented among the subgroups. There were no strong associations with either comorbid autoimmune diseases or neoplasm.[89,94] Malignancy was identified during the evaluation in only 9% plus an additional 4% had a prior remote history of cancer (thymoma or lymphoma). Of those with cancer identified during the workup, about 60% were in the PERM/SPS group, with half being thymoma. Other current cancers included lymphoma, breast cancer, and small-cell lung cancer.[94]

Routine ancillary neurological testing in anti-GlyR mediated disorders appears to be nonspecific. MRI is typically uninformative, with nonenhancing T2/FLAIR hyperintense lesions seen in a minority of patients (7%; 13/189). EEG abnormalities are infrequently associated with anti-GlyR encephalitis cases (5%; 10/189). Of the 42 cases with epileptic seizures, only 21% showed either slowing (four cases) or epileptiform activity (five cases) on EEG.[94] Swayne et al.'s review, unfortunately, did not comment on CSF abnormalities. Carvajal-Gonzalez et al. 2014[91] reported CSF findings in 30 (of 52) anti-GlyR encephalitis cases, with 60% showing any abnormality, specifically 43% with pleocytosis, 13% with elevated protein, and 20% with oligoclonal bands. A larger study by Blinder and Lewerenz[67] confirmed these anti-GlyR encephalitis CSF abnormalities, with lymphocytic pleocytosis in 29% (18/62), elevated protein in 24% (15/62), and oligoclonal bands in 22% (14/62) (immunoglobulin [IgG] index was not reported). Although previous studies suggested anti-GlyR antibody titers tend to be higher in the CSF than the serum,[15,95] as noted above, the relationship between and relative clinical importance of serum and CSF levels of anti-GlyR is complicated and has not yet been fully elucidated.[96] Interestingly, whereas most antibodies against synaptic cell-surface or extracellular antigens are identified by both specific cell-based assays (CBAs) and the pattern of staining on IHC with animal (often rodent) brain slices, for anti-GlyR antibodies, only CBAs and not IHC appears to work.[97] According to a large literature review, the false-positive rate of anti-GlyR antibodies in healthy controls is just over 1%.[98] Based on 187 cases, Swayne et al. 2018[92,94] found that subjects response rates to immunotherapy were substantial/complete in 49%, partial in 38%, and none in 13%.

Please see Tables 21.1 and 21.2 for a summary of many other AEs with movement disorders and psychiatric features due to other extracellular and synaptic autoantibodies.

Antibodies Against Intracellular Nuclear/Cytoplasmic Antigens

Autoimmune/paraneoplastic neurological disorders targeting intracellular antigens—nuclear and cytoplasmic proteins—differ from extracellular synaptic and/or cell-surface encephalitis in several important respects, including but not limited to associations with malignancy, response to therapy, and mechanism of pathology. Given the limited accessibility autoantibodies have to intracellular antigens, many of these antibodies are thought to be associated with a cytokine and/or T-cell-mediated immune response as evidenced by lymphocytic infiltration and neuronal structure damage.[2]

The nomenclature for the intracellular antigens and their associated antibodies is complicated. The nomenclature used to name antibodies and/or their target intracellular antigens depends on the preference of the research group discovering them and historical factors. Further complicating the issue is that some identical target antigens discovered by separate groups were named with differing nomenclature (e.g., Hu = ANNA-1; Ri = ANNA-2; Yo = PCA-1).

Protocols for the testing for intracellular antibodies are somewhat laboratory specific. The highest sensitivity and specificity of a test result can be achieved by cross-validation with different test methods. Typically, tissue-based assay (TBA) screening is conducted whereby immunohistochemistry is performed on brain sections looking for specific staining patterns. If TBA has a distinct staining pattern, a line assay is performed whereby purified recombinant proteins (e.g., paraneoplastic antigens such as Hu, Ri, Yo, and others) are applied on blot strips and incubated with the patient's serum or CSF. Cut-off values for low and high anti-Hu titers are laboratory specific. Only high titers are clearly associated with the presence of a neurological syndrome, the vast majority of which are paraneoplastic.

Antineuronal Nuclear Antibody (ANNA)

In 1933, Weber and Hill[99] reported a case of subacute progressive sensory neuronopathy with complete degeneration of the posterior columns in association with a lung oat cell carcinoma. A year later, Greenfield[100] coined the term "subacute spinocerebellar degeneration" to describe the disorder. In 1949, Guichard and Vignon[101] first used the term "paraneoplastic syndrome" (PNS) to describe polyneuritis in a patient with a metastatic uterine mesenchymal tumor. In 1958, Brain and Henson[102] suggested that the disorders were linked via an immunological disturbance, a theory confirmed a short time later by Wilkinson and Zeromski.[103] They identified the first antineuronal nuclear antibody (ANNA). The ANNA was later determined not to be a single antibody but were of several types.[104] Different ANNA antibodies have since been associated with a wide variety of distinct and overlapping clinical disorders.

Naming of these antibodies has been inconsistent. Historically, many research groups identifying paraneoplastic neurological syndromes used elements of the name of the first or an early patient or the primary discoverer of the antibody/antigen, often using the first two letters of the last name (e.g., Hu, Ri, Yo, Tr, etc.). Later, there was an attempt to change the classification to descriptive nomenclatures, such as ANNA-1 (anti-Hu) and Purkinje cell cytoplasmic autoantibody type 1 (PCA-1 also known as anti-Yo).[104,105] The literature has yet to settle on consistent nomenclature for these types of earlier identified antibodies, but new antibodies are usually named based on their target antigen.

Hu (ANNA-1)
Anti-Hu (named after the first two letters of the patient's last name) paraneoplastic syndrome was first identified in 1985 in two patients with SCLC and subacute sensory polyneuropathy.[106] Three years later, the pathogenesis was confirmed to be an IgG-mediated process that targeted intracellular nuclear antigens in a patient with paraneoplastic encephalomyelitis (PEM), paraneoplastic sensory neuropathy (PSN), bulbar/cerebellar dysfunction,

myelopathy, limbic encephalitis, and autonomic dysfunction.[107] Later, anti-Hu was classified as a subtype of ANNA and a new classification system was proposed to describe ANNA subtypes depending on the reactivity pattern on different animal tissues, whereby anti-Hu became ANNA-1.[108] The literature has yet to settle on consistent nomenclature for this and several other antibodies but in the remainder of this chapter we use the term "anti-Hu."

Since the anti-Hu antibody was first recognized, it has been associated with a wide variety of neurological disturbances, including, but not limited to, limbic encephalitis,[109] PEM,[110] brainstem encephalitis,[111] opsoclonus-myoclonus,[112] and paraneoplastic cerebellar degeneration (PCD).[113] In the Dalmau et al. 1992[114] series of 71 serologically confirmed anti-Hu cases associated with PEM/PSN, neurological manifestations preceded tumor detection in 83% of patients. Multifocal involvement was more frequent than unifocal (73% vs. 27%). In this cohort, the most frequent neurological manifestations observed at the time of diagnosis included PSN (59%), PEM (41%), brainstem dysfunction (32%), cerebellar dysfunction (25%), autonomic dysfunction (28%), and lower motor neuron impairment (14%). Clinically, it is important to note that patients with sensory neuropathy or neuronopathy, such as anti-Hu PSN, may appear to have a primary movement disorder, which is in fact secondary to a loss of sensory input causing trouble in coordinating or maintaining motor function. Thus, these patients may appear to have chorea, athetosis or ataxia but it is of sensory origin.

Regarding its oncological associations, anti-Hu antibodies are by far most commonly associated with lung cancer, especially SCLC, but can occur in patients with various extrathoracic cancers.[115,116] In a 2001 study of 200 patients with anti-Hu-associated PEM, 84% ($n = 167$) had confirmed neoplasm, of whom 86% ($n = 144$) had lung cancer, mostly SCLC, and the remaining 14% had extrathoracic cancers, including prostate, breast, gastrointestinal, bladder, or ovarian cancer.[110] The Dalmau et al. 1992[114] series reported the disorder was slightly more frequent in women (55%) and had a median age at onset of 60 years (range 4–83). Although subsequent literature has confirmed anti-Hu PNS typically presents in later adulthood, there remains debate regarding the sex ratios, with a European study finding a male to female ratio of 3:1[110] and a US study finding essentially the opposite with a male to female ratio of about 1:2.[117] Cancer risk factors may differ based on sex in different populations.[115,118] Anti-Hu antibodies can also occur in patients with SCLC and other cancers without a neurological syndrome.[119,120]

The diagnostic workup for anti-Hu encephalitis/PNS includes MRI, CSF, EEG, and a neoplasm screening. In a 2011 retrospective case series by Rudzinski et al.,[121] of 28 anti-Hu seropositive patients with at least one EEG and MRI, 15 (54%) patients had focal MRI abnormalities, and 12 had sufficient T2/FLAIR hyperintense lesions restricted to the medial temporal lobes to suggest limbic encephalitis. Eighty-six percent ($n = 24$) of patients had an abnormal EEG, with about 2/3 ($n = 19$) having focal abnormalities. Forty-three percent ($n = 12$) of all patients had focal abnormalities on both EEG and MRI, with half ($n = 6$) showing abnormalities on EEG that localized to regions other than those found on MRI.[121] Unfortunately, this study did not elaborate on CSF abnormalities nor whether antibody testing was performed on serum or CSF. The Dalmau et al. 1992[114] case series reported partial CSF studies in 56 of 71 patients. Among the 50 patients with CSF protein tested, 72% had elevated protein >50 mg/dl and 34% had >100 mg/dl. Among the 17 patients in whom oligoclonal bands were tested, 71% ($n = 12$) were positive.

As with other autoantibody-mediated neurological syndromes with intracellular antigens, the prognosis of anti-Hu PNS has historically been poor. In the Graus et al.,[110] 2001 study of 200 patients with anti-Hu-associated PEM, the median survival was 11.8 months, with only 20% reaching a 3-year survival. A more recent case series and literature review, however, suggests that early diagnosis, immunotherapy, and treatment of the tumor can improve prognosis.[115] The most effective treatment for improving anti-Hu PNS symptoms is treating the associated tumor itself. Thus, the early diagnosis of a PNS, as well as any associated tumors, is imperative.

Ri (ANNA-2)

The original description of anti-Ri PNS was described in 1988 as a stereotyped form of paraneoplastic opsoclonus-myoclonus syndrome (OMS) in seven patients.[122] Since its initial recognition, the clinical phenotype has expanded to include a more heterogeneous multisystem presentation.

Two reasonably large retrospective anti-Ri cohorts have been published, one in 2003 from the United States (Mayo Clinic) with 28[123] and a more recent one from France in 2020 with 36[124] well-characterized cases. The French study identified four reportedly mutually exclusive patterns at clinical onset: cerebellar syndrome (39%), isolated tremor (25%), oculomotor disturbances (17%), and a mixture of other symptoms (19%).[124] The US study reported of the same three predominant neurological syndromes but did not note if they were mutually exclusive: cerebellar syndrome (64%), oculomotor disturbances (43%), and tremor (21%). Both cohorts reported that most cases evolved over a span of six months, unlike most other forms of PNS, which tend to develop faster.[123] The French cohort noted a subacute presentation in 61%, chronic/progressive presentation in 28%, and acute presentation in 11% of cases (defined as acute if developing in <1 week; subacute: between 1 week and 3 months; progressive: >3 months). Additionally, they reported that the clinical progression is often stepwise (78%), beginning with a subacute cerebellar syndrome, followed by symptoms suggestive of brainstem involvement (e.g., oculomotor dysfunction) and subsequent basal ganglia dysfunction (e.g., tremor, dystonia,). The US study did not comment on the frequency of subacute presentations nor on the natural progression. Both studies noted a variety of movement disorders, with the French cohort having myoclonus (28%), cervical or oromandibular dystonia (17%), and parkinsonism (17%)[124] and the US study reporting gait instability (86%), opsoclonus-myoclonus (60%), myelopathy (36%), opsoclonus (36%), myoclonus (32%), oromandibular dystonia and/or laryngospasm (25%), cervical dystonia (7%), parkinsonism (7%), and chorea (4%).

Demographics were similar between both cohorts. Women were more commonly affected than men (2:1), with a median age of onset was 66 years (range 47–87 years) and 65 (range 55–75 years) for French and US cohorts, respectively.[123,124]

Although both cohorts had a very high rate of oncological association, the frequencies of cancer types were slightly different. Of the 92% of the French cohort with cancer, breast cancer was the most common (67%), followed by lung (6%), and other types in the remaining cases (bladder cancer, mediastinal seminoma, and cancer without available histology).[124] Of the 86% of the US cohort with cancer, lung (54%) and breast (38%) were most common, with one case each of cervical and bladder cancer. The French study also conducted a literature review of 55 anti-Ri cases from 27 studies, including the 2003 US cohort, and compared them to their cohort, finding no significant difference in demographics, clinical features, or types of cancers but did find that the cohort from the literature had a lower rate of cancer (72%).[124]

CSF analysis was similar in both cohorts, typically showing at least one marker of inflammation. The French cohort had pleocytosis in 36%, increased protein in 68%, and oligoclonal bands in 80% of patients; only a single patient had normal CSF for all three parameters. Of the 19 patients in the US cohort who had CSF data available, 42% had mild lymphocytic pleocytosis in 42%, 37% had elevated protein, all had negative cytology, and they did not report oligoclonal bands nor comment on the co-occurrence of these CSF markers among patients.[123,124]

Brain imaging was similar and rarely abnormal in both cohorts. Of the 33 patients (92%) in the French study with available brain MRI results, 6 (18%) were abnormal; T2 abnormalities were found in five cases in the brainstem and in one in the globus pallidus.[124] Of the 21 patients (75%) in the US cohort with brain MRI results, four (19%) were abnormal; T2 abnormalities were present in two cases in the pons, a third case in the right insular cortex, and the fourth case in the medial temporal lobes, uncus, hemispheric white matter, and pons, with some gadolinium enhancement.[123]

Though the prognosis of anti-Ri PNS is poor, historically the literature has suggested that patients with anti-Ri PNS have a better response to treatment in comparison to anti-Hu.[123,125] Of the 17 patients in the US cohort with longitudinal follow-up data, following treatment (radiation, chemotherapy, surgery, and/or steroids in various combinations or alone) 76% improved neurologically (follow-up range 3–84 months), yet 53% (9/17) of these patients died by their last follow-up appointment (range 3–72 months).[123] The French cohort also had a relatively poor outcome. Within 12 months of disease onset, the median score on the modified Rankin Scale (mRS) was 4 (i.e., nonambulatory and assistance with most activities of daily living) and 50% of patients had died by 36 months.[124] Early treatment of anti-Ri associated cancer can variably lead to dramatic improvement, emphasizing the importance of early diagnosis, cancer identification and treatment.

Paraneoplastic Cerebellar Degeneration (PCD)

Subacute cerebellar ataxia in a patient with a known cancer is often due to metastatic invasion or other cancer complications, such as infection, coagulopathy, metabolic/nutritional deficits, or side effects of treatment.[125] When direct tumor- and treatment-related causes have been excluded, however, the patient is considered to suffer from PCD. Brouwer[126] first described PCD in 1919, but the association of cerebellar ataxia and cancer was not recognized until 1938.[127] Trotter et al.[128] first described autoantibodies reactive with cerebellar Purkinje cells in a patient's serum with Hodgkin's lymphoma and PCD. Although we have discussed antibodies above that sometimes can present with PCD, in this section we will focus on the entity of PCD, highlighting antibodies that often present with this syndrome. PCD is a heterogeneous group of related disorders that differ in their associated antibody, antigen, neoplasms, and prognosis. Diagnosis often relies on the clinical history, antibody testing, and sometimes imaging.[129,130] At least nine specific paraneoplastic antineuronal antibodies have been associated with PCD. In a Netherlands retrospective cohort of 137 PNS cases, with documented high titers (≥400) of antineuronal antibodies, 36% had PCD with the following breakdown of associated antibodies: anti-Yo (38%), anti-Hu (32%), anti-Tr (14%), anti-Ri (12%), and anti-mGluR1 (4%). Among the entire PNS cohort (n = 137), 100% of those with anti-Yo, anti-Tr, and anti-mGluR1, as well as 86% of anti-Ri, but only 18% of anti-Hu, antibodies had PCD.[125]

Greenlee and Brashear[131] first described what was later called anti-Yo (also called CDR2, CDR62, or PCA-1) associated PCD in 1983 as a high-titer antibody that targeted Purkinje cells in two patients with ovarian cancer. Anti-Yo was named based on the first initials of the last name of an index patient in a subsequent cohort described in 1985.[132-134] In a case series of 48 patients with anti-Yo-associated PCD, all patients presented with a subacute pancerebellar syndrome. Additional symptoms included dysarthria, nystagmus (primarily downbeat), mild long-tract (e.g., pyramidal) involvement, peripheral neuropathy, dysphagia, diplopia, vertigo, and cognitive impairment.[135] Patients typically presented in their 60s. Malignancy was detected in more than 90% of anti-Yo positive PCD patients, with breast and gynecological malignancies being the most common.[130,136] As anti-Yo is almost exclusively associated with breast or gynecological cancers, perhaps it is not unexpected that nearly all patients are female.[137]

The anti-Tr (also known as Delta/notch-like epidermal growth factor-related receptor [DNER]) antibody was first described in 1976 by Trotter et al.[128] in a woman with subacute PCD and Hodgkin's lymphoma. Anti-Tr was later named for Dr. Trotter.[138] The clinical presentation is often subacute ataxia with variable ALE and/or paraneoplastic optic neuropathy (PON). Anti-Tr is almost exclusively found in patients with Hodgkin's lymphoma (90%), with the remaining patients having no identifiable cancer or less commonly another form of lymphoma.[139,140] PCD precedes the diagnosis of neoplasm in most patients. Anti-Tr presents predominantly in males, with a male to female ratio of 3:1, and a median age of onset of 61 years (range, 14 to 75 years).[139]

Other ancillary testing is generally unrevealing for PCDs. Brain MRI is typically uninformative, although some case reports have described cerebellar atrophy and cerebellar/extracerebellar inflammation abnormalities.[141,142] In a review of 55 patients with anti-Yo-associated PCD, of whom 42 had CSF analysis, 83% had abnormalities, with 62% (26/42) having lymphocytic pleocytosis (> 6 WBC/mm^3) and 52% (22/42) elevated protein (48–106 mg/dl). Of the 14 patients with IgG index data, 86% (12/14) had elevated IgG index, and of the seven patients with oligoclonal band testing, 86% (6/7) were elevated.[135] In a review of 28 patients with anti-Tr-associated PCD of whom 22 had CSF analysis, 59% had mild CSF pleocytosis (median 50 WBC per dL; range 14 to 150), and they did not report protein, IGG index, or oligoclonal bands.[139]

In a retrospective review of 50 cases of PCD with high titers (≥400) of antineuronal antibodies, the functional outcome seemed to vary based on the associated antibody.[143] The vast majority of patients with anti-Yo (79%), anti-Hu (75%) and anti-Tr (57%) PCD became bedridden. Subjects with anti-Ri, however, have a better prognosis, with 83% retaining their ability to walk. The median survival of each group was as follows: anti-Hu 7, anti-Yo 13, anti-Ri greater than 69, and anti-Tr greater than 113 months. Although the majority of cases remain severely impaired despite immunotherapy, some literature suggests that if patients are diagnosed and treated early enough, some symptoms of PCD can respond to treatment of the cancer and immunotherapy.[144]

CV2/CRMP5 Antibodies

In a 1996 paper on 45 cases of suspected PNS (negative serology for anti-Hu, anti-Ri, or anti-Yo), 11 cases were identified with collapsin response-mediator protein 5 (CRMP5)/CV2 antibodies in association with lung cancer (7/11), uterine sarcoma (2/11), and malignant thymoma (2/11).[8]

A 2018 literature review of 314 cases of seropositive anti-CV2/CRMP5[9] divided this PNS into two categories: those with neuropathy (42%) and those without (50%) at the time of diagnosis, excluding 26 cases (8%) due to lack of sufficient documentation. The 156 cases without neuropathy typically had a mixed clinical presentation: 24% encephalitis, 23% cerebellar ataxia, 17% myelopathy, 15% myasthenia gravis, 11% chorea or choreoathetosis with encephalopathy, 8% optic neuritis with/without retinopathy, and 3% LEMS. The clinical presentation of the 132 cases with neuropathy at diagnosis was predominated by neuropathy/radiculopathy, although 20% of these cases had co-occurring anti-Hu antibodies, which could have explained those cases of neuropathy. The paper did not specify whether seropositivity was serum or CSF. The remaining 105 anti-CV2/CRMP5 cases with neuropathy and without anti-Hu seropositivity, had moderate to severe neuropathic pain in 79% of cases, and painful axonal polyradiculoneuropathy in 65% of cases. Other neurologic accompaniments included cerebellar ataxia (21%), myelopathy (19%), and optic neuritis and/or retinitis (11%).

The frequent association of anti-CV2/CRMP5 with anti-Hu, and less commonly other intracellular antinuclear, autoantibodies at times has obscured specific syndromic classification for anti-CV2/CRMP5 and at times called into question whether anti-CV2/CRMP5 antibodies had a defined syndrome, which it clearly does. Perhaps the most thorough attempt to address this issue was a study[145] comparing 37 patients with only anti-CV2/CRMP5 to 324 patients with only anti-Hu antibodies. Anti-CV2/CRMP5 PNS was more frequently associated with cerebellar ataxia, chorea, uveitis/retinitis, and myasthenic syndrome (LEMS or MG). In contrast, anti-Hu was more frequently associated with dysautonomia, brainstem encephalitis, and peripheral neuropathy. Similar to anti-Hu, almost all (92%) of anti-CV2/CRMP5 cases were associated with a neoplasm, 62% (21/34) being small cell lung cancer.[9,145] Unlike anti-Hu, anti-CV2/CRMP5 is more often associated with malignant thymoma (15%).[9,145] Another study by Dubey et al.[9] comparing 105 anti-CV2/CRMP5 and 37 anti-Hu neuropathy cases, also confirmed that although these antibodies caused somewhat overlapping syndromes, they also have clear differences.[9]

Other ancillary testing is generally unrevealing. Various case reports and smaller case series have shown MRI T2/FLAIR symmetric hyperintensities in the caudate and putamen or in other cases, in the medial temporal lobes, all without accompanying diffusion abnormalities (as might be seen in prion disease).[145,146] One case with chorea showed FDG-PET hypometabolism in the bilateral caudate nuclei, similar to Huntington's disease.[146] The EEG may or may not display epileptic foci in temporal lobes with focal or generalized slow activity.[145] In the 2018 literature review of 314 cases,[9] CSF analysis of 25 cases with isolated seropositive anti-CV2/CRMP5 showed mild pleocytosis (WBC >4/dL) in just over ½ (52%) (with 92% showing protein elevation (>50 mg/dL).[9] Data on IgG index and oligoclonal bands is lacking in published cohorts.[9,146]

One study suggested the age and sex distribution are similar between both anti-Hu and anti-CV2/CRMP5 groups with a 3:1 male to female predominance and mean ages of about 63+/-11.[145] Another study, however, on 105 anti-CV2/CRMP5 cases associated with neuropathy found females to be slightly predominant (54%).[9] Median survival appears to be much longer in in patients with anti-CV2/CRMP5 than in patients with anti-Hu or in patients with both antibodies (48 versus 12 versus 18 months, respectively).[145]

Antibodies Against Intracellular Synaptic Antigens

A third controversial group of antibody-related brain disorders is antibodies that target intracellular synaptic proteins, such as glutamic acid decarboxylase (GAD65 or GAD67) and amphiphysin. GAD65/67 and amphiphysin are nonintrinsic membrane proteins. They are concentrated in either nerve terminals or more widely distributed throughout the neuron and are associated with the protein complexes of synaptic vesicles on the cytoplasmic surface of neurons. The pathological mechanism of this form of autoimmunity is theorized to result from an antibody-mediated disruption of synaptic vesicle fusion and reuptake. Whether a T-cell-mediated pathogenic mechanism is more important than antibody-mediated mechanisms remain a topic of debate.[2]

Glutamic Acid Decarboxylase

Stiff-person syndrome (SPS) was first described in 1956 and later named in 1958.[147,148] Before 1988, there was a strong suspicion that SPS had an immunologic origin given the high prevalence of comorbid diabetes (up to 35%) and other concomitant autoimmune diseases (vitiligo, celiac sprue, rheumatologic diseases).[149,150] Accordingly, when anti–glutamic acid decarboxylase (GAD) antibodies were first documented in association with SPS in 1988,[151] the association was relatively unquestioned. Controversy would later arise regarding anti-GAD's diagnostic utility given that the antibody is present in low titers in 1% of healthy people and 80% of people with type 1 diabetes mellitus.[152] Currently, it is generally accepted that it requires high titers (greater than 2000 U/mL) of anti-GAD antibodies to be considered the cause of neurological conditions such as SPS, epilepsy, and limbic encephalitis.[153,154] Accordingly, when examining a patient with a neurological disorder with anti-GAD seropositivity, clinicians should keep in mind that elevated titers of serum anti-GAD antibodies alone do not necessitate a diagnosis.[118,153]

Anti-GAD SPS is the most common and classical presentation of this antibody-mediated autoimmune disorder. SPS is characterized by an increased tone of the axial and limb musculature, with superimposed muscle spasms leading to lumbar hyperlordosis and gait impairment. SPS is grouped into the SPS-plus clinical spectrum, which includes progressive encephalomyelitis with rigidity and myoclonus (PERM).[83] In a literature review[83] of 69 autoimmune SPS-spectrum cases from the literature, of 66 cases (96%) in which serum anti-GAD antibody testing was documented i88% (58/66) had anti-GAD positivity; the second-most common antibody was GlyR, followed by several other miscellaneous antibodies. The mean age of all SPS cases, at least 84% of whom were anti-GAD, was 44 (range 1 to 78 years) with about two-thirds in their 40s–60s, and two-thirds were female. To the best of our knowledge, malignancy associated with anti-GAD SPS (without comorbid autoantibodies) remains a rare phenomenon in the literature aside from a few case reports.[83]

Anti-GAD cerebellar ataxia (CA) is the second-most common neurological syndrome associated with positive serum anti-GAD after SPS.[155] In a retrospective cohort[156] of 34 cases of anti-GAD CA compared to 28 cases of anti-GAD SPS, all anti-GAD CA cases presented with a pancerebellar syndrome with about one-quarter (26%) presenting with coexisting SPS. Additional symptoms included gait ataxia in 91%, limb ataxia in 74%, dysarthria in 70%, and nystagmus in 59%, and 26% reported episodes of transient brainstem dysfunction (vertigo, nystagmus, or dysphagia). The demographic features were similar between anti-GAD CA and anti-GAD SPS groups. The median age of onset was 58 years (range 33–80 years) and 56 years (range 19–77), and the percent female was 82% and 93% for the anti-GAD CA and SPS groups, respectively. Cancer was uncommon in both anti-GAD groups, detected in 12% (4/34) of the CA cases (thymoma, endometrial carcinoma, breast cancer, and myelodysplastic syndrome) and essentially none of the SPS cases. Two other neurological syndromes less commonly associated with high-titer anti-GAD antibodies are encephalopathy and/or epilepsy.[157] Unfortunately, we are unaware of any studies that have systematically characterized the MRI and/or EEG abnormalities associated with anti-GAD SPS or CA. In the retrospective review[158] of 19 cases of anti-GAD associated with epilepsy, MRI brain abnormalities included cortical/subcortical parenchymal T2 hyperintensity (58%), parenchymal atrophy (47%), and/or abnormal hippocampal signal (26%) on their first or follow-up MRI (Figure 21.4). The majority of subjects had focal onset complex partial seizures, often originating in the temporal lobes on EEG (17/19; 89%) of which 58% (11/19) were bilateral.[158] Unfortunately, there appears to be a paucity of studies on MRI, CSF, and other ancillary testing in anti-GAD SPS, CA, and encephalopathy syndromes. In the retrospective cohort of 34 cases of anti-GAD CA,[156] of the 74% (25/34) with long-term follow-up, 80% (20/25) received immunotherapy as follows: 10 IVIG; 9 IV methylprednisolone either alone (4) or in combination with IVIg (4) or rituximab (1); and one oral prednisone. Six months following the start of therapy, 50% of treated patients showed clinical improvement (≥1 point decrease on mRS) that persisted in 35% until their last appointment. Thus, patients with anti-GAD CA have some, but limited, improvement with immunotherapy.

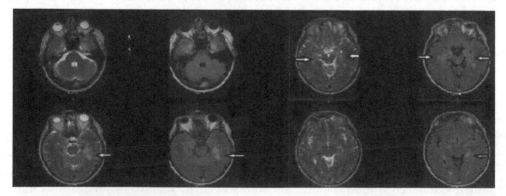

Figure 21.4 Anti-GAD encephalitis brain MRI.

Legend: 59-year-old man presented with transient sensory disturbance, fatigue, dizziness, and anxiety that progressed over a number of weeks to amnesia, confusion, eye twitching, and seizure. MRI brain demonstrates T2 hyperintensities and signal changes in bilateral hippocampi, anterior subtemporal regions as two small areas in the left mesial temporal regions. There was a mild degree of swelling in these areas without any restricted diffusion and no contrast enhancement.

Source: Mansoor S, Murphy K. Anti-GAD-associated limbic encephalitis: an unusual clinical manifestation from northwest of Ireland. *Egypt J Neurol Psychiatry Neurosurg*. 2020;56(1):23. doi:10.1186/s41983-020-0160-1.

Amphiphysin

In 1993, antiamphiphysin PNS was first identified in a woman with SPS and breast carcinoma.[159] Subsequent cohorts have expanded the associated neurological impairments and oncological associations. In a retrospective cohort of 63 patients seropositive for antiamphiphysin, the majority of subjects were female (60%), and the mean age of onset was 64 (range 46–87 years of age). Neurological manifestation at diagnosis included neuropathy (53%: 55% of women, 48% of men), partial SPS/PERM (29%: 39% of women, 12% of men), full criteria SPS (8%; 10% of women, 4% of men), encephalopathy/encephalitis (30%), myelopathy (27%), cerebellar syndrome (29%), myoclonus (10%), and LEMS (8%). The specificity of antiamphiphysin clinical symptomatology is unfortunately obscured given its frequent (68%) association with one or more coexisting autoantibodies.[159, 160]

Antiamphiphysin-associated pure SPS (without PERM) is rare (<10% of SPS cases) in comparison to anti-GAD-[161] and anti-GlyR-associated SPS.[93,96] Unlike anti-GAD-associated SPS, which typically presents with a stiffness that predominantly affects the thoracolumbar musculature, antiamphiphysin SPS typically presents with a pattern of stiffness that is more broadly distributed and more likely to involve the arms and neck. Additionally, whereas anti-GAD-associated SPS is uncommonly cancer-associated, antiamphiphysin SPS is frequently associated with cancer, particularly breast and SCLC.[161,162] Unfortunately, we are not aware of any formal comparisons of anti-Gly SPS with anti-GAD and antiamphiphysin in the literature, but anti-Gly SPS appears to have similar features as anti-GAD SPS (stiffness predominantly affects thoracolumbar musculature and has a low association with malignancy),[93] but has a stronger association with supratentorial dysfunction such as epilepsy.[96] Please see the section "Glycine Receptor α1" for further details distinguishing anti-Gly SPS from other types of SPS.

Regarding ancillary testing, in a retrospective cohort of antiamphiphysin-associated neurological disorders, only 7% (2/27) of subjects with brain MRIs were reported as abnormal.[160] In the same cohort, of 28 cases with CSF analysis, 61% were abnormal, with either pleocytosis (46%; 13/28), elevated protein (36%, 10/28), and/or oligoclonal bands (18%, 5/28). Unfortunately, this review did not document how many patients had multiple CSF abnormalities.[160]

Autoimmune Associated Disorders—Not Associated With Antibodies or of Controversial or Unclear Etiology

Suspected Autoimmune Syndromes Without Clearly Identified Antibodies

In some cases, an autoimmune or even antibody-mediated movement disorder and/or encephalitis is suspected despite extensive commercially available antibody testing (and even IHC on animal brain slices done in a commercial or research lab) being negative. In such cases, it should be determined if the patient satisfies consensus criteria for possible autoimmune encephalitis (see Box 21.1 Section A).[118]

Box 21.1 Diagnostic Criteria[118]

A. Diagnosis of *possible* autoimmune encephalitis

Diagnosis can be made when all three of the following criteria have been met:

1. Subacute onset (rapid progression of less than 3 months) of working memory deficits (short-term memory loss), altered mental status,* or psychiatric symptoms
2. At least one of the following:
   - New focal CNS findings
   - Seizures not explained by a previously known seizure disorder
   - CSF pleocytosis (white blood cell count of more than five cells per mm³)
   - MRI features suggestive of encephalitis†
3. Reasonable exclusion of alternative causes**

*Altered mental status defined as decreased or altered level of consciousness, lethargy, or personality change. †Brain MRI hyperintense signal on T2-weighted fluid-attenuated inversion recovery sequences highly restricted to one or both medial temporal lobes (limbic encephalitis), or in multifocal areas involving gray matter, white matter, or both compatible with demyelination or inflammation.

**CNS infections, Septic encephalopathy, Metabolic encephalopathy, Drug toxicity, Cerebrovascular disease, Neoplastic disorders, Creutzfeldt-Jakob disease, Epileptic disorders, Rheumatologic disorders (e.g., lupus, sarcoidosis, other), Kleine-Levin, Reye syndrome(children), Mitochondrial diseases, Inborn errors of metabolism (children).

B. Diagnostic criteria for *definite* autoimmune limbic encephalitis.

Diagnosis can be made when all four* of the following criteria have been met:

1. Subacute onset (rapid progression of less than 3 months) of working memory deficits, seizures, or psychiatric symptoms suggesting involvement of the limbic system
2. Bilateral brain abnormalities on T2-weighted fluid-attenuated inversion recovery MRI highly restricted to the medial temporal lobes†
3. At least one of the following:
   - CSF pleocytosis (white blood cell count of more than five cells per mm³)
   - EEG with epileptic or slow-wave activity involving the temporal lobes
4. Reasonable exclusion of alternative causes (See Graus et al. 2016, appendix[118])

*If one of the first three criteria is not met, a diagnosis of definite limbic encephalitis can be made only with the detection of antibodies against cell-surface, synaptic, or onconeural proteins.

†[118]Fluorodeoxyglucose (¹⁸F-FDG) PET can be used to fulfill this criterion. Results from studies from the past 5 years suggest that ¹⁸F-FDG-PET imaging might be more sensitive than MRI to show an increase in FDG uptake in normal-appearing medial temporal lobes.

C. Diagnostic criteria for Hashimoto's encephalopathy.

Diagnosis can be made when all six of the following criteria have been met:

1. Encephalopathy with seizures, myoclonus, hallucinations, or stroke-like episodes
2. Subclinical or mild overt thyroid disease (usually hypothyroidism)
3. Brain MRI normal or with nonspecific abnormalities
4. Presence of serum thyroid (thyroid peroxidase, thyroglobulin) antibodies*
5. Absence of well-characterized neuronal antibodies in serum and CSF
6. Reasonable exclusion of alternative causes

*There is no disease-specific cutoff value for these antibodies (detectable in 13% of healthy individuals)

D. Criteria for autoantibody-negative but probable autoimmune encephalitis.

Diagnosis can be made when all four of the following criteria have been met:

1. Rapid progression (less than 3 months) of working memory deficits (short-term memory loss), altered mental status, or psychiatric symptoms
2. Exclusion of well-defined syndromes of autoimmune encephalitis (e.g., typical limbic encephalitis, Bickerstaff's brainstem encephalitis, acute disseminated encephalomyelitis)
3. Absence of well-characterized autoantibodies in serum and CSF, and at least two of the following criteria:
   - MRI abnormalities suggestive of autoimmune encephalitis*
   - CSF pleocytosis, CSF-specific oligoclonal bands or elevated CSF IgG index, or both*
   - Brain biopsy showing inflammatory infiltrates and excluding other disorders (e.g., tumor)
4. Reasonable exclusion of alternative causes

*Some inherited mitochondrial and metabolic disorders can present with symmetric or asymmetric MRI abnormalities and CSF inflammatory changes resembling an acquired autoimmune disorder.

Autoimmune-Mediated Movements Disorders Associated With Other Syndromes or Conditions

Systemic Lupus Erythematosus

Systemic lupus erythematosus (SLE or "lupus") is a chronic autoimmune disease characterized by multisystem organ involvement and thus has a wide array of clinical manifestations.[163]

The first known description of SLE was by Hippocrates (460–375 BC),[164] though modern understanding of the disease began in the late-1950s with the discovery of antinuclear antibodies and recognition that SLE was an autoimmune process. Additional antibodies associated with SLE were described subsequently, including anti-Smith (Sm), anti-Sjögren's syndrome-related antigen A (SSA/Ro), anti-Sjögren's syndrome-related antigen B (SSB/La), and anti-phospholipid antibodies—namely anticardiolipin antibody (aCL), lupus anticoagulant (LA), and anti-β_2 glycoprotein 1 antibody (β_2GP1).[165–167]

SLE overwhelmingly affects women, with a female to male ratio of about 4:1, and the peak prevalence occurs between the ages 40 to 49 in women and 60 to 69 in men.[168–170] Although the clinical presentation of SLE is highly variable, multiorgan dysfunction is typical and may include mucocutaneous, vascular, cardiac, pulmonary, gastrointestinal, renal, and ophthalmologic involvement. SLE may have neurological and neuropsychiatric manifestations, including cognitive dysfunction, stroke, seizure, headache, neuropathy, mood disorder, and psychosis.[170,171] Movement disorders are less common, occurring in less than 7% of patients,[172] with chorea being the most common movement disorder and typically associated with an anticardiolipin (aCL) antibody.[173–175] Rarely, parkinsonism, ataxia, tremor, focal dystonia, or tics may occur.[172,176]

The pathogenesis of SLE is complex and multifactorial, evidenced by the presence of multiorgan involvement and a broad range of clinical presentations. The exact mechanism remains unclear, though evidence has implicated anti-DNA immune complex formation, complement activation, and an underlying genetic predisposition to the disease.[177–180]

Hashimoto's Encephalopathy

Hashimoto's encephalopathy (HE), also sometimes referred to as steroid-responsive encephalopathy associated with autoimmune thyroiditis (SREAT), was first described in 1966 by Brain et al.[181] HE typically presents as subacute encephalopathy with seizures, myoclonus, hallucinations, or stroke-like episodes. Subclinical or mild thyroid disease is often present with a notable elevation of serum anti-thyroperoxidase (TPO) and/or thyroglobulin (TG) antibodies.[118] Other common clinical features of HE include transient aphasia, tremor, myoclonus, ataxia, sleep disturbance, headache, motor or sensory deficits, persecutory delusions, and depression.[182,183] Females are disproportionately affected, with a female to male ratio of about 4:1, and the age of onset is typically around 45–55 years.[183]

Laboratory evaluation for HE is often nonspecific, which is one of the problems with this diagnosis. CSF analysis often demonstrates elevated protein or sometimes mild pleocytosis.[183] EEG reveals diffuse slowing consistent with encephalopathy in the majority of cases. Epileptiform activity is found in fewer than 20% of cases.[183] Brain MRI is typically normal, though some patients have reported subcortical white matter T2 hyperintensities or enhancement of the meninges.[184]

For several reasons, this diagnosis is very controversial, and many experts feel that it is overdiagnosed. First, these antibodies are found in about 13% of the normal population and even higher in older, particularly female, adults.[118] Second, there is no compelling evidence that the TPO or TG antibodies are causative of neuronal dysfunction in vitro or when given exogenously in vivo to animals. Third, many cases historically diagnosed as HE in retrospect were due to other anti–central nervous system antibodies that had not been detected either because they were not tested or were not yet discovered, and therefore assays were not yet available. Despite many referrals for this suspected entity to our neurobehavior and autoimmune encephalopathy clinics, we have not diagnosed a case in more than a decade. We often find another cause, less commonly another antibody-mediated syndrome and more commonly we find the patient does not meet the definition of definite autoimmune encephalopathy (see Box 21.1 Section B) and has a neurodegenerative disorder. When considering this diagnosis, we, therefore, recommend having a broad differential and ensuring the patient meets strict consensus criteria for HE.[118]

Pediatric Autoimmune Neuropsychiatric Disorders Associated With Streptococcal Infections (PANDAS) and Pediatric Acute-Onset Neuropsychiatric Syndrome (PANS)

In the late-1990s, Swedo et al.[185,186] reported a group of children, typically between three years of age and the onset of puberty, who developed sudden-onset obsessive-compulsive disorder (OCD) and tic disorders following group A streptococcal (GAS) infection. Other neurologic abnormalities, particularly choreiform movements, were also common. This entity was initially termed *pediatric autoimmune neuropsychiatric disorders associated with streptococcal infections* (PANDAS) but has since been described more broadly as a *pediatric acute-onset neuropsychiatric syndrome* (PANS) as other infectious causes, notably mycoplasma pneumoniae, influenza, Epstein-Barr virus, and *Borrelia burgdorferi*, have been associated with PANDAS-like symptoms.[187] Diagnostic criteria for PANS were proposed in 2012[188] and include prepubertal, sudden onset of OCD or severely restricted food intake and at least two supporting features (anxiety, emotional lability, depression, irritability, aggression, oppositional behavior, developmental regression, ADHD-like symptoms, memory deficits, sensory or motor abnormalities, and somatic symptoms).[187]

Evidence of a pathophysiological mechanism leading to symptoms of PANDAS/PANS is inconclusive and very controversial.[189] Some experts suspect that the etiology of PANDAS/PANS is similar to that of Sydenham chorea; GAS infection gives rise to antineuronal antibodies that target the basal ganglia,[190] though the evidence is unclear. The controversial Cunningham Panel™—measuring levels of autoantibodies directed against D1 receptors (D1R), D2^{Low} receptors (D2LR), lysoganglioside GM1, and tubulin as well as calcium-dependent calmodulin protein kinase II (CaMKII) activation–was introduced in 2013 in the United States to aid in the diagnosis of autoimmune neuropsychiatric disease,[191] but its diagnostic value is highly questionable.[191-196] In our experience and that of many of our autoimmune neurology colleagues, it has many false positives, and we do not use it. When evaluating a patient for suspected PANS, it is critical to apply the criteria for autoimmune encephalitis or movement disorders and make sure to consider other possible etiologies, autoimmune or otherwise.

Approach to Antibody Testing

The approach to antibody testing for autoimmune movement disorders, particularly with psychiatric features, often includes conditions with encephalitis, and thus, we discuss testing for both. Suspicion of autoimmune encephalitis or movement disorder begins with a clinical history suggestive of subacute/rapid syndrome evolution, evidence of CNS dysfunction, and the exclusion of key differential diagnoses (see Box 21.1 Section A).[118,197] Mimics of autoimmune encephalitis should be excluded if possible before immunotherapy begins (unless the clinical and ancillary testing are pathognomonic of a syndrome), particularly if conditions that could be aggravated by, such as infections, or made more difficult to diagnose, such as lymphoma, are possible. Usually, a detailed clinical and family medical history, complete general and neurological examination, routine blood and CSF analysis, and brain MRI, including contrast and diffusion sequences, are sufficient to rule out common mimics. For AE, the most frequent differential diagnoses are herpes simplex virus encephalitis and other CNS infections. Previous reviews have addressed the differential diagnosis of infectious encephalitis.[3,118]

Diagnosing autoimmune-mediated encephalitis and movement disorders is often complicated by several factors, such as the availability and cost, as well as which fluid (CSF vs. blood) has the highest diagnostic accuracy for certain antibody testing. We recommend using broad panels of autoantibodies based on the predominant syndrome(s) (e.g., ataxia, chorea, encephalopathy, etc.), although in cases with virtually pathognomonic syndromes (e.g., anti-NMDAR and anti-LGI1 encephalitis) or symptoms (FBDS in anti-LGI1, Morvan's in anti-CASPR2), sending for specific antibodies is not unreasonable (Table 21.1). Various assays are used to detect antibodies, each with different advantages and shortcomings (Figure 21.1).

One confusing aspect is how to define a positive test. Currently, testing methods vary significantly between laboratories. Screening procedures in the most highly regarded commercial laboratories often include a screening of serum and/or CSF with immunohistochemistry on animal brain slices (usually a rodent, but some labs also use a monkey brain depending on the clinical syndrome), followed by Western blots, radioimmunoassays, and/or CBAs. For many antibodies, the staining pattern on animal brain slices is virtually pathognomonic allowing one to go directly to a second, confirmatory, test, such as a CBA. CBAs usually use human embryonic kidney (HEK) cells and test the sample on two sets of cells, one that does not (negative control) and another that does express the antigen of interest (positive control); the test is positive if the sample of interest is positive (i.e., fluoresces) only on the cell line expressing the antigen.[6] If results from different methods are conflicting, some laboratories may then test the sample on live cultured neurons or glia (depending on the antigen target) to assess the pattern of staining.[35] An advantage of CBAs is that as living, nonfixed cells, express the antigen in its natural three-dimensional state, whereas IHC on brain tissue and Western blots express denatured proteins.

When possible, antibody testing for autoimmune encephalitis should be performed on both CSF and serum samples, as some antibodies have higher sensitivity in one tissue. Importantly, false positives occur with these assays, even CBAs, albeit less commonly, which is why it is important to be cautious about overreliance on these test results and to ensure the positive test result is consistent with the syndrome. The clinical syndrome should meet the criteria for an antibody-mediated neurological process (see Box 21.1 Section A), be consistent with the antibody identified, and have confirmatory testing by another method (Figure 21.5).[197] Criteria for diagnosing autoantibody-negative but probable autoimmune-mediated disorders are shown in Box 21.1 Section D; in such cases that are clinically convincing for an autoimmune etiology, treatment for an autoimmune condition might be considered. Even in the rapidly evolving era of antibody-mediated syndromes, bedside assessment and clinical judgment remain paramount.

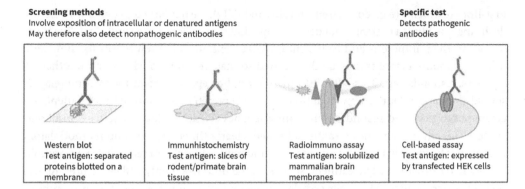

Figure 21.5 The different test systems for antibody detection.

Legend: HEK = human embryonic kidney cell.

Source: Balint B, Vincent A, Meinck H-M, Irani SR, Bhatia KP. Movement disorders with neuronal antibodies: syndromic approach, genetic parallels and pathophysiology. *Brain*. 2018;141(1):13–36. doi:10.1093/brain/awx189.

Treatment

Current treatment recommendations are based largely on retrospective series and expert opinion.[197] The current approach includes immunotherapy as well as identification and re-moval of any immunologic trigger, such as neoplasm, if present. For paraneoplastic cases, early cancer treatment is often vital in mitigating long-term morbidity and improving the overall outcome.[14,63,198]

The clinical benefit of immunomodulatory treatment varies not only between the category of antibody type (i.e., intracellular vs. extracellular antigen) but also the specific antibody. Responsiveness to immunomodulatory treatment is generally as follows: extracellular or cell-surface antigen >> intracellular cytoplasmic surface of a synaptic protein antigen (e.g., GAD, amphiphysin) >> intracellular antigen targets (Table 21.1). Furthermore, the stage of disease matters; patients with active disease (e.g., symptoms still progressing or active central nervous system inflammation, such as CSF pleocytosis or MRI hyperintensities) respond better than those later in the disease course.[14,199]

Unfortunately, there are no large, randomized controlled trials comparing treatments for these antibody-mediated AE and movement disorders.[200] Therefore, current treat-ment recommendations are largely based on expert clinical opinion, observational studies, or consensus opinion, which include comprehensive algorithms.[118,201,202] Perhaps the largest set of observational data from is anti-NMDAR encephalitis. In the Titulaer et al.[63] multi-institutional observational study of 577 cases of anti-NMDAR encephalitis, 53% of patients responded to first-line immunotherapy (steroids, IVIg, or plasma exchange alone or combined) or tumor removal, resulting in improvement within four weeks. Of the 47% of patients who failed first-line therapy, those who underwent more aggressive immunosup-pression with a second-line agent (e.g., rituximab or cyclophosphamide) had significantly better outcomes than those who did not. If a patient is responsive to treatment, the continu-ation of these treatments is recommended.[14,199] For anti-LGI1 AE encephalitis, the first-line therapy with the best treatment response appears to be high-dose steroids (e.g., 1 gm/day IV methylprednisolone for five days), which is often followed by a slow oral steroid taper over weeks to months or monthly IV steroid pulses.[201] Some experts recommend combining first-line treatments (e.g., concurrent steroids and IVIg), particularly if patients with AE are declining quickly. If a patient is not declining quickly, we prefer to use a single first-line treatment and then, if there is an insufficient improvement, to wait a few weeks to allow for a delayed response before trying another second so that we know to which immunotherapy a patient responds best. This latter information can be very important for treating relapses should they occur. Our review of anti-GABA$_A$ encephalitis cases showed that patients receiving both first- and second-line immunotherapies seemed to lead to better overall outcomes. Though the current literature is limited, clearly timely use of immunomodulatory therapy has been shown to improve outcomes and reduces the risk of relapses.[14] For example, in anti-LGI1 disease, early treatment, such as at the time when only FBDS are present, can prevent progression to AE.[203] Nevertheless, first- or second-line treatment even months or occasionally years after onset can lead to improvement in some cases.[1] As relapses can occur, varying depending on the antibody, maintenance therapy with steroid-sparing agents, such as mycophenolate mofetil, azathioprine, or rituximab, is usually recommended, typically for one to a few years, as tolerated.[118,201,202]

Regardless of the specific syndrome, prompt immunotherapy has been associated with a favorable outcome as spontaneous clinical improvement is uncommon. Though the classic course of autoimmune encephalitis is typically monophasic, relapses may occur, particularly after immunotherapy is reduced or discontinued. Regular tumor surveillance, usually every six months for up to four years, for patients with antibodies that are more often associated with cancer[204] is of the utmost importance as the relapse rate, and prognosis often depends on the tumor status and corresponding autoimmune encephalitis subtype.[4,14,63,204]

Conclusion

The field of autoimmune/antibody-mediated AE with movement disorders and neuropsychiatric features is ever-expanding. Clinicians need to be aware of these conditions in order to know when to consider and test for them, as many are treatable if not reversible. Improved awareness and understanding of these disorders will help with early identification and prompt treatment, thereby reducing long-term morbidity and mortality.

References

1. Irani SR, Gelfand JM, Al-Diwani A, Vincent A. Cell-surface central nervous system autoantibodies: clinical relevance and emerging paradigms. *Ann Neurol.* 2014;76(2):168–184. https://doi.org/10.1002/ana.24200

2. Lancaster E, Dalmau J. Neuronal autoantigens—pathogenesis, associated disorders and antibody testing. *Nat Rev Neurol.* 2012;8(7):380–390. https://doi.org/10.1038/nrneurol.2012.99

3. Dalmau J, Armangué T, Planagumà J, et al. An update on anti-NMDA receptor encephalitis for neurologists and psychiatrists: mechanisms and models. *Lancet Neurol.* 2019;18(11):1045–1057. https://doi.org/10.1016/S1474-4422(19)30244-3

4. Gadoth A, Pittock SJ, Dubey D, et al. Expanded phenotypes and outcomes among 256 LGI1/CASPR2-IgG–positive patients. *Ann Neurol.* 2017;82(1):79–92. https://doi.org/10.1002/ana.24979

5. Pittock SJ, Kryzer TJ, Lennon VA. Paraneoplastic antibodies coexist and predict cancer, not neurological syndrome. *Ann Neurol.* 2004;56(5):715–719. https://doi.org/10.1002/ana.20269

6. Balint B, Vincent A, Meinck H-M, Irani SR, Bhatia KP. Movement disorders with neuronal antibodies: syndromic approach, genetic parallels and pathophysiology. *Brain.* 2018;141(1):13–36. https://doi.org/10.1093/brain/awx189

7. Ricken G, Schwaiger C, De Simoni D, et al. Detection methods for autoantibodies in suspected autoimmune encephalitis. *Front Neurol.* 2018;9: 841. https://doi.org/10.3389/fneur.2018.00841

8. Honnorat J, Antoine JC, Derrington E, Aguera M, Belin MF. Antibodies to a subpopulation of glial cells and a 66 kDa developmental protein in patients with paraneoplastic neurological syndromes. *J Neurol Neurosurg Psychiatry.* 1996;61(3):270–278. https://doi.org/10.1136/jnnp.61.3.270

9. Dubey D, Lennon VA, Gadoth A, et al. Autoimmune CRMP5 neuropathy phenotype and outcome defined from 105 cases. *Neurology.* 2018;90(2):e103–e110. https://doi.org/10.1212/WNL.0000000000004803

10. Buckley C, Oger J, Clover L, et al. Potassium channel antibodies in two patients with reversible limbic encephalitis. *Ann Neurol.* 2001;50(1):73–78. https://doi.org/10.1002/ana.1097

11. Dalmau J, Tüzün E, Wu H, et al. Paraneoplastic anti-N-methyl-D-aspartate receptor encephalitis associated with ovarian teratoma. *Ann Neurol.* 2007;61(1):25–36. https://doi.org/10.1002/ana.21050

12. Thieben MJ, Lennon VA, Boeve BF, Aksamit AJ, Keegan M, Vernino S. Potentially reversible autoimmune limbic encephalitis with neuronal potassium channel antibody. *Neurology.* 2004;62(7):1177–1182. https://doi.org/10.1212/01.wnl.0000122648.19196.02

13. Vincent A, Buckley C, Schott JM, et al. Potassium channel antibody-associated encephalopathy: a potentially immunotherapy-responsive form of limbic encephalitis. *Brain.* 2004;127(Pt 3):701–712. https://doi.org/10.1093/brain/awh077

14. Dalmau J, Graus F. Antibody-mediated encephalitis. Ropper AH, ed. *N Engl J Med.* 2018;378(9):840–851. https://doi.org/10.1056/NEJMra1708712

15. McKeon A, Martinez-Hernandez E, Lancaster E, et al. Glycine 0. *JAMA Neurol.* 2013;70(1):44–50. https://doi.org/10.1001/jamaneurol.2013.574

16. Collingridge GL, Isaac JTR, Wang YT. Receptor trafficking and synaptic plasticity. *Nat Rev Neurosci.* 2004;5(12):952–962. https://doi.org/10.1038/nrn1556

17. Rao VR, Finkbeiner S. NMDA and AMPA receptors: old channels, new tricks. *Trends Neurosci.* 2007;30(6):284–291. https://doi.org/10.1016/j.tins.2007.03.012

18. Thompson J, Bi M, Murchison AG, et al. The importance of early immunotherapy in patients with faciobrachial dystonic seizures. *Brain.* 2018;141(2):348–356. https://doi.org/10.1093/brain/awx323

19. Gutman GA, Chandy KG, Grissmer S, et al. International Union of Pharmacology. LIII. Nomenclature and molecular relationships of voltage-gated potassium channels. *Pharmacol Rev.* 2005;57(4):473–508. https://doi.org/10.1124/pr.57.4.10

20. Dodson PD, Forsythe ID. Presynaptic K+ channels: electrifying regulators of synaptic terminal excitability. *Trends Neurosci.* 2004;27(4):210–217. https://doi.org/10.1016/j.tins.2004.02.012

21. Rudy B, Maffie J, Amarillo Y, et al. Voltage Gated Potassium Channels: Structure and Function of Kv1 to Kv9 Subfamilies. In: *Encyclopedia of Neuroscience.* Elsevier; 2009:397–425. https://doi.org/10.1016/B978-008045046-9.01630-2

22. Shillito P, Molenaar PC, Vincent A, et al. Acquired neuromyotonia: Evidence for autoanti-bodies directed against K+ channels of peripheral nerves. *Ann Neurol.* 1995;38(5):714–722. https://doi.org/10.1002/ana.410380505

23. Hart IK, Waters C, Vincent A, et al. Autoantibodies detected to expressed K+ channels are implicated in neuromyotonia. *Ann Neurol.* 1997;41(2):238–246. https://doi.org/10.1002/ana.410410215

24. Hart IK, Maddison P, Newsom-Davis J, Vincent A, Mills KR. Phenotypic variants of auto-immune peripheral nerve hyperexcitability. *Brain.* 2002;125(8):1887–1895. https://doi.org/10.1093/brain/awf178

25. Lee EK, Maselli RA, Ellis WG, Agius MA. Morvan's fibrillary chorea: a paraneoplastic man-ifestation of thymoma. *J Neurol Neurosurg Psychiatry.* 1998;65(6):857–862. https://doi.org/10.1136/jnnp.65.6.857

26. Liguori R, Vincent A, Clover L, et al. Morvan's syndrome: peripheral and central nervous system and cardiac involvement with antibodies to voltage-gated potassium channels. *Brain.* 2001;124(12):2417–2426. https://doi.org/10.1093/brain/124.12.2417

27. Irani SR, Alexander S, Waters P, et al. Antibodies to Kv1 potassium channel-complex proteins leucine-rich, glioma inactivated 1 protein and contactin-associated protein-2 in limbic en-cephalitis, Morvan's syndrome and acquired neuromyotonia. *Brain.* 2010;133(9):2734–2748. https://doi.org/10.1093/brain/awq213

28. Lai M, Huijbers MGM, Lancaster E, et al. Investigation of LGI1 as the antigen in limbic encephalitis previously attributed to potassium channels: a case series. *Lancet Neurol.* 2010;9(8):776–785. https://doi.org/10.1016/S1474-4422(10)70137-X

29. Petit-Pedrol M, Sell J, Planagumà J, et al. LGI1 antibodies alter Kv1.1 and AMPA receptors changing synaptic excitability, plasticity and memory. *Brain.* 2018;141(11):3144–3159. https://doi.org/10.1093/brain/awy253

30. Ohkawa T, Fukata Y, Yamasaki M, et al. Autoantibodies to epilepsy-related LGI1 in limbic encephalitis neutralize LGI1-ADAM22 interaction and reduce synaptic AMPA receptors. *J Neurosci.* 2013;33(46):18161–18174. https://doi.org/10.1523/JNEUROSCI.3506-13.2013

31. Fukata Y, Lovero KL, Iwanaga T, et al. Disruption of LGI1–linked synaptic complex causes abnormal synaptic transmission and epilepsy. *Proc Natl Acad Sci.* 2010;107(8):3799–3804. https://doi.org/10.1073/pnas.0914537107

32. Zhou Y-D, Lee S, Jin Z, Wright M, Smith SEP, Anderson MP. Arrested maturation of excitatory synapses in autosomal dominant lateral temporal lobe epilepsy. *Nat Med.* 2009;15(10):1208–1214. https://doi.org/10.1038/nm.2019

33. Binks SNM, Klein CJ, Waters P, Pittock SJ, Irani SR. LGI1, CASPR2 and related antibodies: a molecular evolution of the phenotypes. *J Neurol Neurosurg Psychiatry.* 2018;89(5):526–534. https://doi.org/10.1136/jnnp-2017-315720

34. van Sonderen A, Schreurs MWJ, Wirtz PW, Sillevis Smitt PAE, Titulaer MJ. From VGKC to LGI1 and Caspr2 encephalitis: The evolution of a disease entity over time. *Autoimmun Rev.* 2016;15(10):970–974. https://doi.org/10.1016/j.autrev.2016.07.018

35. van Sonderen A, Thijs RD, Coenders EC, et al. Anti-LGI1 encephalitis: clinical syndrome and long-term follow-up. *Neurology.* 2016;87(14):1449–1456. https://doi.org/10.1212/WNL.0000000000003173

36. Li W, Wu S, Meng Q, et al. Clinical characteristics and short-term prognosis of LGI1 antibody encephalitis: a retrospective case study. *BMC Neurol.* 2018;18(1):1–8. https://doi.org/10.1186/s12883-018-1099-z

37. Celicanin M, Blaabjerg M, Maersk-Moller C, et al. Autoimmune encephalitis associated with voltage-gated potassium channels-complex and leucine-rich glioma-inactivated 1 antibodies—a national cohort study. *Eur J Neurol.* 2017;24(8):999–1005. https://doi.org/10.1111/ene.13324

38. Irani SR, Pettingill P, Kleopa KA, et al. Morvan syndrome: clinical and serological observations in 29 cases. *Ann Neurol.* 2012;72(2):241–255. https://doi.org/10.1002/ana.23577

39. Finke C, Prüss H, Heine J, et al. Evaluation of cognitive deficits and structural hippocampal damage in encephalitis with leucine-rich, glioma-inactivated 1 antibodies. *JAMA Neurol.* 2017;74(1):50–59. https://doi.org/10.1001/jamaneurol.2016.4226

40. Loane C, Argyropoulos GPD, Roca-Fernández A, et al. Hippocampal network abnormalities explain amnesia after VGKCC-Ab related autoimmune limbic encephalitis. *J Neurol Neurosurg Psychiatry.* 2019;90(9):965–974. https://doi.org/10.1136/jnnp-2018-320168

41. Szots M, Blaabjerg M, Orsi G, et al. Global brain atrophy and metabolic dysfunction in LGI1 encephalitis: a prospective multimodal MRI study. *J Neurol Sci.* 2017;376:159–165. https://doi.org/10.1016/j.jns.2017.03.020

42. Kotsenas AL, Watson RE, Pittock SJ, et al. MRI findings in autoimmune voltage-gated potassium channel complex encephalitis with seizures: one potential etiology for mesial temporal sclerosis. *Am J Neuroradiol.* 2014;35(1):84–89. https://doi.org/10.3174/ajnr.A3633

43. Miller TD, Chong TT-J, Aimola Davies AM, et al. Focal CA3 hippocampal subfield atrophy following LGI1 VGKC-complex antibody limbic encephalitis. *Brain.* 2017;140(5):1212–1219. https://doi.org/10.1093/brain/awx070

44. Bellen HJ, Lu Y, Beckstead R, Bhat MA. Neurexin IV, Caspr and paranodin—novel members of the neurexin family: encounters of axons and glia. *Trends Neurosci.* 1998;21(10):444–449. https://doi.org/10.1016/S0166-2236(98)01267-3

45. Bhat MA, Rios JC, Lu Y, et al. Axon-glia interactions and the domain organization of myelinated axons requires neurexin iv/Caspr/paranodin. *Neuron.* 2001;30(2):369–383. https://doi.org/10.1016/S0896-6273(01)00294-X

46. Boyle MET, Berglund EO, Murai KK, Weber L, Peles E, Ranscht B. Contactin orchestrates assembly of the septate-like junctions at the paranode in myelinated peripheral nerve. *Neuron.* 2001;30(2):385–397. https://doi.org/10.1016/S0896-6273(01)00296-3

47. Zhou L, Messing A, Chiu SY. Determinants of excitability at transition zones in Kv1.1-deficient myelinated nerves. *J Neurosci.* 1999;19(14):5768–5781. https://doi.org/10.1523/JNEUROSCI.19-14-05768.1999

48. Hivert B, Pinatel D, Labasque M, Tricaud N, Goutebroze L, Faivre-Sarrailh C. Assembly of juxtaparanodes in myelinating DRG culture: differential clustering of the Kv1/Caspr2 complex and scaffolding protein 4.1B: juxtaparanodal assembly in myelinating culture. *Glia.* 2016;64(5):840–852. https://doi.org/10.1002/glia.22968

49. Pinatel D, Hivert B, Saint-Martin M, et al. The Kv1-associated molecules TAG-1 and Caspr2 are selectively targeted to the axon initial segment in hippocampal neurons. *J Cell Sci.* 2017;130(13):2209–2220. https://doi.org/10.1242/jcs.202267

50. Patterson KR, Dalmau J, Lancaster E. Mechanisms of Caspr2 antibodies in autoimmune encephalitis and neuromyotonia. *Ann Neurol.* 2018;83(1):40–51. https://doi.org/10.1002/ana.25120

51. Boyko M, Au KLK, Casault C, de Robles P, Pfeffer G. Systematic review of the clinical spectrum of CASPR2 antibody syndrome. *J Neurol.* 2020;267(4):1137–1146. https://doi.org/10.1007/s00415-019-09686-2

52. Binks S, Varley J, Lee W, et al. Distinct HLA associations of LGI1 and CASPR2-antibody diseases. *Brain.* 2018;141(8):2263–2271. https://doi.org/10.1093/brain/awy109

53. Bien CG, Mirzadjanova Z, Baumgartner C, et al. Anti-contactin-associated protein-2 encephalitis: relevance of antibody titres, presentation and outcome. *Eur J Neurol.* 2017;24(1):175–186. https://doi.org/10.1111/ene.13180

54. van Sonderen A, Ariño H, Petit-Pedrol M, et al. The clinical spectrum of Caspr2 antibody–associated disease. *Neurology.* 2016;87(5):521–528. https://doi.org/10.1212/WNL.0000000000002917

55. Dalmau J, Lancaster E, Martinez-Hernandez E, Rosenfeld MR, Balice-Gordon R. Clinical experience and laboratory investigations in patients with anti-NMDAR encephalitis. *Lancet Neurol.* 2011;10(1):63–74. https://doi.org/10.1016/S1474-4422(10)70253-2

56. Tominaga N, Kanazawa N, Kaneko A, et al. Prodromal headache in anti-NMDAR encephalitis: an epiphenomenon of NMDAR autoimmunity. *Brain Behav.* 2018;8(7):e01012. https://doi.org/10.1002/brb3.1012

57. Lejuste F, Thomas L, Picard G, et al. Neuroleptic intolerance in patients with anti-NMDAR encephalitis. *Neurol—Neuroimmunol Neuroinflammation.* 2016;3(5):e280. https://doi.org/10.1212/NXI.0000000000000280

58. Gable MS, Sheriff H, Dalmau J, Tilley DH, Glaser CA. The frequency of autoimmune N-methyl-D-aspartate receptor encephalitis surpasses that of individual viral etiologies in young individuals enrolled in the California Encephalitis Project. *Clin Infect Dis.* 2012;54(7):899–904. https://doi.org/10.1093/cid/cir1038

59. Salovin A, Glanzman J, Roslin K, Armangue T, Lynch DR, Panzer JA. Anti-NMDA receptor encephalitis and nonencephalitic HSV-1 infection. *Neurol Neuroimmunol Neuroinflammation.* 2018;5(4): e458. https://doi.org/10.1212/NXI.0000000000000458

60. Titulaer MJ, McCracken L, Gabilondo I, et al. Late-onset anti-NMDA receptor encephalitis. *Neurology.* 2013;81(12):1058–1063. https://doi.org/10.1212/WNL.0b013e3182a4a49c

61. Viaccoz A, Desestret V, Ducray F, et al. Clinical specificities of adult male patients with NMDA receptor antibodies encephalitis. *Neurology.* 2014;82(7):556–563. https://doi.org/10.1212/WNL.0000000000000126

62. Bacchi S, Franke K, Wewegama D, Needham E, Patel S, Menon D. Magnetic resonance imaging and positron emission tomography in anti-NMDA receptor encephalitis: A systematic review. *J Clin Neurosci.* 2018;52:54–59. https://doi.org/10.1016/j.jocn.2018.03.026

63. Titulaer MJ, McCracken L, Gabilondo I, et al. Treatment and prognostic factors for long-term outcome in patients with anti-NMDA receptor encephalitis: an observational cohort study. *Lancet Neurol.* 2013;12(2):157–165. https://doi.org/10.1016/S1474-4422(12)70310-1

64. Gillinder L, Warren N, Hartel G, Dionisio S, O'Gorman C. EEG findings in NMDA encephalitis—A systematic review. *Seizure.* 2019;65:20–24. https://doi.org/10.1016/j.seizure.2018.12.015

65. Schmitt SE, Pargeon K, Frechette ES, Hirsch LJ, Dalmau J, Friedman D. Extreme delta brush: a unique EEG pattern in adults with anti-NMDA receptor encephalitis. *Neurology.* 2012;79(11):1094–1100. https://doi.org/10.1212/WNL.0b013e3182698cd8

66. Dalmau J, Gleichman AJ, Hughes EG, et al. Anti-NMDA-receptor encephalitis: case series and analysis of the effects of antibodies. *Lancet Neurol.* 2008;7(12):1091–1098. https://doi.org/10.1016/S1474-4422(08)70224-2

67. Blinder T, Lewerenz J. Cerebrospinal fluid findings in patients with autoimmune encephalitis—a systematic analysis. *Front Neurol.* 2019;10:804. https://doi.org/10.3389/fneur.2019.00804

68. Gresa-Arribas N, Titulaer MJ, Torrents A, et al. Antibody titres at diagnosis and during follow-up of anti-NMDA receptor encephalitis: a retrospective study. *Lancet Neurol.* 2014;13(2):167–177. https://doi.org/10.1016/S1474-4422(13)70282-5

69. Lancaster E, Lai M, Peng X, et al. Antibodies to the GABA(B) receptor in limbic encephalitis with seizures: case series and characterisation of the antigen. *Lancet Neurol.* 2010;9(1):67–76. https://doi.org/10.1016/S1474-4422(09)70324-2

70. Petit-Pedrol M, Armangue T, Peng X, et al. Encephalitis with refractory seizures, status epilepticus, and antibodies to the GABAA receptor: a case series, characterisation of the antigen, and analysis of the effects of antibodies. *Lancet Neurol.* 2014;13(3):276–286. https://doi.org/10.1016/S1474-4422(13)70299-0

71. Boronat A, Sabater L, Saiz A, Dalmau J, Graus F. GABA(B) receptor antibodies in limbic encephalitis and anti-GAD-associated neurologic disorders. *Neurology.* 2011;76(9):795–800. https://doi.org/10.1212/WNL.0b013e31820e7b8d

72. Höftberger R, Titulaer MJ, Sabater L, et al. Encephalitis and GABAB receptor antibodies: novel findings in a new case series of 20 patients. *Neurology.* 2013;81(17):1500–1506. https://doi.org/10.1212/WNL.0b013e3182a9585f

73. Dogan Onugoren M, Deuretzbacher D, Haensch CA, et al. Limbic encephalitis due to GABAB and AMPA receptor antibodies: a case series. *J Neurol Neurosurg Psychiatry.* 2015;86(9):965–972. https://doi.org/10.1136/jnnp-2014-308814

74. Qiao S, Zhang Y-X, Zhang B-J, et al. Clinical, imaging, and follow-up observations of patients with anti-GABAB receptor encephalitis. *Int J Neurosci.* 2017;127(5):379–385. https://doi.org/10.1080/00207454.2016.1176922

75. van Coevorden-Hameete MH, de Bruijn MAAM, de Graaff E, et al. The expanded clinical spectrum of anti-GABABR encephalitis and added value of KCTD16 autoantibodies. *Brain.* 2019;142(6):1631–1643. https://doi.org/10.1093/brain/awz094

76. Guo C-Y, Gelfand JM, Geschwind MD. Anti-gamma-aminobutyric acid receptor type A encephalitis: a review. *Curr Opin Neurol.* 2020;33(3):372–380. https://doi.org/10.1097/WCO.0000000000000814

77. Pettingill P, Kramer HB, Coebergh JA, et al. Antibodies to GABAA receptor α1 and γ2 subunits. *Neurology.* 2015;84(12):1233–1241. https://doi.org/10.1212/WNL.0000000000001326

78. Spatola M, Petit-Pedrol M, Simabukuro MM, et al. Investigations in GABAA receptor antibody-associated encephalitis. *Neurology.* 2017;88(11):1012–1020. https://doi.org/10.1212/WNL.0000000000003713

79. Spatola M, Sabater L, Planagumà J, et al. Encephalitis with mGluR5 antibodies. *Neurology.* 2018;90(22):e1964–e1972. https://doi.org/10.1212/WNL.0000000000005614

80. McKay JH, Dimberg EL, Lopez Chiriboga AS. A systematic review of Gamma-aminobutyric acid receptor type B autoimmunity. *Neurol Neurochir Pol.* 2019;53(1):1–7. https://doi.org/10.5603/PJNNS.a2018.0005

81. Si Z, Wang A, Liu J, Zhang Z, Hu K. Typical clinical and imaging manifestations of encephalitis with anti-γ-aminobutyric acid B receptor antibodies: clinical experience and a literature review. *Neurol Sci.* 2019;40(4):769–777. https://doi.org/10.1007/s10072-018-3679-5

82. Hutchinson M, Waters P, McHugh J, et al. Progressive encephalomyelitis, rigidity, and myoclonus: a novel glycine receptor antibody. *Neurology.* 2008;71(16):1291–1292. https://doi.org/10.1212/01.wnl.0000327606.50322.f0

83. Sarva H, Deik A, Ullah A, Severt WL. Clinical spectrum of stiff person syndrome: a review of recent reports. *Tremor Hyperkinetic Mov.* 2016;6:340. https://doi.org/10.7916/D85M65GD

84. Clerinx K, Breban T, Schrooten M, et al. Progressive encephalomyelitis with rigidity and myoclonus: resolution after thymectomy. *Neurology*. 2011;76(3):303–304. https://doi.org/10.1212/WNL.0b013e318207b008

85. Mas N, Saiz A, Leite MI, et al. Antiglycine-receptor encephalomyelitis with rigidity. *J Neurol Neurosurg Psychiatry*. 2011;82(12):1399–1401. https://doi.org/10.1136/jnnp.2010.229104

86. Turner MR, Irani SR, Leite MI, Nithi K, Vincent A, Ansorge O. Progressive encephalomyelitis with rigidity and myoclonus: glycine and NMDA receptor antibodies. *Neurology*. 2011;77(5):439–443. https://doi.org/10.1212/WNL.0b013e318227b176

87. Peeters E, Vanacker P, Woodhall M, Vincent A, Schrooten M, Vandenberghe W. Supranuclear gaze palsy in glycine receptor antibody-positive progressive encephalomyelitis with rigidity and myoclonus. *Mov Disord Off J Mov Disord Soc*. 2012;27(14):1830–1832. https://doi.org/10.1002/mds.25239

88. Damásio J, Leite MI, Coutinho E, et al. Progressive encephalomyelitis with rigidity and myoclonus: the first pediatric case with glycine receptor antibodies. *JAMA Neurol*. 2013;70(4):498–501. https://doi.org/10.1001/jamaneurol.2013.1872

89. Stern WM, Howard R, Chalmers RM, et al. Glycine receptor antibody mediated progressive encephalomyelitis with rigidity and myoclonus (PERM): a rare but treatable neurological syndrome. *Pract Neurol*. 2014;14(2):123–127. https://doi.org/10.1136/practneurol-2013-000511

90. Bourke D, Roxburgh R, Vincent A, et al. Hypoventilation in glycine-receptor antibody related progressive encephalomyelitis, rigidity and myoclonus. *J Clin Neurosci*. 2014;21(5):876–878. https://doi.org/10.1016/j.jocn.2013.07.014

91. Carvajal-González A, Leite MI, Waters P, et al. Glycine receptor antibodies in PERM and related syndromes: characteristics, clinical features and outcomes. *Brain*. 2014;137(8):2178–2192. https://doi.org/10.1093/brain/awu142

92. Martinez-Hernandez E, Ariño H, McKeon A, et al. Clinical and immunologic investigations in patients with stiff-person spectrum disorder. *JAMA Neurol*. 2016;73(6):714. https://doi.org/10.1001/jamaneurol.2016.0133

93. Piquet AL, Khan M, Warner JEA, et al. Novel clinical features of glycine receptor antibody syndrome: a series of 17 cases. *Neurol Neuroimmunol Neuroinflammation*. 2019;6(5):e592. https://doi.org/10.1212/NXI.0000000000000592

94. Swayne A, Tjoa L, Broadley S, et al. Antiglycine receptor antibody related disease: a case series and literature review. *Eur J Neurol*. 2018;25(10):1290–1298. https://doi.org/10.1111/ene.13721

95. Clardy SL, Lennon VA, Dalmau J, et al. Childhood onset of stiff-man syndrome. *JAMA Neurol*. 2013;70(12):1531–1536. https://doi.org/10.1001/jamaneurol.2013.4442

96. Carvajal-González A, Leite MI, Waters P, et al. Glycine receptor antibodies in PERM and related syndromes: characteristics, clinical features and outcomes. *Brain J Neurol*. 2014;137(Pt 8):2178–2192. https://doi.org/10.1093/brain/awu142

97. McCracken LM, Lowes DC, Salling MC, et al. Glycine receptor α3 and α2 subunits mediate tonic and exogenous agonist-induced currents in forebrain. *Proc Natl Acad Sci U S A*. 2017;114(34): E7179–E7186. https://doi.org/10.1073/pnas.1703839114

98. Lang K, Prüss H. Frequencies of neuronal autoantibodies in healthy controls. *Neurol Neuroimmunol Neuroinflammation*. 2017; 4(5):e386. https://doi.org/10.1212/NXI.0000000000000386

99. Weber FP, Hill TR. Short notes and clinical cases: complete degeneration of the posterior columns of the spinal cord with chronic polyneuritis in a case of widespread carcinomatous disease elsewhere. *J Neurol Psychopathol*. 1933;14(53):57–60. https://doi.org/10.1136/jnnp.s1-14.53.57

100. Greenfield JG. Subacute spino-cerebellar degeneration occuring in elderly patients. *Brain*. 1934;57(2):161–176. https://doi.org/10.1093/brain/57.2.161

101. Guichard A, Vignon G. La polyradiculonévrite cancéreuse métastatique; paralysies multiples des nerfs craniens et rachidiens par généralisation microscopique d'un épithélioma du colutérin. *J Med Lyon*. 1949;30(700):197–207.

102. Brain R, Henson RA. Neurological syndromes associated with carcinoma: the carcinomatous neuromyopathies. *Lancet Lond Engl*. 1958;2(7054):971–975. https://doi.org/10.1016/s0140-6736(58)90471-9

103. Wilkinson PC, Zeromski J. Immunofluorescent detection of antibodies against neurones in sensory carcinomatous neuropathy. *Brain*. 1965;88(3):529–583. https://doi.org/10.1093/brain/88.3.529

104. Lennon VA. Paraneoplastic autoantibodies: the case for a descriptive generic nomenclature. *Neurology*. 1994;44(12):2236–2240. https://doi.org/10.1212/wnl.44.12.2236

105. Dalmau J, Posner JB. Neurologic paraneoplastic antibodies (anti-Yo; anti-Hu; anti-Ri): the case for a nomenclature based on antibody and antigen specificity. *Neurology*. 1994;44(12):2241-2246. https://doi.org/10.1212/wnl.44.12.2241

106. Graus F, Cordon-Cardo C, Posner JB. Neuronal antinuclear antibody in sensory neuronopathy from lung cancer. *Neurology*. 1985;35(4):538–543. https://doi.org/10.1212/wnl.35.4.538

107. Anderson NE, Budde-Steffen C, Wiley RG, et al. A variant of the anti-Purkinje cell antibody in a patient with paraneoplastic cerebellar degeneration. *Neurology*. 1988;38(7):1018--1026. https://doi.org/10.1212/wnl.38.7.1018

108. Lennon VA. Anti-Purkinje cell cytoplasmic and neuronal nuclear antibodies aid diagnosis of paraneoplastic autoimmune neurological disorders. *J Neurol Neurosurg Psychiatry*. 1989;52(12):1438–1439. https://doi.org/10.1136/jnnp.52.12.1438

109. Xu L, Hu J, Chen Q. Two cases of paraneoplastic limbic encephalitis associated with small cell lung cancer and a literature review. *Exp Ther Med*. 2015;9(2):335–340. https://doi.org/10.3892/etm.2014.2142

110. Graus F, Keime-Guibert F, Reñe R, et al. Anti-Hu-associated paraneoplastic encephalomyelitis: analysis of 200 patients. *Brain J Neurol*. 2001;124(Pt 6):1138–1148. https://doi.org/10.1093/brain/124.6.1138

111. Vigliani M-C, Novero D, Cerrato P, et al. Double step paraneoplastic brainstem encephalitis: a clinicopathological study. *J Neurol Neurosurg Psychiatry*. 2009;80(6):693–695. https://doi.org/10.1136/jnnp.2008.145961

112. Morales La Madrid A, Rubin CM, Kohrman M, Pytel P, Cohn SL. Opsoclonus-myoclonus and anti-Hu positive limbic encephalitis in a patient with neuroblastoma. *Pediatr Blood Cancer*. 2012;58(3):472–474. https://doi.org/10.1002/pbc.23131

113. Huemer F, Melchardt T, Tränkenschuh W, et al. Anti-Hu antibody associated paraneoplastic cerebellar degeneration in head and neck cancer. *BMC Cancer*. 2015;15:996. https://doi.org/10.1186/s12885-015-2020-4

114. Dalmau J, Graus F, Rosenblum MK, Posner JB. Anti-Hu-associated paraneoplastic encephalomyelitis/sensory neuronopathy: a clinical study of 71 patients. *Medicine (Baltimore)*. 1992;71(2):59–72. https://doi.org/10.1097/00005792-199203000-00001

115. Li J, Lin W. Various clinical features of patients with anti-Hu associated paraneoplastic neurological syndromes: An observational study. *Medicine (Baltimore)*. 2018;97(18):e0649. https://doi.org/10.1097/MD.0000000000010649

116. Pignolet BS, Gebauer CM, Liblau RS. Immunopathogenesis of paraneoplastic neurological syndromes associated with anti-Hu antibodies: a beneficial antitumor immune response going awry. *Oncoimmunology*. 2013;2(12):e27384. https://doi.org/10.4161/onci.27384

117. Lucchinetti CF, Kimmel DW, Lennon VA. Paraneoplastic and oncologic profiles of patients seropositive for type 1 antineuronal nuclear autoantibodies. *Neurology*. 1998;50(3):652–657. https://doi.org/10.1212/wnl.50.3.652

118. Graus F, Titulaer MJ, Balu R, et al. A clinical approach to diagnosis of autoimmune encephalitis. *Lancet Neurol*. 2016;15(4):391–404. https://doi.org/10.1016/S1474-4422(15)00401-9

119. Graus F, Dalmou J, Reñé R, et al. Anti-Hu antibodies in patients with small-cell lung cancer: association with complete response to therapy and improved survival. *J Clin Oncol Off J Am Soc Clin Oncol*. 1997;15(8):2866–2872. https://doi.org/10.1200/JCO.1997.15.8.2866

120. Senties-Madrid H, Vega-Boada F. Paraneoplastic syndromes associated with anti-Hu antibodies. *Isr Med Assoc J IMAJ*. 2001;3(2):94–103.

121. Rudzinski LA, Pittock SJ, McKeon A, Lennon VA, Britton JW. Extratemporal EEG and MRI findings in ANNA-1 (anti-Hu) encephalitis. *Epilepsy Res*. 2011;95(3):255–262. https://doi.org/10.1016/j.eplepsyres.2011.04.006

122. Budde-Steffen C, Anderson NE, Rosenblum MK, et al. An antineuronal autoantibody in paraneoplastic opsoclonus. *Ann Neurol*. 1988;23(5):528–531. https://doi.org/10.1002/ana.410230518

123. Pittock SJ, Lucchinetti CF, Lennon VA. Anti-neuronal nuclear autoantibody type 2: paraneoplastic accompaniments. *Ann Neurol*. 2003;53(5):580–587. https://doi.org/10.1002/ana.10518

124. Simard C, Vogrig A, Joubert B, et al. Clinical spectrum and diagnostic pitfalls of neurologic syndromes with Ri antibodies. *Neurol Neuroimmunol Neuroinflammation*. 2020;7(3): e699. https://doi.org/10.1212/NXI.0000000000000699

125. Shams'ili S, Grefkens J, de Leeuw B, et al. Paraneoplastic cerebellar degeneration associated with antineuronal antibodies: analysis of 50 patients. *Brain*. 2003;126(6):1409–1418. https://doi.org/10.1093/brain/awg133

126. Brouwer B. Beitrag zur Kenntnis der chronischen diffusen Kleinhirnerkrankungen. *Neurol Centralbl*. 1919;38:674–682.

127. Brouwer B, Biemond A. Les affections parenchymateuse du cervelet et leur signification du point de vue de l'anatomie et de la physiologie de cet organe. *J Belge Neurol Psychiat*. 1938;38:691–757.

128. Trotter JL, Hendin BA, Osterland CK. Cerebellar degeneration with Hodgkin disease: an immunological study. *Arch Neurol*. 1976;33(9):660–661. https://doi.org/10.1001/archneur.1976.00500090066014

129. Posner JB. Anti-Hu autoantibody associated sensory neuropathy/encephalomyelitis: a model of paraneoplastic syndrome. *Perspect Biol Med*. 1995;38(2):167–181. https://doi.org/10.1353/pbm.1995.0043

130. Venkatraman A, Opal P. Paraneoplastic cerebellar degeneration with anti-Yo antibodies—a review. *Ann Clin Transl Neurol*. 2016;3(8):655–663. https://doi.org/10.1002/acn3.328

131. Greenlee JE, Brashear HR. Antibodies to cerebellar Purkinje cells in patients with paraneoplastic cerebellar degeneration and ovarian carcinoma. *Ann Neurol*. 1983;14(6):609–613. https://doi.org/10.1002/ana.410140603

132. Jaeckle KA, Graus F, Houghton A, Cardon-Cardo C, Nielsen SL, Posner JB. Autoimmune response of patients with paraneoplastic cerebellar degeneration to a Purkinje cell cytoplasmic protein antigen. *Ann Neurol*. 1985;18(5):592–600. https://doi.org/10.1002/ana.410180513

133. Dalmau J, Posner JB. Neurological paraneoplastic syndromes. *Springer Semin Immunopathol*. 1996;18(1):85–95. https://doi.org/10.1007/BF00792611

134. Furneaux HF, Reich L, Posner JB. Autoantibody synthesis in the central nervous system of patients with paraneoplastic syndromes. *Neurology*. 1990;40(7):1085–1091. https://doi.org/10.1212/wnl.40.7.1085

135. Peterson K, Rosenblum MK, Kotanides H, Posner JB. Paraneoplastic cerebellar degeneration. I. A clinical analysis of 55 anti-Yo antibody-positive patients. *Neurology.* 1992;42(10):1931–1937. https://doi.org/10.1212/wnl.42.10.1931

136. Graus F, Delattre JY, Antoine JC, et al. Recommended diagnostic criteria for paraneoplastic neurological syndromes. *J Neurol Neurosurg Psychiatry.* 2004;75(8):1135–1140. https://doi.org/10.1136/jnnp.2003.034447

137. Sutton IJ, Fursdon Davis CJ, Esiri MM, Hughes S, Amyes ER, Vincent A. Anti-Yo antibodies and cerebellar degeneration in a man with adenocarcinoma of the esophagus. *Ann Neurol.* 2001;49(2):253–257. https://doi.org/10.1002/1531-8249(20010201)49:2<253::aid-ana47>3.0.co;2-3

138. Graus F, Dalmau J, Valldeoriola F, et al. Immunological characterization of a neuronal antibody (anti-Tr) associated with paraneoplastic cerebellar degeneration and Hodgkin's disease. *J Neuroimmunol.* 1997;74(1-2):55–61. https://doi.org/10.1016/s0165-5728(96)00205-6

139. Bernal F, Shams'ili S, Rojas I, et al. Anti-Tr antibodies as markers of paraneoplastic cerebellar degeneration and Hodgkin's disease. *Neurology.* 2003;60(2):230–234. https://doi.org/10.1212/01.wnl.0000041495.87539.98

140. Geromin A, Candoni A, Marcon G, et al. Paraneoplastic cerebellar degeneration associated with anti-neuronal anti-Tr antibodies in a patient with Hodgkin's disease. *Leuk Lymphoma.* 2006;47(9):1960–1963. https://doi.org/10.1080/10428190600678082

141. McHugh JC, Tubridy N, Collins CD, Hutchinson M. Unusual MRI abnormalities in anti-Yo positive "pure" paraneoplastic cerebellar degeneration. *J Neurol.* 2008;255(1):138–139. https://doi.org/10.1007/s00415-007-0682-9

142. Rees JH. Paraneoplastic cerebellar degeneration: new insights into imaging and immunology. *J Neurol Neurosurg Psychiatry.* 2006;77(4):427. https://doi.org/10.1136/jnnp.2005.082339

143. Shams'ili S, Grefkens J, de Leeuw B, et al. Paraneoplastic cerebellar degeneration associated with antineuronal antibodies: analysis of 50 patients. *Brain J Neurol.* 2003;126(Pt 6):1409–1418. https://doi.org/10.1093/brain/awg133

144. Hasadsri L, Lee J, Wang BH, Yekkirala L, Wang M. Anti-yo associated paraneoplastic cerebellar degeneration in a man with large cell cancer of the lung. *Case Rep Neurol Med.* 2013;2013:725936. https://doi.org/10.1155/2013/725936

145. Honnorat J, Cartalat-Carel S, Ricard D, et al. Onco-neural antibodies and tumour type determine survival and neurological symptoms in paraneoplastic neurological syndromes with Hu or CV2/CRMP5 antibodies. *J Neurol Neurosurg Psychiatry.* 2008;80(4):412–416. https://doi.org/10.1136/jnnp.2007.138016

146. Vernino S, Tuite P, Adler CH, et al. Paraneoplastic chorea associated with CRMP-5 neuronal antibody and lung carcinoma. *Ann Neurol.* 2002;51(5):625–630. https://doi.org/10.1002/ana.10178

147. Moersch FP, Woltman HW. Progressive fluctuating muscular rigidity and spasm ("stiff-man" syndrome); report of a case and some observations in 13 other cases. *Proc Staff Meet Mayo Clin.* 1956;31(15):421–427.

148. Asher R. A woman with the stiff-man syndrome. *Br Med J.* 1958;1(5065):265–266.

149. Dalakas MC. Stiff person syndrome: advances in pathogenesis and therapeutic interventions. *Curr Treat Options Neurol.* 2009;11(2):102–110. https://doi.org/10.1007/s11940-009-0013-9

150. Ali F, Rowley M, Jayakrishnan B, Teuber S, Gershwin ME, Mackay IR. Stiff-person syndrome (SPS) and anti-GAD-related CNS degenerations: protean additions to the autoimmune central neuropathies. *J Autoimmun.* 2011;37(2):79–87. https://doi.org/10.1016/j.jaut.2011.05.005

151. Solimena M, Folli F, Denis-Donini S, et al. Autoantibodies to glutamic acid decarboxylase in a patient with stiff-man syndrome, epilepsy, and type I diabetes mellitus. *N Engl J Med.* 1988;318(16):1012–1020. https://doi.org/10.1056/NEJM198804213181602

152. Meinck HM, Faber L, Morgenthaler N, et al. Antibodies against glutamic acid decarboxylase: prevalence in neurological diseases. *J Neurol Neurosurg Psychiatry.* 2001;71(1):100–103. https://doi.org/10.1136/jnnp.71.1.100

153. Saiz A, Blanco Y, Sabater L, et al. Spectrum of neurological syndromes associated with glutamic acid decarboxylase antibodies: diagnostic clues for this association. *Brain.* 2008;131(Pt 10):2553–2563. https://doi.org/10.1093/brain/awn183

154. McKeon A, Tracy JA. GAD65 neurological autoimmunity. *Muscle Nerve.* 2017;56(1):15–27. https://doi.org/10.1002/mus.25565

155. Hadjivassiliou M, Martindale J, Shanmugarajah P, et al. Causes of progressive cerebellar ataxia: prospective evaluation of 1500 patients. *J Neurol Neurosurg Psychiatry.* 2017;88(4):301–309. https://doi.org/10.1136/jnnp-2016-314863

156. Ariño H, Gresa-Arribas N, Blanco Y, et al. Cerebellar ataxia and glutamic acid decarboxylase antibodies: immunologic profile and long-term effect of immunotherapy. *JAMA Neurol.* 2014;71(8):1009–1016. https://doi.org/10.1001/jamaneurol.2014.1011

157. Kuo Y-C, Lin C-H. Clinical spectrum of glutamic acid decarboxylase antibodies in a Taiwanese population. *Eur J Neurol.* 2019;26(11):1384–1390. https://doi.org/10.1111/ene.14005

158. Fredriksen JR, Carr CM, Koeller KK, et al. MRI findings in glutamic acid decarboxylase associated autoimmune epilepsy. *Neuroradiology.* 2018;60(3):239–245. https://doi.org/10.1007/s00234-018-1976-6

159. De Camilli P, Thomas A, Cofiell R, et al. The synaptic vesicle-associated protein amphiphysin is the 128-kD autoantigen of stiff-man syndrome with breast cancer. *J Exp Med.* 1993;178(6):2219–2223. https://doi.org/10.1084/jem.178.6.2219

160. Pittock SJ, Lucchinetti CF, Parisi JE, et al. Amphiphysin autoimmunity: paraneoplastic accompaniments. *Ann Neurol.* 2005;58(1):96–107. https://doi.org/10.1002/ana.20529

161. Murinson BB, Guarnaccia JB. Stiff-person syndrome with amphiphysin antibodies. *Neurology.* 2008;71(24):1955–1958. https://doi.org/10.1212/01.wnl.0000327342.58936.e0

162. Antoine JC, Absi L, Honnorat J, et al. Antiamphiphysin antibodies are associated with various paraneoplastic neurological syndromes and tumors. *Arch Neurol.* 1999;56(2):172–177. https://doi.org/10.1001/archneur.56.2.172

163. Fava A, Petri M. Systemic lupus erythematosus: diagnosis and clinical management. *J Autoimmun.* 2019;96:1–13. https://doi.org/10.1016/j.jaut.2018.11.001

164. Smith CD, Cyr M. The history of lupus erythematosus: from Hippocrates to Osler. *Rheum Dis Clin North Am.* 1988;14(1):1–14.

165. Cervera R. Antiphospholipid syndrome. *Thromb Res.* 2017;151 Suppl 1:S43–S47. https://doi.org/10.1016/S0049-3848(17)30066-X

166. Mallavarapu RK, Grimsley EW. The history of lupus erythematosus. *South Med J.* 2007;100(9):896–898. https://doi.org/10.1097/SMJ.0b013e318073c9eb

167. Wenzel J, Gerdsen R, Uerlich M, Bauer R, Bieber T, Boehm I. Antibodies targeting extractable nuclear antigens: historical development and current knowledge. *Br J Dermatol.* 2001;145(6):859–867. https://doi.org/10.1046/j.1365-2133.2001.04577.x

168. Aringer M, Costenbader K, Daikh D, et al. 2019 European League Against Rheumatism/American College of Rheumatology classification criteria for systemic lupus erythematosus. *Arthritis Rheumatol.* 2019;71(9):1400–1412. https://doi.org/10.1002/art.40930

169. Johnson AE, Gordon C, Palmer RG, Bacon PA. The prevalence and incidence of systemic lupus erythematosus in Birmingham, England: relationship to ethnicity and country of birth. *Arthritis Rheum.* 1995;38(4):551–558. https://doi.org/10.1002/art.1780380415

170. Unterman A, Nolte JES, Boaz M, Abady M, Shoenfeld Y, Zandman-Goddard G. Neuropsychiatric syndromes in systemic lupus erythematosus: a meta-analysis. *Semin Arthritis Rheum.* 2011;41(1):1–11. https://doi.org/10.1016/j.semarthrit.2010.08.001

171. Hanly JG, Kozora E, Beyea SD, Birnbaum J. Nervous system disease in systemic lupus erythematosus: current status and future directions. *Arthritis Rheumatol.* 2019;71(1):33–42. https://doi.org/10.1002/art.40591

172. Baizabal-Carvallo JF, Bonnet C, Jankovic J. Movement disorders in systemic lupus erythematosus and the antiphospholipid syndrome. *J Neural Transm.* 2013;120(11):1579–1589. https://doi.org/10.1007/s00702-013-1023-z

173. Avcin T, Benseler SM, Tyrrell PN, Cucnik S, Silverman ED. A followup study of antiphospholipid antibodies and associated neuropsychiatric manifestations in 137 children with systemic lupus erythematosus. *Arthritis Rheum.* 2008;59(2):206–213. https://doi.org/10.1002/art.23334

174. Orzechowski NM, Wolanskyj AP, Ahlskog JE, Kumar N, Moder KG. Antiphospholipid antibody-associated chorea. *J Rheumatol.* 2008;35(11):2165–2170. https://doi.org/10.3899/jrheum.080268

175. Sanna G, Bertolaccini ML, Cuadrado MJ, Khamashta MA, Hughes GRV. Central nervous system involvement in the antiphospholipid (Hughes) syndrome. *Rheumatology.* 2003;42(2):200–213. https://doi.org/10.1093/rheumatology/keg080

176. Baizabal-Carvallo JF, Jankovic J. Autoimmune and paraneoplastic movement disorders: An update. *J Neurol Sci.* 2018;385:175–184. https://doi.org/10.1016/j.jns.2017.12.035

177. Choi J, Kim ST, Craft J. The pathogenesis of systemic lupus erythematosus—an update. *Curr Opin Immunol.* 2012;24(6):651–657. https://doi.org/10.1016/j.coi.2012.10.004

178. Trouw LA, Groeneveld TWL, Seelen MA, et al. Anti-C1q autoantibodies deposit in glomeruli but are only pathogenic in combination with glomerular C1q-containing immune complexes. *J Clin Invest.* 2004;114(5):679–688. https://doi.org/10.1172/JCI21075

179. Valle RR, Eaton RB, Schnneider G, Schur PH. Complement activation by antibodies to DNA in systemic lupus erythematosus measured by enzyme immunoassay. *Clin Immunol Immunopathol.* 1985;34(3):345–354. https://doi.org/10.1016/0090-1229(85)90183-7

180. Munroe ME, James JA. Genetics of lupus nephritis: clinical implications. *Semin Nephrol.* 2015;35(5):396–409. https://doi.org/10.1016/j.semnephrol.2015.08.002

181. Brain L, Jellinek EH, Ball K. Hashimoto's disease and encephalopathy. *Lancet Lond Engl.* 1966;2(7462):512–514. https://doi.org/10.1016/s0140-6736(66)92876-5

182. Castillo P, Woodruff B, Caselli R, et al. Steroid-responsive encephalopathy associated with autoimmune thyroiditis. *Arch Neurol.* 2006;63(2):197–202. https://doi.org/10.1001/archneur.63.2.197

183. Laurent C, Capron J, Quillerou B, et al. Steroid-responsive encephalopathy associated with autoimmune thyroiditis (SREAT): characteristics, treatment and outcome in 251 cases from the literature. *Autoimmun Rev.* 2016;15(12):1129–1133. https://doi.org/10.1016/j.autrev.2016.09.008

184. Vernino S, Geschwind M, Boeve B. Autoimmune encephalopathies. *The Neurologist.* 2007;13(3):140–147. https://doi.org/10.1097/01.nrl.0000259483.70041.55

185. Swedo SE, Leonard HL, Mittleman BB, et al. Identification of children with pediatric autoimmune neuropsychiatric disorders associated with streptococcal infections by a marker

associated with rheumatic fever. *Am J Psychiatry*. 1997;154(1):110–112. https://doi.org/10.1176/ajp.154.1.110

186. Swedo SE, Leonard HL, Garvey M, et al. Pediatric autoimmune neuropsychiatric disorders associated with streptococcal infections: clinical description of the first 50 cases. *Am J Psychiatry*. 1998;155(2):264–271. https://doi.org/10.1176/ajp.155.2.264

187. Chang K, Frankovich J, Cooperstock M, et al. Clinical evaluation of youth with pediatric acute-onset neuropsychiatric syndrome (PANS): recommendations from the 2013 PANS Consensus Conference. *J Child Adolesc Psychopharmacol*. 2015;25(1):3–13. https://doi.org/10.1089/cap.2014.0084

188. Swedo S.E., Leckman J.F., Rose N.R. (2012) From Research Subgroup to Clinical Syndrome: Modifying the PANDAS Criteria to Describe PANS (Pediatric Acute-onset Neuropsychiatric Syndrome). *Pediatr Therapeut* 2(2):113. doi:10.4172/2161-0665.1000113

189. Chiarello F, Spitoni S, Hollander E, Matucci Cerinic M, Pallanti S. An expert opinion on PANDAS/PANS: highlights and controversies. *Int J Psychiatry Clin Pract*. 2017;21(2):91–98. https://doi.org/10.1080/13651501.2017.1285941

190. Cunningham MW, Cox CJ. Autoimmunity against dopamine receptors in neuropsychiatric and movement disorders: a review of Sydenham chorea and beyond. *Acta Physiol*. 2016;216(1):90–100. https://doi.org/10.1111/apha.12614

191. Shimasaki C, Frye RE, Trifiletti R, et al. Evaluation of the Cunningham Panel™ in pediatric autoimmune neuropsychiatric disorder associated with streptococcal infection (PANDAS) and pediatric acute-onset neuropsychiatric syndrome (PANS): changes in antineuronal antibody titers parallel changes in patient symptoms. *J Neuroimmunol*. 2020;339:577138. https://doi.org/10.1016/j.jneuroim.2019.577138

192. Hesselmark E, Bejerot S. Biomarkers for diagnosis of pediatric acute neuropsychiatric syndrome (PANS): sensitivity and specificity of the Cunningham Panel. *J Neuroimmunol*. 2017;312:31–37. https://doi.org/10.1016/j.jneuroim.2017.09.002

193. Hesselmark E, Bejerot S. Corrigendum to biomarkers for diagnosis of pediatric acute neuropsychiatric syndrome (PANS): sensitivity and specificity of the Cunningham Panel [J. Neuroimmunol. 312. (2017) 31–37]. *J Neuroimmunol*. 2017;313:116–117. https://doi.org/10.1016/j.jneuroim.2017.11.001

194. Bejerot S, Hesselmark E. The Cunningham Panel is an unreliable biological measure. *Transl Psychiatry*. 2019;9(1):1–2. https://doi.org/10.1038/s41398-019-0413-x

195. Frye RE, Shimasaki C. Reliability of the Cunningham Panel. *Transl Psychiatry*. 2019;9(1):1–2. https://doi.org/10.1038/s41398-019-0462-1

196. Bejerot S, Klang A, Hesselmark E. The Cunningham Panel: concerns remain. *Transl Psychiatry*. 2019;9: 224. https://doi.org/10.1038/s41398-019-0562-y

197. Ganesh A, Wesley SF. Practice current: when do you suspect autoimmune encephalitis and what is the role of antibody testing? *Neurol Clin Pract*. 2018;8(1):67–73. https://doi.org/10.1212/CPJ.0000000000000423

198. Höftberger R, van Sonderen A, Leypoldt F, et al. Encephalitis and AMPA receptor antibodies. *Neurology*. 2015;84(24):2403–2412. https://doi.org/10.1212/WNL.0000000000001682

199. Rosenfeld MR, Dalmau J. Paraneoplastic neurologic syndromes. *Neurol Clin*. 2018;36(3):675–685. https://doi.org/10.1016/j.ncl.2018.04.015

200. Dubey D, Britton J, McKeon A, et al. Randomized placebo-controlled trial of intravenous immunoglobulin in autoimmune LGI1/CASPR2 epilepsy. *Ann Neurol*. 2020;87(2):313–323. https://doi.org/10.1002/ana.25655

201. McKeon A. Immunotherapeutics for autoimmune encephalopathies and dementias. *Curr Treat Options Neurol.* 2013;15(6):723–737. https://doi.org/10.1007/s11940-013-0251-8

202. Shin Y-W, Lee S-T, Park K-I, et al. Treatment strategies for autoimmune encephalitis. *Ther Adv Neurol Disord.* 2018;11:1756285617722347. https://doi.org/10.1177/1756285617722347

203. Irani SR, Michell AW, Lang B, et al. Faciobrachial dystonic seizures precede Lgi1 antibody limbic encephalitis. *Ann Neurol.* 2011;69(5):892–900. https://doi.org/10.1002/ana.22307

204. Titulaer MJ, Lang B, Verschuuren JJ. Lambert–Eaton myasthenic syndrome: from clinical characteristics to therapeutic strategies. *Lancet Neurol.* 2011;10(12):1098–1107. https://doi.org/10.1016/S1474-4422(11)70245-9

Index

For the benefit of digital users, indexed terms that span two pages (e.g., 52–53) may, on occasion, appear on only one of those pages.

Note: Tables, figures, and boxes are indicated by *t*, *f*, and *b* following the page number